D0700237

DIVING MEDICINE

Second Edition

ALFRED A. BOVE, M.D.

Chief, Section of Cardiology
Temple University Hospital
Philadelphia, Pennsylvania

JEFFERSON C. DAVIS, M.D.

Hyperbaric Medicine, P.A.
San Antonio, Texas

1990
W. B. SAUNDERS COMPANY

HARCOURT BRACE JOVANOVICH, INC.

Philadelphia, London, Toronto, Montreal, Sydney, Tokyo

W. B. SAUNDERS COMPANY
Harcourt Brace Jovanovich, Inc.

The Curtis Center
Independence Square West
Philadelphia, PA 19106

Library of Congress Cataloging-in-Publication Data

Diving medicine / [edited by] Alfred A. Bove, Jefferson C. Davis—2nd ed.

p. cm.

ISBN 0–7216–2934–2

1. Submarine medicine. I. Bove, Alfred A. II. Davis, Jefferson C. (Jefferson Carroll), 1932–1989.

[DNLM: 1. Diving. 2. Naval Medicine. QT 260 D618]

RC1005.D583 1990

616.9′8022—dc19

DNLM/DLC
for Library of Congress 89–5907
CIP

Sponsoring Editor: Tom Mackey

Production Manager: Frank Polizzano

Manuscript Editor: Keryn Lane

Illustration Coordinator: Joan Sinclair

Indexer: Diana Witt

DIVING MEDICINE ISBN 0–7216–2934–2

Printed in the United States of America.

Last digit is the print number: 9 8 7 6 5 4 3 2

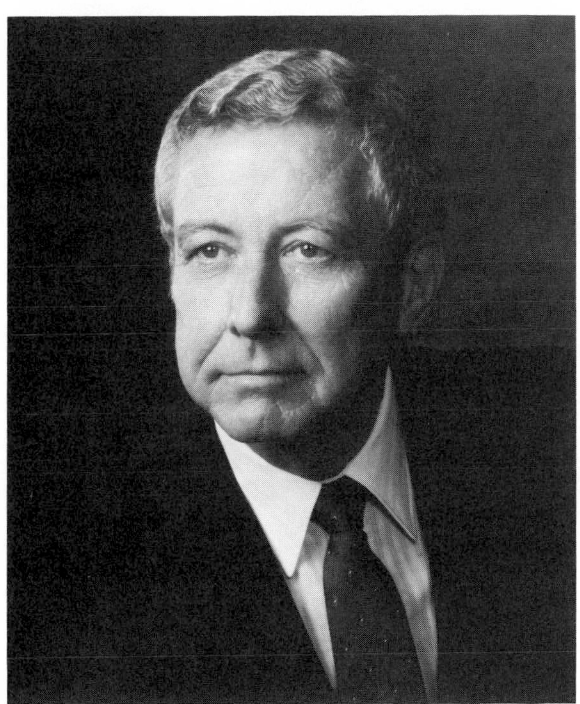

Dr. Jefferson C. Davis died in July of 1989 just at the time that this book was completed. In place of a dedication, Dr. Theodore R. Struhl, a close friend and colleague, has provided the following.

IN MEMORIAM

Jefferson C. Davis was a world-renowned scientist, researcher, and physician in the fields of Diving Medicine, Aerospace Medicine, and Hyperbaric Oxygen. His untimely death at the age of 56 leaves a void that will be extremely difficult to fill. Dr. Davis accomplished in his short life what many others could not achieve in many lifetimes.

I am proud and privileged to have known Jefferson Davis as a doctor, as a diver, as a diving buddy, and as a close personal friend for so many years. He will be sorely missed by his friends, his colleagues, his wife Helen, and his sons. May his dedication to diving medicine, which has advanced to its current state because of his efforts, be continued in his memory by his many colleagues in diving medicine.

THEODORE R. STRUHL, M.D., F.A.C.S., F.I.C.S.
Senior Surgeon, Mount Sinai Medical Center
Miami, Florida

Contributors

ARTHUR J. BACHRACH, PH.D.

Retired Head, Environmental Stress Department, Naval Medical Research Institute; Adjunct Professor of Medical Psychology (retired), Uniformed Services University of the Health Sciences, 1972–1987, Bethesda, Maryland.

Human Performance Under Water

PETER B. BENNETT, PH.D., D.SC.

Associate Professor of Neurobiology, Duke University; Professor of Anesthesiology and Senior Director, F. G. Hall Hyperbaric Center, Duke University Medical Center, Durham, North Carolina.

Inert Gas Narcosis and HPNS

ALFRED A. BOVE, M.D., PH.D.

Bernheim Professor of Medicine, Chief of Cardiology, Temple University Medical School, Philadelphia, Pennsylvania.

Mixed Gas Diving; Diving in the Elderly and the Young; Cardiovascular Disorders and Diving; Physical Examination of Divers

MARK E. BRADLEY, M.D, M.P.H.

Assistant Professor, Department of Epidemiology and Preventive Medicine, University of Maryland School of Medicine, Baltimore, Maryland.

Pulmonary Barotrauma

JAMES M. CLARK, M.D., PH.D.

Clinical Associate Professor of Pharmacology, University of Pennsylvania School of Medicine, Philadelphia, Pennsylvania.

The Toxicity of Oxygen, Carbon Monoxide, and Carbon Dioxide

JEFFERSON C. DAVIS, M.D.

Hyperbaric Medicine, P.A., San Antonio, Texas.

Treatment of Decompression Sickness and Arterial Gas Embolism; Medical Evaluation for Diving

A. J. DUTKA, M.D.

Head, Medicine Division, Diving Medicine Department, Naval Medical Research Institute; Assistant Professor, Department of Neurology, Uniformed Services University of Health Sciences, Bethesda, Maryland.

Pathophysiology of Decompression Sickness

CARL EDMONDS, M.B., M.R.C.P. (Lond), F.R.A.N.Z.C.P., F.R.A.C.P., F.A.C.O.M., Dip D.H.M., M.R.C.Psych

Consultant in Diving Medicine, North Shore Medical Centre; Director, Diving Medical Centre, Sydney, Australia.

Marine Animal Injuries

GLEN H. EGSTROM, Ph.D.

Professor of Kinesiology, University of California at Los Angeles, Los Angeles, California.

Diving Equipment; Human Performance Under Water

JOSEPH C. FARMER, Jr., M.D., F.A.C.S.

Associate Professor, Division of Otolaryngology, Department of Surgery, Duke University Medical Center; Attending Physician, Duke University Medical Center, Durham, North Carolina.

Ear and Sinus Problems in Diving

EDWARD T. FLYNN, Jr., M.D.

Head, Diving Medicine Department, Naval Medical Research Institute, Bethesda, Maryland.

Medical Supervision of Diving Operations

T. J. R. FRANCIS, M.Sc. M.B.

Royal Navy Exchange Medical Officer, Naval Medical Research Institute, Bethesda, Maryland.

Pathophysiology of Decompression Sickness

HUGH D. GREER, M.D.

Associate Clinical Professor of Medicine (Neurology), University of Southern California; Staff Neurologist, Santa Barbara Medical Foundation Clinic, and Cottage Hospital, Santa Barbara, California.

Neurological Consequences of Diving

J. M. HALLENBECK, M.D.

Professor, Department of Neurology, Uniformed Services University of Health Sciences; Chief, Neurology Service, National Naval Medical Center, Bethesda, Maryland.

Pathophysiology of Decompression Sickness

SUK KI HONG, M.D., Ph.D.

Professor of Physiology, State University of New York at Buffalo, Buffalo, New York.

Breath-Hold Diving

ERIC P. KINDWALL, M.D.

Associate Professor of Surgery (Hyperbaric Medicine), Division of Plastic and Reconstructive Surgery and Department of Emergency Medicine, Medical College of Wisconsin; Chief of Hyperbaric Medicine, Froedert Memorial Lutheran Hospital, Milwaukee, Wisconsin.

A Short History of Diving and Diving Medicine

Foreword

Knowledge of this comprehensive and systematic text will be of immense value in the prevention of diving accidents and, when an accident does occur, in the provision of specific therapy for what could otherwise be a perplexing situation. So wrote Al Behnke in his foreword to the first edition of this book, and his remarks remain equally true for this revised edition.

The boundaries of diving medicine do not change; a new reader must fully understand the physics and physiology of diving and the interaction between man, his equipment, and the environment before embarking on the clinical aspects of this uniquely challenging specialty. However, the recipients of all this attention, the diving population, have changed. There are relatively fewer of the fit young males for whose benefit the navies of the world developed diving procedures and decompression tables. These young men have become outnumbered by an increasing population of recreational divers of both sexes, of almost any age, and with a lesser degree of general physical and medical fitness. Sports divers and, for that matter, diving scientists, civilian divers associated with waterways and hydroelectric schemes, and divers of the civil public services, such as the police, are also now distributed almost homogeneously inland away from the open sea. The diver has changed with the years in other ways. He is more knowledgeable about the physiology and medicine of diving and has a natural concern for health and safety implications, particularly allegations about possible long-term effects of diving. All this leads to a new perspective, which is the underlying theme of this textbook—the clinical practice of diving medicine.

In the years that have passed since the publication of the first edition, many scientific papers have been published, each in its own way advancing our understanding about man in the sea, and much practical experience has been gained. This knowledge has been reviewed, assessed, and, where appropriate, incorporated into the revised text. Such developments, together with a wider distribution among the community of diving, have led to the reinforcement of what is essential in a textbook of medicine: sections that are orientated to practical clinical problems. The best examples are of particular importance to the practicing diving physician and relate to the need to make decisions concerning the fitness of an individual to take up, to continue, or to resume the sport of diving. For professional divers there are necessarily strict criteria regarding fitness to dive and returning to diving after illness or injury. For sports divers who can choose if, when, and how to dive, there are, however, no such rules. Indeed, the requirement for an annual medical examination has yet to be universally recognized by sports diving authorities. Thus for the doctor who is asked by his or her patient, "Can I dive? . . ." this book provides invaluable guidance in relation to the many medical conditions that may interact with the underwater environment.

This book is particularly instructive about the problems that may occur in association with real diving situations, and it is available for reference when needed.

But a textbook that meets all of these objectives should not be exclusively for physicians. As Osler's textbook of medicine held the interest of the informed layman, so, wrote Al Behnke in the first edition, this text reveals the panorama of hyperbaric and undersea medical science. The second edition upholds the high standards set previously by Dick Strauss and not only takes the contents further into the interpretation of recent developments, but also widens the scope so that it will be especially useful for the physician who may have divers among his patients but who himself is not a diver.

DAVID H. ELLIOTT, O.B.E., F.R.C.P., D.PHIL.

Preface

The new edition of *Diving Medicine* is intended to provide a practicum on diving medicine which can be used by the physician involved in the care of divers. We were concerned most with commercial and sport diving because many physicians in medical practice encounter patients with acute or chronic illness who are divers or who wish to dive. In our encounters with physicians, we found them lacking a compendium of diving medicine that could be used as a reference for patient care.

To provide such a work and still retain the initial flavor of the first edition of *Diving Medicine,* we organized the initial chapters to provide the physiological background for understanding the effects of the diving environment on the healthy diver and on the patient with acute or chronic illness who is a diver or who wishes to become a diver. Physiology in diving must be linked with equipment for life support under water; thus a chapter contributed by Dr. Egstrom is devoted to diving equipment. This chapter concentrates on sport diving equipment because sport divers are most commonly seen in private practice and because the technology in commercial diving changes rapidly.

We have attempted to incorporate knowledge recently developed on women, the elderly, and the young. Although little formal research has been done in these areas, data on exercise, endocrine function, and growth effects have been extrapolated from published literature.

The most significant change is the addition of chapters dealing with various medical disorders. The classic diving disorders are covered in several chapters, but also provided are discussions on common pulmonary, neurological, cardiac, and other medical disorders that may interact with the diving environment. These chapters provide the data needed to produce informed decisions regarding diving in subjects with medical illnesses.

A chapter on dangerous and toxic marine animals was considered a requisite addition. Dr. Edmonds has provided an excellent review of this subject.

Requirements for medical clearance to dive are given in two chapters. One is devoted to sport divers, the other to commercial divers. These are complemented by suggested history and physical examination forms provided in an appendix.

Each of the chapters has been written by an experienced diving physician or scientist with established and well-recognized experience in his or her particular area. The chapters on diving physiology and physics are written by scientists who have contributed extensively to the literature of diving physiology. The clinical chapters have been written by physicians recognized nationally and internationally for their expertise in diving and hyperbaric medicine.

The result is a thorough, up-to-date text on diving medicine that can serve the practicing physician who sees divers occasionally as well as the diving medical officer who deals with divers on a daily basis.

We wish to acknowledge the contributions of the experts who wrote chapters for this text and to express our gratitude for sharing their knowledge with us. We also want to thank our secretaries for their invaluable assistance in the typing and the communications that are essential to a work of this kind.

Our goal of improving the health of divers and the safety of diving hopefully will be advanced with this text.

ALFRED A. BOVE, M.D., PH.D.
JEFFERSON C. DAVIS, M.D.

Contents

Chapter 1

A Short History of Diving and Diving Medicine

ERIC P. KINDWALL

Man's first entry into the sea was through breath-hold diving, undoubtedly to harvest shellfish and to retrieve lost tools or utensils. From early history we find that breath-hold divers accomplished such prodigious amounts of work that they became economically important. In many areas of the world, commercial pearl and pearl-shell diving still rely on the breath-hold diver to a great extent. Depths of 60 to 80 feet are common, and commercial breath-hold diving has been done to depths of 100 feet.

Even the salvage of treasure has been accomplished using the free diver. In 1680, Sir William Phipps recovered some £ 200,000 in sterling silver from a wrecked Spanish galleon in the Carribean, and the "fishing up of the wrecked plate ships at Vigo Bay" cited by Stevenson in *Treasure Island* was accomplished by naked divers.

The depths that can be reached by the breath-hold diver are dependent on two factors. The first is how long the diver can hold his breath without the CO_2 level in the blood forcing him to breathe (breath-hold breaking point). The second is the relationship between the diver's total lung capacity and his residual volume. As pressure is increased on the lung, its volume is decreased, and even with a thoracic blood shift to fill some of the space, lung squeeze will occur, somewhere in excess of 150 to 200 feet. However, certain exceptional individuals with a high tolerance for CO_2 who have practiced breath-hold diving have set extraordinary depth records. A record of 247 feet was set in 1967 by Robert Croft, a U.S. Navy submarine engineman and escape training tower instructor. Subsequently, Jacques Mayol, a Frenchman, set the current record of 282 feet in 1973, surfacing fully conscious (see Chapter 6).

BELL DIVING

The use of the diving bell, which consists of trapped air in an inverted container, was the next method employed to extend working time on the bottom.

The diving bell is first mentioned in a French manuscript of 1250 A.D., which has a fanciful illustration of Alexander the Great descending in the diving bell at the Seige of Tyre in 332 B.C. It is highly unlikely that Alexander ever did go down in a diving bell, but he was shrewd enough to use military divers (free swimmers) for destroying enemy vessels.

The first modern records of diving bells used in practical salvage start in the 1640's, when Von Treileben used a primitive bell for salvaging 42 cannons from the sunken Swedish ship of the line *Vasa* which lay in 132 feet of water in Stockholm Harbor. The bell, shaped like a truncated cone, had no air supply other than that contained within the bell. Divers would descend to the bottom in the bell, swimming from the bell to the wreck to attach lines to the objects to be salvaged and returning to the bell for a breath of fresh air between excursions. Bell divers soon learned the air at the top of the bell was more breathable than that at the bottom, after they had been working for some period under water. CO_2 is slightly heavier than air, and as it accumulated the CO_2 became more concentrated along the surface of the water toward the bottom of the bell. There is no report of decompression sickness among Von Treileben's submarine workers, but it is extremely possible that by working at those depths, especially if several dives a day were made, that they could have absorbed enough nitrogen into their systems to have caused decompression sickness. It is amazing the amount of work that was accomplished by those early bell divers; in 1960, a single remaining bronze cannon was recovered from the same wreck by a helmeted deep-sea diver. Even with all of the advantages of modern equipment and a 150-ton floating crane, it took the diver 1½ days to remove the gun.

The next recorded note of a diving bell dates to 1690 when Halley (discoverer of the comet) devised a successful bell with the first system for renewing air within the bell while it was on the bottom. Lead-weighted barrels carried fresh air down to the occupants of the bell. Halley's bell was somewhat cumbersome and heavy, but we have records that it was used to depths of 60 feet. It is unlikely that any practical salvage was carried out with it.

The first modern practical diving bell was invented by Smeaton in 1790 with a workable force pump to continuously refresh the air in the bell. This bell or caisson was the forerunner of all modern types. It was first used in Ramsgate Harbor, England, for breakwater construction. Caissons are still used for the construction of bridge piers in much the same manner that Smeaton used his.

SURFACE SUPPLIED DIVING GEAR

The object of having a man free to walk around the bottom without having to hold his breath or return to the safety of a diving bell was first realized when Augustus Siebe invented his diving dress. Siebe was a German coppersmith working in London. In 1819, he devised a diving rig that consisted of a copper helmet riveted to a leather jacket. The diver entered the dress through the open waist and then thrust his arms into the sleeves with his head protruding into the helmet. There was no control over the amount of air entering the helmet, and the excess air bubbled out around the diver's waist. Other inventors had tried their luck at similar designs, but apparently Siebe's diving dress was accepted because of his extremely reliable and successful force pump that produced the necessary compressed air. Siebe's original rig was used for successful salvage work on the sunken British war ship, *The Royal George*, and was used by divers on many other important projects. It had one disadvantage in that if the diver were to lie down or turn upside down, the dress quickly filled with water and he was likely to drown. Nevertheless, much useful salvage was accomplished with this primitive apparatus.

However, Siebe was a constant innovator, and by 1837 he had produced an improved design. This consisted of a full suit that was waterproofed and could be bolted to a breastplate and helmet. Since the suit covered the diver's entire body, he was able to work in any position. Valves were provided for admitting varying amounts of air to the diving suit as needed, and an air exhaust valve was provided in the helmet. The 1837 Siebe closed dress design proved itself so successful that it has remained essentially unchanged to the present day for classical deep-sea diving. The United States Navy Mark V deep-sea diving suit, which was in use by the Navy until the mid 1980's, is almost an exact copy of Siebe's original 1837 design, except for some refinements in materials and improvements in the valves. Navy instruction with the Mark V ceased in 1982, and it was officially replaced by the Mark XII in 1986. It is still used, however, by a number of commercial harbor divers.

The classical deep-sea diving suit remained unchallenged until approximately 1945 when a lightweight diving mask for work down to depths of 90 to 100 feet was introduced. This was designed by a Milwaukee diver, Jack Browne, and was manufactured for the U.S. Navy. It subsequently became widely used among commercial divers especially in the Gulf of Mexico. It was also at the end of World War II when the self-contained underwater breathing apparatus (scuba) first made its appearance outside of occupied France. It had been invented in 1943 by Emile Gagnon and Jacques Cousteau. The Cousteau-Gagnon patent had at its heart a demand regulator that automatically delivered only the amount of air the diver needed at any depth to which he dived. This simple, but ingenious, device presaged the current boom in sport diving and also was adapted for a number of commercial applications. Since 1960, there have been many advances made in deep-sea diving equipment with the use of more modern helmets made of space age materials, hot water–heated suits for thermal protection, and the use of the diving bell in combination with the diving suit.

DECOMPRESSION SICKNESS

Our first hint as to the etiology of decompression sickness was provided in 1670 by Sir Robert Boyle when he produced symptoms of decompression sickness in a snake that had been placed in a vacuum chamber. He was prompted to write: "I once observed a Viper furiously tortured in our Exhausted Receiver . . . that had manifestly a conspicuous Bubble moving to and fro in the waterish humour of one of its eyes." Thus, Boyle noted that rapid reduction of ambient pressure may result in the production of bubbles in the tissues of the body.

The first description of the symptoms of decompression sickness in humans was provided by Triger in 1841. The victims in this case were coal miners who worked in mines pressurized to keep out the water. Triger noticed that some men suffered cramps and pains in their muscles after leaving compressed air, and apparently their symptoms were treated vigorously with alcohol given both internally and rubbed on externally. We have no other report as to how they later fared.

In 1854, Pol and Watelle began to study the phenomenon of decompression sickness. They noticed that this disease was always associated with leaving the compressed air environment. They wrote, "one pays only on leaving." They also noted that a return to compressed air alleviated the symptoms. They pointed out that young men of 18 who had "not reached their greatest mature physical strength" suffered less from decompression sickness symptoms than those in their mid 30's "who were in their prime." The first scientific approach to the problem of decompression sickness was begun by the French physiologist Paul Bert, when he published his monumental book *Barometric Pressure* in 1878. Bert was able to demonstrate that bubbles associated with symptoms of decompression sickness were formed during rapid decompression and, furthermore, that these bubbles consisted mainly of nitrogen. Bert also discovered that oxygen is toxic when breathed under pressure; the convulsions that occur when oxygen is breathed for any period of time at pressures greater than 33 feet have been termed the "Paul Bert effect."

The word "bends" as a synonym for decompression sickness came into being during the construction of the piers for the Brooklyn Bridge. The fashionable ladies of the era had an affected posture for walking called "the Grecian bend." Workers emerging from the caisson, limping with symptoms of decompression sickness, were chided by their fellows for "doing the Grecian bend." This was later shortened to simply "the bends" and subsequently became legitimized by use.

By the turn of the century, even though the etiology of decompression sickness was known to be nitrogen bubbles evolving within the body and that the symptoms could be relieved by returning to increased pressure, there were no decompression schedules that could be followed to minimize the possibility of decompression sickness occurring. Since the Royal Navy consistently used divers in its routine operations, it commissioned J.S. Haldane to work out a set of decompression schedules that could be written down in tabular form and followed by its fleet divers. In 1908, Haldane published the first set of practical, though empirical, decompression schedules. In his work, Haldane demonstrated that the body could tolerate a two-to-one reduction in ambient pressure without symptoms. All common decompression schedules in use since have been based on Haldane's method.

The Haldanian schedules were found to be quite realistic over their middle range; but divers soon found that it was possible to "cut corners" on short, shallow dives without risking bends and that on long, deep dives, the Haldane tables were not conservative enough. Haldane's tables were modified empirically over the years to solve these problems. Haldane must also receive the credit for developing the concept of half-time tissues; he realized that all of the tissues of the body absorb nitrogen at varying rates, depending on their vascularity and the types of tissue involved. Recognizing that this was a spectrum that probably went from seconds to hours, he arbitrarily chose to recognize the existence of 5-, 10-, 20-, 40-, and 75-minute half-time tissues for mathematical convenience in calculating nitrogen uptake and elimination. He assumed that nitrogen uptake and elimination occurred at equal rates and that the longest half-time tissue in the body was probably 60 minutes. He therefore assumed that the body would essentially achieve total saturation in 6 hours. However, he made his longest tissue 75 minutes just to be on the safe side. Since that time, the U.S. Navy standard air decompression tables have been based on a 12-hour period for total saturation, and the exceptional exposure air tables have been based on a 24-hour time period for total saturation. Even longer tissue half-times have been developed for saturation diving.

INCREASING DEPTHS AND EXPERIMENTS WITH HELIUM-OXYGEN BREATHING

In 1915, the United States Submarine F-4 sank in 306 feet of water off Honolulu, Hawaii. The U.S. Navy was anxious to recover the submarine and bodies of its crew, and thus diving operations were commenced. Frank Crilley, in that year, set a world depth record of 306 feet by descending to the submarine and attaching a large hawser to it. The pressures at such depths are enormous, having been enough to completely crush the sides of the submarine and to reveal the outlines of the diesel engines beneath. The fact that Crilley was able to dive to this depth and return to the surface alive, using the primitive decompression schedules then employed, was an astounding feat. Perhaps Crilley's size had something to do with it, as he weighed only 127 pounds. Three hundred feet is still about the extreme limit for compressed air diving; the nitrogen narcosis at that depth renders all but the most experienced divers incapable of any kind of useful work. The current U.S. Navy maximum operating depth for compressed air diving is 190 feet.

Because air seems to have a limit of approximately 300 feet, the physiologist Elihu Thompson wrote a letter to the Bureau of Mines in 1919 suggesting that helium mixed with oxygen might be used as a diving gas. Because helium is so much lighter than nitrogen, he thought that, with the decreased breathing resistance, permissible diving depth might be doubled. Nitrogen narcosis was still not understood in 1919. The British Admiralty, along with the United States Bureau of Mines, began experimenting with helium oxygen mixtures and thought that bends might be avoided because nitrogen was no longer in the breathing mixture. However, since Royal Navy divers developed severe decompression sickness after breathing helium, even when decompressed on conservative air decompression schedules, they concluded that it was unsafe as a diving gas and ceased further experiments. The U.S. Navy Experimental Diving Unit, which had worked with the Bureau of Mines on helium, also abandoned its studies of helium in 1924 because helium seemed to produce decompression sickness more quickly than when compressed air was breathed. In Admiral Momsen's words, experimentation with helium diving was "put very much on the back burner." Because of the necessity to dive to great depths on occasion for military operations, Damant extended the original Haldane air schedules to 320 feet in 1930.

NEW DEVELOPMENTS

Occasionally, divers returning to the surface from trivial depths (less than 33 feet) suffered sudden incapacitation. This was thought to be due to a capricious form of decompression sickness, and indeed the U.S. Navy reported two cases of "unusual decompression sickness in 16 feet of water" in the mid 1930s. Both of these cases proved fatal, but the mechanism of death was not understood. Submarine escape training began in the U.S. Navy at the beginning of the 1930's, and occasionally even with the use of the Momsen lung, trainees would develop severe distress or die quickly after surfacing. Further investigation revealed that death in these cases was due to over-distention of the lungs, with subsequent rupture and escape of air into the pulmonary veins. From the pulmonary veins, the air bubbles were directed to the left heart and thence to the brain. Cerebral air embolism became recognized for the first time. When it was understood that air bubbles in the brain were the cause of the symptoms and that nitrogen alone was not involved, immediate recompression to 165 feet became the standard treatment, and the victims of air embolism were treated as though they had severe decompression sickness. Most of them survived when immediately recompressed, and eventually recompression chambers were installed at the top of the submarine escape training towers in New London, Connecticut, and in Honolulu to handle such cases.

Meanwhile, Albert R. Behnke, a U.S. Navy Submarine Medical Officer and an outstanding scientist, became interested in the problem of mental deterioration when the divers exceeded depths of 150 feet. Using mixtures of gases other than nitrogen, he demonstrated that heavier inert gases produce more narcosis and that nitrogen produces mental deterioration in air diving. Behnke also demonstrated that high levels of CO_2 contribute to nitrogen narcosis but that nitrogen itself is the culprit. He showed that the narcotic potency of any inert gas is predicated on its oil-water solubility ratio and, like the aliphatic anesthetics, followed the Meyer-Overton hypothesis for predicting anesthetic effect.

HELIUM REVISITED AND NEW DEPTH RECORDS SET

In 1937, Edgar End, a 26-year-old intern at the Milwaukee County General Hospital, thought that helium could be used successfully to avoid nitrogen narcosis. He was undeterred by the fact that both the British Admiralty and the U.S. Navy Experimental Diving Unit had been unable to adapt helium successfully for diving. By doing some original calculations, he developed a set of helium decompression schedules that he believed would be compatible with this rapidly diffusing gas. Together with Max Gene Nohl, a friend and a Milwaukee diver, End breathed helium/oxygen in an old recompression chamber located at the Milwaukee County Emergency Hospital. The two men found that they could surface safely from depths of 100 feet after various exposures breathing helium. Using Nohl's self-contained suit, they conducted a series of open water dives in Lake Michigan to increasing depths until finally, Frank Crilley's record was broken and a new world depth record of 420 feet was set in December of 1937 diving from a Coast Guard cutter off of Port Washington, Wisconsin. Nohl surfaced safely without signs of decompression sickness. After End and Nohl proved that helium could be used successfully for deep diving, the Navy stepped up its own interest in helium/oxygen experimentation. By 1939, a series of helium/oxygen decompression schedules that had been developed by Behnke were ready. The helium/oxygen equipment had been sent to a warehouse at Kittery, Maine for field testing in the summer of 1939 when the submarine *U.S.S. Squalus* operating out of Portsmouth, New Hampshire sank off the Isle of Shoals in 240 feet of water.

The submarine was quickly located, and the first dive was made on compressed air. The downhaul cable to the torpedo room hatch had parted, and a compressed air diver was too confused to replace it. A diver breathing helium then went down and accomplished the task with ease. Some 36 men were rescued from the submarine using the McCann Rescue Bell, and then the actual salvage of the submarine was carried out using the new helium/oxygen schedules and equipment. Over 100 helium dives were made on the *Squalus*, and it is remarkable that with this first venture in deep water with a new gas, not a single diver was killed or seriously injured. For the next 20 years the U.S. Navy was to be the only user of helium/oxygen diving (as the United States had the only readily available sources of helium), and all Navy submarine rescue vessels were equipped with helium/oxygen diving gear.

In 1945, Jack Browne, the son of a Milwaukee automobile dealer, had become interested in diving and believed that a practical diving mask could be more useful than the heavy and cumbersome standard deep-sea dress. He devised a triangular-shaped mask, and in a wet test tank at the Diving Equipment and Supply Company in Milwaukee, Wisconsin, descended to a new world depth record of 550 feet. The decompression schedules for this dive were worked out by Edgar End with some modifications by Behnke, who was also present.

It was also in 1945 that the Swedish engineer Arne Zetterström investigated the possibilities of using a mixture of hydrogen and oxygen for diving. Hydrogen-oxygen is nonexplosive when the oxygen percentage is less than 4 per cent. Zetterström reached a depth of 526 feet in the Baltic Sea in August, 1945, and the hydrogen-oxygen mixture was perfectly satisfactory as a breathing mix. Unfortunately, he was killed on ascent due to a winch accident that had nothing to do with his breathing mixture. Hydrogen diving was not attempted again until the 1970's, when Peter Edel in New Orleans began experimenting with gas on a contract from the U.S. Navy.

DEVELOPMENT OF TREATMENT TABLES FOR DECOMPRESSION SICKNESS

There have been many schools of thought as how to best treat a diver stricken with bends. Some believed that the diver should be returned to his original working pressure; others held that he should be taken to his depth of relief; still others thought that the treatment pressure should be the depth of relief plus 1 atm. Then there were many schemes for gradually reducing the pressure on the diver so that he would not sustain decompression sickness during his ascent in the treatment chamber. The U.S. Navy in 1944 and 1945 studied all of these methods and soon promulgated the U.S. Navy Air Recompression Tables 1–4. These tables represented a nine-fold improvement over previous recompression procedures and became the world standard of treatment for the next 20 years. They embodied the concept that the diver should be taken to depth of relief plus 1 atm as a minimum, with a 6-atm maximum, as a trade-off between maximally compressing any offending bubbles and causing too much nitrogen narcosis and too much extension of subsequent decompression time. For serious symptoms, they provided a "12-hour soak," sometimes known as the "overnight soak," at the 30-foot stop on return to the surface so that all tissues could theoretically be equilibrated to 30 feet. Following Haldanian theory, decompression to the surface could then be safely made without exceeding a two-to-one ratio for any tissue. However, to be cautious, several more hours were taken to decompress from 30 feet. Tables 1 through 4 proved themselves fairly successful when used to treat decompression sickness stemming from dives carried out on standard Navy schedules. Air was used as the breathing medium throughout the tables, but oxygen was later introduced for use in the shallower stops. The shortest of the air tables, Table 1A took 6 hours and 13 minutes, and Table 4 took 38 hours. The length of these schedules did not make them popular with divers but represented the only escape from unbearable pain, paralysis, or both.

In 1947, Edgar End, still active in the diving field, began treating caisson workers in Milwaukee with oxygen, using the rationale that gaseous nitrogen was the cause of the patients' symptoms and that the addition of more nitrogen to the patients' tissues when taken to great depth only prolonged treatment time. He generally treated his patients for one to two hours at 30 pounds (67 feet) and then decompressed them. His experience with some 250 cases was excellent, but his data using this method remained unpublished.

Since 1947, no diver or compressed air worker has been treated for bends in Milwaukee with compressed air treatment; only oxygen has been used.

SATURATION DIVING

When a diver goes to depth under water, the inert gas or gases breathed—whether nitrogen, helium, or even hydrogen—begin going into solution in his tissues. After many hours at a given depth, probably in excess of 24 hours, no more gas enters the diver's tissues and a state of equilibrium is reached. His tissues are then totally saturated. After that time the decompression obligation is the same whether the diver stays under water for two days or two weeks. This is commercially useful as the diver does not waste time every day decompressing.

The first intentional saturation dive was carried out by Edgar End and Max Nohl in Milwaukee, Wisconsin at the County Emergency Hospital recompression chamber on December 22, 1938 when they spent 27 hours at 101 feet breathing air. They decompressed fairly successfully, taking about 5 hours with only Nohl experiencing decompression sickness. These bends symptoms were treated with moderate pressures of air with complete relief.

Practical saturation diving was first conceived in 1957 by the late Captain George Bond of the U.S. Navy when working in the Submarine Medical Research Laboratory in New London, Connecticut. Captain Bond (then Commander Bond) envisioned undersea laboratories located at various depths down to 600 feet on the continental shelf. He calculated that by breathing helium, scientists could work at full sea pressure in these laboratories studying physiology, submarine geology, and marine biology for prolonged periods of time. They could then be transferred under pressure by submarine vehicle to a shallower habitat where they could continue their studies while decompressing. Several habitats would be used, each one at a shallower depth, so that finally the scientist could emerge with minimal decompression after completing his tour of study which might last weeks.

It was first necessary to demonstrate that animals could tolerate saturation exposures. These research efforts were termed Project Genesis and, after further work at the Experimental Diving Unit in Washington under the direction of R. D. Workman, saturation decompression schedules were devised for humans. These were later tested in the open sea on Projects Sealab 1 and 2. Meanwhile in 1962, Ed Link saturated a diver for 24 hours at a depth of 200 feet in the Mediterranean. Captain Jacques Cousteau also established saturation habitats in his "Con Shelf" series.

In 1965 commercial saturation diving began when Westinghouse, using their Cachelot diving system, worked at 200 feet on the Smith Mountain Dam in Virginia to replace faulty trash racks. Divers were saturated for periods of up to five days on this job. Since that time saturation has become commonplace, especially in oil field work, where periods of saturation up to two weeks are routine, and one-month saturations have occurred.

COMMERCIAL HELIUM DIVING

With the advent of offshore oil production, diving services were required in deep water, and this need became acute, especially on the West Coast of the United States. Diving companies usually hired local abalone divers to handle various odd jobs associated with drilling rigs; but when pressures of 250 feet were reached, the compressed air equipment used by the commercial divers caused nearly prohibitive nitrogen narcosis. Dan Wilson, an abalone diver from California, decided that helium-oxygen was necessary. In 1962, using a Japanese abalone deep-sea diving dress and a special oronasal mask, he made the first modern civilian helium dive to a depth of 420 feet. Within a year, he was contracting helium-oxygen diving services to oil companies in the Santa Barbara area.

On the Gulf Coast the oil rigs were also moving into deeper water, and Edel calculated the first helium-oxygen schedules for use in the Gulf in 1963. With the demand for deep-sea commercial diving accelerating rapidly, new helium equipment was developed by civilians, and commercial helium diving capabilities soon outstripped those of the U.S. Navy. Bell diving also came into vogue to deliver the commercial diver to the work site.

In all fairness to the U.S. Navy, it must be stated that in the early 1960's, those responsible for Navy budgeting could not identify the operational necessity for deeper helium diving or improved helium diving equipment. It was only in the early 1970's that the U.S. Navy again became active in doing frontline research in this area.

LOW PRESSURE OXYGEN TREATMENT OF DECOMPRESSION SICKNESS

By 1964, the Navy noted that the failure rate for bends treatment Tables 1 through 4 began to rise sharply. This was because the Navy was called upon to treat more civilian scuba divers who had failed to observe any kind of standard decompression schedules. In the year 1964 alone the failure rate on the initial recompression for serious symptoms had risen to 47.1 per cent. Workman and Goodman of the U.S. Navy Experimental Diving Unit reinvestigated the use of oxygen under low pressure as the primary treatment modality for decompression sickness. Oxygen had been suggested by Behnke in 1939 as a promising treatment method after starting with a brief excursion to 6 atm absolute. After three years of work, the U.S. Navy promulgated the low pressure oxygen Tables 5 and 6 on August 22, 1967. At the same time, treatment Tables 5A and 6A for treatment of air embolism were published. The treatment times required for decompression sickness were drastically reduced, and the maximum depth of treatment was only 60 feet (26.7 psig). Table 5 took only 135 minutes and had a failure rate on the initial recompression of only 1 per cent. For serious symptoms and recurrences, Table 6 took only 285 minutes, and the failure rate on the initial recompression fell to only 3.6 per cent. The use of Tables 1 through 4 has now been nearly abandoned. Continued experience with the low pressure oxygen tables revealed frequent recurrences of decompression sickness with the shorter Tables 5 and 5A, and these also either have been abandoned or have seen limited use.

More recent animal research by Leitch and others has shown that little or no advantage is gained by going to 165 feet (6 ata) breathing air on Table 6A in the treatment of embolism, and in fact it may do more harm than good. For this reason, most facilities now use mixed gas containing 50 per cent oxygen-nitrogen or helium-oxygen instead of air with the 6-ata treatment depth. The importance of using high partial pressures of oxygen in treatment of bubble-related diving disorders has been well established.

NEW PRESSURE RECORDS

In the mid 1960's, Hannes Keller, a Swiss experimental diver, reached a depth of 1000 feet in the open sea using a proprietary blend of gases, and the race for increasing depth was on. In 1970, the British reached a depth of 1500 feet in a dry chamber using helium-oxygen as the breathing mixture at the Royal Navy Physiological Laboratory at Alverstoke, England. A new phenomenon appeared called the high pressure nervous syndrome or HPNS. It was discovered that rapid compressions to depths in excess of 500 feet could bring on uncontrollable shaking and nausea in the divers breathing helium. Bennett found that slow compressions could be used to minimize this problem, and the 1970 British dive was accomplished using several days to reach maximum depth.

The French were in strong competition with the British. Using slow compression, they set a record of 1700 feet in the dry chamber in 1971. Again in 1972 the French set a new record of 2001 feet in the dry chamber at the Comex Company. The U.S. Navy, using its Mark 1 deep-sea diving system, set an open sea depth record of 1010 feet off Catalina Island in June of 1972. Today commercial work has been done in excess of 1300 feet. The current pressure record is 2250 feet set in 1981 at Duke University by Peter Bennett. He used a mixture of 10 per cent nitrogen in his blend of helium-nitrogen-oxygen to minimize HPNS. It was Bennett who discovered that adding nitrogen back to the gas mixture could alleviate most of the clinical symptoms of HPNS. This finding enabled compression to 1000 feet in less than half an hour without symptoms.

RECENT DEVELOPMENTS

Universities with oceanography programs took an interest in diving, and civilian saturation diving for research purposes gained ascendency in the late 1960's and the early 1970's. The U.S. Navy, along with other agencies of the government, sponsored the Tektite series of saturation dives to depths of 50 feet in the Caribbean. The Tektite divers breathed normoxic nitrogen-oxygen mixtures. Hydrolab was established by the Perry Submarine Company off Freeport, Grand Bahama, at depths of 42 and 60 feet. Dozens of scientists have been saturated for periods of up to two weeks in this habitat breathing compressed air. The Puerto Rican International Underwater Laboratory (PRINUL) was built with a saturation capability to 100 feet. The Tektite 2 series saw the first all-woman team of aquanauts carry out scientific research while saturated. Saturation on air deeper than about 60 feet cannot be carried out because of primary oxygen toxicity considerations. Deeper than that, mixed gas with a lesser partial pressure of oxygen must be used.

Tri-gas mixtures became of interest commercially in the 1960's, and André Galèrne of International Underwater Contractors pioneered their use. These mixes consist of helium, nitrogen, and oxygen and are being used commercially more and more. Neon and helium have been used experimentally. The French have successfully experimented with mixtures of hydrogen and helium and reached depths in the open sea greater than 1500 feet in March 1988.

Commercial contracts for deep diving have become more sophisticated, and by 1974 contracts called for diving services to depths of 1500 feet in support of off-shore oil production, if needed.

While studies to define limits and protect divers exposed to increasing hydrostatic pressure continue, another development has been the use of "one-atmosphere diving systems" for deep diving. These are basically submarines with manipulators to allow the operator to work at great depth while the interior is maintained at 1 ata and environmental control systems maintain safe physiological parameters. They range from armored one-person 1-ata suits (e.g., Jim, WASP, and so forth) to submersibles, which allow for more than one occupant.

FUTURE RESEARCH

Diving depths to 3000 feet are now being considered with tri-gas mixes. Hydrogen as a diving gas is under active investigation by Comex in France, and the blood changes in decompression sickness are beginning to be quantified. The first symposium on blood changes in bends was conducted in Toronto in 1973.

At the present time more attention is being paid to the study of the actual elimination curves of inert gas during decompression, but empiricism (using computer data) is relied on more than mathematical models for devising decompression tables. Future research will undoubtedly provide answers to the exact mechanism of inert gas elimination from the body and what the tolerable limits of tissue trauma may be during this process.

Chapter 2

Diving Physics

LEE H. SOMERS

Man naturally exists within a relatively narrow range of environmental parameters. Outside of this narrow range nearly all unusual experiences encountered in diving, both pleasant and unpleasant, stem directly or indirectly from the great differences in physical properties and characteristics which exist between the gaseous and liquid media. Some apparent differences include:

- water has a much higher density and viscosity
- optical and acoustical properties differ
- water has a higher degree of heat conductivity than air
- gases breathed under increased pressure have varied physiological effects.

In order to understand the basic principles of diving and to function safely in the underwater environment, the diver must be familiar with certain aspects of the science of physics which deal with pressure and density relative to liquids and gases. A knowledge of the physical environment is also essential to the physician involved with the care of divers.

This chapter will not undertake a complete orientation to elementary physics. Rather, it will review the pertinent physical principles necessary for a fundamental understanding of the diving environment. Certain aspects such as light and vision underwater, propagation of sound underwater, and thermal factors will also be addressed.

TERMINOLOGY AND SYMBOLS

Terminology and symbol abbreviations used are based on those commonly used by divers in the United States. Units of measure are generally expressed in both the U.S. Customary System and the International Metric System (in parentheses). Symbols for common units of measure are given in Table 2–1; conversions for these units are given in Table 2–2.

PRESSURE

Pressure is the amount of force applied per unit of area. In diving, pressure units commonly used are pounds per square inch (psi or lb/in^2),

TABLE 2–1. Symbols for Common Units of Measure

SYMBOL	UNIT
cf (ft^3)	cubic feet
cfm (ft^3/min)	cubic feet per minute
scf	standard cubic feet
scfm	standard cubic feet per minute
acfm	actual cubic feet per minute
psi (lb/in^2)	pounds per square inch
psig	pounds per square inch, gauge
psia	pounds per square inch, absolute
fsw	feet sea water
fpm	feet per minute
atm	atmospheres
ata	atmospheres absolute
l	liters
cu m (m^3)	cubic meters
cm	centimeter
cu cm (cm^3)	cubic centimeter
gm/cm^2	grams per square centimeter
cm Hg	centimeters mercury
mm Hg	millimeters mercury
kg	kilograms
gm	grams
m	meter
°C	degrees Celsius
°F	degrees Fahrenheit
°R	degrees Rankine
°K	degrees Kelvin

TABLE 2–2. Conversion Table for Units of Pressure

1 pound per square inch (psi)	= 2.31 ft of fresh water
	= 2.25 ft of sea water
	= 0.068 atm
	= 2.036 in Hg
	= 70.3 gm/cm^2
	= 0.0703 kg/cm^2
	= 5.17 cm Hg
1 atmosphere (atm)	= 14.696 psi
	= 29.92 in Hg
	= 33.9 ft of fresh water
	= 33 ft of sea water
	= 1.033 kg/cm^2
	= 1.013 bars
	= 760 mm Hg
1 foot of sea water (fsw)	= 0.445 psi
1 gram per square centimeter (gm/cm^2)	= 0.394 in of fresh water
	= 0.001 kg/cm^2
	= 1 cm of fresh water
1 kilogram per square centimeter (kg/cm^2)	= 1000 gm/cm^2
	= 10 m of fresh water
	= 9.75 m of sea water
	= 73.56 cm Hg
	= 14.22 psi
	= 32.8 ft of fresh water
	= 28.96 in of mercury

kilograms per square centimeter (kg/cm^2), and atmospheres (atm). One *atmosphere* is the amount of pressure or force exerted on all bodies or structures by the earth's atmosphere. At sea level, atmospheric pressure is equal to 14.7 psi or 1.03 kg/cm^2. At higher elevations, the atmospheric pressure is less.

Hydrostatic pressure is the force resulting from the weight of water (or any fluid) acting upon a body or object immersed in the water. Like atmospheric pressure, it is equal in all directions at a specific level or depth. The pressure increases as the diver descends at a rate of 0.445 psi per foot (or 1 kg/cm^2 per 9.75 meters) in sea water and at 0.432 psi per foot (or 1 kg/cm^2 per 10 meters) in fresh water.

Absolute pressure exerted on a submerged body is the sum of the atmospheric pressure and the hydrostatic pressure. It is measured in pounds per square inch absolute (psia) and kilograms per square centimeter (kg/cm^2) absolute. Ambient pressure refers to the presence surrounding or encompassing the body or object and is usually expressed in absolute pressure terms.

Gauge pressure refers to the difference between the pressure being measured and the atmospheric pressure. Most gauges are calibrated to read zero at normal atmospheric pressure. Gauge pressure is converted to absolute pressure by adding 14.7 psi (1.03 kg/cm^2).

For every 33 feet that the diver descends in sea water (34 feet in fresh water), there is a pressure increase of 1 atm (14.7 psi or 1 kg/cm^2). Thus, at 99 fsw, the absolute pressure is equal to four atmospheres (58.8 psia or 4 kg/cm^2 absolute).

In a mixture of gases, the proportion of the total pressure contributed by a single gas in the mixture is called the *partial pressure*. The partial pressure contributed by a single gas is in direct proportion to its percentage of the total volume of the mixture. It is the partial pressure that determines the amount of dissolved gas in tissues. Concentration of gas in tissues is an important factor in decompression sickness and in nitrogen narcosis.

BUOYANCY

Any object placed in a liquid will either float or sink depending on the density of the object relative to the density of the liquid. The principle of buoyancy was first stated by Archimedes, who established that "any object wholly or partially immersed in a liquid is buoyed up by a force equal to the weight of the liquid displaced by the object" (Fig. 2–1). The buoyant force of a fluid depends upon its density (weight per unit volume). Pure water, with a density of 62.4 lb/ft^3 (1 g/cm^3), has a slightly less buoyant force than sea water, which has a density of 64 lb/ft^3 (1.025 g/cm^3). If an object

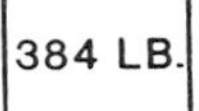

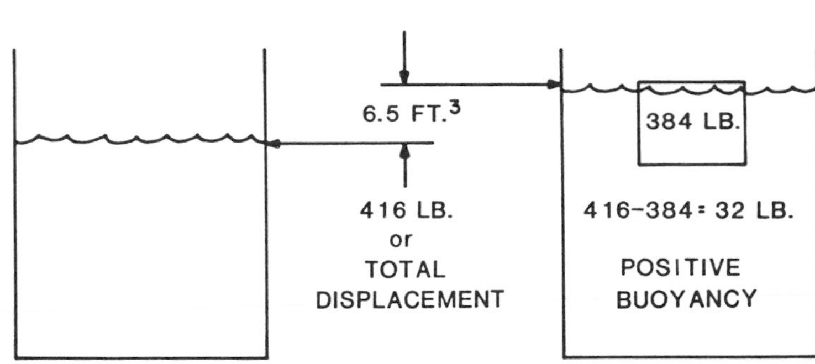

FIGURE 2–1. Archimedes' principle of buoyancy is illustrated by this example.

floats, it is said to be positively buoyant, if it sinks, it is negatively buoyant. Neutral buoyancy, or a state of hydrostatic balance, is achieved when the weight of the water displaced equals the weight of the object when totally submerged. An object in a state of neutral buoyancy neither sinks nor floats.

Since this slight density difference exists between fresh water and sea water, the diver tends to float more easily in the ocean than in a fresh water lake or pool. Sea water increases buoyancy by approximately 3 per cent of the body weight over what it would be in fresh water. When a diver properly weighted for fresh water plans to dive in the ocean, the weight belt will have to be increased by several pounds.

Buoyancy is an extremely important factor in diving. During underwater swimming with scuba, the diver strives to maintain a state of neutral buoyancy. If the diver is negatively buoyant, he will have to exert considerable effort to counteract the sinking or downward movement. This can cause unnecessary fatigue and can inhibit the diver's ascent. Excessive positive buoyancy is equally undesirable in that the diver must exert a considerable amount of effort to counteract the upward movement and maintain a given depth level. The scuba diver's buoyancy control situation is further complicated by diving suit compression-expansion, air supply utilization, and breathing characteristics. Lung inflation-deflation can have a significant effect on buoyancy. Buoyancy compensation procedures and equipment are important considerations in diving safety.

DIVING GASES

Air is comprised of nitrogen (79.1 per cent), oxygen (20.9 per cent), carbon dioxide (0.033 per cent), and various inert and rare or trace gases. It may also contain water vapor and suspended or dissolved solids.

Nitrogen, the main component of air, is colorless, odorless, tasteless, and inert (in its free state). Under increased pressures, it is selectively soluble in various body tissues and acts as an intoxicant or anesthetic on the central nervous system.

Oxygen, the only gas capable of supporting life, is colorless, odorless, and tasteless in its free state. Under high pressures, oxygen has toxic effects on the body.

Carbon dioxide, a natural waste product of metabolism, is colorless and tasteless in normal concentration. It is the principal respiratory stimulant to respiration. High concentrations are toxic to humans and will produce unconsciousness with subsequent death.

Other gases important to the diver are carbon monoxide and helium. *Carbon monoxide* is highly poisonous, and all possible measures must be taken to prevent its contamination of the diver's air supply. It is the product of incomplete combustion of fossil fuels. *Helium* is colorless, odorless, tasteless, inert, lightweight, nontoxic, and nonexplosive. During the last two decades, helium has become the major inert gas substituted for nitrogen in deep-diving breathing media. Narcotic effects of helium are relatively limited, and breathing resistance due to lower density is significantly reduced. However, helium does conduct heat about five times as rapidly as air.

In comparison to a liquid or solid, air, as any gas, has a very low density, is compressible, and its behavior is governed by simpler laws of physics. Air weighs only about 0.081 lb/ft^3 at 0°C or 0.075 lb/ft^3 at 20°C.

GAS LAWS

The physical behavior of ideal gases (nitrogen, oxygen, helium) is subject to three closely interrelated factors—temperature, pressure, and volume. A change in one of these three factors, such as an increase in temperature, must result in measurable change in the other factors. The kinetic behavior of any one ideal gas will be the same for all ideal gases or mixtures of gases. The temperature, pressure, and volume relationships are useful for diving gases conveniently expressed in terms of the behavior of an ideal gas. In working with gas laws, all pressures are expressed in terms of absolute pressure, all temperatures are in terms of absolute temperature, and all units used in the equation should be in one system of measure. The gas laws of direct concern to divers are Boyle's law, Charles' law, Dalton's law, and Henry's law.

Boyle's Law

Boyle's law states that if the temperature of a fixed mass of gas is kept constant, the relationship between the volume and pressure will vary in such a way that the product of the pressure and volume will remain constant. Mathematically, PV = K where P is absolute pressure, V is volume, and K is a constant. The temperature and mass are constant. Thus, at a constant temperature and mass, the volume of a gas is inversely proportional to the pressure exerted on that gas. Consequently, when the pressure is doubled, the volume is reduced to one half of the original volume. This relationship is graphically illustrated in Figure 2–2. Two different states of a gas at the same temperature may be denoted by subscripts 1 and 2. Using this type of notation, Boyle's law may also be written:

$$P_1V_1 = P_2V_2.$$

To illustrate Boyle's law, let us assume that a closed flexible container of air (i.e., a rubber balloon) with a volume of 1 cf at the surface is submerged to a depth of 33 fsw. Using the above formula,

$$\begin{aligned} P_1V_1 &= P_2V_2 \\ 1 \times 1 &= 2\,V_2 \\ 0.5\text{ cf} &= V_2 \end{aligned}$$

where P_1 is atmospheric pressure, V_1 is the volume at P_1 or 1 cf, P_2 is the pressure at 33 fsw in atmospheres, and V_2 is the volume at 33 fsw. Note that the volume is changed by 50 per cent.

In order to illustrate a very important factor in diving, let us now submerge the same flexible container from 33 to 66 fsw. Using the formula,

$$\begin{aligned} P_1V_1 &= P_2V_2 \\ 2 \times .5 &= 3\,V_2 \\ 0.33\text{ cf} &= V_2 \end{aligned}$$

observe that the change between 33 fsw and 66 fsw is much less than the surface and 33 fsw, a change of only 0.17 cf compared with 0.5 cf. Understanding this relationship is important to the diver because it illustrates that sudden changes in depth while in shallow water can be far more hazardous than equivalent changes in depth in deep water.

The pressure-volume relationship can be much more dramatically illustrated in terms of an emergency ascent. As a part of a training exercise and, possibly, in actual diving, a diver will have to make an emergency swimming ascent from some given depth. For discussion purposes, let us assume that the diver must ascend from a depth of 66 fsw. While at 66 fsw the diver breathes air from scuba delivered at ambient pressure of 3 ata, so that a pressure balance exists between the body and the surrounding environment. Assuming normal size and capacity lungs, the diver fills them to about 5 liters on each breath. As the diver ascends, the ambient pressure is reduced and the air volume in the lungs increases. As long as the diver continues to breathe during a normal ascent or continuously exhales during an emergency ascent and maintains a pressure balance with the surrounding environment, there should be no problem. However, if the diver holds his breath, the lungs attempt to function like a closed flexible container. During ascent from 66 fsw to 33 fsw, the volume of air in the lungs will increase from 5 liters to 7.5 liters; from 33 fsw to the surface, this volume will double. The implications are clear. The lungs will rupture if the diver holds his breath. The serious implications of lung rupture or barotrauma will be discussed later (see Chapter 16).

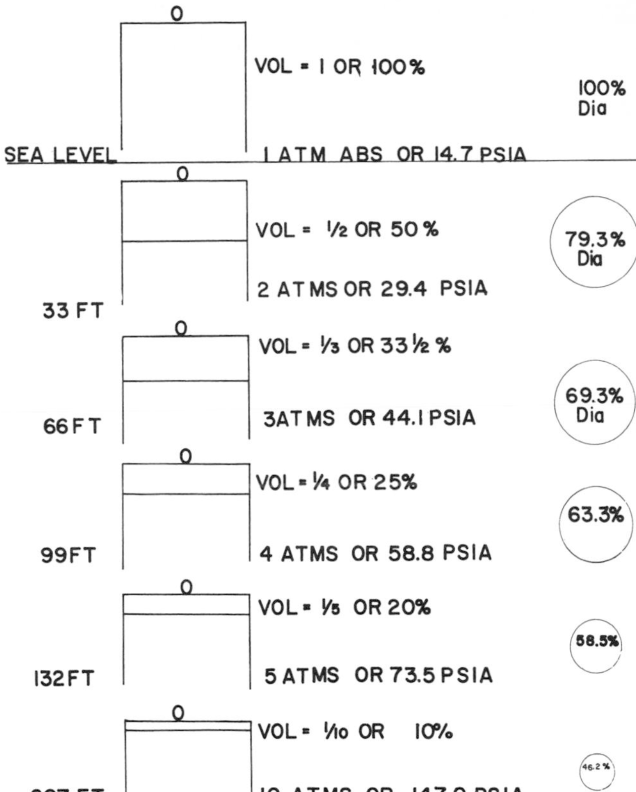

FIGURE 2–2. Gas volume and bubble diameter as a function of depth—Boyle's law.

One can easily see the seriousness of sudden pressure changes in shallow water. Improper, rapid ascent from 10 fsw can cause serious lung damage with subsequent air embolism, a potentially fatal pressure-related injury. Ten feet of sea water is swimming-pool depth.

Charles' Law

Charles' law states that if the pressure of a fixed mass of gas is kept constant, the volume of the gas will vary directly with the absolute temperature. Conversely, if the volume is restrained in a rigid container (such as a scuba air cylinder), the pressure will vary directly with the absolute temperature. The formula is expressed as:

$$PV = RT$$

where P is absolute pressure, V is volume, T is absolute temperature, and R is a universal constant for all gases.

Boyle's and Charles's laws demonstrate that for any gas the factors of temperature, volume, and pressure are so interrelated that a change in any of these factors must be balanced by a corresponding change in one or both of the others. The *general gas law* is a convenient combination of these two laws in predicting the behavior of a given quantity of gas when changes may be expected in any or all of the variables. These relationships for an ideal gas can be expressed as:

$$\frac{PV}{T} = K$$

where K is a constant. Two states of the gas may be denoted with subscripts:

$$\frac{P_1V_1}{T_1} = \frac{P_2V_2}{T_2}$$

To illustrate gas behavior using the general gas law, let us examine the effects of temperature change on a scuba cylinder. A standard 71.2 cf scuba cylinder is filled to 3000 psig in chilled water at 45°F. The cylinder is transported to a tropical beach where it is placed directly in the sun. The cylinder temperature is measured at 140°F following a long exposure to the direct sun. What has happened to the air in the cylinder? Applying the general gas law, we can compare the cylinder under two conditions—the chilled water tank and the tropical beach. First, the volume of the rigid cylinder remains unchanged so $V_1 = V_2$. This factor can be eliminated from the problem. The variables, therefore, are temperature and pressure. Mathematically,

$$\frac{P_1}{T_1} = \frac{P_2}{T_2}$$

where P_1 equals absolute pressure at the time the cylinder was charged (3000 psig + 14.7 psi = 3015 psia), T_1 equals the absolute temperature of the cylinder when charged (45°F + 460° = 505°F), T_2 equals the absolute temperature of the cylinder on the beach (140°F + 460° = 600°R*), and P_2 is the unknown.
Substituting the values in the equation,

$$\frac{3015 \text{ psia} \times 600°\text{R}}{505°\text{R}} = P_2$$

$$3582 \text{ psia} = P_2$$

$$3567 \text{ psig} = P_2$$

Under the new environmental condition, direct sunlight on the beach, the cylinder is significantly overpressure.

Dalton's Law

In diving, one generally works with a mixture of gases rather than with a single pure gas. The concept of partial pressure is explained by Dalton's law, which states that the total pressure exerted by a mixture of gases is the sum of the pressures that would be exerted by each gas if it were to occupy the total volume. Partial pressure computations are useful for understanding diving physiology and are necessary for mixed-gas diving. The partial pressure (pA) of a given gas in a mixture may be calculated by the formula,

$$pA = P_t V_{\%}$$

where P_t is the total pressure of the gas mixture (absolute) and $V_{\%}$ is the percentage of gas A by volume in the mixture. Hence, the partial pressure of oxygen in the atmosphere at sea level is:

$$pO_2 = 14.7\ (0.21) \text{ or } 3.1 \text{ psi}$$

The partial pressure of nitrogen and oxygen in air is given in Table 2–3.

Henry's Law

Gas is soluble in a liquid, and absorption by a liquid is governed by Henry's law, which states that the amount of a gas that will dissolve in a liquid at a given temperature is directly proportional to the partial pressure of that gas. The "amount" refers to number of molecules or mass of the gas. When gas is in solution, its actual volume is negligible, and there is no volumetric increase in the amount of liquid. Henry's law simply expresses the effect of partial pressure on the amount of gas that will dissolve in a liquid. Solubility is also dependent on the type of liquid and temperature. For example, the solubility of nitrogen in oil or fat is about five times its solubility in water at the same pressure. The lower the temperature, the higher the solubility. This explains why a warm bottle of carbonated beverage forms bubbles more actively than does a cold one.

Gas diffusion refers to the intermingling of gas molecules. In diving, Henry's and Dalton's laws are considered when dealing with the diffusion of gas in the human body under pressure. The difference between the partial pressure (or tension) of a gas dissolved in a liquid and its outside partial pressure will cause the gas to diffuse in or out of the liquid and control the rate of diffusion. This pressure differential is frequently called a diffusion gradient. If a

*Convert the temperature from degrees Fahrenheit to its absolute equivalent in degrees Rankine, °R = °F + 460°.

TABLE 2–3. Absolute and Partial Pressures of Nitrogen and Oxygen in Air at Various Depths

	Absolute Pressure			Partial Pressure*			
				Nitrogen		Oxygen	
Depth (ft)	*atm*	*mm Hg*	*psi*	*mm Hg*	*psi*	*mm Hg*	*psi*
0 (surface)	1	760	14.7	600	11.6	160	3.1
33	2	1520	29.4	1200	23.2	320	6.2
66	3	2280	44.1	1800	34.8	480	9.3
99	4	3040	58.8	2400	46.4	640	12.4
132	5	3800	73.5	3000	58.0	800	15.5
165	6	4560	88.2	3600	69.6	960	18.6

*Approximate air composition values of 79 per cent nitrogen and 21 per cent oxygen.

gas-free liquid is exposed to a gas, the inward gradient is high, and the rate at which gas molecules will migrate into the liquid is high. As the gas tension in the liquid increases, the net rate of diffusion decreases and eventually stops when equilibrium is attained, at which point the gas tensions in the liquid and outside of the liquid are equal. The liquid is then considered to be saturated for a given pressure and gas. The subjects of gas solubility and diffusion are important in the study of decompression sickness and nitrogen narcosis.

Surface equivalent is another notation that frequently appears in the discussion of diving theory. Calculation of surface equivalent (SE) can be expressed algebraically as:

$$SE = \frac{p_D}{1} \times 100\%$$

where p_D is the partial pressure at depth expressed in atmospheres, and 1 is one atmosphere surface pressure. The term surface equivalent and its significance can best be explained by examining a hypothetical air contamination situation. Surface air contaminated with 2 per cent CO_2 (pCO_2 = 0.02 atm) is breathed by a diver at a depth of 132 fsw (5 ata). The partial pressure of the CO_2 in the inspired gas at depth is therefore 0.1 atm (0.02 atm × 5 atm). This partial pressure converts to a surface equivalent percentage:

$$SE = \frac{0.1 \text{ atm}}{1.0 \text{ atm}} \times 100\% = 10\%.$$

Normally, 2 per cent carbon dioxide causes only a slight increase in respiration; however, a diver breathing 10 per cent concentration may exhibit signs of mental confusion, irrationality, drowsiness, and pending unconsciousness.

In this case, the term surface equivalent is used to imply that the concentration and physiological effect of a gas at a given partial pressure at depth is the same as would be experienced at "x" per cent breathing on the surface. Although it is a commonly used term, surface equivalent is often misinterpreted, and it is preferable to use the more exact form of expressing partial pressure in units of pressure (atm, mm Hg, and so forth).

LIGHT AND VISION

Underwater vision is of major concern to the diver. In order to complete a task or observe the surrounding environment, the diver must be equipped to see as clearly as possible. The human eye needs light in order to see. What is actually seen by the eye is an image created by the reflection of light from the subject being viewed. Underwater light is affected by many factors that directly influence the diver's ability to see and interpret images. The major factors include:

- *turbidity:* particles in the water that obscure vision by obstructing light rays
- *diffusion:* the scattering of the light rays by the water molecules and particulate matter
- *absorption:* the property that alters color and intensity of light; light is absorbed and transformed to heat
- *refraction:* the bending of a light ray as it passes from one medium to another
- *reflection:* the angle at which the light rays strike the water's surface; some enter the water and others are reflected.

Turbidity is a primary limiting factor that affects the diver's safety and performance. Solar light does not penetrate much beyond 1650 feet even under the most ideal conditions of water transparency. In clear water the luminous energy (or ambient light) is reduced to about one-fourth surface value at 16 feet, one-eighth surface value at 50 feet, and one-thirteenth surface value at 130 feet. In clear water, enough light generally remains for vision down to 400 feet. However, in very turbid waters such as are found near some coastal areas or in many inland lakes, underwater visibility may be severely reduced at shallow depths. These waters contain large quantities of suspended materials such as sedimentary particles, biological matter (plankton), and chemical pollutants. Under these conditions, the light rays are partially or totally obstructed.

Any time there is a significant decrease in the level of ambient light, the eye must adapt accordingly. As light level rapidly decreases, the eye must transform from a day vision light sensory mode to a night vision light sensory mode. Although most of the dark adaptation occurs within the first 10 minutes, the complete process may require about 30 minutes depending on light level differentials. The diver generally descends much more rapidly than the adaptation process can take place. The process is further changed by the absorption of light at greater depths, low underwater light levels in late afternoon or early morning when the sun is at a lower angle, and the turbidity state of the water. This adaptation process accounts, in part, for the apparent loss of perceived light as the diver goes deeper. It also accounts for the fact that the diver may sense an increase in ambient light level after remaining on the bottom for 20 to 30 minutes.

The color quality of the light also changes with increasing depth. The color of the water itself is influenced by the color of the sky, the quality and nature of suspended materials in the water, and the water depth. Water in the open ocean appears blue for the same reason that the sky is blue. This is caused by scattering of light rays by water molecules and by tiny particles suspended in the water. Blue, being of short wave length, is scattered more effectively than light of longer wave length (such as red). Although the water is commonly a shade of blue in open ocean, it may appear as various shades of green, brown, or brownish-red near shore as a result of material contained in the water.

Colors under water are modified with depth because the wave lengths of the visible spectrum are progressively absorbed and filtered out by the water. The process starts almost as soon as the light enters the water. The water acts as a blue filter that intensifies with depth. Although many factors affect the color absorption, in average clear water, all red colors are gone at a depth of about 30 feet, yellows at 75 feet, and only blues and greens are visible below 100 feet. At these depths the marine life and submarine features take on a rather drab bluish-grey appearance. Naturally, the color spectrum can be replaced using artificial light.

The angle that the light rays from the sun strike the water significantly affects the light intensity under water. When the sun is high in the sky at mid-day, as much as 97 per cent of the light rays striking the surface of calm clear water may enter the water. As the angle of the sun relative to the water's surface decreases, as in the early morning or late afternoon, more and more light is reflected back into the atmosphere. There is still sufficient light to see under water even at dusk and dawn, since light is scattered back into the water from the atmosphere.

As the sun rises in the morning, nearly all of the light rays are reflected off the water's surface until the sun reaches 48.6° (measured from the vertical); this is the critical angle of sunlight penetration. As the sun continues to rise, a larger percentage of the rays enter the water. The same critical angle applies to internal light. A ray of light directed upward toward the under surface of the water at an angle of greater than 48.6° is totally reflected back into the water instead of being partially reflected into the atmosphere. This makes the surface appear as a mirror when the diver is in the proper position.

The roughness of the water's surface (wave motion) constantly changes the reflective and penetrating angles of the sun's light rays. When the surface is rough and the sun is lower than the critical angle, more light is transmitted into the water than it would be on calm surfaces because of excessive diffusion of light at the surface. However, when the sun passes above the critical angle, the rougher the water surface, the greater the reflection back into the atmosphere.

Refraction is another phenomenon associated with light transmission that is significant to the diver. When a light ray is transmitted from a medium of one density into a medium of another, the speed that the ray is traveling is reduced. Reducing speed alters the path angle of the ray. In air, light travels at a speed of 186,000 miles per second; in water the speed is reduced to about 135,000 miles per second. The relative *index of refraction* is therefore the ratio of the speed of light between the two mediums. The air:water index of refraction is approximately 4:3 and varies slightly according to the density of a given body of water.

Consequently, because of this refraction between air and water, objects viewed through a face mask under water appear larger and closer than they actually are (Fig. 2–3). Occasionally novice divers will find themselves reaching for objects that are actually slightly beyond their reach. This modification of depth perception can be compensated for with training and experience.

When the cornea of the human eye interfaces with water rather than air, it loses much of its refractive power because the index of refraction of the cornea is nearly the same as that of water. Consequently, vision is extremely poor and images appear blurred.

PROPAGATION OF SOUND

The average speed of sound under water is about 4900 ft/sec, compared with a speed of less than 1100 ft/sec in air. Sounds such as those produced by striking a steel scuba cylinder with a metal object (e.g., diver's knife) travel relatively long distances and can be heard clearly

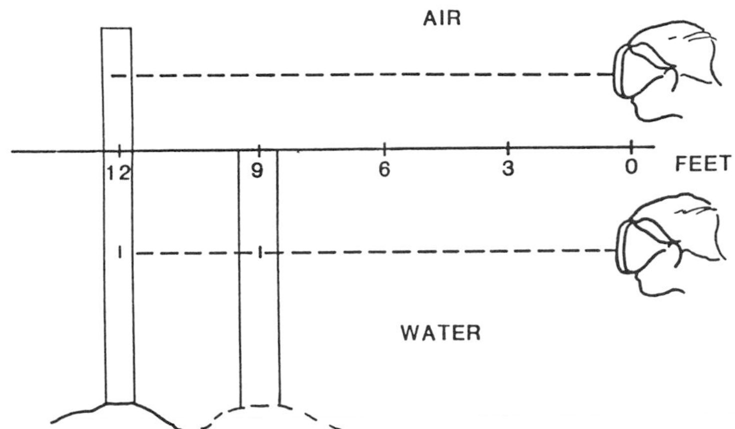

FIGURE 2–3. Refraction between air and water occurs at an index of approximately 4:3. In this example, an object that is 12 ft away appears under water to be only 9 ft away.

by other divers. However, determining the direction of the sound source is not always easy. The faster speed of sound under water almost eliminates the important time delay between near and distant ears detecting the sound, a factor necessary for determining direction.

Although sound moves faster in water, it travels very poorly from air into water. All but about 1/10,000 of the sound is lost during the transition through the air-water interface. Diver-to-diver communication by voice is ineffective under water. Since the human voice originates in the throat, an air environment, most of the sound is lost as it enters the water. As a result, very little intelligible sound ever reaches another diver unless special communication devices are used.

HEAT TRANSFER

Each winter thousands of recreational divers subject themselves to climatic and water conditions equivalent to those found in the polar latitudes. Probably most cold weather diving is conducted in fresh water lakes where the water temperature generally ranges from 33°F to 40°F (.5°C to 4.4°C). About 25 per cent of all civilian diving activities in the United States are conducted in waters with temperatures below 40°F (4.4°C). Undoubtedly, this figure is higher for the vast population of Canadian divers. To further complicate the situation, cold water is present in the deeper northern lakes throughout the entire year.

The body loses heat in several ways when exposed to excessively cold temperatures. An unprotected diver loses heat to the water surrounding him mainly by convection and direct conduction through his skin.

Conduction is the direct molecule to molecule transfer of heat through a substance or through materials that are in contact with each other. The body warms, by conduction or radiation, a thin layer of water or air next to the skin. If the water surrounding the diver is moved by currents, either natural or diver-produced, heat is transferred away from that area surrounding the body by *convection*. Even if the body is left completely still and there is no water movement, convective currents are formed in the heat transfer process. The water next to the body expands slightly as it is warmed by conduction from the body. Therefore, being slightly lighter than the surrounding water, this water rises and colder water replaces it. Thus, convection currents are formed.

The body also loses heat from exposed surfaces through *radiation*. Any warm body or object emits electromagnetic waves, usually in the infrared range. Diver heat loss by radiation is negligible compared with that by convection and conduction. However, the diver is cautioned to protect the uncovered surfaces such as the head, neck, and hands prior to the dive. These areas, where blood supplies are very close to the surface, radiate considerable amounts of heat and may be responsible for serious cooling of the diver prior to entering the water.

Evaporation of perspiration from the skin and of water vapor from the lungs contributes significantly to the amount of heat lost by the body. Although perspiring is not generally a problem faced by the cold water diver, the evaporation of water from the lungs is. Heat lost through respiratory evaporation can also be significant. The magnitude of the problem can be appreciated when one considers that 1/12 oz. (2.5 ml) of evaporated perspiration cools the body approximtely 2°F (0.94°C). Consider the fact that scuba cylinders must be filled with *moisture-free* air. Consequently, with each breath considerable amounts of water vapor and heat are transferred to the expired air. Even under normal conditions, the body loses a significant amount of heat with each exhalation. In cold water diving, a considerable amount of heat is lost with each inhalation; considerable energy is required to heat the cold air that is breathed from the scuba. Breathing of this air under pressure is more likely to produce heat loss than breathing air above water in cold weather, even though the water temperature is not below freezing. When divers use helium-oxygen at deep depths, the heat loss can produce serious clinical hypothermia. Both air and oxy-helium carry more heat when compressed, thus when under pressure, heat loss through breathing gas can become significant. In deep oxy-helium diving, the breathing gas is heated to avoid hypothermia. In scuba diving, breathing air can be cooled below ambient temperature by the cooling effect of gas expansion as it leaves the high pressure cylinder.

Cold water diving produces considerable stress even before concern with breathing resistance, emotional stress, and swimming exertion become important. Although widely studied, all the implications of cold stress on the diver are not clear. However, one thing is clear: To cope with the unusually high stresses involved with working in cold water, the potential diver must be healthy and extremely physically fit.

SUMMARY

The basic principles of physics provide a foundation for understanding the reasons for employing various diving techniques and procedures. They assume particular significance in studying the effects of pressure and the underwater environment upon the human body.

FURTHER READING

Adolfson J, Berghage T: Perception and Performance Underwater. New York, John Wiley & Sons, 1974.

Calhoun F: NAUI Physics for Divers. Montclair, National Association of Underwater Instructors, 1978.

Kuehn L (ed): Thermal Constraints in Diving. Bethesda, Undersea Medical Society, 1981.

Shilling CW, Werts MF, Schandelmeir NR: The Underwater Handbook. New York, Plenum Press, 1976.

U.S. Navy Diving Manual, NAVSEA 0994-LP-001-9010, Chapter 2, 1973.

Webb P (ed): Prolonged and Repeated Work in Cold Water. Bethesda, Undersea Medical Society, 1985.

Chapter 3

Diving Equipment

GLEN H. EGSTROM

Diving equipment evolution has progressed dramatically since the 1950's. The increased use of specialized materials has enhanced engineering design advances and manufacturing programs. There has been a proliferation of full service dive operations throughout the world which are marketing a sophisticated line of products and services to meet the needs of an enlarged diving population. The diver in the 1980's has access to a wide and varied range of equipment (Fig. 3–1). This chapter is meant to provide practical insight into some of the more important considerations of such equipment and its effective use. All divers have the responsibility to know their limitations with whatever equipment they choose. Hopefully, all divers will use equipment as tools rather than as crutches and will be comfortable on each and every dive they undertake. Proper diving preparation includes an effective adaptation to the proper use of such tools within the diving environment.

Proper training in the use of the equipment coupled with knowledge of personal limitations will minimize the risk of a loss of control, which could lead to injury or death.

MASKS

The purpose of the mask is to provide an air pocket that permits the eye to focus and thus allows the diver to see clearly under water. The size of the air pocket can vary from that within a special contact lens to goggles, masks, and even helmets. Problems are related to visual distortion, restricted visual fields, pressure-volume changes with attendant discomfort, and occasional irritation from chemical or bacteriological sources.

Visual distortions are the result of variations in the distance from the mask lens to the eye. The index of refraction of water is 1.333 due to its increased density, while air has an index of 1. This difference results in light rays being shortened in water causing the diver to perceive objects closer and larger than they really are. For example, an object 4 feet away will appear to be 3 feet away if one views it directly forward with the mask lens perpendicular to the line of vision. As the line of vision moves across the flat lens, however, the distortion of the object being viewed is increased and appears larger.

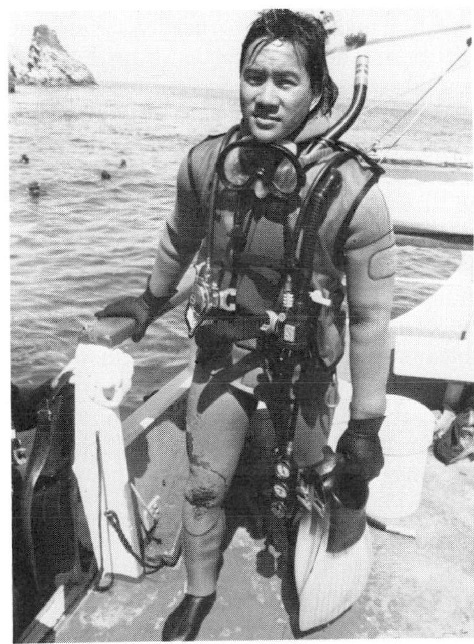

FIGURE 3–1. Fully dressed scuba diver wearing wetsuit, buoyancy compensator jacket, and tank. Fins are removed for mobility on ship's deck.

Divers adapt readily to this problem and, with experience, learn to adjust their hand-eye coordination and spatial-visual judgments accurately.

Restrictions of the visual field through the mask are annoying and are largely a function of the distance of the lens from the eye, the size of the nose, and dimensions of the lens and skirt of the mask. Placing the lens close to the eye permits a wider visual field. The size of the nose and the nose pocket found on many masks creates an obstruction in the medial portion of the visual field. Masks with side lenses at corrected angles are popular, but there is always a distorted area where the lens planes change. This can lead to an interesting phenomenon. A fish swimming across the diver's line of vision may be seen out of the side panel, and as it gets closer it may disappear from view or may appear to bend as it comes into view on the front panel. Additionally the newer clear skirts and side windows permit light to come into the mask from the side and reflect off the inside of the lens, causing some loss of acuity. The new hypoallergenic silicone skirts have improved comfort, have decreased irritation of the skin and eyes, and will last significantly longer than natural rubber products.

Cleaning products for the lenses and skirts should be handled with care. Some of the cleaning products leave residue in the mask which may get into the eyes, causing severe irritation and potential damage. Thorough rinsing of the mask prior to use is a fundamental precaution. The fit of the mask to the contours of the face is very important and should be considered carefully before purchase, since tightening the mask strap to make a seal will create discomfort for the diver. The split at the back of the headband should spread the resistive load of the mask over the upper portion of the back of the skull. This will avoid a bad angle of pull on the mask with the attendant symptoms of a mask squeeze normally caused by barotrauma. If a mask leaks, the cause is usually the result of trapped hair or the edge of the hood; making a seal by assuring smooth contact with the skin is much more effective than tightening the strap excessively.

Individuals with serious visual problems should use care when diving with contact lenses since they can be washed out of the eye with ease if the mask is flooded without warning. Lenses with appropriate corrections can be placed in masks quite easily and offer an alternative for the diver. Attempting to insert eyeglasses into masks will prove to be unsatisfactory and is not recommended.

FINS

Fins (Fig. 3–2) are worn to increase the surface area of the foot and to provide a greater resistive surface to improve propulsion so that the diver can overcome the resistance developed by the diving equipment. Fins can be found to meet the needs of virtually any diver. The development of long flexible fins for competitive fin swimming and the use of new lightweight materials for better thrust and durability have added a new dimension to diving efficiency.

One criterion for evaluating fins involves comfort, both in the footpocket and in the stress on the leg muscles during use under diving conditions. Leg length and strength must also be considered, since weak muscles on a long leg may result in the inability to effectively use an otherwise excellent fin configuration. Weak hip rotational muscles, for example, may permit the hip to rotate during the thrust phase of the kick, resulting in the fin turning on the edge and slicing through instead of flexing and providing thrust.

Fin studies conducted at UCLA have consistently demonstrated that individual variation in the ability to use fins effectively dictates which fin may be superior for an individual at a given level of conditioning. A study of nine popular fins was conducted during which nine subjects were asked to use each fin in random order on two occasions in a blind test under three work

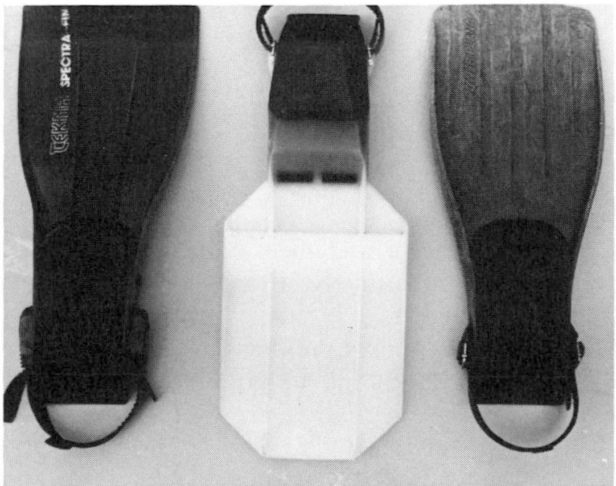

FIGURE 3–2. Examples of several types of diving fins.

loads. The subjects were experienced divers ranging from 5′5″ to 6′4″ in height. The data revealed that the longer, narrower fins tended to be slightly more efficient than the shorter, wider fins and that fins with vents, regardless of their direction, were not superior to those without vents. The longer, less flexible fins required stronger leg muscles and delivered higher levels of thrust when they could be operated without rapid fatigue. It is clear that divers should condition themselves to be able to use fins effectively. This may require working with fins of increasing rigidity over a period of time in order to develop the necessary strength and endurance to support the work load imposed by the stronger fins. Cramping and discomfort may be due to poor adaptation to a particular fin.

Kicking style may also be an important factor since it is important to apply resistance in the direction opposite to the swimmer's intended path. When using a drag dominant kick, whereby the fin works primarily as a paddle, the vector of force at 90° of flexion of the knee is primarily to the rear (Fig. 3–3). At full extension of the knee, the vector of force is perpendicular to the desired path of travel. Thus when the legs cross the forward, thrust is reduced essentially to zero. This identifies the deeper, slower kick as more efficient than the rapid, shallow kick often used by novice divers. When using a lift dominant kick, such as a sculling type kick, the fins respond more like propeller blades or wings directing the resistance to the rear while the leg is nearly straight. The power from this type of kick comes from the powerful rotator muscles of the hip joint; the fins sweep through the water rather than paddle against it. Since different functional muscle groups work in each case, it can be very helpful to become proficient in both types of kicking style in order to provide relief from fatigue.

Each new pair of fins will require a period of breaking in while the diver is adapting to the new work load, and it is not wise to take a new, stronger fin and immediately use it on a strenuous dive. Progressive increases in the work load will result in the development of comfort and efficiency with new fins.

SNORKELS

Snorkel tubes used for easier breathing while swimming on the surface have evolved from simple tubes open at both ends to devices that offer purge valves, swivel mouthpieces, advanced materials, and improved design of mouthpieces (Fig. 3–4). An adequate snorkel should permit the diver to work relatively hard on the surface without encountering resistance that would significantly impair the ventilatory demand of increased work of breathing and produce discomfort. Long, small-diameter tubes with unnecessary bends or internal corrugations are undesirable and may lead to intolerable respiratory distress.

Self-draining snorkels have reduced the amount of water the diver must move in order

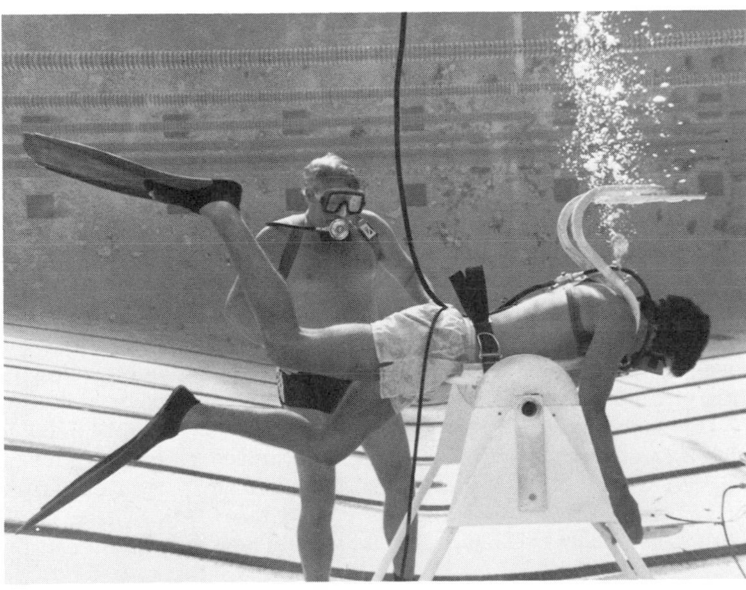

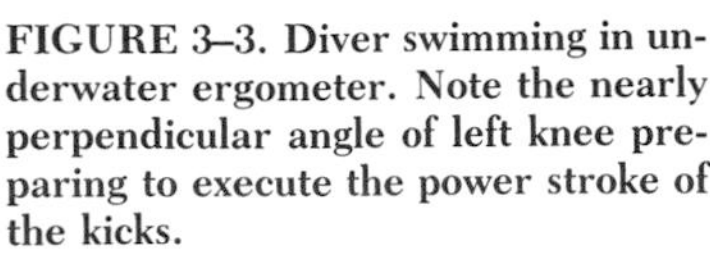

FIGURE 3–3. Diver swimming in underwater ergometer. Note the nearly perpendicular angle of left knee preparing to execute the power stroke of the kicks.

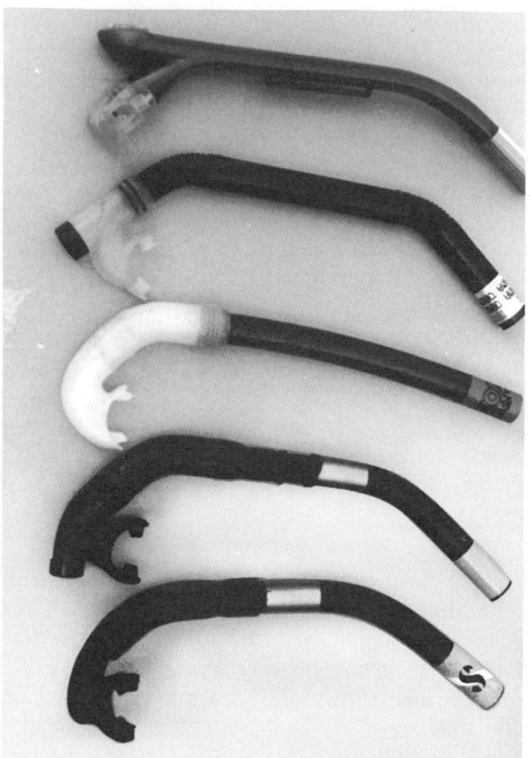

FIGURE 3–4. Examples of several snorkels. Note that some snorkels are designed with alternative purge valves.

to clear the snorkel. These devices contain an exhaust valve below the water line in order to permit water trapped in the tube to drop to the level of the surrounding water. A sharp pulse of exhalation pressure is then directed against a smaller water column, and water is purged out of the tube with the momentum generated in the water column. The diver must understand that doubling the flow rate of air through the tube will result in the necessity to overcome the square of the resistance to breathing and that the energy cost of this extra effort will be increased approximately eight times. The snorkel must be considered as an extension of the airway and as such should provide minimum resistance to breathing. If the diver feels exceptional respiratory distress, swimming on the back with the snorkel removed from the mouth and, if necessary, the mask removed from the face should be considered, but only after inflation of the buoyancy compensation device.

The snorkel mouthpiece should be placed so that it can have the lip flange of the mouthpiece aligned with the teeth and gums. Blisters can occur as a result of poor alignment, and many of the newer snorkels have a swivel located near the mouthpiece to allow for a comfortable placement.

BREATHING APPARATUS

The constant evolution of breathing apparatus has resulted in devices with a wide variety of minor differences in construction and function. The following discussion will cover the generic types of life support equipment and provide some considerations for effective use. Every diver should understand the basic operation of equipment and should be able to maintain it properly for safe, effective operation.

By far, the most widely used life support equipment is the scuba, or self-contained underwater breathing apparatus, used by recreational, scientific, commercial, and military divers. This type of apparatus permits a diver to move at will through the environment while carrying the entire life support system. Umbilical diving, on the other hand, uses a hose connected to the surface or to a chamber and restricts the diver to the limitations of the restraints involved. The tradeoffs between the systems generally involve consideration of the need for communication, heating, greater gas supply, and increased work loads.

Scuba

Open Circuit

The most common form of scuba is open circuit gear and consists of a tank or tanks of compressed (1800 to 4750 psi) air and a regulator, which will reduce the compressed gas to ambient pressure so the diver can breathe without difficulty (Fig. 3–5). The air in the tank is moved through a first stage of the regulator, where it is reduced to the range of 150 psi and is passed through an intermediate pressure hose to a second stage, located at the mouth, where it will be balanced to the pressure of the surrounding environment and the diver's lungs. The diver exerts a slight negative pressure on a mouthpiece connected to the second stage and causes a nonreturn valve between the intermediate pressure hose and mouthpiece to open, allowing air to flow into the diver's airways. The diver then exhales back through the mouthpiece, and the exhaled breath is exhausted out to the open water through a nonreturn exhaust valve.

There are a variety of ways that this basic system can be configured, and the marketplace

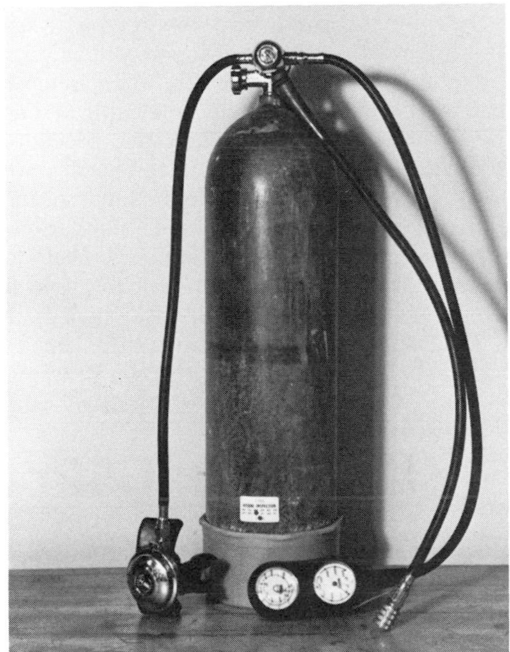

FIGURE 3–5. Typical open circuit scuba apparatus consisting of a pressure cylinder, single stage regulator, underwater tank pressure gauge and depth gauge, and spare hose for connecting to buoyancy device.

contains hundreds of models that offer the diver more or less sophisticated alternatives. Each manufacturer offers variations on the basic theme and competes on the basis of cost, enhanced performance, and design appeal.

The open circuit systems are designed to provide easy breathing with inhalation and exhalation resistances of less than 3 in. of differential water pressure (usually more on the order of 1.5 in.) during normal respiration at sea level. Regulators with resistances above 6 in. of differential pressure are usually in need of maintenance and/or repair. The resistance of breathing can be expected to change as a function of a number of variables, such as respiration rate changes, water depth, temperature variations, and so forth. Resistance characteristics vary with the different regulator designs, and the diver should be encouraged to obtain the most efficient regulator available for the type of diving that is planned. For example, most better regulators have balanced first stages that compensate for changing tank pressures so that the diver will have a consistent breathing resistance regardless of tank delivery pressures. This gives the diver an advantage in terms of breathing work but may produce a disadvantage for the diver who fails to heed the tank pressure gauge. There will not be an increasing breathing resistance when the tank pressures become low, and the diver may not feel the breathing becoming more difficult. As a result, a careless diver at depth may suddenly find that there is insufficient air to make a normal ascent to the surface. Every diver should have thorough knowledge of the capabilities of each piece of equipment, but special attention should be directed to the regulator(s) since its operation is critical on a breath-by-breath basis. Although regulator failure is an extremely rare occurrence, it is a possibility, and every diver should be prepared for such an event.

An integral part of the regulator is the tank pressure gauge and, in most cases, a depth gauge (Fig. 3–5). These devices are commonly worn together, sometimes with bottom timers and compasses attached in a console arrangement. Frequently this somewhat weighty console is left unattached at the distal end, with a range of motion equal to the length of the high pressure hose, and it assumes the characteristics of a martial arts weapon when it gains momentum. It is important to arrange a stable position for the gauges and the alternate air source in order to minimize trauma. The high pressure hose, for example, can be led under the left arm and under the waist strap of the backpack, so that the console hangs down along the left thigh with sufficient length to permit the console to be held up for easy viewing of the instruments. Periodic assessment of the accuracy of the instruments will add a margin of safety to diver performance.

Buddy Breathing

Currently in sport scuba diving there is a move toward the requirement for an alternate air source as a solution to the out-of-air emergency (which can also be precipitated by a poorly managed air supply). This raises an important equipment-related issue. Not only are there a variety of alternate air source configurations (Octopus, Pony bottle, Air II—Fig. 3–6), but buddy breathing from a single air source is a viable alternative. There has been little acceptance of a standardized procedure for any of the alternatives other than buddy breathing, and, as a result, confusion exists. The location of the alternate air source is fixed in the case of buddy breathing and devices like the Air II, which attach to the oral inflation hose on the buoyancy compensator. Octopus and independent systems, such as Pony bottles, are usually

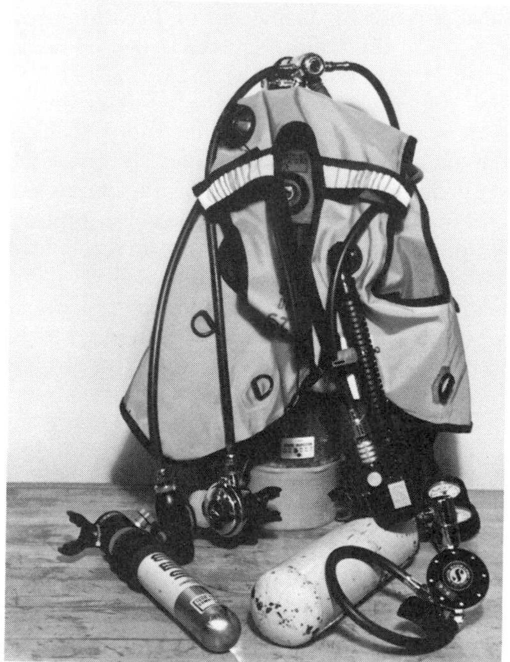

FIGURE 3–6. Clockwise from lower left, independent air supply, octopus, primary regulator, Air II, Pony Bottle.

configured to the whims of the individual. Not uncommonly, hoses connected to mouthpieces permit different locations dependent upon the diver's body position in the water at any given moment. In short, the proliferation of configurations available for solving the out-of-air emergency is limited only by the diver's imagination.

In the face of this dilemma it is possible and perhaps necessary to standardize the donor response to the standard out-of-air signal. The air source should therefore be located in a consistent position on the front of the body, where a single move on the part of the donor would enable the presentation of an air source to the mouth of the person who gave the out-of-air signal.

A procedure to simplify the problem would require all divers to agree that the signal for an out-of-air emergency would be a hand drawn sharply across the throat followed by the "I want to buddy breathe" signal with the hand and fingers motioning toward the mouth. Following this signal, the donor and recipient would link up; the donor would grasp the recipient's shoulder strap with the left hand and the recipient would grasp the donor's shoulder strap with the right hand. At this point the buddy team would be facing each other as the donor immediately passes an air source toward the recipient's mouth and the recipient uses the left hand to guide the donor-controlled air source to the recipient's mouth. Such an agreement by the buddies should be established at a time prior to the dive, when the procedure could be reinforced by careful rehearsal under nonstressful conditions. While the ideal solution would involve a single, simple, standardized equipment procedure, it appears that the equipment variations promoted in the field require a more generalized response, such as the one suggested above. In any event the pre-dive buddy check should include the clarification of the emergency procedures, particularly when diving with a new buddy.

Closed Circuit

A typical closed circuit breathing apparatus consists of a mouthpiece and hoses connected to a breathing bag, a CO_2 absorbent cannister, and a high pressure oxygen supply (Fig. 3–7). The diver inhales oxygen from the breathing bag, and upon exhalation the residual oxygen and the carbon dioxide resulting from the metabolism are routed through a nonreturn valve on the mouthpiece into a cannister containing a carbon dioxide absorbent. From the absorbent cannister the remaining oxygen goes back into the breathing bag, where additional oxygen is

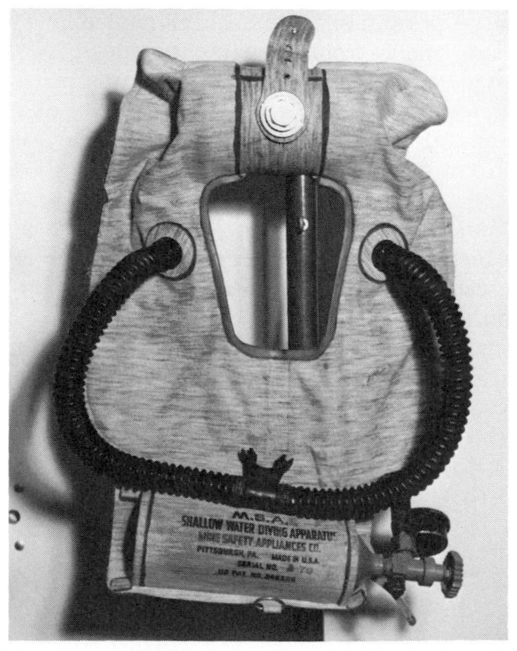

FIGURE 3–7. Closed circuit O_2 device showing breathing bags, oxygen cylinder, and mouthpiece.

added from the high pressure supply, and a full bag of oxygen is once again available for inhalation. The flow of oxygen from the high pressure source may be controlled manually, by fixed flow in simple models, or by automatic sensors that monitor bag volume and keep the bag full at the end of each exhalation. There are also mixed gas rebreathing devices with sensors that monitor the partial pressures of the gases and keep them within safe ranges for the depth. Typically these devices require additional training and care in their use. Depth limitations for pure oxygen are normally 25 fsw or less. The lack of bubbles emanating from rebreathers, linked with a significant reduction in the amount of gas used, gives them their greatest appeal. Depth limitations for pure oxygen and expensive monitoring devices for deeper depths generally limit use of these devices to special diving applications other than sport diving. A high degree of training in the use of each type of device is a fundamental prerequisite for safe diving.

Increased breathing resistance and large dead spaces are common to these systems and generally interfere with the diver's ability to perform heavy work at depth. Carbon dioxide buildup is also a significant threat since the absorbent materials tend to lose efficiency due to channeling of the expired gas through the absorbent material, the accumulation of moisture in the cannister, temperature drops, and carbon dioxide saturation of the absorbent. The use of rebreathing devices in recent years has focused upon military and commercial needs and has not received a great deal of attention in sport diving applications.

Umbilical Diving

The use of umbilical hoses and lines permits the diver to maintain active communication with the surface and to have virtually unlimited supplies of gas, power, and heat. Diving with umbilicals requires highly specialized training and surface support, since the specter of fouled lines and entanglement is always present. A detailed treatment of this topic can be found in the U.S. Navy Diving Manual, the NOAA Civilian Diving Manual, and The University of Michigan Research Diver's Manual, among others.

PERSONAL FLOTATION DEVICES

Personal flotation devices have evolved from small, front-mounted bladders with oral inflation only, to large jacket-type flotation bladders with up to 80 lbs of positive buoyancy (Fig. 3–8). There is considerable controversy regarding the tradeoffs one must consider in the selection, operation, and training needed for personal buoyancy control. The controversy has its roots in the question of the amount of buoyancy needed for adequate control in contrast to the amount needed in an emergency, with concern regarding rapid ascent rates and restricted movements.

A state-of-the-art buoyancy device will have a large bladder arranged in a jacket-like configuration so that substantial amounts of flotation will be placed under the arms and on the front of the chest. Front-mounted "horse collar" vests

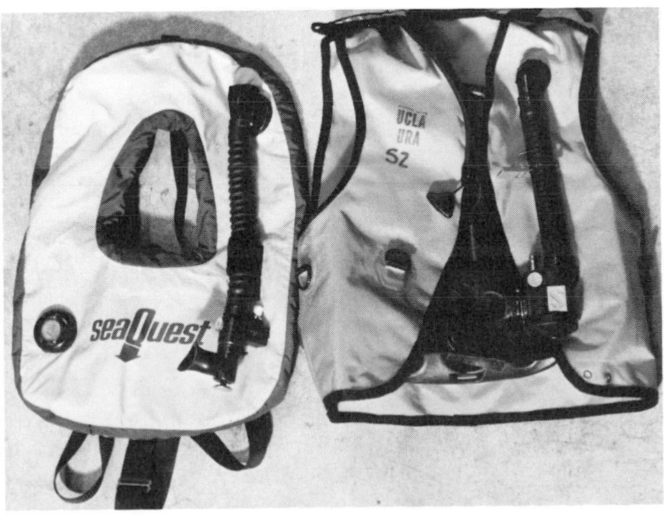

FIGURE 3–8. Horse collar (left) and jacket-type (right) buoyancy compensator.

and back-mounted horseshoe-shaped bladders are still preferred by many, but the trend is definitely toward the jacket configurations.

All of these devices have an oral inflation hose with an option for an automatic inflation device designed to deliver air from the tank directly to the bladder. These automatic devices are not standardized, and their use in an emergency will require each of the buddy team members to become familiar with the strengths and limitations of each other's equipment.

The following considerations are important to the safe use of such devices.

1. The oral inflation hose should be located on the left side and should be long enough to permit easy inflation by the user or the buddy. A Velcro collar on the hose near the mouthpiece with a corresponding attachment surface on the body of the flotation bladder can be useful in keeping the location of the mouthpiece stable during the dive.

2. Proper weighting of the diver is important to minimize adjustments of the device. Improper weighting can result in the need to add air to the bladder in amounts that could lead to loss of control when the air expands rapidly in the bag during the last portion of the ascent. Purging excess air during ascent can become difficult if one waits too long before starting the process. Equalizing the buoyancy device frequently on ascent can become as important as equalizing frequently on descent.

3. The device should be used as a tool rather than as a crutch. More expert divers rarely find it necessary to make major adjustments with the devices. Relying on the device to accommodate for being overweighted is unnecessary and is potentially dangerous. Proper weighting techniques will reduce the need for inflating the bladder to "fine tune" for significant depth changes, surface inflation for long swims, and emergency procedures.

4. Regular maintenance of the autoinflator is an important safety factor and should not be overlooked. Salt water left in the bladder and oral inflation hose can cause increased corrosion and potential malfunctions of the inflation mechanisms. Rinsing thoroughly, externally and internally, after use and checking for leaks are fundamental tasks for the diver who prefers prevention over accident management as a way of life.

5. Single bladder configurations provide less form drag than the double bag types. Remember that increasing the frontal surface area of the diver will increase the swimming resistance dramatically if speed remains constant. The increased resistance in turn will require a dramatic increase in energy production if speed is to be maintained. It is clear that form drag reductions are important to the question of diver efficiency, particularly when currents may be active or divers are making an effort to move rapidly through the water. The deceptive ease with which the diver explores a reef should not be confused with the exponential nature of the work load changes associated with increasing resistance due to increasing speed of movement through the water.

6. Rate of ascent under varying degrees of buoyancy may become a significant factor with larger buoyancy bladders. Since one liter of air displaces 2.2 lbs of water, a buoyancy bladder will be exerting 2.2 lbs of lifting force wherever it is located on the body. Smaller buoyancy compensators will have capacities on the order of 10 liters, while larger devices have capacities in excess of 20 liters. The increased potential for a rapid ascent with greater displacement requires that the diver adjust the air in the vest to a safe controllable level *before* control becomes a problem. Remember the exponential nature of the gas expansion as the diver gets nearer the surface. The rule of equalizing early and often is important on ascent as well as on descent.

7. Neutral buoyancy—the state at which a diver will neither rise nor sink—is obviously a desirable state at any depth. This is especially true at the end of a dive when the bottom time has come close to the decompression limit and the diver wishes to take an optional 10 feet decompression stop. The ability to achieve neutrality at 10 feet on ascent requires that the diver give consideration to the problem before the dive begins in order to avoid serious over- or underweighting.

HYDRODYNAMIC DRAG

Drag is developed in three basic modes while diving: frontal resistance, skin friction, and turbulent or eddy resistance. Drag is the sum of these resistances.

Frontal resistance is the force developed when an object presents a surface to a fluid and attempts either to move through it or to have the fluid move past the object. In either case the resistive force is a function of the frontal surface area, shape, and speed. If the frontal surface area is increased and the speed remains constant, the resistive force increases linearly with a shape function that can be expected to further increase the drag. If the frontal surface area is constant and the speed is doubled, the resistive force is squared. Reducing speed or surface area will reduce frontal resistance dramatically. These relationships emphasize the importance of maintaining a body position aligned with the intended travel path in a head to toe direction. Over- or underweighting results in an upward or downward angle of the body to the intended travel path and dramatically increases frontal surface exposure with significant increases in resistance. Inflating buoyancy compensating devices or adding equipment to the body will also result in increased frontal surface area. Streamlining efforts can effectively reduce this factor.

Skin friction is the force that develops as fluid particles pass over the body and exert frictional drag on the body. Viscosity, shape of the body, and speed are important considerations. Laminar flow of water over the surface of the diver is nearly impossible, but flaps, straps, lumps, and bumps can be reduced by smoothing the body surface.

Eddy resistance, or turbulent flow, usually results when the smooth flow of water passing over the body is disrupted by an irregularity and the water flow develops "eddies." In conditions where water passes over squared off areas such as the end of the tank or the back of the head when the neck is hyperextended, the turbulence creates resistance that slows the diver's forward progress. Divers being towed by boats or diver propulsion vehicles are faced with the prospect of the loss of their masks if they inappropriately position their heads and permit turbulent flow to develop on the edge of the mask. The mask is pulled off rather than being pushed off.

These drag producing factors become more important as the speed of water flow over the body increases. It is the exponential nature of the increase which is frequently not well understood. Divers who go downstream of the boat and then attempt to swim upcurrent to return to the boat at the end of the dive may fail simply because they cannot produce the force necessary to overcome the additional resistance caused by the current.

THERMAL PROTECTION

Man is a homeotherm who, in modern times, is basically designed for operation in subtropical environments where thermal neutrality can be maintained with a minimal involvement of thermoregulatory mechanisms. When he enters water, which has a conductive heat capacity 25 times that of air, there are rapid, large scale changes that take place in order to protect the body's core temperature from dangerous levels of change. Since the comfort range for humans is on the order of +/− 1°C of core temperature, and since a gain or loss of 3 to 4°C in the core temperature can result in a medical emergency, it becomes apparent that additional thermal protection is necessary under most prolonged diving conditions.

Circumstances whereby body metabolism is unable to keep up with heat lost to the environment put the diver on the path to clinical hypothermia. Protective garments have been developed to increase the length of time that the diver can remain within the safe range of core temperature.

The most common protective garment is the wetsuit (Fig. 3–9), which uses a layer of gas-impregnated rubber as the insulating boundary to trap water next to the diver's skin. The water stores heat, and a well-fitted wetsuit holds it in position. Unfortunately, the wetsuit compresses as the diver descends in the water column, and insulative protection is reduced with greater

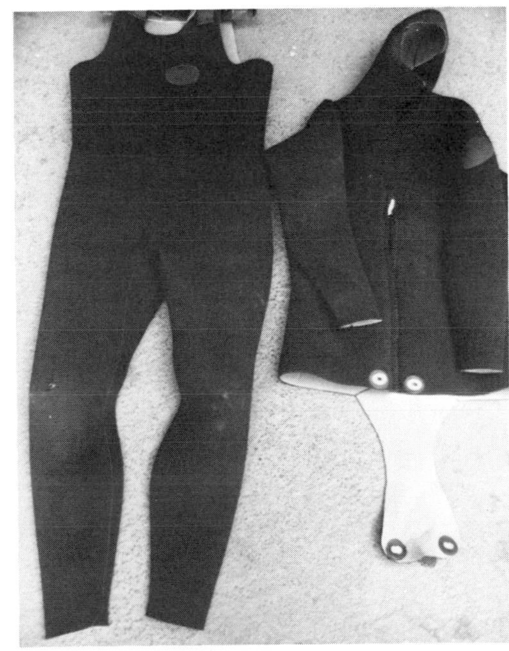

FIGURE 3–9. Typical scuba wetsuit constructed of closed cell neoprene rubber foam. Suit thickness is based on the degree of thermal protection needed.

PERFORMANCE DECREMENTS IN COLD WATER

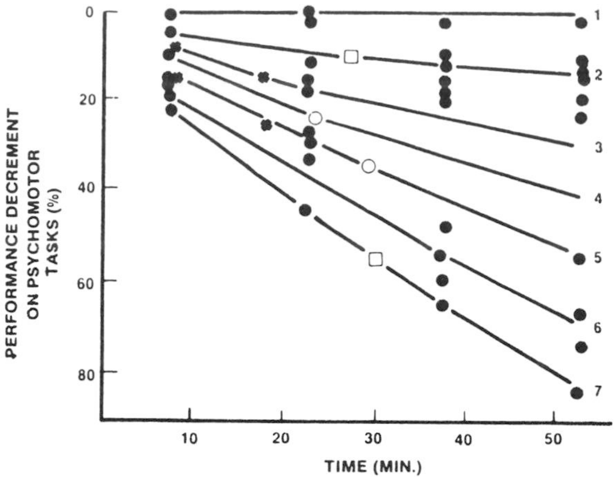

PROPER DECREMENT CURVE

TYPE TASK	WATER TEMPERATURE 70	60	50	40
FINE DIGITAL MANIPULATION	1	5	6	7
SIMPLE ASSEMBLY	1	2	4	6
GROSS BODY & POWER MOVE	1	2	2	3

● STANG · WIENER (1970)
● BOWEN (1968)
○ WELTMAN & EGSTROM, ET AL. (1970)
□ WELTMAN & EGSTROM, ET AL. (1971)

FIGURE 3–10. Upper graph shows percentage of reduction in performance. Numbers to the right indicate conditions of measurement described in the lower graph. (See text for interpretation.)

depths. The graph shown in Figure 3–10 provides information that can be used as a guideline for anticipating the effects of cold water on diver performance. The data on the graph reflect the temperature effects on a diver wearing a ¼-in. neoprene wetsuit with hood, booties, and gloves. The numbers under the temperature readings reflect the appropriate decrement curve for listed motor skills. For example, after diving in 60°F water for 50 minutes, fine digital manipulation would be expected to be degraded by over 50 per cent (Fig. 3–10).

The improvement of wetsuit materials has led to improvement of its insulating value and less compressible materials reduce the loss of protection at depth. Wetsuit material has been used to develop a type of dry suit that fits much like a wetsuit but contains seals at the neck, wrist, and ankles which prevent water from entering the suit. These suits offer better thermal protection but usually provide less mobility for the diver.

Dry suits have become more popular in recent years due to improvements in fit and mobility. Comfortable insulating undergarments, effective valve mechanisms, and better seals have also added to value. However, dry suits require additional training in their proper use before they can be used safely and effectively. Newer dry suits are sometimes called shell suits since they provide a waterproof outside covering suit over an inner insulating garment. These suits provide considerably improved thermal protection over the other two types of thermal protective garments but have range of motion restrictions and potential control difficulties. It is recommended that such suits be used with an independent buoyancy control system following a thorough training program during which the diver becomes skilled in the operation of the entire diving system. Using the shell suit as a buoyancy control system may result in difficulties with an internal air bubble, which will move to the portion of the suit closest to the surface of the water. Such a bubble can be sufficiently large to cause serious control problems. Divers cannot afford to lose control.

The equipment that a diver wears and uses should fit like a second skin and should be considered part of the body. Specific training and development of adequate levels of strength and endurance to meet the demands of the environment should enable the diver to concentrate on the dive rather than on survival. An uncomfortable diver is likely to be at a greater risk for loss of control.

Chapter 4

Mechanisms and Risks of Decompression

RICHARD D. VANN

Animal experiments by Paul Bert during the nineteenth century and autopsies of divers and caisson workers by Leonard Hill and others at the beginning of the twentieth century led to the conclusion that decompression sickness is caused by bubbles of inert gas in the blood and tissues.[1-5] The variety and severity of the symptoms depend upon bubble volume and location. Unconsciousness and death can result from bubbles in the brain, dyspnea from bubbles in the pulmonary arteries, and paralysis from bubbles in the spinal cord. The causes of the minor forms of decompression sickness are less clear, but muscle and joint pain appear to be due to bubbles in ligaments, fascia, periosteum, muscle spindles, and nerve sheaths. More recently, bubbles have been recognized to have biochemical as well as mechanical effects.[6]

DISSOLVED INERT GAS EXCHANGE

Perfusion-Limited Inert Gas Exchange

The first quantitative attempt to describe inert gas exchange was made in 1897 by Zuntz.[7] Zuntz assumed that cardiac output was distributed evenly throughout the body, nitrogen in blood mixed instantaneously with nitrogen in tissue, and nitrogen solubilities in blood and tissue were equal. With these assumptions, nitrogen exchange was completely determined by blood flow and tissue volume.

"Well-stirred" tissues of this nature are known as *perfusion limited.* Their gas exchange properties are defined by a characteristic *half-time* during which the difference between the arterial and tissue nitrogen tensions is reduced to half its initial value. This concept is illustrated in Figure 4–1 in which the x-axis is time in half-time units, and the y-axis is the difference in the arterial and tissue nitrogen tensions expressed as a percentage of the initial difference. At zero time, the nitrogen saturation is zero. After one half-time, tissue is half saturated, and after two half-times, it is three-quarters saturated. With each additional half-time, the dif-

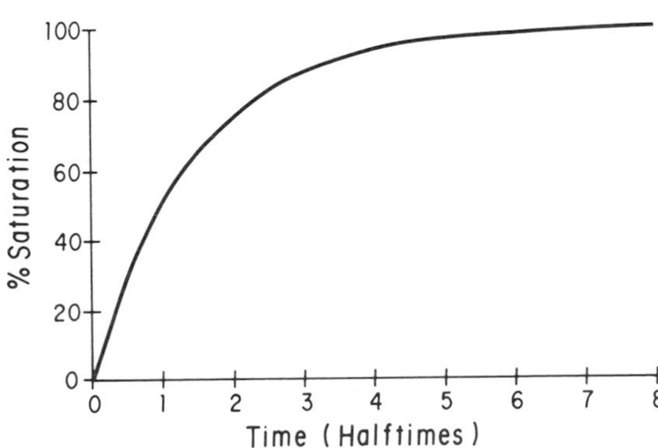

FIGURE 4–1. Percentage of nitrogen saturation in a well-stirred Haldane tissue as a function of time. Nitrogen saturation is expressed as the percentage difference between the arterial and tissue or venous tension. Time is in half-time units. The difference between the arterial and tissue tensions is reduced by half with each unit of time.

ference between the tissue and arterial tensions is reduced by half.

Using the same assumptions as Zuntz, Haldane estimated the total body half-time of nitrogen to be 23 min.[8] He pointed out, however, that there are tissues with shorter and longer half-times because blood flow is not evenly distributed, and nitrogen is more soluble in fat than in lean tissue. Haldane selected tissue half-times of 5, 10, 20, 40, and 75 min to represent the whole body.

Figure 4–2 shows the responses of these tissues to a 15-min dive at 168 fsw.[8] The x-axis is time in minutes, and the y-axis is the absolute pressure in atmospheres (ata). The solid line is the dive profile with decompression stages at 60, 40, 30, 20, and 10 feet of seawater (fsw). The dashed lines are the nitrogen tensions in the five tissues. The 5-min tissue responds rapidly to pressure change, while the 75-min tissue absorbs nitrogen slowly and retains it for a long time. According to Haldane's theory for safe decompression, bubble formation and decompression sickness could be avoided if no tissue tension were ever allowed to exceed twice the absolute pressure.

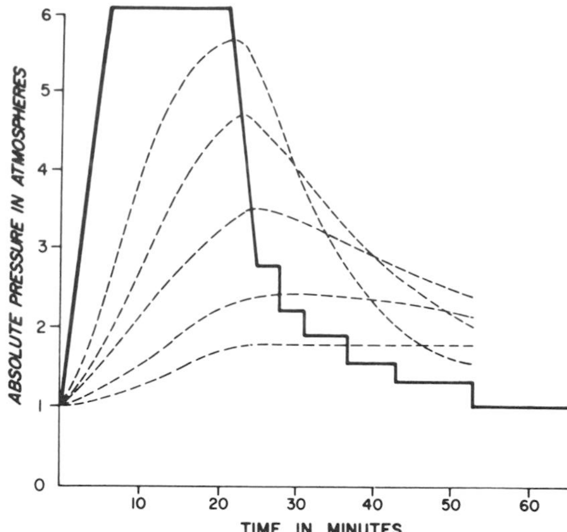

FIGURE 4–2. The responses of five Haldane tissues *(broken lines)* having 5-, 10-, 20-, 40-, and 75-min half-times to a 20-min dive at 168 fsw *(solid line)*. Decompression is conducted in stages according to the Haldane rule that no tissue tension should ever exceed twice the absolute pressure. (From Boycott AE, Damant GCC, Haldane JS: The prevention of compressed air illness. J Hyg 8:342–443, 1908, by permission of Cambridge University Press.)

Diffusion-Limited Inert Gas Exchange

Recent studies have demonstrated that except for avascular tissues such as bone or eye, perfusion is the primary determinant of dissolved inert gas exchange. Diffusion can have secondary effects, however, which make gas exchange slower than in well-stirred Haldane tissues.

Figure 4–3A shows inert gas diffusing between adjacent well-stirred tissues that are perfused at different rates or that have different inert gas solubilities.[9–13] Such intertissue diffusion might be significant in decompression, for example, where a slowly exchanging fat deposit acts as an inert gas reservoir for an adjacent rapidly exchanging lean tissue that is sensitive to decompression injury.

Figure 4–3B demonstrates how inert gas diffusing between adjacent arterioles and venules can be shunted around tissue. Arteriovenous diffusion shunts have been observed for oxygen[14–16] and would reduce the exchange rate of a highly diffusible gas like helium relative to a less diffusible gas like nitrogen.[17, 18]

Diffusion between closely spaced capillaries is generally so rapid that virtually no radial concentration gradients can exist. If the capillaries are very long, however, axial concentration gradients can develop in surrounding tissue because of the large longitudinal diffusion distances (Fig. 4–4). Such gradients act to reduce the rate of inert gas exchange.[19, 20]

UNDISSOLVED INERT GAS EXCHANGE

The Oxygen Window

Diffusion has only secondary effects on inert gas exchange as long as the gas remains dissolved. When bubbles form, however, inert gas becomes isolated from the circulation and cannot be removed by blood flow until it diffuses back into tissue. The speed of diffusion is determined by the difference between the nitrogen partial pressure in the bubble and the nitrogen tension in tissue. This difference is a direct result of the metabolic conversion of oxygen, a relatively insoluble gas, into carbon dioxide, which is some 21 times more soluble. Haldane understood this mechanism but did not need it in his theory for safe decompression, which assumed that decompression sickness and bubble formation occurred simultaneously.[8]

The effect of exchanging oxygen for carbon dioxide on dissolved gas tension is illustrated in

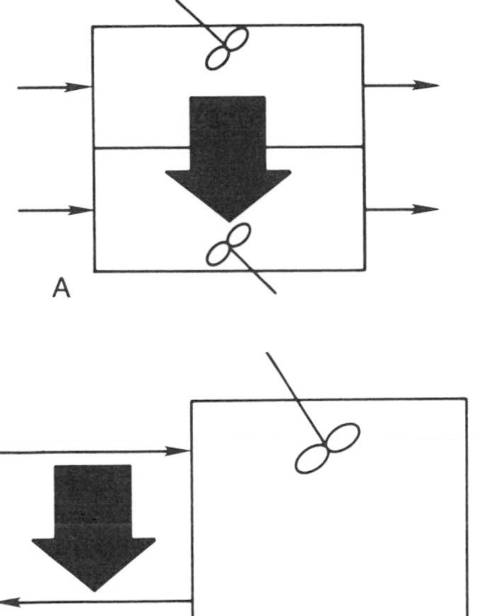

FIGURE 4–3. *A*, Inert gas diffusion between adjacent tissues that have different inert gas solubilities or perfusion rates. *B*, Inert gas diffusion between adjacent arterioles and venules. This causes a diffusion shunt that allows inert gas to bypass the tissue.

Figure 4–5. The x-axis is dissolved gas tension in torr; the y-axis is gas content in ml gas per 1000 ml blood. The steeper line shows the relationship between carbon dioxide tension and content. The slope of this line is the carbon dioxide solubility. The other line represents the same relationship for oxygen. Its gradual slope reflects a lower oxygen solubility.

Suppose, as indicated by Point 1 in Figure 4–5, that the oxygen tension were 100 torr. This corresponds to an oxygen content of 3 ml oxygen per 1000 ml blood (Point 2). If each oxygen molecule were exchanged for a carbon dioxide molecule (Point 3), there would be no change in the dissolved gas volume, but the tension would fall to 4.7 torr (Point 4). This is because carbon dioxide is more soluble than oxygen.

The exchange of oxygen for carbon dioxide which occurs in tissue is illustrated in Table 4–1 for an air-equilibrated diver at sea level. In the lung, the sum of the alveolar partial pressures is normally near 760 torr. The sum of the arterial gas tensions is slightly less, largely because of ventilation-perfusion inequalities. Since the diver is equilibrated with atmospheric nitrogen, the alveolar, arterial, and venous nitrogen tensions are equal. Metabolism, however, causes the oxygen tension to fall from 95 torr in the arterial blood to 40 torr in the venous blood, while the arterial carbon dioxide rises from 40 torr to a venous level of 45 torr. The 55-torr fall in oxygen tension accompanied by the 5-torr rise in carbon dioxide tension are due to the solubility difference between oxygen and carbon dioxide with a small contribution from a respiratory quotient of less than one. Summing the venous tensions, the total dissolved gas tension is equal to 701 torr or 59 torr less than the absolute pressure.

TABLE 4–1. Alveolar, Arterial, and Venous Gas Tensions

	Alveolar (torr)	Arterial (torr)	Venous (torr)
CO_2	40	40	45
O_2	104	95	40
H_2O	46	46	46
N_2	570	570	570
Total	760	751	701

The gas tensions in Table 4–1 are shown as bar graphs in Figure 4–6. The bar on the left presents gases in a diver's lungs at sea level. Dalton's law of partial pressures requires that the sum of these gases be 1 ata. The bar on the right represents the gases in the diver's tissues whose sum is less than 1 ata because of the oxygen for carbon dioxide exchange.

In Figure 4–7, the diver is breathing air at 33 fsw. The bar graphs on the left show the gases in his lungs and tissue upon arrival at depth. The oxygen and nitrogen partial pressures in his lungs have increased to make the sum of all gases equal to the absolute pressure of 2 ata, but his tissues have absorbed no additional nitrogen. The bar graphs on the right show the lungs and tissues after nitrogen equil-

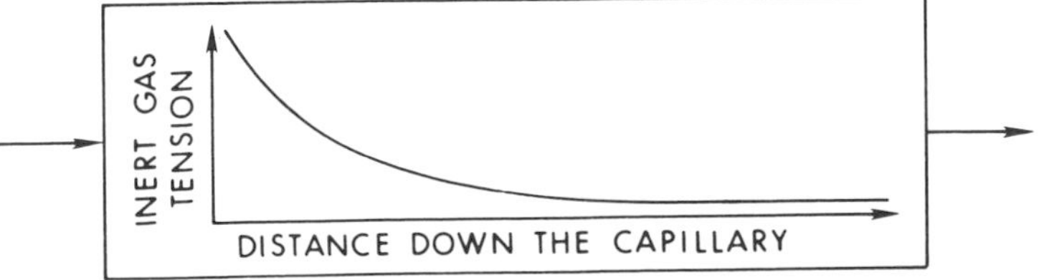

FIGURE 4–4. Inert gas concentration gradients in a tissue having long parallel capillaries. These gradients reduce the inert gas exchange rate and are the result of large axial diffusion distances.

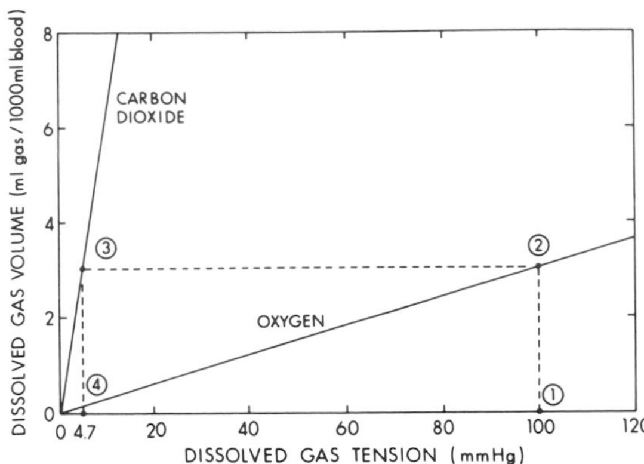

FIGURE 4–5. The effects of exchanging oxygen for carbon dioxide on dissolved gas tension. When oxygen is converted into carbon dioxide, the gas tension falls from 100 to 4.7 torr, but the dissolved gas volume or content remains unchanged because carbon dioxide is more soluble than oxygen.

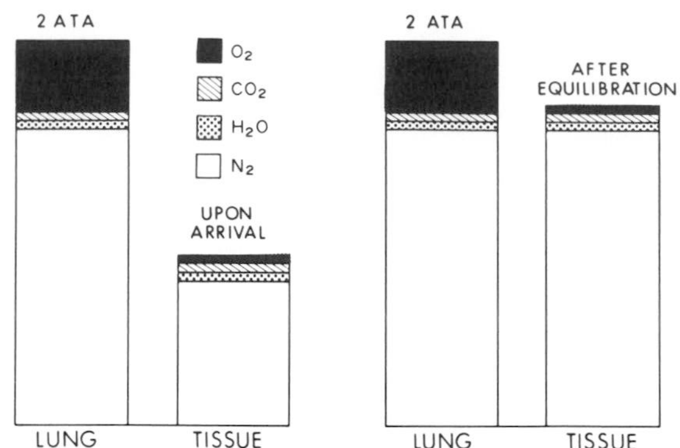

FIGURE 4–7. Gases in the lungs and tissues of an air breathing diver at 33 fsw. Initially, the tissue nitrogen tension is the same as in Figure 4–6, but after sufficient time at depth tissue nitrogen equilibrates with the 2 ata of air in the lung.

ibration. The tissue nitrogen tension now equals the alveolar nitrogen partial pressure.

Now, as shown in Figure 4–8, the diver returns to sea level, and bubbles form in his tissues. By Dalton's law, the sum of the partial pressures in the bubble is 1 ata. The water vapor pressure is constant, and the oxygen and carbon dioxide partial pressures are controlled to tissue levels. Since the nitrogen tension in tissue is elevated, nitrogen diffuses both into the bubble and into the blood. Nitrogen that diffuses into the blood and remains dissolved is carried to the lungs and is eliminated harmlessly, but nitrogen diffusing into the bubble causes it to expand.

Expanding bubbles may cause clinical decompression sickness. If so, the diver is placed on 100 per cent oxygen and is recompressed to 60 fsw where the absolute pressure is 2.82 ata in the bubble and lung (Fig. 4–9). Metabolism soon returns the oxygen and carbon dioxide in the bubble to their tissue levels. This raises the nitrogen partial pressure in the bubble, and nitrogen diffuses rapidly out of the bubble because of the large concentration gradient. Momsen[9] called this gradient the *partial pressure vacancy*; Hills[21] called it the *inherent unsaturation*; and Behnke[22, 23] called it the *oxygen window*.

Diffusion Gradients Around Bubbles

Figure 4–10 shows the effects of the oxygen window upon the concentration gradients of oxygen, nitrogen, or helium around a bubble.[24]

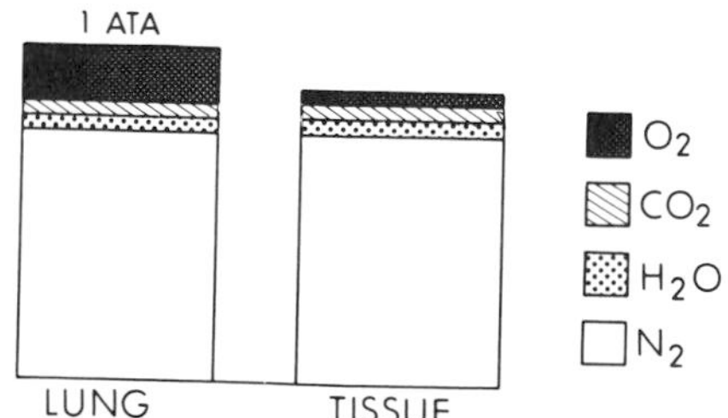

FIGURE 4–6. Gases in the lungs and tissues of an air breathing diver at sea level. The metabolic exchange of oxygen for carbon dioxide results in a total tissue gas tension that is less than the ambient pressure. This difference is the *oxygen window*.

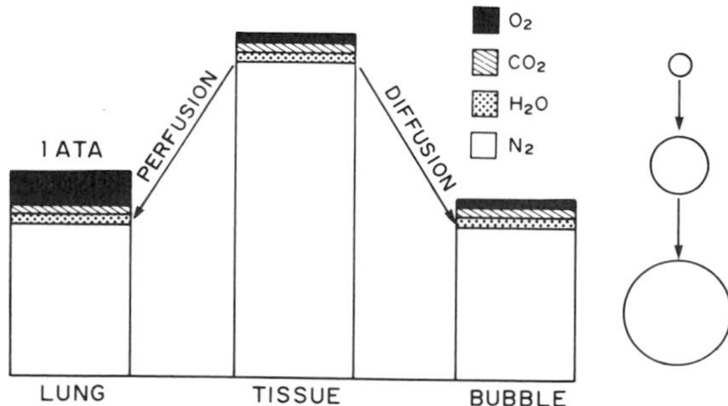

FIGURE 4–8. Bubble formation and growth after decompression from 33 fsw to sea level. The bubble grows by inward diffusion of supersaturated nitrogen from tissue. Dissolved nitrogen also is carried to the lungs by the circulation.

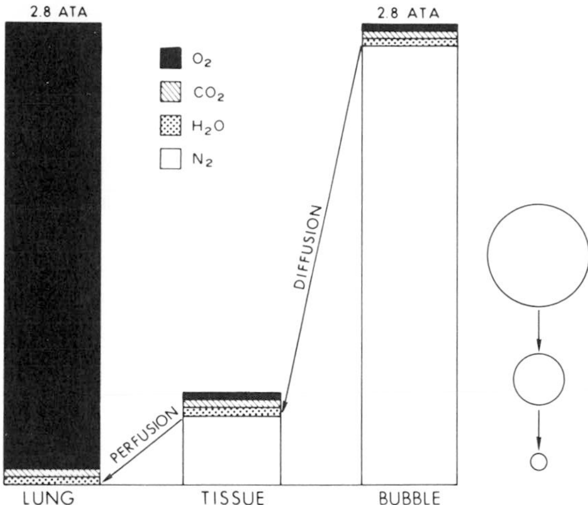

FIGURE 4–9. A diver who develops decompression sickness and is recompressed to 60 fsw while breathing 100 per cent oxygen. The sum of the partial pressures of all gases in the bubble increases to 2.82 ata, but outward diffusion of excess oxygen and carbon dioxide reduces their partial pressures to tissue levels. Since oxygen, carbon dioxide, and water vapor are controlled to their tissue values, the nitrogen partial pressure must rise until the sum of all partial pressures equals 2.82 ata. The oxygen window is the concentration gradient between nitrogen in the bubble and in the tissue down which nitrogen diffuses. The size of the oxygen window increases as the tissue nitrogen tension is reduced by perfusion.

The oxygen gradient is steepest because it is metabolically consumed. Helium and nitrogen extend further into tissue than oxygen because they are not consumed and are eliminated only by perfusion. The nitrogen gradient is steeper than the helium gradient because nitrogen is less diffusible than helium. This makes helium more available for removal by the circulation. Since an inert gas in a bubble must diffuse back into tissue before removal, its elimination after decompression is slower than its uptake at depth.[25–27]

BUBBLE FORMATION

Gas Nuclei

Studies by Hills[27] and Powell[28] suggest that only 5 or 10 per cent of the inert gas absorbed during normal diving is released as bubbles after decompression. While this may seem a small fraction, it agrees with both in vitro and in vivo observations that bubble formation is not widespread and is limited to discrete nucleation sites, whose number fluctuates with changing environmental and physiological conditions.

These phenomena are illustrated in observations of bubble formation under the transparent shells of shrimp. Table 4–2 shows the results of experiments by Daniels, who decompressed shrimp from sea level to altitude.[29] Bubble formation rose with increasing altitude as additional nucleation sites were recruited to about 3.5 bubbles per shrimp (Table 4–2, Lines 1 to 4). When the shrimp were hydrostatically compressed for 2 min to 201 ata prior to altitude exposure (Table 4–2, Line 5), bubble formation fell to 0.5 bubbles per shrimp. Nucleation sites that can be deactivated in this manner are known as *gas nuclei* and are believed to contain free gas that is dissolved by hydrostatic pressure.[30–32] With a 24-hour sea level recovery period between pressure treatment and altitude exposure, bubble formation returned to its initial level, indicating that gas nuclei were reactivated or created (Table 4–2, Line 6). Evans and Walder found that bubble formation increased when shrimp were exercised after pressure treatment but before altitude exposure.[33] McDonough and Hemmingsen observed decreased bubble formation in various immobilized marine animals and suggested that exercise caused bubble formation through a mechanism known as *tribonucleation.*[34–37]

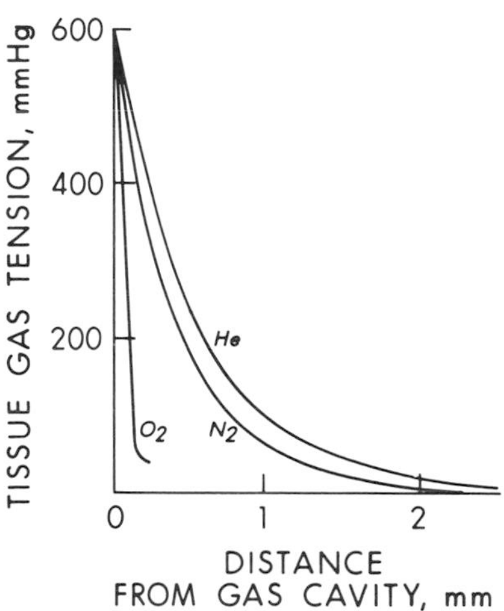

FIGURE 4–10. Dissolved gas concentration gradients around a bubble filled with oxygen, nitrogen, or helium. The oxygen concentration gradient is steepest because oxygen is metabolized in tissue as it diffuses out of the bubble. Nitrogen and helium are metabolically inert and are removed from tissue only by perfusion. Helium extends further into tissue than nitrogen because it diffuses more quickly. (Redrawn from Van Liew HD: Coupling of diffusion and perfusion in gas exit from subcutaneous pockets in rats. Am J Physiol 214:1176–1185, 1968.)

TABLE 4–2. Bubble Formation in Shrimp Decompressed to Altitude After Hydrostatic Pressure Treatment

	RECOVERY PERIOD	HYDROSTATIC PRESSURE TREATMENT	15 MIN ALTITUDE EXPOSURE	BUBBLES PER SHRIMP
1.	—	—	27,500 ft (0.33 ata)	0.0
2.	—	—	33,500 ft (0.25 ata)	0.5
3.	—	—	42,000 ft (0.17 ata)	3.2
4.	—	—	53,000 ft (0.10 ata)	3.5
5.	—	200 ata for 2 min	53,000 ft (0.10 ata)	0.5
6.	24 hrs	200 ata for 2 min	53,000 ft (0.10 ata)	3.2

Data from Daniels S, Eastaugh KC, Paton WDM, Smith EB: Micronuclei and bubble formation: A quantitative study using the common shrimp, crangon. *In* Bachrach AJ, Matzen MM (eds): Underwater Physiology. 8th ed. Bethesda, Undersea Medical Society, 1984.

Tribonucleation

Tribonucleation causes bubble formation as a result of large negative pressures generated by viscous adhesion between surfaces separating in liquid.[38–40] These negative pressures, which can be hundreds of atmospheres or more, place the liquid in tension and may cause either spontaneous (de novo) bubble formation or bubble formation from gas nuclei.

Bubbles created by tribonucleation can persist[41] and act as gas nuclei for later bubble formation. The lifetime of such a nucleus is determined by the rate at which it dissolves. Mechanisms that stabilize a nucleus against surface tension can prolong its lifetime. Proposed stabilization mechanisms include gas in hydrophobic crevices[30] and surface active shells around bubbles.[42, 43] Such shells have been observed surrounding bubbles in sea water.[44]

While it is unclear whether stabilization mechanisms play a significant role in decompression sickness, the evidence strongly suggests that the creation and destruction of gas nuclei are in dynamic equilibrium. If exercise shifts this equilibrium toward creation, more bubbles form and the risk of decompression sickness increases. The risk decreases, on the other hand, if pressure treatment shifts the balance toward destruction.

The marine animal experiments[29, 33–37] provided evidence for gas nuclei but did not demonstrate their role in decompression sickness. This link was suggested in experiments that pretreated rats at pressure before decompression from a 2-hour exposure at 240 fsw on air (Fig. 4–11).[45] Without pressure treatment, the incidence of decompression sickness was 83 per cent. With a brief pressure treatment at 600 fsw, the decompression sickness incidence was 74 per cent, and with a 1000 fsw pressure treatment, the incidence decreased to 64 per cent. Thus, pressure treatment reduced decompression sickness in rats as well as eliminated gas nuclei in marine animals.

MECHANISMS OF DECOMPRESSION SICKNESS

Joint Pain

The sites of bubble formation in divers are less mysterious than might be expected. Cracking sounds in joints are caused by collapsing bubbles formed by tribonucleation during the

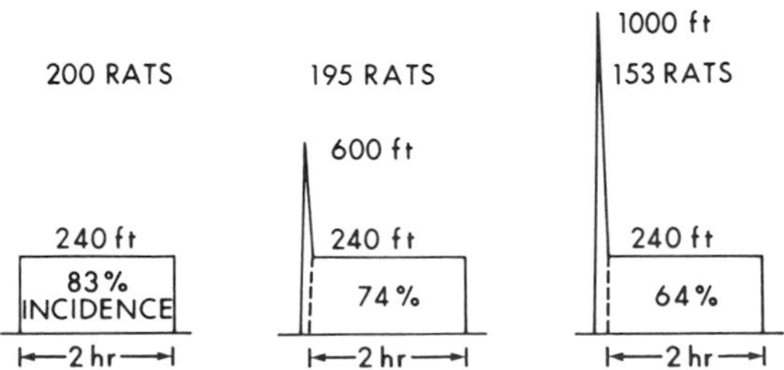

FIGURE 4–11. Decompression sickness in rats subjected to pressure treatment before a 2-hr exposure at 240 fsw on air. The incidence of decompression sickness decreased from 83 per cent with no pressure treatment, to 74 per cent after a 600 fsw treatment, and to 64 per cent after a 1000 fsw treatment, suggesting that preexisting gas nuclei are responsible for the bubbles that cause decompression sickness in rats. (From Vann RD: Decompression theory and application. *In* Bennett PB, Elliott DH (eds): The Physiology and Medicine of Diving. London, Bailliere Tindall, 1982.)

separation of joint surfaces.[41, 46] Tribonucleation occurs in marine animals despite the lack of mammalian joint structure and may occur during the relative motion of tendons, ligaments, and bones. The collapse of a bubble with an associated sound is known as *vaporous cavitation*.[47] As the dissolved gas content increases or the hydrostatic pressure decreases, a transition occurs from vaporous to *gaseous cavitation*, which is soundless and leaves a stable bubble.

Gas-filled joints have been detected after diving or during altitude exposure by radiographs and by the presence of crepitus.[48–51] Ferris and Engle reported that gas in joint capsules was asymptomatic, while gas in perivascular and periarticular tissues was frequently accompanied by pain.[48] This gas appeared radiographically as discrete, round bubbles in the popliteal fat pad behind or lateral to the neck of the femur or as a fine longitudinal streaking along tendon or muscle bundles in the popliteal fossa. In stereoscopic studies, these regions appeared as ribbon-like shadows apparently in the fascial planes and along tendons. With recompression, both crepitus and shadows disappeared but reappeared upon immediate decompression.

Thomas and Williams found gas in the knee joints of all subjects exposed to an altitude of 20,000 feet.[52] Gas accumulations as large as 50 to 75 ml were sometimes present at higher altitudes but were not always accompanied by pain (Fig. 4–12A). Joint aspiration showed this gas to be in approximate equilibrium with gases in the blood. Knee radiographs of 27 subjects having moderate to severe pain at 35,000 feet revealed irregular collections of gas in periarticular tissues as well as small discrete bubbles and streaking along fascial planes and tendons (Fig. 4–12B). Bubbles and pain were associated in 46 of 74 observations (62 per cent), while streaking and pain were associated in 47 of 62 observations (76 per cent).

Besides joint pain, acute altitude exposure often produced recurrent, transient, sharp pains of moderate intensity in the hands and feet.[48] These pains were accompanied by crepitus in the tendon sheaths. Palpation of the tendon sheaths revealed bubbles that, when milked away, often relieved the pain. Ferris and Engle cite such observations to argue that decompression pain is of extravascular rather than of intravascular origin.

Spinal Decompression Sickness and the Vacuum Phenomenon

After the limbs, the most common site of decompression sickness is the spinal cord. Spinal symptoms are generally manifested as disturbances of the sensory and motor systems ranging from " pins and needles" and marginal

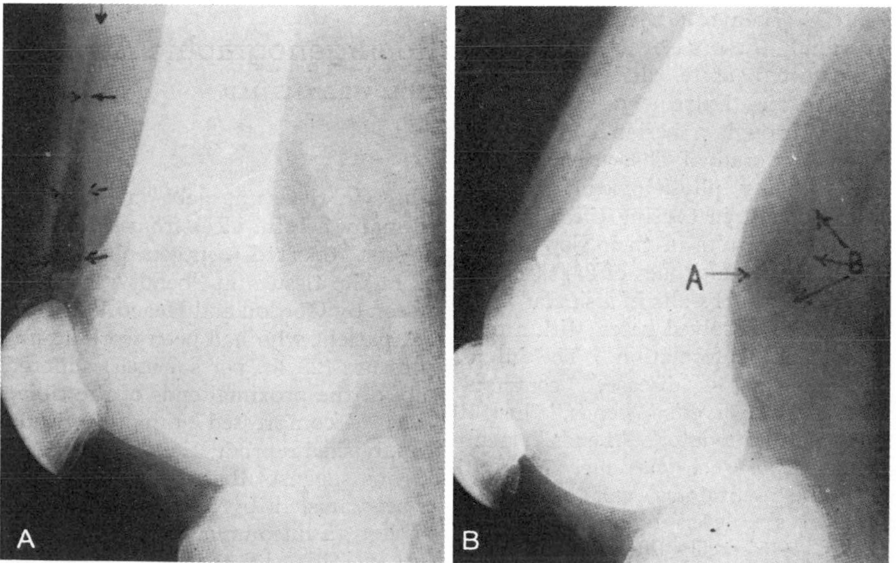

FIGURE 4–12. *A*, **A large volume of gas in the suprapatellar bursa of a subject who had no pain after 28 min at 38,000 feet of altitude.** *B*, **Discrete and irregular bubbles (A) posterior to the distal end of the shaft of the femur. The wavy streak of gas (B) appears to lie in a facial plane or along a tendon. The subject had moderately severe pain after three sets of deep-knee bends during 10 min at 35,000 feet. (From Thomas SF, Williams OL: High altitude joint pains (bends): Their roentgenographic aspects. Radiology 44:259–261, 1945.)**

weakness to total loss of sensation and paralysis.[53] The legs are most frequently affected.

The spinal lesions responsible for these symptoms are presumably caused by bubbles whose origin may be in the normal occurrence of free gas in the spine at sea level (Fig. 4–13).[54] This was first observed by Fick in 1910 and is now known as the *vacuum phenomenon*.[55, 56] Fick ascribed the vacuum phenomenon to reduced pressure in the joints as a result of movement, a mechanism currently recognized as tribonucleation.[38, 39, 41] The vacuum phenomenon is associated with aging joints, injury, or structural pathology and is frequently seen in intervertebral discs[57–59] but also has been observed in the epidural space surrounding the spinal cord.[60] Ford found the gas in a lumbar disc to be 90 to 92 per cent nitrogen.[16]

Unlike joint pain, spinal decompression sickness appears to be an intravascular rather than an extravascular phenomenon owing to the peculiar nature of the spinal circulation.[6] The venous plexus of the spinal cord is like a lake into which tributaries flow. It is valveless, under low pressure, and subject to the intrathoracic pressure changes accompanying respiration. These factors result in low blood flow of variable direction. Bubbles and bubble-induced thrombi are particularly likely to obstruct the venous plexus leading to ischemic spinal damage.

TABLE 4–3. Precordial Doppler Bubble Grading Scale

Grade 0	No bubbles
Grade I	Occasional bubbles
Grade II	Bubbles in less than half cardiac periods
Grade III	Bubles in all cardiac periods
Grade IV	Continuous bubbles

Data from Spencer MP: Decompression limits for compressed air determined by ultrasonically detected blood bubbles. J Appl Physiol 40:227–235, 1976.

Intravascular Bubbles and Doppler Bubble Detection

Intravascular bubbles are commonly observed after decompression, but their origin is obscure, since blood is highly resistant to bubble formation.[30, 40, 62, 63] The prevalence of bubbles in and around joints suggests that intravascular bubbles may have an extravascular beginning. The cavitation damage that accompanies tribonucleation in mechanical systems is severe enough to erode steel[64] and might cause capillary damage in vivo. A blood-gas interface introduced into a damaged capillary could initiate a continuous stream of intravascular bubbles, much like bubbles in beer grow and escape from a seed bubble on a glass. Observations that bubbles are usually present in blood draining from limbs affected by altitude decompression sickness support this hypothesis.[65]

In contrast to the lazy circulation of the spinal cord, most of the venous circulation carries bubbles directly to the right heart where a Doppler ultrasonic bubble detector can be used to convert the bubble signals into sounds.[28] These sounds are graded according to a scale such as that shown in Table 4–3.[66]

The relationship between decompression sickness and the Doppler bubble grade is shown in Figure 4–14 for subsaturation diving, altitude exposure, and saturation diving.[67] The x-axis is the bubble grade, and the y-axis is the incidence of decompression sickness which occurred at each grade. These observations suggest that high Doppler bubble grades, with decompression risks of 30 to 50 per cent, are poor predictors of decompression sickness, while low bub-

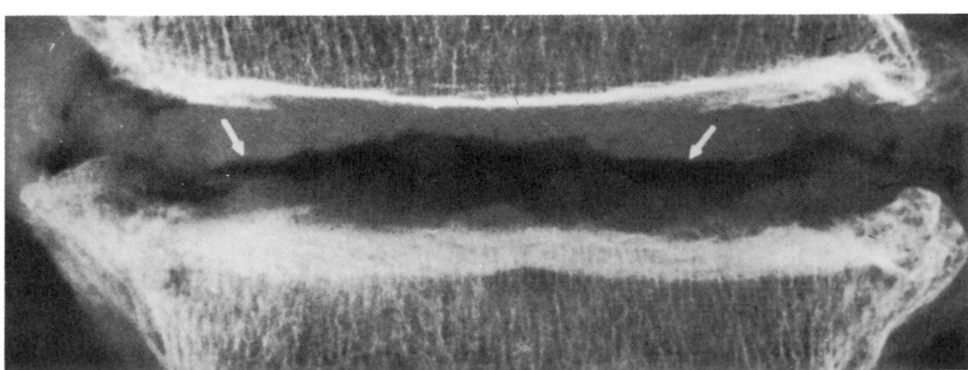

FIGURE 4–13. The vacuum phenomenon in an intervertebral disc. A collection of gas in the discal cleft appears as a radiolucent area *(arrows)*. (From Resnick D, Niwayama I: Diagnosis of Bone and Joint Disorders. Philadelphia, WB Saunders Company, 1981, p 1373.)

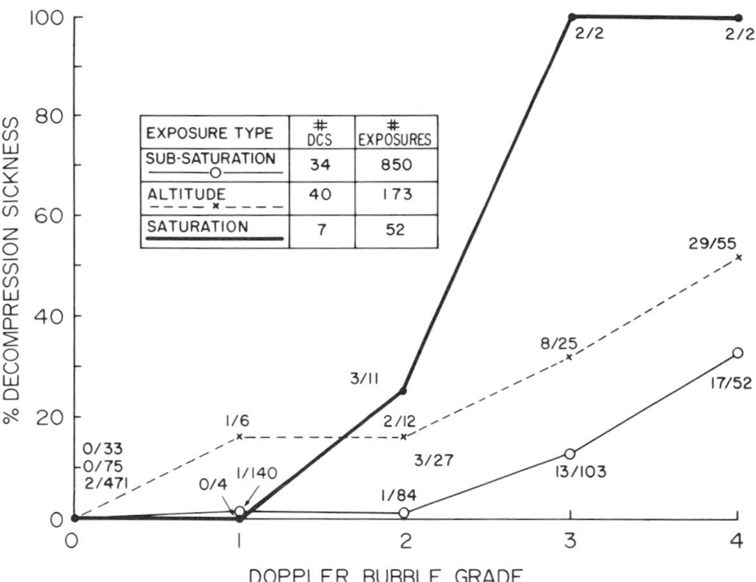

FIGURE 4–14. The relationship between Doppler bubble grade and the incidence of decompression sickness for subsaturation air diving, altitude exposure, and nitrogen-oxygen saturation diving. The risk of decompression sickness is small at low bubble grades and increases at higher grades. Low bubble grades are good predictors of decompression safety, but high grades are poor predictors of decompression sickness.

ble grades are good predictors of decompression safety. A breakdown of 84 decompression incidents (Table 4–4) shows that 87 per cent of all decompression sickness was associated with Grades 2, 3, or 4, and 100 per cent of Type II decompression sickness was associated with Grades 3 or 4.[68] Thus, while Doppler may be unsatisfactory for the early diagnosis of decompression sickness as was once hoped,[69] it can be useful to develop low-risk decompression procedures for which high bubble grades are not permitted.

Pulmonary and Arterial Bubbles

Excessive numbers of venous bubbles cause pulmonary irritation leading to bronchoconstriction and pulmonary decompression sickness (the chokes). At low gas loads, the lungs filter intravascular bubbles well and generally prevent their entry into the arterial circulation. When the filtering capacity of the lungs is exceeded, however, bubbles cross from the pulmonary to the arterial circulation. Sheep with high precordial bubble grades frequently had bubbles in the carotid artery.[28]

The brain and many other tissues appear to be resistant to local bubble formation despite high levels of nitrogen supersaturation,[70] and true cerebral decompression sickness is a rare event.[6] Bubbles can enter the cerebrovascular circulation, however, after arterial gas embolism or when venous bubbles are inadequately filtered or pass through pulmonary shunts or cardiac defects. (Fryer reports that about one quarter of the population have patent foramina ovalae.[71]) Arterial bubbles also can seed other organs and expand as they enter regions supersaturated with inert gas. The brain is particularly vulnerable to such bubbles due to its location and bubble buoyancy.

TABLE 4–4. Precordial Doppler Bubble Grades for 84 Decompression Incidents

	Bubble Grade				
	0	I	II	III	IV
Type I DCS	2	9	11	29	19
Type II DCS	—	—	—	7	7

From Vann RD, Dick AP, Barry PD: Doppler bubble measurements and decompression sickness. Undersea Biomed Res 9(Suppl 1):24, 1982.

Micro-Air Embolism

Serious decompression sickness occasionally occurs inexplicably after dives that are well within the no-decompression exposure limits and that should be too brief to cause trouble. Walder proposed that these unusual events are the results of *micro-air embolism* in which minor damage to lung tissue releases a small number of bubbles into the arterial circulation.[72] This damage might be caused by pulmonary blebs that rupture or by mucus from a recent cold which blocks a terminal bronchiole. The resulting arterial bubbles could cause bubble growth and decompression sickness in tissues that would otherwise be bubble-free.

FACTORS AFFECTING DECOMPRESSION RISK IN HUMANS

Exercise Before Diving

The risk of decompression sickness is determined primarily by depth and bottom time, but any factor affecting bubble formation or inert gas exchange also will influence risk. Increased bubble formation due to exercise before decompression, for example, has been noted in human as well as in animal studies. Heavy weight-lifting accompanied by muscle soreness within 24 hours of diving was associated with high precordial Doppler bubble grades and Type II decompression sickness.[73, 74] Weight-lifting would be expected to increase the frequency of tribonucleation and the vacuum phenomenon. Other forms of pre-exposure exercise have been implicated in unexpected decompression sickness after diving and during altitude exposure.[75, 76]

Adaptation

Conversely, the risk of decompression sickness is reduced by frequent exposure to pressure.[77] Haldane recognized this effect, now known as *adaptation*, and recommended part-time duties for new compressed-air workers.[78] Walder observed that during their first 10 exposures, the incidence of decompression sickness in compressed-air workers fell from 12 to 3 per cent.[79] After 10 days without pressure exposure, the incidence returned to its initial level. Adaptation was specific for each pressure and reoccurred when the working pressure increased.[77]

Some of the unexpected cases of decompression sickness which occur after innocuous dive profiles may be due to the absence of adaptation. First-time divers or infrequent vacation divers who have accumulated free gas in and around their joints as a result of tribonucleation and the vacuum phenomenon may have an elevated susceptibility to decompression sickness. If the free gas were eliminated by hyperbaric oxygen exposure before diving began, this susceptibility might be reduced.

The effects of pre-dive exercise and adaptation are consistent with the proposed dynamic equilibrium between the creation and destruction of gas nuclei. The creation of additional nuclei (vacuum phenomena) by tribonucleation during pre-dive exercise would result in the release of more than the expected 5 to 10 per cent free gas volume upon decompression. Adaptation during repeated compression-decompression cycles, on the other hand, could eliminate some of the nuclei and reduce the gas volume that formed upon decompression. The elimination of nuclei by hyperbaric oxygen exposure might be the most effective way of producing adaptation.

Exercise at Depth

Exercise affects inert gas exchange as well as bubble formation. Exercise at depth accelerates inert gas uptake by elevating perfusion. Behnke and Willmon demonstrated that exercise at sea level increased the whole body gas exchange rates of both nitrogen and helium.[80] Recent studies investigated nitrogen elimination at sea level after short air dives with rest or exercise at depth.[81] Figure 4–15 shows resting nitrogen elimination curves measured at sea level after dives to 130 feet for 10 min. Mean nitrogen elimination 60 min post-dive was 64 per cent greater after the exercising dives than after the resting dives, indicating that exercising divers absorb more nitrogen than resting divers.

By raising the volume of gas absorbed during a dive, exercise at depth increases decompression risk and time needed for safe decompression. Van Der Aue found that resting divers had a decompression risk of 11 per cent, while working divers had a risk of 21 per cent on the same schedules.[82] He also observed that decompression sickness occurred most frequently in parts of the body which were exercised vigorously at depth. (Vigorous exercise may have caused tribonucleation.) In other tests, Van Der Aue reported that air decompression schedules that were safe for resting divers produced 20 to 30 per cent decompression sickness in working divers.[83] Buhlmann found that divers doing light work during helium-oxygen dives required 20 to 40 per cent more decompression time than resting divers.[84]

Recent studies have shown how decompression is affected by 60 min of exercise at 100 fsw with a nitrogen-oxygen breathing mix having an oxygen partial pressure of 0.7 atm.[85] These results are shown in Figure 4–16 in which the x-axis defines the dive conditions, and the y-axis is the decompression time. The number of decompression incidents over the number of trials appears at the top of each bar. Dry, resting

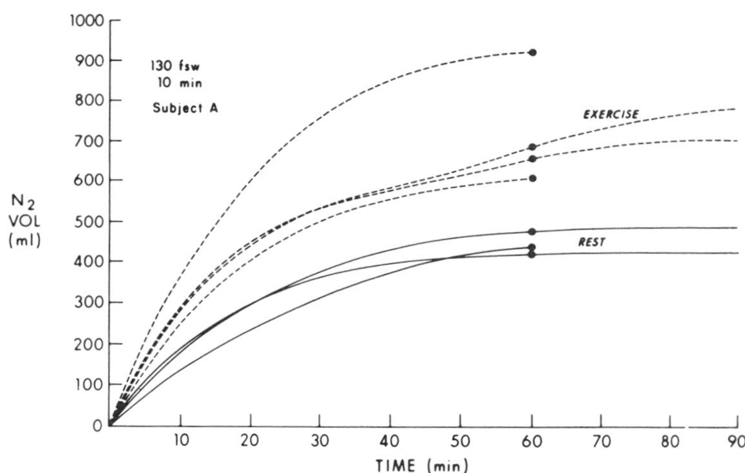

FIGURE 4–15. Respiratory nitrogen elimination curves taken at sea level from a resting subject after 10 min dives to 130 fsw. The subject exercised at depth during dives with elimination curves marked "exercise" *(dashed lines)*. During dives with elimination curves marked "rest" *(solid lines)*, the subject rested at depth. (From Dick AP, Vann RD, Mebane GY, and Feezor MD: Decompression induced nitrogen elimination. Undersea Biomed Res 11(4):369–380, 1984.)

exposures required only 40 min of decompression. In wet trials during which the divers exercised at depth and rested during decompression, both decompression sickness incidence and decompression time increased. After light exercise, 90 min of decompression were required, while 115 min were needed after moderate exercise. The 115-min schedule was insufficient to prevent decompression sickness after heavy exercise. Thus, a wet dive with heavy exercise at depth and resting decompression can require more than three times the decompression time of a dry, resting dive.

The safety of a decompression schedule is determined not only by the total stop time but also by the distribution of this time over depth. Stops too deep or too long are ineffective in eliminating excess inert gas and may cause additional gas uptake. Stops too shallow or too short can promote extensive bubble growth, which must be reduced by extra decompression time before the surface can be safely approached.

Exercise After Decompression

In the early days of decompression diving, U.S. Navy and Royal Navy divers routinely exercised during decompression as it was believed that exercise would accelerate inert gas elimination and increase decompression safety.[8, 86] When subsequent altitude and diving experiments showed that exercise increased the severity and incidence and reduced the onset time of decompression sickness, Van Der Aue recommended that exercise during or after decompression be avoided.[87, 88]

Van Der Aue applied his prohibition to both kinds of exercise, despite the fact that the early studies only investigated exercise after decompression, because the two forms of exercise were thought to have the same effects. Exercise

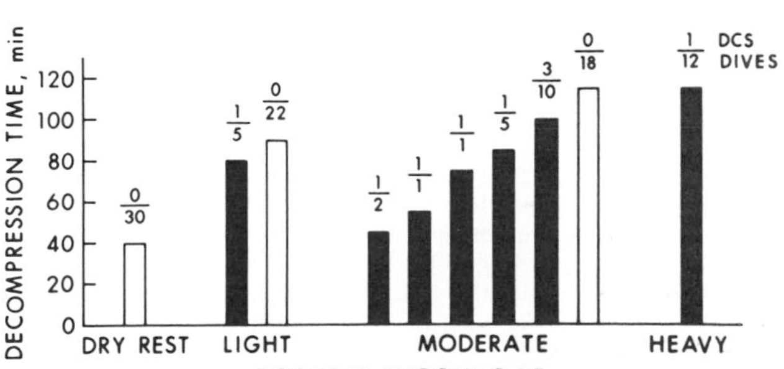

FIGURE 4–16. The effect of exercise at depth on decompression time and the incidence of decompression sickness. For a given workload at depth, the incidence of decompression sickness decreased as the decompression time was extended. Higher workloads required longer decompression times. (From Vann RD: Decompression theory and application. *In* Bennett PB, Elliott DH: The Physiology of Diving and Compressed Air Work. 3rd ed. London, Bailliere Tindall, 1982, pp 352–382.)

after decompression, however, causes increased bubble formation when the body is supersaturated with inert gas as a result of tribonucleation. These bubbles are eliminated slowly since gas in the bubbles is isolated from the circulation.

This effect is illustrated in Figure 4–17 in which the rate of krypton elimination from a subject's hand increased upon recompression from an altitude of 38,000 feet to sea level.[89] Thus, exercise after decompression should be avoided.

Exercise During Decompression

If extensive supersaturation and bubble formation do not occur during decompression, it is reasonable to suppose that exercise would accelerate inert gas elimination. Balke provided evidence to this effect in showing that exercise during oxygen breathing prior to altitude exposure delayed the onset of altitude decompression sickness.[90]

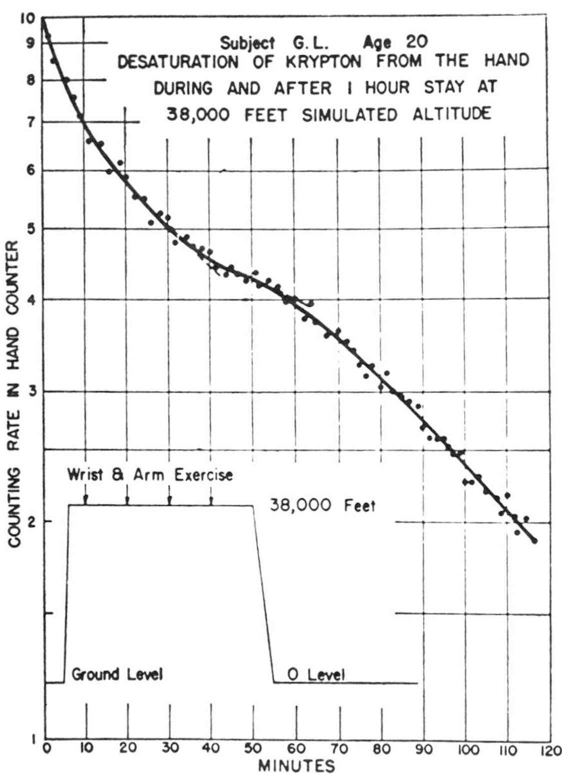

FIGURE 4–17. The effect of altitude decompression on the rate of krypton elimination from a subject's hand. The elimination rate increased upon recompression to sea level. (From Tobias CA, Jones HB, Lawrence JH, Hamilton JG: The uptake and elimination of krypton and other inert gases by the human body. J Clin Invest 28:1375–1385, 1949. Reproduced from the *Journal of Clinical Investigation* by copyright permission of the American Society for Clinical Investigation.)

The hypothesis that exercise during decompression could improve decompression safety and reduce decompression time was tested during dives to 100 and 150 fsw in which divers breathed 0.7 atm oxygen in nitrogen and performed light exercise for 60 min at depth and either rested or continued exercise during decompression.[85] Exercise during decompression reduced the incidence of decompression sickness and allowed shorter decompression stops. After the 100-fsw dive, one-third less stop time was needed with light exercise instead of rest during decompression. After the 150-fsw dive, stops were unreasonably long with resting decompression but were practical with exercise.

Thermal Effects

Exercise during decompression may exert part of its effect by warming a diver and preventing the decreased perfusion that accompanies hypothermia.[91] This would reduce decompression risk and stop time because warm divers eliminate nitrogen more rapidly than cold divers.[92]

As with exercise, however, the phase of the dive determines the effect that the thermal state will have upon decompression. A diver who is cold during decompression will *eliminate* less nitrogen while a diver who is cold at depth will *absorb* less nitrogen. Divers who were cold at depth during no-decompression diving were shown to have fewer intravascular bubbles than warm divers.[93] A diver who absorbs additional nitrogen at depth because he is warm will have an increased risk of decompression sickness. Divers in hot water suits are more likely to develop decompression sickness than colder divers in wet suits.[94] In trials of surface decompression with the divers in the water at depth and in a dry chamber during decompression, the incidence of decompression sickness was greater in warm water than in cold water.[83] Divers who are cold during or after decompression have a greater incidence of decompression sickness than warm divers because they eliminate nitrogen less effectively.[95, 96]

Individual Susceptibility

Much of the variability of decompression sickness is a result of differences in individual susceptibility. Fryer, for example, found that of 2199 subjects exposed twice at an altitude of

28,000 feet, 95.2 per cent had no problems, while 4.3 per cent developed decompression sickness once and 0.5 per cent twice.[71] Paton and Walder followed 376 compressed-air workers during 40,000 exposures in which the mean incidence of decompression sickness was 0.87 per cent.[97] Fifty-five per cent of this population had an incidence of below the mean, 11 per cent had an incidence equal to the mean, 6 per cent had twice the mean incidence, and 10 per cent had five times the mean incidence. The remaining 18 per cent had an incidence 28 times the mean, but as these workers quit after only a few exposures, their incidence is not reliable.

Susceptibility to decompression sickness is known to increase with age and obesity. Gray estimated that a 28-year-old man was twice as susceptible to altitude decompression as an 18-year-old, and a 70-inch-tall, 196-lb man was twice as susceptible as a 126-lb man of the same height.[98] Gray found that the best correlation with susceptibility occurred when both age and body type were considered together. Dembert observed that Navy divers who had the greatest skinfold thickness developed decompression sickness nine times more often than thinner divers.[99]

The effect of obesity on decompression risk is readily explained by the high nitrogen solubility in fat which causes increased nitrogen absorption and bubble growth. This was pointed out by Haldane[8] and has been demonstrated frequently in later years. The increased decompression risk with age is probably related to a more frequent occurrence of the vacuum phenomenon which accompanies the degeneration of aging joints.[57–60] Indeed, the vacuum phenomenon is more likely whenever joint surfaces are of eccentric fit,[41] and an eccentric joint configuration might predispose an individual to decompression sickness regardless of age.

RISK AND SAFETY IN DECOMPRESSION

No-Decompression Diving

Decompression risk has become easier to assess since introduction of the method of maximum likelihood.[100] This statistical technique can be applied to binary data, such as the presence or absence of decompression sickness, and has, for the first time, allowed objective analysis of decompression experience.

Maximum likelibood was applied to 1998 air and nitrogen-oxygen no-decompression dives in which there were 136 cases of decompression sickness for an overall incidence of 6.8 per cent.[101] These dives are shown in Figure 4–18 in which the x-axis is bottom time in min, and the y-axis is depth in fsw. The crosses represent at least one decompression incident, and the

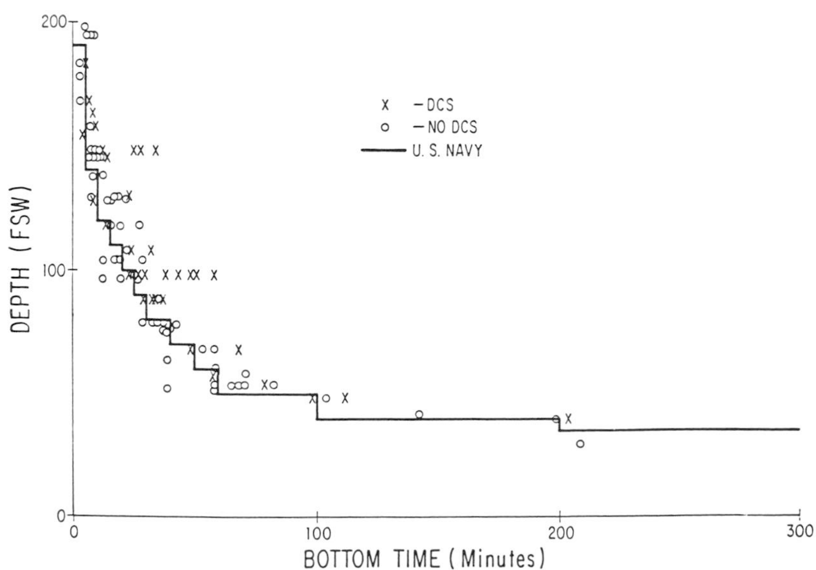

FIGURE 4–18. The results of 1998 air or nitrogen-oxygen no-decompression dives.[101] An "X" represents at least one incident of decompression sickness and an "O" at least one safe dive. The solid line is the U.S. Navy no-decompression exposure limit.[102]

circles represent at least one safe dive. The solid line defines the U.S. Navy no-decompression exposure limits.[102] All dives were included in the analysis whether wet, dry, warm, cold, working, or resting, and no consideration was given to whether the divers had exercised before, during, or after diving or were adapted to decompression by frequent diving.

Analysis of these data by maximum likelihood allows the decompression risk to be estimated for any no-decompression dive. Dives with estimated risks of 1 and 5 per cent are shown as curves in Figure 4–19. Each point on these curves represents the depth and bottom time of a no-decompression dive, which has a predicted risk of 1 or 5 per cent. A 100-min dive to 50 fsw, for example, has a predicted risk of 1 per cent. The Navy no-decompression exposure limits and shorter limits proposed by Huggins are also shown.[103] For dives from 190 to 130 feet, the Navy limits had risks of between 0.5 and 2 per cent. For dives from 120 to 50 feet, the risks fell between 2 and 3 per cent, and for shallower dives, the risks were between 5 and 7 per cent. Huggins' shorter limits reduced the risks to between 0.2 and 2 per cent.

Table 4–5 shows the estimated bottom times for no-decompression dives at 50 and 100 fsw at risks of 1, 2, and 3 per cent. At 50 feet, increasing the risk from 1 to 2 per cent adds 21 min to the allowable bottom time. A 3 per cent risk allows an additional 15 min. At 100 feet, increasing the risk from 1 to 2 per cent adds 5 min, and to 3 per cent, another 4 min. These and other risk estimates[104] apply to the mean behavior of a relatively large diver population and assume that all divers are equally likely to develop decompression sickness. In reality, the risk to a given diver on a specific day depends upon his individual susceptibility and cannot be predicted with certainty.

TABLE 4–5. The Effect of Bottom Time on Decompression Risk for No-Decompression Dives

	Bottom Times at Indicated Decompression Risk (%)		
Depth	**1%**	**2%**	**3%**
50 fsw	69 min	90 min	105 min
100 fsw	16 min	21 min	25 min

From Vann RD: DCS risk and no-stop air diving. Undersea Biomed Res 12(Suppl 1):30, 1985.

Closely related to no-decompression diving, particularly in sport diving, are repetitive and multilevel dives. Several sets of tables exist for these forms of diving, and more are under development, but little information is available on their effectiveness. Limited studies conducted by Thalmann at the Navy Experimental Diving Unit indicate that the Navy repetitive dive tables are overly conservative for some no-decompression dives but not conservative enough for some decompression dives.[105]

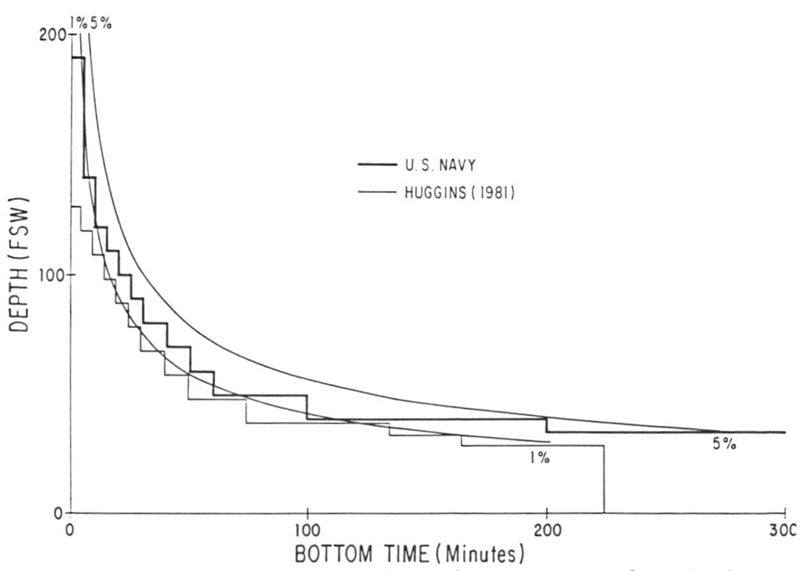

FIGURE 4–19. Predicted risks of decompression sickness for no-decompression air diving.[101] The curves represent 1 per cent and 5 per cent decompression risks. The U.S. Navy no-decompression exposure limits[102] and Huggins shorter exposure limits[103] are also shown.

Decompression Computers

The ultimate solution for multilevel, repetitive diving is the diver-worn decompression computer. This concept is nearly 40 years old, and a number of working models have been manufactured or evaluated,[106–113] but not until recently has the hardware been available to build reasonably reliable instruments.[114–117] These instruments incorporate a mathematical model of the decompression process which must be safe over a wide range of dive profiles. Such a model has not been easy to develop. A decompression computer should be tested under controlled conditions over its expected range of use before it is sold, but just as tests of a new drug cannot cover all possibilities, even decompression trials cannot ensure infallibility.

Because there are no published records documenting the use of decompression computers, it is difficult to draw firm conclusions concerning their safety. Some divers use them extensively and report significant safe increases in repetitive dive bottom times. There have been a few decompression incidents involving computers, however, as would be expected in the wide employment of any decompression procedure. Eight of these cases reported to the Divers Alert Network[118] are presented in Table 4–6. All divers were male, and the computers used appeared to function properly and to have been employed correctly. Table 4–6 shows that six cases involved decompression dives (the 40-year-old diver made cautionary stops), seven involved repetitive dives, seven involved divers older than 30, and eight involved dives to 100 fsw or deeper. If Table 4–6 has a message, it is that divers over the age of 30 who make repetitive decompression dives deeper than 100 fsw are the most likely to develop decompression sickness when decompression computers are used.

Decompression Diving

Even when the number of decompression incidents is known, the decompression risk cannot be estimated without knowledge of how many dives were made. Indeed, risk estimates are difficult to obtain for any decompression

TABLE 4–6. Decompression Incidents Reported to the Divers Alert Network (DAN) After Dives with Decompression Computers

	DIVE PROFILE				SYMPTOMS			
Age	Depth (fsw)	Bot. Time (min)	Dec. Time (min)	Surf. Int. (min)	Onset	Description	TREATMENT	COMMENT
34	136 133	29 19	30 9	180 —	In water	Arm and shoulder pain	None	Decomp. dives previous 2 days
23	120 96	25 22	21 11	180 —	15 min post dive	Arm and shoulder pain	Table 6A: Minor residual stiffness	—
33	174 174	27 18	60 77	240 —	In water	Headache, limb pain, and fatigue	Table 5: Full relief	Untreated symptoms 2 days ago
59	96 90–50	23 22	ND ND	145 —	45 min post dive	Neck and shoulder—pain and numbness	None: Resolved after 1 hr	—
36	108 70	48 30	17 ND	95 —	5 min post dive	Arm pain and tingling; lost dexterity	Table 5: Mild residual stiffness	Hard work on 2nd dive
40	105 40 30	18 55 60	5 3 3	53 161 —	22 hrs post dive in plane	Foot, hand, and cheek—cold and numb	None: Resolved after 24 hrs	1 to 2 ND dives/day previous 6 days
39	140 140 120 100 120	5 5 30 5 5	ND ND 28 ND ND	30 30 60 25 —	5 min post dive	Shoulder pain	Table 6	—
37	224	Unknown		—	In water	Apnea, paralysis, and severe pain	Multiple HBO: Residual paralysis	No problems on similar dives

TABLE 4–7. Estimated Decompression Risks and Safe Decompression Times for U.S. Navy Standard Air Decompression Schedules

	Depth (fsw)	Bottom Time (min)	USN Dec. Time[102] (min)	Est. Risk[104] (%)	Est. Safe Decomp. Time[105] (min)
1.	60	100	15	2–4	—
2.	80	70	24	3	—
3.	100	40	17	0.5	—
4.	60	180	57	11–16	171
5.	80	120	74	10–14	222
6.	150	40	60	5	120
7.	190	30	63	5	60
8.	150	60	113	12–15	>339
9.	190	40	103	9–11	>309

procedure. The U.S. Navy standard air decompression tables[102] are widely quoted, for example, but little information has been available on their safety until the recent tests by Thalmann[105] and the maximum likelihood analysis by Weathersby.[104] Navy schedules with decompression times ranging from 10 to 30 min have estimated decompression risks of 1 to 3 per cent as shown in Table 4–7. Long dives, such as 180 min at 60 fsw or 120 min at 80 fsw, have estimated risks of 10 to 16 per cent and require triple the decompression time specified by the Standard Air Tables. Deeper and shorter dives, such as 40 min at 150 fsw or 30 min at 190 fsw, have estimated risks of 5 per cent and require double the standard decompression time. Longer dives, such as 60 min at 150 fsw or 40 min at 190 fsw, have estimated risks of 9 to 15 per cent and are not safe even with triple the standard decompression time.

Tables requiring longer decompressions than the U.S. Navy Standard air decompression tables have been published in recent years. The Royal Navy Physiological Laboratory (RNPL) air diving tables,[119, 120] developed from the conservative Blackpool compressed air tables,[121] are very long and have a good reputation for safety,[122] although the results of their use are not readily available. The new Canadian Armed Forces tables[123] are shorter than the RNPL tables and were developed in a careful series of laboratory trials[124–127] but have not yet been field tested.

Increasing the decompression time reduces, but does not eliminate, the risk of decompression sickness. Figure 4–20 shows decompression schedules from seven sources for a 20-min air dive to 200 fsw.[8, 102, 119, 128–130] The longest of these schedules, from the RNPL table, was used after a dry chamber dive to 190 fsw.[85] Decompression sickness occurred, despite the schedule's length, when a diver restricted the

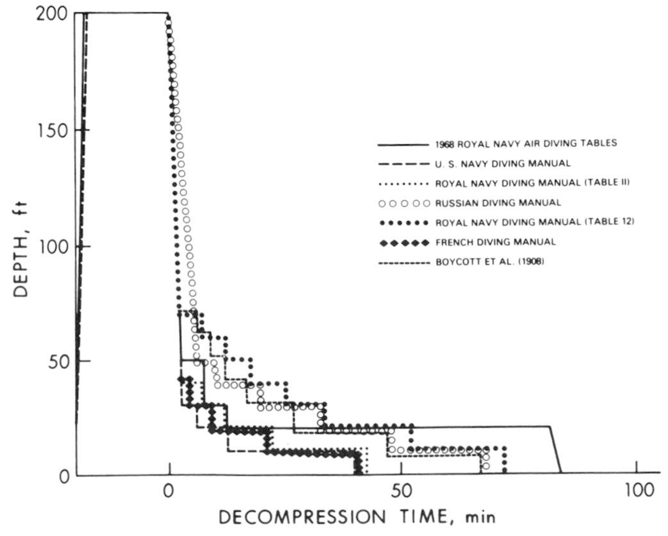

FIGURE 4–20. Seven decompression schedules for a 20-min air dive at 200 fsw. An incident of decompression sickness occurred on the longest of these schedules after a 190 fsw dive during which a diver restricted the circulation to his arm during a nap at the 20 fsw stop. (From Vann RD: Decompression theory and application. *In* Bennett PB, Elliott DH: The Physiology of Diving and Compressed Air Work. 3rd ed. London, Bailliere Tindall, 1982, pp 352–382.)

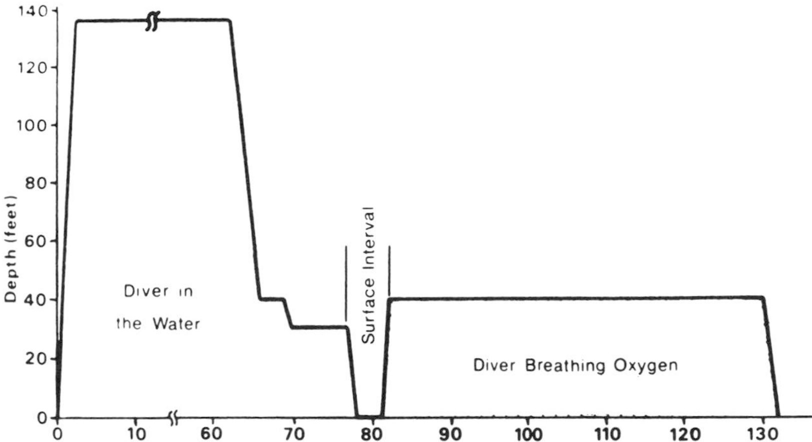

FIGURE 4–21. The U.S. Navy method for surface decompression using oxygen. The diver is removed from the water after his 30 fsw stop and is recompressed within 5 min to 40 fsw in a surface chamber where he breathes 100 per cent oxygen. (From U.S. Navy Diving Manual, NAVSEA 0994-LP-001-9010, January 1979.)

circulation to one arm during a nap at the 20-fsw stop. Once again, physiological factors, particularly when normal function is impaired, significantly affect decompression risk.

Oxygen

Extended bottom times are sometimes necessary in military, commercial, or scientific diving or in compressed-air work[131] but not in recreational diving. This problem is best solved by the careful use of oxygen. An elevated oxygen partial pressure reduces nitrogen absorption at depth and accelerates bubble elimination during decompression (see Oxygen Window section). Both factors decrease the decompression time. Raising the oxygen partial pressure from 0.7 to 1.4 atm reduces decompression time from 90 to 20 min after a 60-min nitrogen-oxygen dive to 100 fsw and from over 195 min to 100 min after a 60-min dive to 150 fsw.[85]

Oxygen is also effective in surface decompression (Fig. 4–21) during which the diver is removed from the water after his 30-fsw stop and is recompressed to 40 fsw in a surface chamber while breathing 100 per cent oxygen.[102] Bubbles that form during the brief surface interval are eliminated by the large oxygen window at 40 fsw in a manner similar to the 60-fsw oxygen treatment tables (see Fig. 4–9). Surface decompression and oxygen breathing, however, introduced hazards not present in air diving and should not be used without proper training and equipment.

SUMMARY

Because of the many environmental and biological factors affecting bubble formation and inert gas exchange, it should not be surprising that decompression sickness is unpredictable and that the safety of a dive is determined by more than just depth and time. Unfortunately, depth and time are the only parameters that can be measured conveniently and must be used to best advantage to estimate the limits of diving safety.

Decompression and other diving hazards make an occasional accident inevitable. While such accidents may be statistically rare, they must be anticipated because their consequences can be both physically and financially devastating.[132] Communications should be available for notifying an accident response system such as the Divers Alert Network,[118] adequate ground or water transportation should be pre-arranged, oxygen should be on-hand for surface use, and recompression facilities should be available within a reasonable distance. Equally important, initial diver training should teach that there are no depth-time limits that confer immunity from decompression sickness or from diving accidents in general. Only with these precautions can the greatest diving safety be assured.

REFERENCES

1. Bert P: Barometric Pressure: Researches in Experimental Physiology. Bethesda, Undersea Medical Society, 1978.

2. Keays FL: Compressed air illness, with a report of 3,692 cases. Dept Med Publ Cornell Univ Med Coll 2:1–55, 1909.
3. Erdman S: Aeropathy or compressed air illness among tunnel workers. JAMA 49(20):1665–1670, 1907.
4. Hill L: Caisson sickness and the physiology of work in compressed air. London, Arnold, 1912.
5. Levy E: Compressed-air illness and its engineering importance with a report of cases at the East River tunnels. Department of the Interior, Bureau of Mines, Tech. Paper 285. Washington DC, Government Printing Office, 1922.
6. Hallenbeck JM, Andersen JC: Pathogenesis of the decompression disorders. *In* Bennett PB, Elliott DH (eds): London, Bailliere Tindall, 1982, pp 435–460.
7. Kety SS: The theory and applications of the exchange of inert gas at the lungs and tissues. Pharmacol Rev 3:1–41, 1951.
8. Boycott AE, Damant GCC, Haldane JS: The prevention of compressed air illness. J Hyg 8:342–443, 1908.
9. Momsen CB: Report on use of helium-oxygen mixtures for diving. NEDU Report 2–42, AD728758, 1942.
10. Perl W, Lesser GT, Steele JM: The kinetics of distribution of the fat-soluble inert gas cyclopropane in the body. Biophys J 1:111–135, 1960.
11. Hempleman HV: 1963. Tissue inert gas exchange and decompression sickness. *In* Lambertsen CJ, Greenbaum LJ Jr (eds): Proceedings of the 2nd Symposium of Underwater Physiologists, NAS-NRC Publ. 1181, Washington, DC, 1963, pp 6–13.
12. Perl W, Rackow H, Salanitre E, et al: Intertissue diffusion effect for inert fat-soluble gases. J Appl Physiol 20:621–627, 1965.
13. Crone C, Garlick D: The penetration of inulin, sucrose, mannitol, and tritiated water from the interstitial space in muscle into the vascular system. J Physiol 210:387–404, 1970.
14. Aukland K, Akre S, Lerrand S: Arteriovenous countercurrent exchange of hydrogen gas in skeletal muscle. Scand J Clin Lab Invest 19 (Suppl 99):72, 1967.
15. Sejrsen P, Tonnesen KH: Inset gas diffusion method for measurement of blood flow using saturation techniques. Circ Res 22:679–693, 1968.
16. Duling BR, Berne RM: Longitudinal gradients in periarteriolar oxygen tension. Circ Res 27:669–678, 1970.
17. Piiper J, Meyer M: Diffusion-perfusion relationships in skeletal muscle: Models and experimental evidence from inert gas washout. Adv Exp Med Biol 169:457–465, 1984.
18. Piiper J, Meyer M, Scheid P: Dual role of diffusion in tissue gas exchange: Blood-tissue equilibration and diffusion shunt. Adv Exp Med Biol 180:85–94, 1984.
19. Perl W, Chinard FP: A convection-diffusion model of indicator transport through an organ. Circ Res 22:273–298, 1968.
20. Tepper RS, Lightfood EN, Baz A, Lanphier EH: Inert gas transport in the microcirculation: Risk of isobaric supersaturation. J Appl Physiol 46 (6):1157–1163, 1979.
21. Hills BA: A thermodynamic and kinetic approach to decompression sickness. Ph.D. Thesis. Libraries Board of South Australia, University of Adelaide, 1966.
22. Behnke AR: The isobaric (oxygen window) principle of decompression. *In* Transcripts of the 3rd Annual Conference of the Marine Technology Society, San Diego, 1967.
23. Behnke, AR: Early quantitative studies of gas dynamics in decompression. *In* Bennett PB, Elliott DH (eds): The Physiology and Medicine of Diving and Compressed Air Work. 2nd ed. London, Bailliere Tindall, 1975, pp 392–416.
24. Van Liew HD: Coupling of diffusion and perfusion in gas exit from subcutaneous pockets in rats. Am J Physiol 214:1176–1185, 1968.
25. Hempleman HV: The unequal rates of uptake and elimination of tissue nitrogen gas in diving procedures. RNPL Reports 5/60, 1960.
26. D'Aoust BG, Smith KH, Swanson HT: Decompression-induced decrease in nitrogen elimination rate in awake dogs. J Appl Physiol 41:348–355, 1976.
27. Hills BA: Effect of decompression per se on nitrogen elimination. J Appl Physiol 45:916–921,1978.
28. Powell MR, Spencer MP, von Ramm OT: Ultrasonic surveillance of decompression. *In* Bennett PB, Elliott DH (eds): The Physiology of Diving and Compressed Air Work. 3rd ed. London, Bailliere Tindall, 1982, pp 404–434.
29. Daniels S, Eastaugh KC, Paton WDM, Smith EB: Micronuclei and bubble formation: A quantitative study using the common shrimp, crangon cragnon. *In* Bachrach AJ, Matzen MM (eds): Underwater Physiology VIII. Bethesda, Undersea Medical Society, 1984.
30. Harvey EN, Barnes DK, McElroy WD, et al: Bubble formation in animals. I. Physical factors. J Cell Comp Physiol 24(1):1–22, 1944.
31. Hayward ATJ: The role of stabilized gas nuclei in hydrodynamic cavitation inception. J Phys [D] 3:574–579, 1970.
32. Yount DE, Strauss RH: Bubble formation in gelatin: A model for decompression sickness. J Appl Physics 47(11):model for decompression sickness. J Appl Physics 47(11):5081–5089, 1976.
33. Evans A, Walder DN: Significance of gas micronuclei in the aetiology of decompression sickness. Nature 222:251–252, 1969.
34. McDonough PM, Hemmingsen EV: Bubble formation in crustaceans following decompression from hyperbaric gas exposures. J Appl Physiol 56(2):513–519, 1984.
35. McDonough PM, Hemmingsen EV: Bubble formation in crabs induced by limb motions after decompression. J Appl Physiol 57(1):117–122, 1984.
36. McDonough PM, Hemmingsen EV: A direct test for the survival of gaseous nuclei in vivo. Aviat Space Environ Med 56:54–56, 1985.
37. McDonough PM, Hemmingsen EV: Swimming movements initiate bubble formation in fish decompressed from elevated gas pressures. Comp Biochem Physiol 81A(1):209–212, 1985.
38. Hayward ATJ: Tribonucleation of bubbles. Br J Appl Phys 18:641–644, 1967.
39. Campbell J: The tribonucleation of bubbles. Br J Appl Phys Ser. 2, 1:1085–1088, 1968.
40. Ikels KG: Production of gas bubbles in fluids by tribonucleation. J Appl Physiol 28:524–527, 1970.
41. Unsworth A, Dowson D, Wright V: "Cracking joints," a bioengineering study of cavitation in the metacarpophalangeal joint. Ann Rheum Dis 30:348–357, 1971.

42. Fox FE, Herzfeld KF: Gas bubbles with organic skin as cavitation nuclei. J Acoust Soc Am 26(6):984–989, 1954.
43. Yount DE: Skins of varying permeability: A stabilization mechanism for gas cavitation nuclei. J Acoust Soc Am 65:1429–1439,1979.
44. Johnson BD, Cooke RC: Generation of stabilized microbubbles in seawater. Science 213:209–211, 1981.
45. Vann RD, Grimstad J, Nielsen CH: Evidence for gas nuclei in decompressed rats. Undersea Biomed Res 7(2):107–112, 1980.
46. Roston JB, Haines RW: Cracking in the metacarpophalangeal joint. J Anat 81:165–173, 1947.
47. Strasberg M: Onset of ultrasonic cavitation in tap water. J Acoust Soc Am 31(2):163–176, 1959.
48. Ferris EB, Engle GL: The clinical nature of high altitude decompression sickness. *In* Fulton JF (ed): Decompression sickness. Philadelphia, WB Saunders Company, 1951, pp 4–52.
49. Bradley ME, Vorosmarti J: Hyperbaric arthralgia during helium-oxygen dives from 100 to 850 fsw. Undersea Biomed Res 1(2):151–167, 1974.
50. Hanson R de G, Vorosmarti J, Harrison JAB: Gas-filled joints after oxy-helium saturation dive. Br Med J 3:154, 1974.
51. Bondi KR, Miller DA, Knight DR, Harvey CA: Joint crepitation after chamber air dives to 188 fsw. Undersea Biomed Res. 4(1):89–94, 1977.
52. Thomas SF, Williams OL: High altitude joint pains (bends): Their roentgenographic aspects. Radiology 44:259–261, 1945.
53. Elliott DH, Kindwall EP. Manifestations of the decompression disorders. *In* Bennett PB, Elliott DH (eds): The Physiology and Medicine of Diving and Compressed Air Work. 2nd ed. London, Bailliere Tindall, 1982, pp 461–472.
54. Resnick D, Niwayama I: Diagnosis of Bone and Joint Disorders. Philadelphia, WB Saunders Company, 1981, p 1373.
55. Magnusson W: Uber die bedingungen des hervortretens der wirklichen gelenkspalte auf dem rontgenbilde. Acta Radiologica 18:733–741, 1937.
56. Fuiks DM, Grayson CE: Vacuum pneumarthrography and the spontaneous occurrence of gas in the joint spaces. J Bone Joint Surg 32A(4):933–938, 1950.
57. Marr JT: Gas in intervertebral discs. Am J Roentgenol 70:804–809, 1953.
58. Gershon-Cohen J, Schraer H, Sklaroff DM, Blumberg N: Dissolution of the intervertebral disk in the aged normal. Radiology 62:383–387, 1954.
59. Ford LT, Goodman FG: X-ray studies of the lumbosacral spine. South Med J 59:1123–1128, 1966.
60. Gulati AN, Weinstein ZR: Gas in the spinal canal in association with the lumbosacral vacuum phenomenon: CT findings. Neuroradiology 20:191–192, 1980.
61. Ford LT, Gilula LA, Murphy WA, Gado M: Analysis of gas in vacuum lumbar disc. Am J Roentgenol 128:1056–1057, 1977.
62. Darwin E: Experiments on animal fluids in the exhausted receiver. Philos Trans 64:344–349, 1774.
63. Hemmingsen BB, Steinberg NA, Hemmingsen EA: Intracellular gas supersaturation tolerances of erythrocytes and resealed ghosts. Biophys J 47:491–496, 1985.
64. Plesset MS: On cathodic protection in cavitation damage. J Basic Eng Dec:808–820, 1960.
65. Waligora JM, Horrigan DJ, Conklin J, Hadley AT III: Verification of an altitude decompression sickness prevention protocol for Shuttle operations utilizing a 10.2 psi pressure stage. NASA JSC Report of Jan. 30, 1984.
66. Spencer MP: Decompression limits for compressed air determined by ultrasonically detected blood bubbles. J Appl Physiol 40:227–235, 1976.
67. Vann RD: A comprehensive strategy for saturation decompression with nitrogen-oxygen. *In* Workshop on Decompression from NITROX Saturation Diving. Undersea Medical Society and NOAA. Philadelphia, University of Pennsylvania Institute for Environmental Medicine, January 8–9, 1985.
68. Vann RD, Dick AP, Barry PD: Doppler bubble measurements and decompression sickness. Undersea Biomed Res 9(1, Suppl):24, 1982.
69. Pearson R: Early diagnosis of decompression sickness. Undersea Medical Society Report July 30, 1977.
70. Spencer MP, Powell MR: The etiology of convulsions after hyperbaric exposures. Undersea Biomed Res 4(1):A23, 1977.
71. Fryer DI: Subatmospheric Decompression Sickness in Man. Slough, England, Technivision Services, Library of Congress Catalog Card No. 69–19960, 1969.
72. Walder DN: 1973. Man in the deep—Part 1. Oceans 2000. 3rd World Congress of Underwater Activities. BSCA/CMAS, 1973, pp 24–25.
73. Vann RD: Mk XV decompression trials at Duke: A summary report. Final Report on ONR Contract N00014-77-C-0406, 1982.
74. Nishi RY, Eatock BC, Buckingham IP, Ridgewell BA: Assessment of decompression profiles by ultrasonic monitoring. Phase III: No-decompression diving. DCIEM Report No. 82-R-38, 1982.
75. Hughes JS, Eckenhoff RG: Spinal cord decompression sickness after standard U.S. Navy air decompression. Milit Med 151:166–168, 1986.
76. Piwinski SE, Mitchell RA, Goforth GA, et al: A blitz of bends: Decompression sickness in four students after hypobaric chamber training. Aviat Space Environ Med 57:600–602, 1986.
77. Walder DN: The prevention of decompression sickness. *In* Bennett PB, Elliott DH (eds): The Physiology and Medicine of Diving and Compressed Air Work. 2nd ed. London, Bailliere Tindall, 1975, pp 456–470.
78. Rubenstein CJ: Role of decompression conditioning in the incidence of decompression sickness in deep diving. NEDU Report No. 12–68, 1968.
79. Walder DN: Adaptation to decompression sickness in caisson work. *In* Proceedings of the 3rd International Biometerology Congress. Oxford, 1968, pp 350–359.
80. Behnke AR, Willmon TL: Gaseous nitrogen and helium elimination from the body during rest and exercise. Am J Physiol 131:619–626, 1941.
81. Dick AP, Vann RD, Mebane GY, Feezor MD: Decompression induced nitrogen elimination. Undersea Biomed Res 11(4):369–380, 1984.
82. Van Der Aue OE, Brinton ES, Kellar RJ: Surface decompression: Derivation and testing of decompression tables with safety limits for certain depths and exposures. NEDU Report 5-45, 1945.
83. Van Der Aue OE, Kellar RJ, Brinton ES, et al: Calculation and testing of decompression tables for air dives employing the procedure of surface decompression and the use of oxygen. U.S. Navy Experimental Diving Unit Report 13–51, 1951.

84. Buhlmann AA: Decompression theory: Swiss practice. *In* Bennett PB, Elliott DH (eds): The Physiology and Medicine of Diving and Compressed Air Work. 2nd ed. London, Bailliere Tindall, 1975, pp 348–365.
85. Vann RD: 1982. Decompression theory and application. *In* Bennett PB, Elliott DH (eds): The Physiology of Diving and Compressed Air Work. 3rd ed. London, Bailliere Tindall, 1982, pp 352–382.
86. Ellsberg E: On the Bottom. New York, Dodd, Mead, 1929.
87. Henry FM. The role of exercise in altitude pain. Am J Physiol 145:279–284, 1945.
88. Van Der Aue OE, Kellar RJ, Brinton ES: The effect of exercise during decompression from increased barometric pressures on the incidence of decompression sickness in man. U.S. Navy Experimental Diving Unit Report 8-49, 1949.
89. Tobias CA, Jones HB, Lawrence JH, Hamilton JG: The uptake and elimination of krypton and other inert gases by the human body. J Clin Invest 28:1375–1385, 1949.
90. Balke B: Rate of gaseous nitrogen elimination during rest and work in relation of the occurrence of decompression sickness at high altitude. USAF School of Aviation Medicine Project No. 21-1201-0014, Report No. 6, Oct, 1954.
91. Bazett HC, Love L, Newton M, et al: Temperature changes in blood flowing in arteries and veins in man. J Appl Physiol 1:3–19, 1948.
92. Balldin UI: Effects of ambient temperature and body position on tissue nitrogen elimination in man. Aerosp Med 44(4):365–370, 1973.
93. Dunford R, Hayward J: Venous gas bubble production following cold stress during a no-decompression dive. Undersea Biomed Res 8:41–49, 1981.
94. Long RW: 1981. Final workshop general discussion. *In* Kuehn LA (ed): Thermal Constraints in Diving. Undersea Medical Society Workshop, UMS Publ. 44 WS(TC). April 1, 1981, p 413.
95. Balldin UI: The Preventive effect of denitrogenation during warm water immersion on decompression sickness in man. Proceedings of 1st Annual Scientific Meeting of the European Undersea Biomedical Society, Stockholm. Forsvarsmedicin 9:239–243, 1973.
96. Mekjavic IB, Kakitsuba N: The effect of peripheral temperature on the formation of venous gas emboli (VGE). 9th International Symposium on Underwater and Hyperbaric Physiology. Kobe, Sept, 16–20, 1986.
97. Paton WDM, Walder DN: Compressed air illness. Special Report Medical Research Council No. 281. London: HMSO, 1954.
98. Gray JS: Constitutional factors affecting susceptibility to decompression sickness. *In* Fulton JF (ed): Decompression sickness. Philadelphia, WB Saunders Company, 1951, pp 182–191.
99. Dembert ML, Jekel JF, Mooney LW: Health risk factors for the development of decompression sickness among U.S. Navy divers. Undersea Biomed Res 11(4):395–406, 1984.
100. Weathersby PK, Homer LD, Flynn ET: On the likelihood of decompression sickness. J Appl Physiol 57(3):815–825, 1984.
101. Vann RD: DCS risk and no-stop air diving. Undersea Biomed Res 12 (1, Suppl):30, 1985.
102. U.S. Navy Diving Manual, NAVSEA 0994-LP-001-9010, January 1979.
103. Huggins KE: New no-decompression tables based on no-decompression limits determined by Doppler ultrasonic bubble detection. Michigan Sea Grant College Program Publication No. MICHU-SG-81-205, 1981.
104. Weathersby PK, Survanshi SS, Homer LD, et al: Statistically based decompression tables. I. Analysis of standard air dives: 1950–1970. NMRI 85-16, 1985.
105. Thalmann ED: Air tables revisited: Development of a decompression computer algorithm. Undersea Biomed Res 12(1 Suppl):A90, 1985.
106. Searle WF Jr: Foxboro Decomputer Mark I. NEDU Evaluation Report 7-57, 1957.
107. Workman RD: Evaluation of a decompression computer developed for divers. NEDU Evaluation Report 1-63, 1963.
108. Stubbs RA, Kidd DJ: Computer analogues for decompression. 3rd Symposium on Underwater Physiology 1967, Chapter 26, pp 300–311.
109. Bares WA: Optimum diving profiles. Biomed Sci Instrum 10:29–32, 1974.
110. Borom MP, Johnson LA: Decompression meter for scuba diving utilizing semipermeable membranes. Aerosp. Med 45:135–142, 1974.
111. Howard RS: The single pneumatic resistor decompression meter and Albano's theory of decompression. Mar Technol Soc J 11:5–7, 1977.
112. Howard RS, Bradner H, Schmitt K: Theory of evaluation of the single pneumatic resistor decompression computer. Med Biol Eng 14:570–579, 1976.
113. Gibbs G: Decompression meters: Past—present—future. NAUI News Feb/Mar:10–11, 1986.
114. Jennings KE: Decometer: A microprocessor-based decompression computer for divers. ASME 77-WA/OCE-8, 1977.
115. Nishi RY: Real-time decompression monitoring by computers. DCIEM Report No. 78×27, 1978.
116. Bassett B: The diver's edge. Skin Diver 32(7):84–87, 1983.
117. Hass H: High technology approach to decompression calculation. Skin Diver 32(8):30–31, 1983.
118. Bennett PB: The United States National Diving Accident Network. EMT J 5(5):323–327, 1981.
119. Royal Navy Diving Tables, Royal Navy Physiological Laboratory, Alverstoke, 1968.
120. CIRIA Underwater Engineering Group: RNPL metric air diving tables. Report UR7, 1976.
121. CIRIA Underwater Engineering Group: Medical code of practice for work in compressed air. Report 44, 1982.
122. Hempleman HV: Decompression theory: British practice. *In* Bennett PB, Elliott DH (eds): The Physiology and Medicine of Diving and Compressed Air Work. 2nd ed. Baltimore, Williams and Wilkins, 1975, 331–347.
123. Lauckner GR, Nishi RY: Decompression tables and procedures for compressed air diving based on the DCIEM 1983 decompression model. DCIEM Report No. 84-R-74, 1984.
124. Nishi RY, Kisman KE, Buckingham IP, et al: XDC-2 digital decompression computer: Assessment of decompression profiles by ultrasonic monitoring, Phase I: 36-54 MSW. DCIEM Report No. 80-R-32, 1980.

125. Nishi RY, Eatock BC, Buckingham IP, Masurel G: XDC-2 digital decompression computer: Assessment of decompression profiles by ultrasonic monitoring, Phase II: 30–75 MSW. DCIEM Report No. 81-R-02, 1981.
126. Nishi RY, Eatock BC, Buckingham IP, Ridgewell BA: Assessment of decompression profiles by ultrasonic monitoring. Phase III: No-decompression diving. DCIEM Report No. 82-R-38, 1982.
127. Nishi RY, Lauckner GR, Eatock BC, Hewitt JT: Oxygen decompression techniques for compressed air diving using the XDC-2 decompression computer programmed with the Kidd-Stubbs 1971 model. DCIEM Report No. 84-R-19, 1984.
128. Royal Navy Diving Manual, Ministry of Defence B.R. 2806, March, 1972.
129. French Navy Diving Manual—Bulletin Official du Ministere du Travail, Fascicule Special No. 74-48 bis, Mesures particulares de protection applicables aux scaphandriers, 14 Juin 1977.
130. Shikanov YP (ed): Russian Diving Manual—Handbook for Divers. Joint Publications Research Service (JPRS) 60691, NTIS Springfield, VA, 4 December 1973.
131. Downs GJ, Kindwall EP: Aseptic necrosis in caisson workers: A new set of decompression tables. Aviat Space Environ Med 57:569–574, 1986.
132. Tzimoulis PJ: Don't risk a $30,000 mistake. SDM editorial. Skin Diver 87:6, 1986.

Chapter 5

Mixed Gas Diving

ALFRED A. BOVE *and* J. MORGAN WELLS

Although air has been the standard gas for divers for many years, extensions of depth and time for diving have generated a need for gas mixtures other than air.[1] These may be various mixtures of nitrogen and oxygen[2]; mixtures of helium and oxygen; trimixes of oxygen, nitrogen, and helium[3]; or experimental gas mixtures such as hydrogen-oxygen and neon-oxygen. All of these mixtures provide advantages over air under specific conditions and have been used in either operational or experimental diving.

The term "mixed gas" refers to breathing media other than air or oxygen. The most commonly used gas mixtures are nitrogen-oxygen (nitrox), helium-oxygen (heliox), and helium-nitrogen-oxygen (trimix). Appropriate inspired oxygen partial pressure (pO_2) is a key factor in mixed gas diving. The inspired pO_2 must be maintained lower than 1.6 bar to avoid central nervous system oxygen toxicity and above 0.16 bar to prevent hypoxia. During long saturation dives the inspired pO_2 must be maintained below 0.5 bar to avoid pulmonary oxygen toxicity. Air can be used during saturation excursions from an undersea habitat or saturation chamber, provided pulmonary and central nervous system oxygen tolerance limits are not exceeded and depths are not in the range to produce nitrogen narcosis.

NITROGEN-OXYGEN (NITROX)

Air has been used as a breathing gas since the beginning of diving. Diving bells using compressed air were described in the sixteenth century.[4] Its principal advantage is that it is readily available and inexpensive to compress into cylinders or to use directly from compressors with surface-supplied equipment.[4] It is not the "ideal" breathing mixture because of the decompression obligation accrued by breathing nitrogen at increased partial pressure, and because of the narcotic effects of nitrogen at increased pressure.

Mixtures of oxygen and nitrogen that contain less oxygen than the usual proportions of air (21 per cent oxygen, 79 per cent nitrogen) provide protection from oxygen toxicity with moderately deep diving (>130 feet) and are useful in saturation exposures during which divers are subjected to increased ambient pressure for days.[5] With such exposures, oxygen partial pressure may be high enough to cause pulmonary toxicity after prolonged exposure (see Chapter 8). To prevent oxygen toxicity, the pO_2 must be reduced to levels between 0.2 and 0.35 bar. To achieve this pO_2, nitrox mixtures with reduced oxygen percentage are used. Nitrox mixtures are designed to provide a pO_2 of 0.3 to 0.35 bar at saturation depth. Table 5–1 shows typical nitrox mixtures for shallow habitat saturation exposures. Numerous shallow habitat saturation exposures have been carried out during the past two decades. These ranged in depth from 30 fsw to 140 fsw[6] and employed normoxic nitrox mixes or air.[5] In these studies no evidence of pulmonary oxygen toxicity was found in exposures up to 30 days.[7]

When exposing saturation divers to normoxic nitrox mixtures, care must be taken to prevent exposure to mixtures that contain dangerously low levels of oxygen. Such exposures can occur in nitrox mixtures of less than 15 per cent oxygen at 1 ata. Nitrox saturation dives begin with air if the dive is shallow (e.g., 40 fsw, where pO_2 = 0.44 bar); one technique used to establish a safe pO_2 is to allow the oxygen to be consumed in the habitat to the percentage

TABLE 5–1. Characteristics of Nitrox Mixtures Used for Habitat Saturation Diving

SAT. DEPTH *fws*	SAT. PRESS *bar abs*	O_2-AIR *%*	pO_2-AIR *bar abs*	O_2-NITROX *%*	pO_2-NITROX *bar abs*
40	2.21	21	0.46	13.6	0.3
60	2.82	21	0.59*	10.6	0.3
80	3.42	21	0.72*	8.8	0.3
100	4.03	21	0.85*	7.4	0.3
120	4.64	21	0.97*	6.5	0.3
140	5.24	21	1.10*	5.7	0.3

*Air cannot be used at these depths because of pulmonary oxygen toxicity.

required by replacing atmospheric gas with small amounts of 100 per cent nitrogen.[8] Once a normoxic concentration is established in the habitat, oxygen is replenished to match consumption and maintain pO_2 at the decided concentration. More commonly, the chamber is compressed to about 16 fsw with air to achieve a pO_2 of 0.35 bar, then the remainder of the compression is done with nitrogen. Carbon dioxide must also be removed in this closed environment. This is usually done with a carbon dioxide absorbent such as lithium hydroxide.

Two nitrox mixing patterns are shown in Figure 5–1. In the left panel is depicted a typical nitrox mixing pattern for a small habitat with two divers saturated at 66 feet for several days. In this example pO_2 will fall from the initial 0.6 bar to 0.3 bar over 41 hours as the two aquanauts consume oxygen. During this period consumed oxygen is replaced by nitrogen to achieve the desired mixture. Once a 10 per cent oxygen mixture is established, oxygen is replenished as consumed and carbon dioxide is scrubbed from the atmosphere. The right panel of Figure 5–1 shows a more typical procedure. Air is used for compression to 16 fsw (0.30 bar O_2). The remainder of the compression is with 100 per cent nitrogen. Consumed oxygen is replaced by adding air or oxygen. Normoxic nitrox mixtures create problems with narcosis at depths greater than 120 fsw, and helium is commonly used below that depth.

Decompression

Although a benefit is achieved with normoxic nitrox (pO_2 between 0.21 and 0.35 bar) with regard to pulmonary oxygen toxicity in saturation dives, a greater decompression debt is incurred owing to the increased partial pressure of nitrogen. The increased nitrogen partial pressure results in greater tissue content of nitrogen than is achieved when breathing air. Using normoxic mixtures for short duration (subsaturation) dives would result in significant increases in decompression time with little advantage in lung protection from oxygen. In saturation diving, however, the longer decompression time is tolerable as an alternative to pulmonary oxygen toxicity. Extension of decompression time for saturation diving can be accounted for in operational planning.

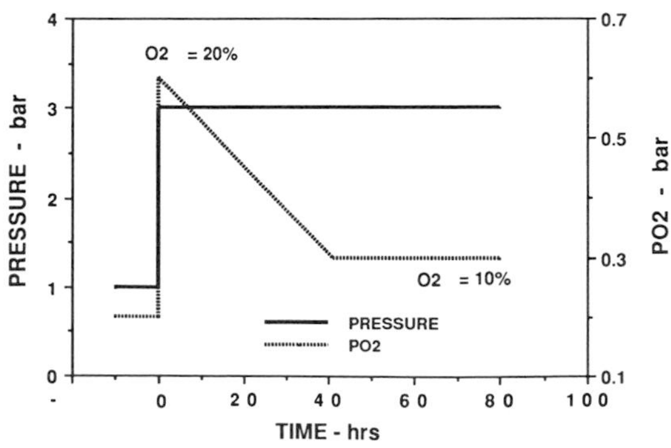

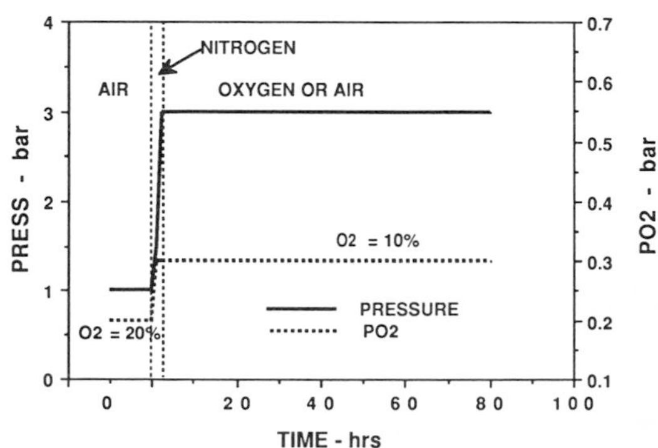

FIGURE 5–1. Two methods for changing nitrogen and oxygen concentrations in a saturation diving habitat. In the left panel, divers descend to 3 bar pressure (66 fsw) in the chamber, and breathe down the oxygen concentration until it reaches 0.3 bar and 10 per cent concentration. Nitrogen is added to replace consumed oxygen until the desired percentage of oxygen is achieved. In the right panel, the diving habitat is compressed to 0.3 bar pO_2 (16.5 fsw) with air, then compression is continued with 100 per cent nitrogen to achieve 66 fsw (3 bar) depth. Air or oxygen is added to maintain the 10 per cent O_2 environment.

Oxygen-Enriched Nitrox

Recently, interest has been expressed in nitrox mixtures that have increased oxygen partial pressure. Mixtures of 30 per cent oxygen, for example, contain a reduced partial pressure of nitrogen and, compared with air dives at the same depth, result in less nitrogen content of tissues. The mixture thus confers a decompression safety factor if standard air decompression procedures are followed, or longer dive times can be achieved at the same depth because the nitrogen partial pressure is equivalent to partial pressures of nitrogen at shallower depths with air. Figure 5–2 illustrates equivalent nitrogen partial pressures for actual depth with several oxygen-enriched nitrox mixtures.

The decompression procedure that must be followed when nitrox is used is based on the concept of equivalent air depth (EAD). This procedure equates the inspired nitrogen pressure of a nitrox mixture at one depth to that of air at another depth—the EAD. This procedure has been used for over 20 years with semiclosed and closed-circuit mixed gas underwater breathing apparatus. Such equipment is both very expensive and complicated. In recent years, nitrox use in open-circuit diving equipment has increased significantly. The following equation is used to calculate the EAD:

$$\text{EAD} = [\frac{(1 - \text{fiO}_2)}{0.79} \times (\text{D} + 33)] - 33$$

where fiO_2 = decimal fraction of oxygen in the mixture and D = depth in feet. For example, using 32 per cent oxygen, 68 per cent nitrogen, and a depth of 130 feet,

$$[\frac{(1 - .32)}{0.79} \times (130 + 33)] - 33$$

EAD = 107.3 fsw.

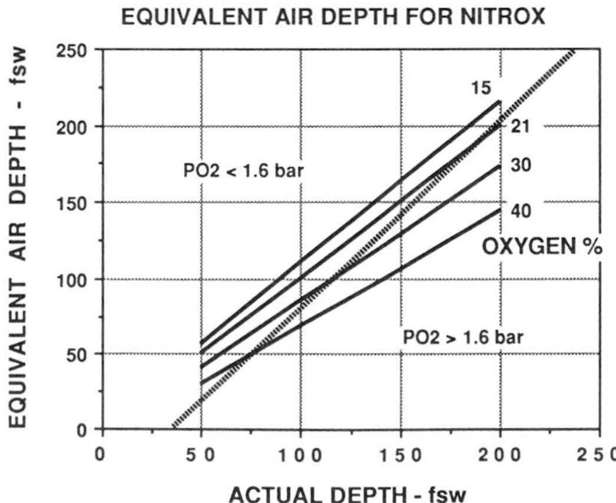

FIGURE 5–2. Equivalent air depths when using oxygen-enriched nitrox at several concentrations of oxygen. Equivalent depth is less than actual depth for mixes with greater than 21 per cent oxygen. The diagonal dotted line identifies the boundary for safe oxygen partial pressure (<1.6 bar). When diving with enriched nitrox mixtures, depth should not exceed the intersection of the dotted line and the mixture line.

Using the next deeper standard air decompression table (110 fsw), the diver would be able to descend to a depth of 130 feet and follow no-decompression limits or decompress as if the dive were made to 110 feet. The no-decompression time for an air dive to 130 feet (U.S. Navy standard decompression tables) is 10 minutes, while 20 minutes would be available using a 32 per cent oxygen nitrox mixture. A standard nitrox mixture containing 32 per cent oxygen has been adopted by the National Oceanic and Atmospheric Administration (NOAA) to avoid the computation errors and oxygen limitation problems often encountered during EAD calculations. This standard mixture is known as NOAA nitrox I (NNI); 130 feet is the maximum depth to which this mixture can be used without exceeding oxygen limits. No-decompression limits for several gas mixtures are shown in Table 5–2.

Although longer bottom times can be achieved with oxygen-enriched nitrox, two serious problems can arise when using these mixtures. There is a real risk of acute central nervous system oxygen toxicity when those mixtures are used improperly in operational diving. The acceptable maximum oxygen partial pressure to prevent acute oxygen toxicity during diving (U.S. Navy standards) is 1.6 bar (20 fsw with 100 per cent oxygen). With a 40 per cent oxygen mixture, this level is achieved at 4.4 bar (113 fsw). Divers using enriched-oxygen nitrox must be aware of the potential for acute oxygen toxicity, which is usually manifest by a seizure with deeper dives (Fig. 5–2). An underwater seizure is a catastrophic event that is likely to cause death of the diver and risks others who attempt rescue.

TABLE 5–2. No-Stop Times for Dives from 40 to 120 fsw, Using Several Gas Mixtures

FSW →	40	60	80	100	120
Air	200	60	40	25	15
He (0.7)	390	133	51	29	18
N_2 (0.7)	367	74	39	27	19
NN1 (32%)	310	100	59	40	25

Helium and nitrogen are mixed to constitute 70 per cent, with oxygen the remaining 30 per cent. NN1 is NOAA nitrox 1, a 32 per cent oxygen mixture. Time is given in minutes.

A second problem with oxygen-enriched nitrox is the need for precise mixing of the gases to establish known concentrations of oxygen and nitrogen. Increased pO_2 nitrox mixtures are readily made by adding air to oxygen under pressure. Gas proportions in these mixtures are often determined by calculating partial pressures. Although this technique is theoretically capable of determining exact gas partial pressures, inaccuracy of gauges and manifolds often results in mixtures that deviate from calculated values. These mixtures should be analyzed for gas content by independent gas analysis to be certain of oxygen safety limits and to determine an equivalent depth for calculation of decompression schedules. Errors in gas composition that produce errors of 5 to 10 fsw in equivalent depth will result in improper decompression and can increase risk for decompression sickness. Divers using oxygen-enriched breathing gas must be familiar with the complexities of partial pressure tables and calculate new decompression schedules based on the nitrogen partial pressure of the breathing gas. It should be obvious that dive computers, often used for air decompression, cannot be used with oxygen-enriched nitrox because their gas kinetic models are based on the usual nitrogen concentrations found in air. Meters should become available for use with nitrox.

HELIUM-OXYGEN (HELIOX)

Helium-oxygen gas mixtures were studied in the 1930's by Behnke and Willmon,[9] and End described a deep heliox dive in 1938. These investigators were searching for an inert gas that could eliminate the problem of narcosis found with air breathing below 150 fsw. Operational diving was limited to depths shallower than 150 feet in the early twentieth century due to severe narcosis produced by air breathing.[10] The laboratory studies of Behnke and Willmon were tested operationally when the submarine *Squalus* sank in 240 fsw.[11] Recovery of the submarine and rescue of the crew were accomplished using surface-supplied helium-oxygen diving. At the completion of this operation, heliox diving was established as the method for deep diving (below 150 fsw). The clarity of thought and the manual dexterity retained on helium at depths below 200 fsw were praised by divers at the time as a major advance.

Since this early experience with helium, diving to depths greater than 2000 fsw has been accomplished with this gas mixture, and extensive research on its effect has been conducted (see Chapters 4, 7, and 23). The ability of helium to prevent narcosis is most likely based on lipid-water partition coefficients and lipid solubility.[12] The low solubility of helium in lipid appears to contribute to its non-narcotic properties.[13–15] The lack of narcotic effects of this gas unmasked a new diving disorder—the high pressure nervous syndrome (HPNS)—which appears to result from direct pressure effects on excitable cells and a complete lack of narcotic effect of helium (see Chapter 7 for further discussion).

Surface-Supplied Heliox Diving

Surface-supplied heliox diving remains useful for single survey and rescue dives or for short duration working dives for which surface decompression can be used to shorten in-water decompression time. Current practice is to use saturation diving with heliox for diving projects below 150 fsw when a large amount of dive time is needed (e.g., 40 or more man-hours). Surface-supplied helium diving is an extension of surface-supplied air diving and as such follows many of the operational procedures developed for air diving. Important differences, however, do exist between air and heliox surface-supplied diving.

Because heliox mixtures vary in oxygen content as a function of diving depth to avoid oxygen toxicity, tables for decompression from surface-supplied dives are based on helium partial pressure and not on actual depth. The U.S. Navy helium-oxygen decompression tables illustrate the fundamental principles of mixed gas diving and oxygen decompression. The arrangement of the tables is such that the partial pressure of helium (pHe) in the breathing medium (not depth) and time are the factors that determine decompression obligation. To select an appropriate decompression schedule, the pressure (expressed in feet of seawater absolute, fswa) of the dive is multiplied by the fraction of helium (fiHe) in the breathing medium to determine the partial pressure of helium. For example,

$$\text{Depth} = 200 \text{ fsw}, fiO_2 = 0.2, fiHe = 0.8$$
$$(200 + 33) \times .80 = 187 \text{ pHe (fswa)}$$

A helium partial pressure table of 190 fswa would then be the appropriate decompression schedule for this dive, and the actual time of the dive would be used to determine decompression obligation.

Standard heliox partial pressure tables are available in the U.S. Navy Diving Manual.[16] Many commercial diving corporations use alternate helium partial pressure tables that often are proprietary. Tables for helium-air decompression are also available. Decompression schedules for heliox are determined for the depth of dive and for the partial pressure of helium achieved in the dive, which depends on the percentage of helium and the depth. Most heliox decompression schedules require a switch to 100 per cent oxygen at 50 fsw and usually incorporate surface decompression with oxygen to reduce total in-water time. During ascent and decompression stops, the helium-oxygen mixture is breathed until 50 fsw is reached, at which point the breathing medium is changed to oxygen. Oxygen breathing continues throughout the 50 and 40 fsw decompression stops. At the end of the 40 fsw stop the diver is brought directly to the surface. Provisions within the tables also allow for surface decompression (in a chamber) for the latter part of decompression. The surface decompression has several advantages: the diver is in a controlled chamber environment where loss of body heat is prevented, communications are improved, and oxygen toxicity can be detected and treated early. Another advantage is that the diving support vessel can break its moor and get under way rather than remain on station for the total decompression time. Table 5–3 is calculated from the U.S. Navy surface-supplied helium-oxygen decompression tables[16] and shows a typical decompression profile for heliox diving. During the "bottom time" of a dive, the oxygen content of the breathing medium is maintained as high as is allowed by the oxygen partial pressure limits, thereby keeping the partial pressure of helium as low as possible and reducing the rate of helium uptake.

TABLE 5–3. Decompression Profile for a Helium-Oxygen Dive

DEPTH *fsw*	TIME *min*	GAS
110	7	He-O_2
90	2	He-O_2
80	6	He-O_2
70	7	He-O_2
60	10	He-O_2
50	10	O_2
40	87	O_2

Table is calculated for a 250 fsw dive or 30 mins using 16% oxygen in helium and a U.S. Navy MK-12 surface-supplied diving system. Helium partial pressure table for this time-depth and oxygen percentage give a partial pressure table of 244 fsw, which is rounded off to the next highest depth of 250 fsw absolute.

Some commercial diving tables expand even further on the above principles by adding air and nitrox mixtures at various points in the dive profile. If the breathing medium during deep decompression stops of a helium-oxygen dive is changed from helium-oxygen to air at a depth where nitrogen narcosis and oxygen toxicity are not limiting, helium elimination will occur at the maximum possible rate since there will be no helium in the inspired gas. Some nitrogen uptake will occur during this time, and therefore the total tissue insert gas partial pressure will not drop as fast as if oxygen were breathed. However, a more rapid reduction in the total inert gas pressure will occur owing to the physical properties of the gases. On ascent from shallower depths, a nitrox mixture containing more oxygen than air (but with an acceptable pO_2) can be used to reduce the nitrogen in the breathing medium. When the breathing medium at shallow depths ($<$ 50 fsw) is switched to oxygen, both helium and nitrogen will be eliminated at the maximum possible rates. This type of procedure can reduce total ascent time for a particular dive when compared with the U.S. Navy tables and can reduce the quantity of expensive helium required for the dive. Numerous variations of this generic type of dive profile exist in the commercial diving industry. Most decompression schedules for heliox require longer decompression time than that for air. In some no-decompression dives, use of heliox may provide slightly longer bottom times.[16] Table 5–2 illustrates this point with several gas mixtures.

Saturation Diving with Heliox

An important advance in diving technology resulted from the work of Bond,[17] who conducted saturation experiments with heliox.[18] This work demonstrated that divers could spend prolonged periods (weeks) under pressure without serious physiological changes. Working dives using this technique have been conducted at depths over 1000 feet in open sea for periods of up to 3 to 4 weeks. Breathing gases for these saturation dives are mixed with extreme care, since dives of 1000 feet where normoxic mixtures (0.3 to 0.5 bar oxygen) require that oxygen concentrations be held to tolerances of 0.10 per cent to avoid hypoxia and oxygen toxicity. Figure 5–3 shows typical percentage of oxygen in heliox for various depths. Changes of less than 1 per cent at deeper depths can shift the oxygen level to an unsafe proportion.

Typical deep saturation diving operations at

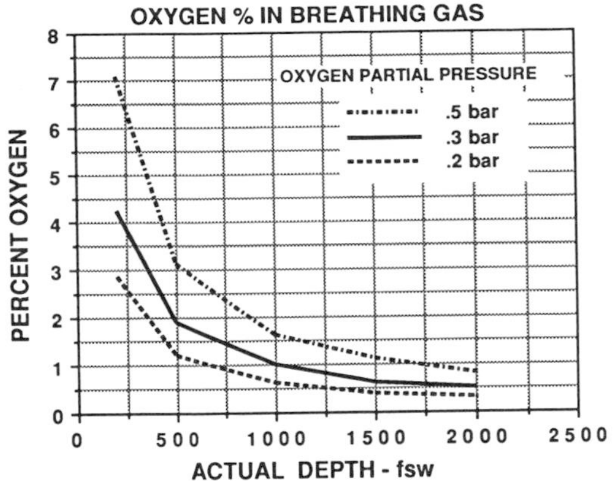

FIGURE 5–3. Oxygen percentage of heliox for deep diving. Three oxygen concentrations are shown, which span the safe pO_2 range for avoiding oxygen toxicity.

present avoid sea floor habitats as originally conceived by Bond and co-workers.[17, 18] Although habitat operations are useful for scientific or exploratory projects, underwater construction, particularly in undersea oil recovery operations in deep water, cannot be supported by underwater habitats. Most working saturation dives are currently conducted using a shipboard chamber (deck decompression chamber [DDC]) and a pressurized transfer chamber (PTC) that delivers divers to the worksite (Fig. 5–4). With this method, divers can be easily supported by a ship's crew through transfer locks on the shipboard chamber for the duration of the dive, then decompress once over several days. The DDC can be supported easily compared with a sea floor habitat. The transfer chamber is mated to the DDC and is pressurized to equalize with the pressure inside the DDC, which is held at the pressure of the worksite. Divers transfer from the habitat chamber to the transfer chamber under pressure. When all hatches are secured, the transfer chamber is detached and lowered to the worksite, where one or more divers can leave the transfer chamber to perform whatever work is needed. Continuous shifts of divers can conduct operations on a 24-hour schedule in prolonged projects.

The Helium Environment

With the frequent use of helium saturation diving, several unique problems were discovered which result from the helium gas. Because of its small molecular size, helium is highly diffusible and can penetrate many pressure seals not affected by nitrogen. Electronic parts, cables, vacuum tubes, and pressure-proof watches are examples of equipment that has been damaged by unexpected penetration of helium. However, design modifications of equipment to be used in heliox environments have eliminated most of the helium diffusion problems.

An amusing but troublesome problem with helium atmospheres is the change in voice which has become characteristic of this environment.[19] The high-pitched "Donald Duck" quality of the voice at first imports humor, which soon reverts to concern for communication with the divers. The voice change induced by helium renders communication difficult and in many cases impossible. Initial efforts to communicate under these conditions depended on memorized responses so that dive supervisors could translate the poorly understood communication.

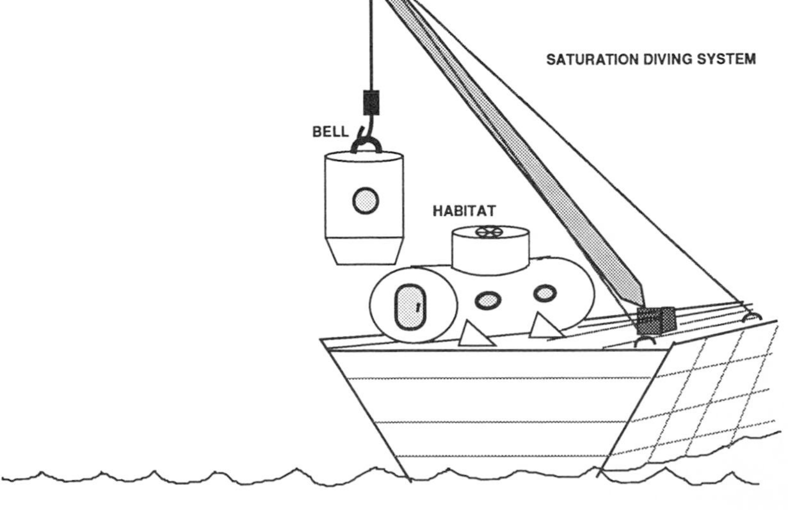

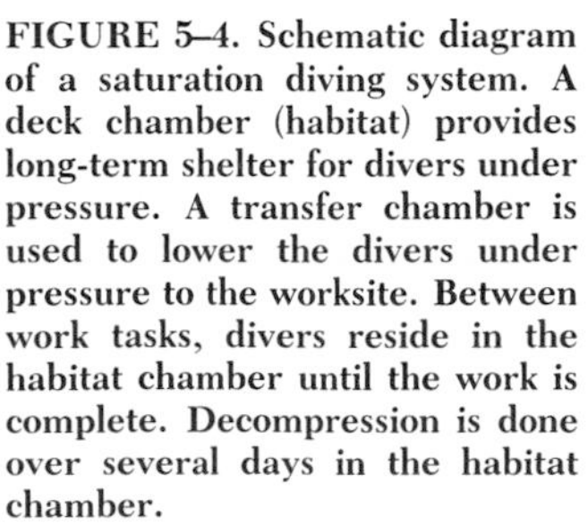
FIGURE 5–4. Schematic diagram of a saturation diving system. A deck chamber (habitat) provides long-term shelter for divers under pressure. A transfer chamber is used to lower the divers under pressure to the worksite. Between work tasks, divers reside in the habitat chamber until the work is complete. Decompression is done over several days in the habitat chamber.

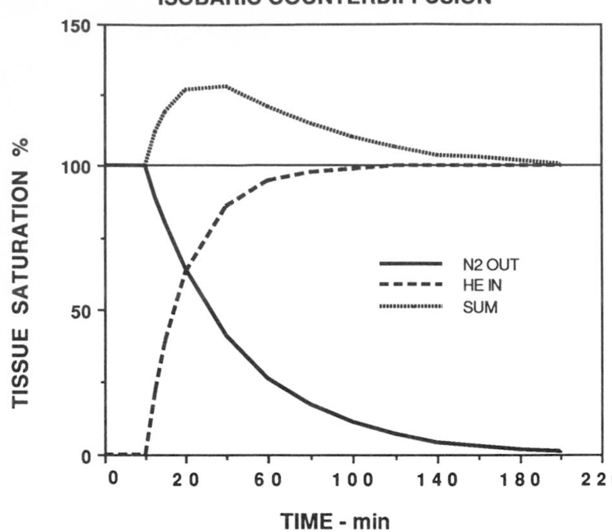

FIGURE 5–5. Tissue gas concentration curves during switching of two breathing gases of differing diffusion rates. The incoming gas diffuses more rapidly than the outgoing gas; a net increase in inert gas concentration curves can cause decompression sickness. Curves shown are typical of a switch from air to heliox at constant pressure.

Electronic voice encoding has significantly improved communications. This technique reconstructs normal voice characteristics by frequency filtering and spectral shifting. The resultant voice, although not ideal, significantly improves communicability of divers conversing in a heliox environment.

Physiological effects of heliox were studied in a series of dives conducted by a joint American-Japanese research team (operation Sea Dragon). Recounting of this work is provided in several papers by Hong and co-workers.[20–22] They noted an increase in basal metabolism in divers living at a depth of 985 fsw. All divers lost weight in spite of increased food consumption[21] and felt cold when ambient temperature fell below 80°F. This latter perception is predictable from the high thermal conductivity of compressed helium. Most divers in a helium environment need several blankets to keep warm when sleeping, even when ambient temperature is near 80°F.[22] Cardiac conduction and contractile force may also be affected by helium. Ask and Tyssebotn[23] recently demonstrated altered cardiac performance in rabbits exposed to 960 fsw helium. Their data show small effects that are likely to be insignificant in humans; however, the finding of an inert gas effect in cardiac tissues is of interest. Helium effects on the central nervous system are discussed in detail in Chapter 7 and will not be repeated here.

HELIUM-NITROGEN-OXYGEN (TRIMIX)

Bennett's discussion of trimix and of the Atlantic series of dives in Chapter 7 provides adequate review of this topic. This gas mix is used at deep depths (over 2000 fsw) to alleviate HPNS.[1, 24, 25] The theoretical basis for this mixture is discussed in Chapter 7. The successful use of this mixture by Bennett and colleagues[26] is an excellent example of basic research applied to operational diving. Reduction of HPNS with trimix was accomplished by the addition of 5 to 10 per cent nitrogen to heliox. The small amount of nitrogen opposes the hyperexcitable state that results from a high pressure helium environment.[26]

Trimix is also used in shallower working dives to reduce the cost of helium and to reduce narcotic effects of nitrogen. In this case, helium is added to air in varying proportions.

HYDROGEN-OXYGEN

Hydrogen offers the potential for minimal narcotic effects based on its solubility.[12, 13, 15] An important operational limitation of hydrogen use, however, is its extreme flammability. Mixtures of hydrogen and oxygen are explosive except in situations where the percentage of oxygen is less than 2 per cent.[27] Mixtures of this type are applicable at depths below 600 fsw (see Fig. 5–3). Gardette, Rostain, and coworkers[27, 28] recently described several successful hydrogen-oxygen dives to 1480 fsw. On such a dive, divers begin with heliox, and at 650 fsw (200 msw) switch to a nonexplosive mixture of hydrogen-helium-oxygen. On return to the surface, the breathing gas is switched back to heliox when a higher percentage of oxygen is required. Gas switching of this kind under pressure can result in decompression sickness from counterdiffusion of gases (see below). Deep hydrogen-oxygen diving eliminates the need for large stores of helium. The use of helium in deep diving and other demands for helium have increased the cost and have reduced the availability of this gas. Hydrogen gas can be obtained from electrolysis of water and is potentially more abundant than helium. Although most current hydrogen diving is experimental, the diminishing supply of helium may make hydrogen-oxygen gas mixes an attractive alternative to helium in the future.

OTHER INERT GASES

Although mixtures containing neon, argon, and xenon[14, 29] have been used experimentally in deep diving exposures, none of these gases are useful because of their narcotic properties and in some cases their increased density, which limits ventilation. These gases are obtained by fractional distillation of liquefied air and are expensive to produce.

ISOBARIC COUNTERDIFFUSION

During the PSIV series of deep dives conducted by Lambertsen and co-workers,[30] gas-containing skin lesions were found in some divers exposed to 1000 fsw pressure breathing a helium-neon-oxygen mixture while in a helium-oxygen environment. These skin lesions were eliminated when the diver was placed in a sealed suit and surrounded by the same gas as the breathing medium.[30] Graves and colleagues[31] reported further observations on this phenomenon and described the diffusion kinetics responsible for the effect. Figure 5–5 shows the mechanism that causes gas phase to form in tissues during switching of gases at fixed ambient pressure. The effect requires that two gases have different diffusion and solubility coefficients, and the gas with the higher coefficient replaces the lower coefficient gas. Under these conditions the high coefficient gas diffuses rapidly into tissue, while the low coefficient gas diffuses out more slowly. Total inert gas concentration will rise and supersaturate tissues. The supersaturation can reach levels that cause gas phase formation and clinical decompression sickness. Counterdiffusion effects can be separated into superficial effects involving the skin and deep effects involving other organs and tissues not affected by the surface interface with the inert gas. Superficial counterdiffusion depends on gas diffusion through the skin and causes bubbles in superficial tissues, including skin and subcutaneous tissue. Deep counterdiffusion occurs in tissues without exposed surfaces and depends on perfusion to supply and remove inert gas. Typical gas switches that cause gas phase formation are air to helium, hydrogen to helium, neon to helium,[32] and, in experimental animals, nitrous oxide to nitrogen.[33] In operational diving, gas switches suspected of causing a counterdiffusion problem are accompanied by a small pressure increase to avoid supersaturation.

Other operational aspects of mixed gas diving, such as excursion from saturation, mixed gas scuba, mixing of gases, and undersea habitats, can be found in references 34, 35, 36, and 37.

REFERENCES

1. Bennett PD, McLeod M: Probing the limits of human deep diving. Philos Trans R Soc Lond B(304):105–117, 1984.
2. Leitch DR, Barnard EEP: Observation on no stop and repetitive air and oxynitrogen diving. Undersea Biomed Res 9:91–112, 1982.
3. Parmentier JL, Harris JL, Bennett PB: Central and peripheral causes of hyperreflexia in humans breathing 50% trimix at 650 M. J Appl Physiol 58:1239–1245, 1985.
4. Bert P: Barometric Pressure (republished). Bethesda, Undersea Medical Society, 1978, pp 355–410.
5. Hamilton RW, Kenyan DJ, Peterson RE: Development of decompression procedures for undersea habitats: Repetitive no-stop and one-stop excursions, oxygen limits and surfacing procedures. *In* Bove AA, Bachrach AJ, Greenbaum LJ (eds): Underwater and Hyperbaric Physiology IX. Bethesda, Underwater and Hyperbaric Medical Society, 1987, pp 197–309.
6. Busch WS, Constraints and considerations for operational scientific diving from a saturation habitat using air and/or nitrox. *In* Bove AA, Bachrach AJ, Greenbaum LJ (eds): Underwater and Hyperbaric Physiology IX. Bethesda, Underwater and Hyperbaric Medical Society, 1987, pp 1165–1180.
7. Cousteau JY: At home in the sea. Natl Geogr 125:465–506, 1964.
8. Miller J (ed): NOAA Diving Manual for Science and Technology, 2nd ed. Washington, DC, US Government Printing Office, 1979.
9. Behnke AR, Willmon TL: Gaseous nitrogen and helium elimination from the body during rest and exercise. Am J Physiol 131:619–626, 1941.
10. Behnke AR: Some early studies of decompression. *In* Bennett PB, Elliott DH (eds): The Physiology and Medicine of Diving and Compressed Air Work (1st Ed). Baltimore, Williams and Wilkins, 1969, pp 226–251.
11. Behnke AR, Willman TL: USS *Squalus*: Medical as-

pects of the rescue and salvage operations and the use of oxygen in deep-sea diving. U.S. Navy Med. Bull 37:629–640, 1939.

12. Smith EB: The role of exotic gases in the study of narcosis. *In* Bennett PB, Elliott DH (eds): The Physiology and Medicine of Diving and Compressed Air Work (1st Ed). Baltimore, Williams and Wilkins, 1969, pp 181–192.
13. Meyer KH: Contributions to the theory of narcosis. Trans Faraday Soc 33:1062–1068, 1937.
14. Miller KW, Paton WD, Smith EB: Site of action of general anesthetics. Nature 206:574–577, 1965.
15. Smith EB: On the science of deep-sea diving. Observations on the respiration of different kinds of air. Undersea Biomed Res 14:347–369, 1987.
16. U.S. Navy Diving Manual, Volume 2: Mixed-gas Diving NAVSFA 0994-LP-001-9020. Washington, DC, U.S. Government Printing Office, 1987, pp 15-3–15-24.
17. Bond G: New developments in high pressure living. Arch Env Health 9:310–314, 1964.
18. Lord G, Bond G, Schaefer K: Breathing under high ambient pressure. J Appl Physiol 21:1833–1838, 1966.
19. Rothman HB, Gelfand R, Hollien H, Lambertsen CJ: Speech intelligibility of high helium-oxygen pressures. Undersea Biomed Res 7:205–275, 1980.
20. Nakayama H, Murai T, Hong SK: Sea Dragon VI. A 7-day dry saturation dive at 31 ata. I. Objectives, design and scope. Undersea Biomed Res 14:377–385, 1987.
21. Shiraki K, Hong SK, Park YS, et al: Sea Dragon VI. A 7-day dry saturation dive at 31 ata. II. Characteristics of diuresis and nocturia. Undersea Biomed Res 14:387–400, 1987.
22. Konda N, Takeuchi H, Nakayama H, Hong SK: Sea Dragon VI. A 7-day dry saturation dive at 31 ata. IV. Circadian analysis of body temperature and renal functions. Undersea Biomed Res 14:413–423, 1987.
23. Ask JA, Tyssebotn I: Effects of 5, 10 and 30 bar as the contractile activity of isolated atrial preparations from the rat heart. *In* Bove AA, Bachrach AJ, Greenbaum LJ (eds): Proceedings of the 9th International Symposium on Underwater and Hyperbaric Physiology. Bethesda, Undersea and Hyperbaric Medical Society, 1987, pp 465–469.
24. Bennett PB, Coggin R, McLeod M: Effect of compression rate on use of Trimix to ameliorate HPNS in man to 686 M (2250 ft). Undersea Biomed Res 9:335–351, 1982.
25. Brauer RW, Johnson DO, Pessotti RL, Redding R: Effects of hydrogen and helium at pressures to 67 atmospheres. Proc Am Soc Exp Biol 25:202, 1968.
26. Bennett PB, Blenkarn GD, Roby J, Youngblood D: Suppression of the high pressure nervous syndrome in human deep dives by He-N_2-O_2. Undersea Biomed Res 1:221–237, 1974.
27. Rostain JC, Gardette-Chauffour MD, Lemaire C, Naquet R: Effects of a H_2-He-O_2 mixture on the HPNS up to 450 msw. Undersea Biomed Res 15:257–270, 1988.
28. Gardette B, Fructus X, DeLauze HG: First human saturation dive at 450 msw: Hydra V. *In* Bove AA, Bachrach AJ, Greenbaum LJ (eds): Proceedings of the 9th International Symposium on Underwater and Hyperbaric Physiology. Bethesda, Undersea and Hyperbaric Medical Society, 1987, pp 375–389.
29. Bennett PB: Performance impairment in deep diving due to nitrogen, helium, neon and oxygen. *In* Lambertsen CJ (ed): Proceedings of the Third Symposium on Underwater Physiology. Baltimore, Williams and Wilkins, 1967, pp 327–340.
30. Lambertsen CJ, Gelfand R, Clark JM (eds): Predictive studies IV. Work capabilities and physiologic effects of He-O_2 excursions to pressures 400-800-1200 and 1600 feet of sea water. Institute for Environmental Medicine Report 78-1. Philadelphia, University of Pennsylvania, 1978.
31. Graves DJ, Idicula J, Lambertsen CJ, Quinn JA: Bubble formation resulting from counter diffusion supersaturation: A possible explanation for isobaric inert gas "urticaria" and vertigo. Phys Med Biol 18:256–264, 1973.
32. Blenkarn GD, Aquadro C, Hills BA, Saltzman HA: Urticaria following sequential breathing of various inert gases at 7 ata: A possible mechanism of gas-induced osmosis. Aerosp Med 42:141–146, 1971.
33. Ranade A, Lambertsen CJ, Noordergraaf A: Inert gas exchange in the middle ear. Acta Otolaryngol (Suppl) 371:1–23, 1980.
34. Miller JW, Koblick IG: Living and Working in the Sea. New York, Van Nostrand-Reinhold, 1984.
35. Shilling CW, Carlston CB, Mathias RA: The Physician's Guide to Diving Medicine. New York, Plenum Press, 1984.
36. U.S. Navy Diving Manual, Volume 1: Air Diving NAVSEA 0994-LP-001-9020. Washington, DC, U.S. Government Printing Office, 1987.
37. U.S. Navy Diving Manual, Volume 2: Mixed Gas Diving NAVSEA 0994-LP-001-9020. Washington, DC, U.S. Government Printing Office, 1987.

Chapter 6

Breath-Hold Diving

SUK KI HONG

There are perhaps millions of people in the world who engage in amateur breath-hold dives for recreation. They are usually equipped with face masks (or goggles) and snorkels and dive to shallow depths for short periods of time. In addition, there are many thousands of professional divers who dive to deeper depths for longer periods for certain underwater activities. The latter group includes Navy divers, women divers of Korea (Hae-Nyo) and Japan (Ama), sponge divers in Greece, and pearl divers in the Tuamotu Archipelago. These divers learn the art of diving through many years of hard training, in order to increase both the depth of diving and the bottom time with minimal risk. In fact, they have attracted considerable interest from many physiologists during the last 30 years and have contributed extensively to the understanding of the physiology of breath-hold diving.

Unlike scuba (self-contained underwater breathing apparatus) diving, a breath-hold diver cannot usually afford to stay under water for more than two minutes. During such a short period of diving time, however, profound changes in certain physiological functions take place. This chapter will mainly deal with the changes in cardiorespiratory functions and the potential hazards associated with breath-hold diving. Because of the high thermal conductivity of water, if the water temperature is below thermoneutral level (about 35°C or 95°F), the body heat balance is also disturbed. However, various physiological problems directly associated with the regulation of body temperature in water are not dealt with in this chapter but are referred to in Chapter 9.

EFFECTS OF IMMERSION IN WATER TO THE NECK

A breath-hold dive is usually preceded by immersion of the body in water to the neck (head-out immersion). In fact, average breath-hold divers are likely to spend more time floating on the water surface (i.e., immersed to the neck) than totally submerged under water. Therefore, it is important to recognize some of the important physiological changes attendant to immersion to the neck.

When a person is in air, the pressure surrounding the body is no different from one region to another and is equal to the pressure within the lungs (Fig. 6–1A). This is no longer true in the case of immersion up to the neck. As illustrated in Figure 6–1B, the body below the neck is now under the influence of the atmospheric pressure (1 ata) plus the hydrostatic pressure, which is directly proportional to the vertical distance from the water surface. Thus, the pressure distribution over the body is no longer uniform. Because the subject still keeps his head above water and breathes the outside air, the intrapulmonary pressure must be equal to 1 ata. Consequently, the subject is forced to engage in "negative pressure breathing." Since the hydrostatic pressure level over the chest is not uniform, it is not easy to calculate exactly the degree of this negative pressure breathing. By studying the magnitude of the shift in the relaxation pressure (or the total respiratory pressure) observed during head-out immersion, the degree of negative pressure breathing is estimated to be approximately 20 cm H_2O.[1]

Primarily due to this intrapulmonary negative

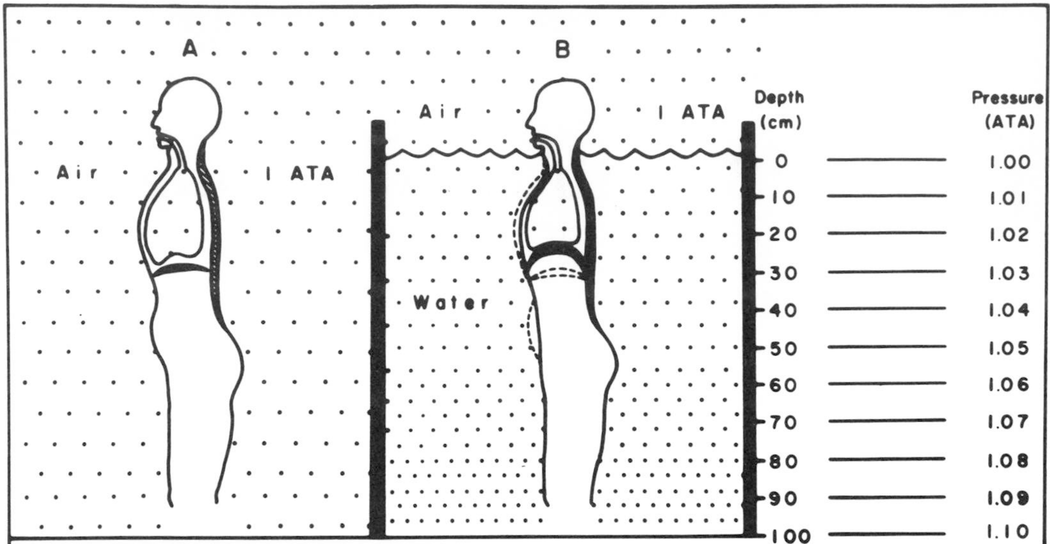

FIGURE 6–1. Distribution of pressure surrounding a man (A) standing in air and (B) immersed in water to the neck. The density of dots reflects the magnitude of pressure. The broken curves over the chest and below the diaphragm in (B) indicate the positions of the chest wall and the diaphragm standing in air.

pressure, coupled with a greater compression of the abdomen by the hydrostatic pressure, the expiratory reserve volume decreases by about 70 per cent during head-out immersion as compared with standing in air.[1–3] In contrast, the vital capacity decreases relatively less during immersion,[3, 4] which indicates an increase in the inspiratory capacity. Several investigators also found a slight, but significant, reduction in residual volume,[2, 4] which they attribute to an increase in the intrathoracic blood volume (see following discussion). More importantly, Hong and colleagues[1] observed a 60 per cent increase in the work (both elastic and dynamic) of breathing during immersion, which is partly due to an increase in the nonelastic airway resistance reported by Agostoni and coworkers.[2]

The end-expiratory intrathoracic pressure, estimated by measurement of the intraesophageal pressure, increases slightly from approximately −5 cm H_2O while standing in air to −2 cm H_2O during immersion.[2, 5] On the other hand, the abdominal pressure below the diaphragm, estimated by the intragastric pressure minus 11 cm H_2O, increases greatly from − 6 cm H_2O in air to + 12 cm H_2O during immersion.[2, 4] These findings indicate an increase in the transdiaphragmatic pressure from nearly zero in air to 14 cm H_2O during immersion. Since venous return is determined by this pressure gradient between the extra- and intrathoracic regions, such an increase in the transdiaphragmatic pressure during immersion is likely to increase venous return. This facilitation of venous return during immersion is further aided by the high density of water which eliminates the usual blood pooling in the peripheral veins in air. (In this respect, a state of immersion in water is analogous to a gravity-free state.) Moreover, the temperature of water in which divers are immersed is usually much lower than thermoneutral (35°C or 95°F), e.g., 26°C or 80°F, even in subtropical Hawaii; hence, one would expect a strong peripheral vasoconstriction in water. This would also bring about a further increase in the central blood volume at the expense of the peripheral volume.

The magnitude of the increase in the intrathoracic blood volume during head-out immersion has been indirectly estimated to be in the order of 500 ml.[1, 6] Arborelius and colleagues,[6] using a dye-dilution technique, reported a 30 per cent increase in the cardiac output and stroke volume during immersion in 34°C water. The same authors also reported an increase in the right atrial pressure from − 2 mm Hg in air to + 16 mm Hg during immersion, which reflects an increase in venous return. The latter observation suggests that the heart (and the intrathoracic blood vessels) is distended as a result of the pronounced blood shift and may be under considerable strain. Fortunately, however, an excessive congestion of the heart during immersion is prevented because of the collapse of the large veins as they enter the chest.[7]

The increase in the intrathoracic blood volume appears to be responsible for so-called immersion diuresis and natriuresis. In a hydropenic subject, both the urine flow and sodium excretion increase four- to five-fold during immersion. Conversely, in a hydrated subject, urine flow increases markedly while sodium excretion increases only slightly during immersion.[8] Typically, these renal responses to immersion are usually, but not always, accompanied by a reduction of the antidiuretic hormone (ADH) and renin-aldosterone level in plasma. Although these endocrine changes, especially the ADH response, were thought to be triggered by the cephalad shift of blood and were held responsible for the renal responses to immersion,[8, 9] more recent data are not consistent with this view. However, it is well beyond the scope of this chapter to comprehensively review the evidence for and against the conventional dogma. It suffices to state that the mechanism underlying this important phenomenon is yet to be understood. In this regard, it is both important and interesting to note that typical renal responses to immersion are considerably attenuated either at night[10] or in endurance-trained athletes.[11] Regardless of the underlying mechanism, the immersion diuresis and natriuresis would eventually lead to a net dehydration, and the immersion technique is clinically used to treat patients with fluid retention.[8] Another important consequence of this increase in intrathoracic circulation during immersion has been reported recently by Balldin and Lundgren.[12] They found that immersion (especially in warm water) enhances the rate of nitrogen elimination during oxygen breathing, which may have some bearing on the risk of decompression sickness.

As mentioned earlier, the abdomen is compressed to a greater degree as compared with the chest during head-out immersion. According to Johnson and colleagues,[5] the intragastric pressure at the end of normal expiration increases from + 5 mm Hg in air to + 20 mm Hg during immersion, while the intraesophageal pressure at the superior limit of the distal esophageal sphincter increases from − 1 to only + 4 mm Hg. Hence, the gastroesophageal pressure gradient increases from 6 mm Hg in air to 16 mm Hg during immersion, thus predisposing the subject to gastric reflux. In fact, pyrosis and regurgitation of gastric contents have been reported by some swimmers. However, in normal subjects who have a competent distal esophageal sphincter, the sphincter pressure also increases by 13 mm Hg during immersion, so that there is no danger of reflux. Drugs that diminish distal esophageal sphincter pressure, and thus its competency, should be avoided during immersion. Individuals with severe gastroesophageal reflux may be at risk from aspiration of gastric contents if occupation or recreation involves water immersion.

In summary, a person immersed in water to the neck is subjected to a reduction in the functional residual capacity, an increased work of breathing, an increase in the intrathoracic (including the heart) blood volume, and dehydration and, in addition, is predisposed to gastric reflux.

ALVEOLAR GAS EXCHANGE DURING BREATH-HOLD DIVING

The basic pattern of alveolar gas exchange during a breath-hold dive is quite different from that during simple breath-holding in air. This is due to the diver undergoing compression during descent, followed by decompression during ascent. Well-trained professional divers hyperventilate mildly, take a deep breath (a lung volume equivalent to about 80 per cent of the vital capacity), close the glottis, and then start a descent. The composition of alveolar gas at this point is given in Figure 6–2, along with that at depth (10 m or 30 ft) and upon return to the surface. These values are taken from studies on Ama divers during actual diving in the ocean.[13]

Typically, the alveolar gas at the very beginning of a dive is comprised of 4 per cent CO_2 (pCO_2 = 29 mm Hg), 17 per cent O_2 (pO_2 = 120 mm Hg), and 79 per cent N_2 (pN_2 = 567 mm Hg), which is only slightly different from the normal composition. During descent, the lung volume decreases due to compression of the chest, which results in increases of partial pressures of O_2, CO_2, and N_2. Since the gas pressures of the mixed venous blood should not change during the first 20 seconds (circulation time) of compression, one would expect diffusion of all three gases from the alveolus to the blood. As shown in Figure 6–2, the concentrations of both O_2 and CO_2 of the alveolar gas obtained when the diver reached the bottom are considerably lower than the corresponding values of the beginning of the dive, which reflects a net transfer of these gases from the alveolus to the blood. The alveolar concentration of N_2 on the bottom and is slightly higher than that before descent, despite the fact that N_2 must also be removed from the alveolus to the blood during descent. This is attributed to

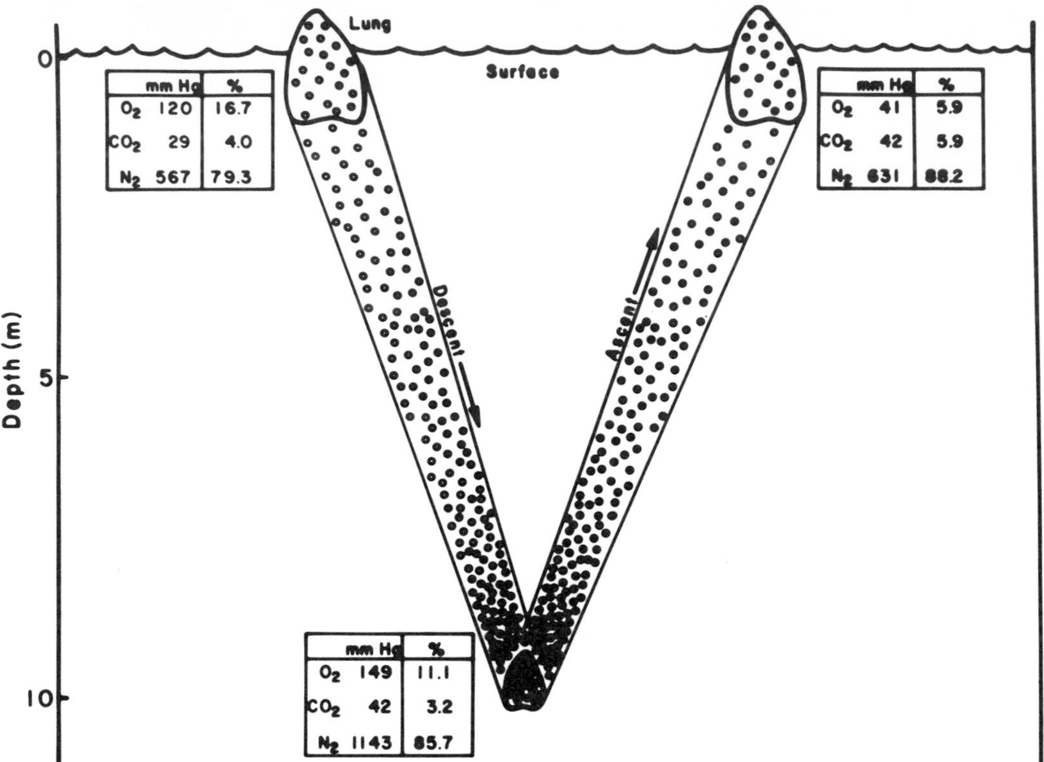

FIGURE 6–2. Alveolar gas composition (%) and pressures immediately before descent *(upper left)*, on the bottom, and immediately after returning to the water surface *(upper right)*. Note a progressive reduction in the lung volume coupled with an increase in the gas density (or pressure) during descent, which are reversed during ascent. (Data on the alveolar gas are from Hong, et al.[13])

a much faster rate of diffusion of CO_2 and O_2 as compared with N_2, which has a very low solubility to blood plasma. As a result of rapid removal of O_2 and CO_2 during compression, the alveolar concentration of N_2 progressively increases during descent.

It is important to note that the pO_2 of alveolar gas on the bottom is as high as 150 mm Hg, which assures an adequate delivery of O_2 to the blood. In other words, as long as the diver is on the bottom, there is a sufficient pO_2 gradient between the alveolus and blood to maintain a continuous diffusion of O_2 into the blood.

Normally, CO_2 is transferred from the blood to the lungs. As just stated, this direction of CO_2 transfer is reversed during descent because the alveolar pCO_2 becomes greater than the mixed venous blood pCO_2 due to compression of the chest. Therefore, large amounts of CO_2 are retained in the blood with a resultant increase in pCO_2. It is interesting to note that the pCO_2 of the arterial blood is now greater than that of mixed venous blood, as long as CO_2 is diffusing into the blood. It is this retention of CO_2, with attendant increase in pCO_2 of the blood, that gives the signal to the diver to return to the surface.

Once the diver leaves the bottom for the surface, the lungs will expand rapidly due to decompression. Consequently, the alveolar pO_2 decreases progressively, thus continuously decreasing the diffusion gradient for O_2. As shown in Figure 6–2, the alveolar concentration of O_2 at the time of return to the surface is only 6 per cent, with pO_2 of 41 mm Hg. The latter value is equal to the pO_2 of the mixed venous blood, which indicates that there is no diffusion gradient for O_2 between the alveolus and the blood at this point, and thus the diver is in a critical state of hypoxia. In fact, the normal direction of O_2 transfer could be completely reversed during ascent if the diver stayed on the bottom longer. Such a reversal of O_2 transfer has indeed been demonstrated.[14] CO_2 retained in the blood during descent (and on the bottom) now leaves the blood for the lungs as alveolar pCO_2 decreases continuously during ascent, and a favorable diffusion gradient between the blood and the alveolus is re-established. However, not all CO_2 retained in the blood during descent (and on the bottom) is eliminated into the lungs during ascent, and the process of excess CO_2 elimination continues even after the return to the surface. A small amount of N_2 that entered the circulation and tissue during descent and on the bottom will also leave slowly, according to the reversed diffusion gradient.

The pattern of alveolar gas exchange during a breath-hold dive as described thus far is distinctly different from that during simple breath-holding in air. In the latter case, the alveolar pO_2 decreases continuously during breath-holding[15] but is higher than that at the end of a breath-hold dive of comparable duration.[13] This is due to the faster removal of alveolar O_2 during descent and on the bottom. Even during simple breath-holding in air, there is a theoretical possibility that the direction of CO_2 transfer could be reversed, but the amount of CO_2 transferred in the reverse direction is much less than that during a breath-hold dive.

Since the amount of N_2 transferred from the alveolus to the circulation during a breath-hold dive is very small, there is no real danger for developing decompression sickness. However, it is theoretically possible to accumulate enough N_2 if the diver repetitively dives to considerable depths with very short surface intervals. In fact, Paulev, by making about 60 breath-hold dives to 20 meters in 5 hours, developed what appeared to be decompression sickness. Each dive lasted about 2.5 min with surface intervals of less than 2 min. He reports: "During the last two hours I had progressive symptoms of nausea, dizziness . . . . Within one-half hour after the end of the diving, I got pains in the left hip joint . . . . Two hours after the end of the diving, severe chest pains began. The paresthesia developed in the right hand together with blurring of the vision. Three hours after the diving, a colleague found me markedly pale and exhausted as in impending shock . . . . As the symptoms were in progress, I was placed in the recompression chamber. At 6 ATA I felt an immediate relief with regard to the dizziness and nausea. In a few minutes the bends and the partial paresis had disappeared . . . ."[16] The pearl divers of the Tuamotu Archipelago make repetitive dives to a depth of 30 to 40 meters (each dive lasting about 1.5 to 2.5 min) for about 6 hours a day during the diving season, and 10 to 30 per cent of divers are known to develop what they call "taravana" (*tara*, to fall; *vana*, crazily) by the end of the day. "Taravana" symptoms include vertigo, nausea, partial or complete paralysis, temporary unconsciousness, and, in extreme cases, death.[17] Although the

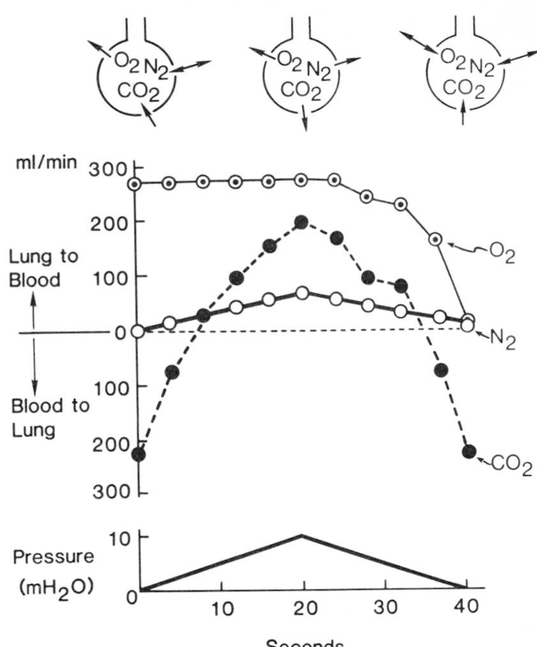

FIGURE 6–3. The rate of alveolar O_2, CO_2, and N_2 exchange during a breath-hold dive to 10 meters. (From Hong SK, Rahn H, Kang DH, et al: Diving pattern, lung volumes, and alveolar gas of the Korean diving women (Ama). J Appl Physiol 18:457–465, 1963.)

etiology of "taravana" is not fully understood, many diving scientists suspect that it may be related to the retention of N_2.

A seemingly complicated pattern of alveolar gas exchange during a breath-hold dive may be summarized as follows: The transfer of O_2 from the lungs to the blood is not disturbed until ascent starts. It is during this ascending phase that the diver could run into a critical state of hypoxia. The normal direction of CO_2 transfer from the blood to the lungs is reversed during descent and on the bottom, which results in a significant retention of CO_2 in the blood (hypercapnia). During ascent, the retained CO_2 is transferred to the lungs. A small amount of N_2 also enters the circulation during the descent, which is reversed during ascent. Based on certain assumptions, the rate of alveolar exchange of O_2, CO_2, and N_2 during a breath-hold dive to 10 meters has been calculated[13] and is shown in Figure 6–3.

DANGER OF EXCESSIVE HYPERVENTILATION BEFORE DIVING

Approximately 7000 deaths by drowning occur yearly in the United States. If we knew the events leading to drowning, lives could be saved. By interviewing swimmers who lost consciousness under water but somehow survived, Craig[18,19] was able to reconstruct events possibly contributing to drowning. He noted that all of the survivors hyperventilated before going under water and also that the swimmers usually noted the urge to breathe but had little or no warning that they were going to "pass out." Most of these survivors also stated that they had some goal in mind or were in competition with others. Based on this and other information, Craig concluded that a combination of hyperventilation, breath-holding, and exercise could lead to loss of consciousness.

Most underwater (breath-hold) swimmers have learned that hyperventilation will increase their breath-holding time. The rate of elimination of CO_2 from the body increases as a function of ventilation and, in fact, the alveolar pCO_2 (and hence arterial blood pCO_2) is inversely proportional to the alveolar ventilation. Therefore, it will take a longer time for blood pCO_2 to reach a breaking point when breath-holding is preceded by excessive hyperventilation, which thereby extends the breath-holding time. However, one has to remember that any extension of breath-holding time is associated with a further reduction in blood pO_2. It is true that hyperventilation slightly increases the level of alveolar and arterial pO_2, but this does not appreciably increase the blood O_2 content because the oxyhemoglobin saturation in the arterial blood is almost 100 per cent during normal ventilation, with the arterial pO_2 being 100 mm Hg. Therefore, the rate of fall in blood pO_2 during breath-holding is about the same with or without preparatory hyperventilation. This is why the alveolar (or arterial blood) pO_2 at breath-hold breaking point is lower with preliminary hyperventilation than without (Table 6–1).

In the case of breath-holding with air at 1 ata, the subject terminates breath-holding as a result of increased pCO_2 coupled with reduced pO_2. In general, the respiratory center (or chemoreceptors) is far more sensitive to a rise in pCO_2 than to a fall in pO_2. However, when the level of pO_2 in the blood decreases to about 50 mm Hg, the ventilation begins to increase rapidly, indicating that the respiratory center is stimulated. Conversely, in case of breath-holding with O_2 at 1 ata, the breath-holding is terminated by the high pCO_2 alone because pO_2 of the blood does not decrease to 50 mm Hg. Therefore, one can hold a breath longer, with a greater accumulation of CO_2, following O_2 breathing than air breathing.

A situation similar to breath-holding with O_2 exists during breath-hold diving. While the diver stays on the bottom with breath held, the urge to breathe (or the signal to return to the surface) will come almost solely from the high pCO_2 of blood, since the blood pO_2 level is maintained high due to compression. Until the pCO_2 reaches a critical level, the diver will stay on the bottom and continuously consume O_2. By then, the diver has barely enough O_2 in the body to return to the surface, as indicated by a very low alveolar pO_2 at the end of the dive (see Fig. 6–2). When a dive is preceded by vigorous hyperventilation, the initial level of blood pCO_2 is lowered; hence, the diver can certainly stay longer on the bottom before the pCO_2 level increases to a critical level. However, remember that the diver's O_2 store in the body is essentially the same with or without vigorous hyperventilation. Therefore, while the diver succeeds in extending the bottom time, the valuable O_2 store is further depleted, thus endangering the safe return to the surface!

The situation just described is further aggravated if the diver is engaged in strenuous activity. It has been shown by many investigators that the level of pCO_2 at the breath-hold breaking point is higher during exercise than at rest

TABLE 6–1. Effects of Hyperventilation on the Breath-Holding (BH) Time and Alveolar Gas Pressure at the Breaking Point in Resting and Exercising Man

MEASUREMENTS	RESTING: Without Hyperventilation	RESTING: With Hyperventilation	EXERCISING: Without Hyperventilation	EXERCISING: With Hyperventilation
BH time (sec)	87	146	62	85
End-tidal pCO_2 (mm Hg)				
Before BH	40	21	38	22
Breaking point	51	46	54	49
End-tidal pO_2 (mm Hg)				
Before BH	103	131	102	130
Breaking point	73	58	54	43

From Craig AB Jr: Causes of loss of consciousness during underwater swimming. J Appl Physiol 16:583–586, 1961.

(Table 6–1). This means that the exercising diver could further extend the bottom time. Since the rate of O_2 consumption increases with exercise, the diver would further deplete the valuable O_2 store more rapidly during this period of extended bottom time. One can, therefore, visualize the occurrence of critical hypoxia leading to loss of consciousness or even to death when a breath-hold dive is combined with vigorous preparatory hyperventilation and a high rate of O_2 consumption.

CARDIOVASCULAR CHANGES DURING BREATH-HOLD DIVING

More than a century ago, Paul Bert of France observed pronounced bradycardia in ducks during diving. Since then, the same phenomenon has been observed in all diving animals. According to Irving and Scholander, this bradycardia is a reflex phenomenon that is accompanied by an intense peripheral vasoconstriction, a drastic reduction in the cardiac output, and a significant reduction of O_2 consumption. In other words, this reflex serves to extend the duration of a breath-hold dive.[20, 21]

Human breath-hold divers also show a distinct bradycardia during dives.[22, 23] As shown in Figure 6–4, the heart rate begins to decrease with the onset of the dive and finally reaches a minimal level in 20 to 30 seconds. Usually the lowest heart rate during a breath-hold dive is equivalent to 60 to 70 per cent of the pre-dive level. Figure 6–4 also indicates that the same heart rate response is observed even during a breath-hold surface swim or a simple breath-hold whole-body immersion at the water surface. Evidently, the response is independent of pressure or physical exercise. In fact, it has been shown subsequently that a breath-hold immersion of the face alone gives rise to the same bradycardial response observed during an actual breath-hold dive,[21] and hence most of the current knowledge on diving bradycardia in humans is derived from such face immersion studies.

As in the case of diving animals, the diving bradycardia in humans is associated with intensive peripheral vasoconstriction.[24, 25] It is, however, generally agreed that the observed bradycardia is not directly coupled to vasoconstriction.[25, 26] The most interesting aspect of diving bradycardia in humans is its dependence on the water temperature. Regardless of whether one is engaged in actual breath-hold

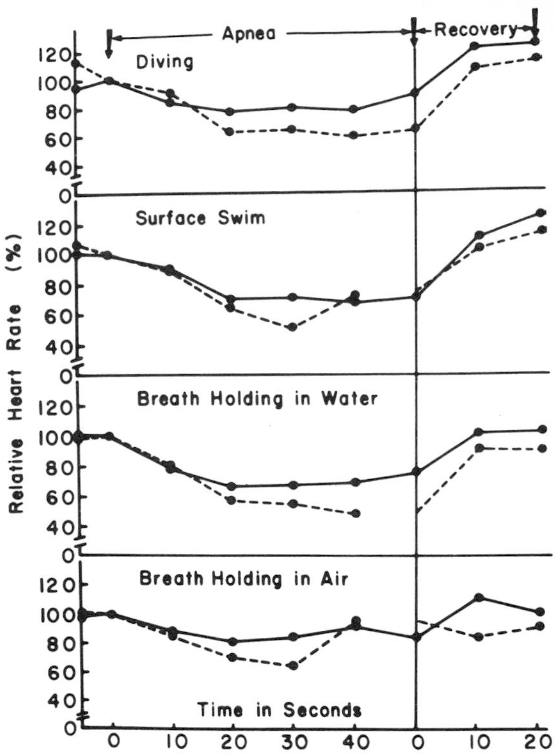

FIGURE 6–4. Relative changes in the heart rate during various breath-hold maneuvers in summer *(solid lines;* water temperature, 27°C) and winter *(broken lines;* water temperature, 10°C). (From Hong SK, Song SH, Kim PK, Suh CS: Seasonal observations on the cardiac rhythm during diving in the Korean Ama. J Appl Physiol 23:18–22, 1967.)

diving or breath-hold face immersion, the degree of bradycardia increases with a decrease in water temperature.[22, 25, 27] However, the relationship between the two variables is not linear, and it is only when the water temperature is below 15°C (59°F) that the degree of bradycardia increases linearly with the reduction in temperature. Moreover, the degree of bradycardia observed during breath-hold face immersion is the same as that during breath-hold whole-body immersion in water of comparable temperature.[28] These findings indicate that the cutaneous cold receptors on the face play a very important role in the development of diving bradycardia. Although some investigators claim that the nasal region is involved in this mechanism, others failed to confirm such findings. The lung volume at the onset of breath-hold face immersion is also known to alter the degree of bradycardia.[25] However, its mechanism is entirely unknown.

A mechanical theory has been proposed by Craig[29, 30] as the alternative to the neural theory just described. His theory is based on the observation that the degree of bradycardia during breath-hold face immersion increases with a decrease in the intrathoracic pressure, and vice versa. This finding has been interpreted to mean that the venous return increases with a decrease in the intrathoracic pressure, which, in turn, decreases the heart rate through a baroreflex mechanism. Undoubtedly, this mechanism is involved in modulating the degree of bradycardia but cannot be considered the sole mechanism for diving bradycardia, because the degree of bradycardia can be still manipulated by changing the face immersion water temperature without changing the intrathoracic pressure.

Recently, a chemical factor has been added to the mechanism. Moore and colleagues[31] observed that the degree of bradycardia is significantly attenuated when a breath-hold face immersion is preceded by a single breath of pure O_2. Other studies[28] support the same conclusion. According to a recent study by Lin and co-workers[32] a 31 per cent reduction in the heart rate induced by breath-hold face immersion (in water of 25°C) represented an arithmetic sum of 19 per cent reduction by the cessation of breathing per se, 18 per cent reduction by hypoxia, and 6 per cent increase by hypercapnia ($19 + 18 - 6 = 31$). This indicates that the hypoxia that develops during the course of breath holding has a major potentiating effect, while hypercapnia has only a minor attenuating effect on breath-hold bradycardia.

The current state of the art concerning the mechanism of diving bradycardia is schematically illustrated in Figure 6–5. The bradycardia is triggered by the act of breath-holding which, through unknown mechanisms, activates the cardioinhibitory center in the central nervous system and then the vagus nerve.[33] This basic response to breath-holding is subjected to either potentiation or attenuation by neural, mechanical, and chemical factors.

Unlike in diving animals, arterial blood pressure seems to increase while cardiac output decreases only slightly during breath-hold face immersion in humans.[27, 34] Moreover, there is no convincing evidence to indicate that there is an O_2 conserving mechanism operating in humans during breath-hold diving.

This dramatic reduction in heart rate, induced by a breath-hold face immersion in cold water has been shown to effectively convert paroxysmal supraventricular tachycardia to normal sinus rhythm.[35] It has also been suggested that the face immersion procedure may offer a useful adjunct to carotid sinus massage and intravenous infusion of vasopressors for the treatment of this arrhythmia.

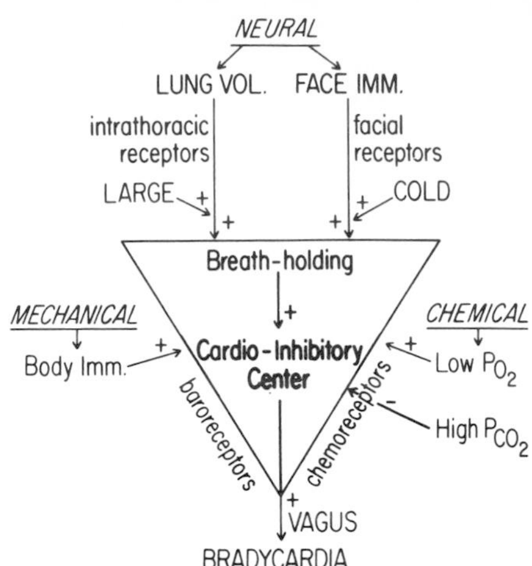

FIGURE 6–5. Schematic model of factors modifying apneic bradycardia: + indicates potentiation; − indicates attenuation of bradycardial responses; triangle symbolizes the different types of stimuli modifying the basic bradycardia accompanying apnea per se. (From Hong SK: Breath-hold diving in man: An overview. *In* Lundgren C, Ferrigno M (eds): Proceedings of Workshop on Physiology of Breath-hold Diving. Bethesda, Undersea Medical Society, 1987, pp 158–173.

One of the most intriguing findings with regard to diving medicine is the occurrence of cardiac arrhythmias during breath-hold diving. This is in contrast to diving animals who display a marked bradycardia but never show any cardiac arrhythmias during diving. In humans, it is common to find various types of arrhythmias even during simple breath-holding. Interestingly enough, the incidence of cardiac arrhythmias during diving also increases significantly when the water temperature is low. In a study conducted on Korean women divers,[22] the incidence of cardiac arrhythmias (e.g., abnormal P waves and nodal rhythms, idioventricular rhythms, premature atrial beats, and premature ventricular beats) is 43 per cent in the summer (water temperature of 27°C or 81°F), as compared with 72 per cent in the winter (water temperature of 10°C or 50°F). It thus appears that diving in cold water is associated with a greater bradycardia and a higher incidence of cardiac arrhythmias. To what extent these changes contribute to fatal diving accidents is yet to be determined.

MAXIMAL DEPTH OF BREATH-HOLD DIVING

Until recently, it was thought that the lung volume decreases continuously during descent until it is reduced to the residual volume measured in air before diving. It was believed that further reduction would cause lung squeeze and that the theoretical maximal depth of a breath-hold dive was the depth at which the lung volume is reduced to the residual volume. For instance, if a diver has a residual volume (RV) of 1.5 liters and his total lung capacity (TLC) is 6.0 liters, Boyle's law tells us that the lung volume will be reduced to the RV at a depth of 30 meters (100 ft or 4 ata).

However, several divers have far exceeded the limit calculated on the basis of the TLC/RV ratio. For instance, Jacques Mayol whose TLC and RV are, respectively, 7.22 and 1.88 liters, dived to a depth of 231 feet. If one assumes that he started the dive with TLC, then the theoretical maximal depth of dive should be 27 meters or 90 feet (TLC/RV = 7.22/1.88 = 3.7 ata or 27 m). Another example may be found in Robert Croft, a U.S. Navy diver, who dived 240 feet (80 m) despite his TLC/RV ratio of 7.0 (= 9.1/1.3; or 60 m equivalent). These records raise questions about the validity of the generally held notion that the maximal depth of a breath-hold dive is determined by the TLC/RV ratio determined in air before diving. There must be additional factors to be considered.

As discussed earlier in this chapter, the intrathoracic blood volume increases during immersion in water to the neck. Although the issue is not completely settled, several investigators[2, 4] reported a significant reduction in the residual volume during immersion. If indeed the residual volume decreases during either head-out immersion or breath-hold diving, one would expect a substantial increase in the TLC/RV ratio. For instance, in the case of Jacques Mayol, if the intrathoracic blood volume increased by 1.0 liter during diving, his residual volume would be reduced from 1.88 to 0.88 liters, thereby increasing the TLC/RV ratio to 8.2 (= 7.22/0.88) and the maximal depth to 72 meters (or 230 ft). In other words, his record depth of 231 feet can be accounted for by a 1.0 liter increase in the intrathoracic blood volume. The most crucial questions is, therefore, "Does the intrathoracic blood volume increase by 1.0 liter during diving?"

There is at least one report related to this question. Schaeffer and co-workers[36] estimated the thoracic blood volume during open-sea dives to 130 feet, by using the impedance plethysmograph, and found that about 1 liter of blood was forced into the thorax. Other evidence for this shift of blood into the thorax during breath-hold diving has been published by Craig.[37] He asked the subject (RV = 2.0 liters) to fully expire and to dive. Surprisingly, the subject dived to a depth of 4.75 meters without developing a significant difference between the ambient pressure at depth and the intrathoracic pressure. These results indicated that the subject's RV must have been compressed from 2.0 liters at the surface to 1.4 liters at depth; also, this change of 0.6 liters could be due to a shift of blood from the peripheral to the central circulation.

These findings indicate that the TLC/RV ratio increases during the dive due to a reduction of RV associated with an increase in the intrathoracic blood volume; hence, the diver can reach a depth considerably deeper than that predicted by the TLC/RV ratio determined at the surface. More recently, several professional divers have reached depths of approximately 100 meters (~300 ft). Obviously, highly trained divers seem to be able to increase the TLC/RV ratio to a level considerably higher than that considered above, most likely by decreasing the RV to a greater extent. Whether this apparent ability to markedly decrease the RV reflects the correspondingly greater degree of blood shift into the thorax during diving is yet to be determined. In this connection, it may be of interest to note that the pliability of the body wall (chest and abdomen) was higher in Japanese Ama as compared with nondivers.[38] Although the anatomical and physiological basis of this physical adaptation is not known at present, it could provide an additional force for increasing the TLC/RV during deep diving.

REFERENCES

1. Hong SK, Cerretelli P, Cruz JC, Rahn H: Mechanics of respiration during submersion in water. J Appl Physiol 27:537–538, 1969.
2. Agostoni E, Gurtner G, Torri G, Rahn H: Respiratory mechanics during submersion and negative pressure breathing. J Appl Physiol 21:251–258, 1966.
3. Hong SK, Ting EY, Rahn H: Lung volumes at different depths of submersion. J Appl Physiol 23:18–22, 1967.
4. Craig AB Jr, Ware DE: Effect of immersion in water on vital capacity and residual volume of the lungs. J Appl Physiol 23:423–425, 1967.
5. Johnson LF, Lin YC, Hong SK: Gastroesophageal dynamics during immersion in water to the neck. J Appl Physiol 38:449–454, 1975.
6. Arborelius M, Balldin UI, Lidja B, Lundgren CEG: Hemodynamic changes in man during immersion with the head above water. Aerosp Med 43:592–598, 1972.
7. Rahn H: The physiological stresses of the Ama. *In* Rahn H (ed): Physiology of Breath-Hold Diving and the Ama of Japan. National Academy of Science, National Research Council Publ 1341, 1965, pp 113–138.

8. Epstein M: Renal effects of head-out water immersion in man: Implications for an understanding of volume homeostasis. Physiol Rev 58:529–581, 1978.
9. Gauer OH, Henry JP, Sieker HO, Wendt WE: The effect of negative pressure breathing on urine flow. J Clin Invest 33:287–296, 1954.
10. Shiraki K, Konda N, Sagawa S, et al: Cardiorenal–endocrine responses to head-out immersion at night. J Appl Physiol 60:176–183, 1986.
11. Claybaugh JR, Pendergast DR, Davis JE, et al: Fluid conservation in athletes: Responses to water intake, supine posture, and immersion. J Appl Physiol 61:7–15, 1986.
12. Balldin UI, Lundgren CEG: Effects of immersion with the head above the water on tissue nitrogen elimination in man. Aerosp Med 43:1101–1108, 1972.
13. Hong SK, Rahn H, Kang DH, et al: Diving pattern, lung volumes, and alveolar gas of the Korean diving women (Ama). J Appl Physiol 18:457–465, 1963.
14. Lanphier EH, Rahn H: Alveolar gas exchange during breath holding with air. J Appl Physiol 18:478–482, 1963.
15. Hong SK, Lin YC, Lally DA, et al: Alveolar gas exchanges and cardiovascular functions during breath holding with air. J Appl Physiol 30:540–547, 1971.
16. Paulev P: Decompression sickness following repeated breath-hold dives. *In* Rahn H (ed): Physiology of Breath-Hold Diving and The Ama of Japan. National Academy of Science, National Research Council, Publ 1341, 1965, pp 211–226.
17. Cross ER: Taravana-diving syndrome in the Tuamotu diver. *In* Rahn H (ed): Physiology of Breath-Hold Diving and the Ama of Japan. National Academy of Science, National Research Council, Publ 1341, 1965, pp 207–219.
18. Craig AB Jr: Underwater swimming and loss of consciousness. JAMA 176:255–258, 1961.
19. Craig AB Jr: Causes of loss of consciousness during underwater swimming. J Appl Physiol 16:583–586, 1961.
20. Irving L, Scholander PF, Grinnel SW: The regulation of arterial blood pressure in the seal during diving. Am J Physiol 135:557–566, 1942.
21. Scholander PF: Physiological adaptation to diving in animals and man. Harvey Lect 57:93–110, 1961–62.
22. Hong SK, Song SH, Kim PK, Suh CS: Seasonal observations on the cardiac rhythm during diving in the Korean Ama. J Appl Physiol 23:18–22, 1967.
23. Scholander PF, Hammel HT, LeMessurier H, et al: Circulatory adjustment in pearl divers. J Appl Physiol 17:184–190, 1962.
24. Brick I: Circulatory responses to immersing the face in water. J Appl Physiol 21:33–36, 1966.
25. Song SH, Lee WK, Chung YA, Hong SK: Mechanisms of apneic bradycardia in man. J Appl Physiol 27:323–327, 1969.
26. Murdaugh HV Jr, Cross CE, Millen JE, et al: Dissociation of bradycardia and arterial constriction during diving in the seal *Phoca vitulina*. Science 162:364–365, 1968.
27. Kawakami Y, Natelson BH, DuBois AB: Cardiovascular effects of face immersion and factors affecting diving reflex in man. J Appl Physiol 23:964–970, 1967.
28. Moore TO, Lin YC, Lally DA, Hong SK: Effects of temperature, immersion, and ambient pressure on human apneic bradycardia. J Appl Physiol 33:36–41, 1972.
29. Craig AB Jr: Heart rate responses to apneic underwater diving and to breath holding in man. J Appl Physiol 18:854–862, 1963.
30. Craig AB Jr: Effects of submersion and pulmonary mechanics on cardiovascular function in man. *In* Rahn H (ed): Physiology of Breath-Hold Diving and the Ama of Japan. Washington, DC, National Academy of Science, National Research Council, Publ 1341, 1965, pp 295–302.
31. Moore TO, Elsner R, Lin YC, et al: Effects of alveolar P_{O_2} and P_{CO_2} on apneic bradycardia in man. J Appl Physiol 34:795–798, 1973.
32. Lin YC, Shida KK, Hong SK: Effects of hypercapnia, hypoxia and rebreathing on heart rate response during apnea. J Appl Physiol 54:166–171, 1983.
33. Hong SK: Breath-hold bradycardia in man: An overview. *In* Lundgren C, Ferrigno M (eds): Proceedings of Workshop on Physiology of Breath-hold Diving. Bethesda, Undersea Medical Society, 1987, pp 158–173.
34. Hong SK, Moore TO, Seto G, et al: Lung volumes and apneic bradycardia in divers. J Appl Physiol 29:172–176, 1970.
35. Gooden BA: The diving response in clinical medicine. Aviat Space Environ Med 53:273–276, 1982.
36. Schaefer KE, Allison RD, Dougherty JH, et al: Pulmonary and circulatory adjustment determining the limits of depths in breath-hold diving. Science 162:1020–1023, 1968.
37. Craig AB Jr: Depth limits of breath-hold diving. (An example of Fennology.) Respir Physiol 5:14–22, 1968.
38. Kobayashi S, Ogawa T, Adachi C, et al: Maximal respiratory pressure and pliability of the body wall of the Japanese Ama. Acta Med Biol 18:249–260, 1971.

Chapter 7

Inert Gas Narcosis and HPNS

PETER B. BENNETT

This book discusses many of the medical problems associated with diving as summarized in Figure 7–1. It is apparent that two problems—nitrogen narcosis (or better, inert gas narcosis) and the high pressure nervous syndrome (HPNS)—appear as major limitations. The former is likely to occur in scuba divers or in other divers breathing compressed air deeper than 100 feet (4 atm abs or ata). The latter is found only in very deep diving to depths greater than 500 feet (16 ata) when divers are usually breathing oxygen-helium.

At first glance there seems to be little connection between these two conditions, since they have very different signs and symptoms. However, it will become clear in this chapter that there is, in fact, a very close relationship between them, although they are in a sense opposites. It will not be possible to consider all of the research in past and recent years in any detail here. This can be obtained elsewhere.[1–10] The relevance of these problems to our knowledge of the mechanism of anesthesia is also described elsewhere.[10–12]

NITROGEN NARCOSIS

The condition known as nitrogen narcosis was first observed as long ago as 1935 when a Frenchman, Junod, noted that when breathing compressed air "the functions of the brain are activated, imagination is lively, thoughts have a peculiar charm and in some persons, symptoms of intoxication are present." Green[13] is perhaps the first American to have noted narcosis. At 160 feet (5.8 ata), he reported sleepiness, hallucinations, and impaired judgment, which he believed required an immediate return to atmospheric pressure.

The Royal Navy carried out a thorough investigation[14] when it was found that during 17 of 58 dives between 200 and 350 feet (7 and 11.6 ata) a condition resulting in "semi–loss of consciousness" occurred. The condition was regarded as serious, since the diver would continue to give all the normal hand signals at depth but after decompression could not remember any of the events that took place under water.

Much speculation about the possible cause resulted, but it was not until 1935 that Behnke and co-workers[15] correctly attributed the narcosis as due to the raised partial pressure of nitrogen in the compressed air. They characterized the narcosis as "euphoria, retardment of the higher mental processes and impaired neuromuscular coordination."

Signs and symptoms start to be noticed at about 100 feet (4 ata) and become increasingly more severe the greater the depth. Laughter, loquacity, and a light-headed sensation may be apparent with feelings of stimulation and excitement. With increased effort at self-control, it may be possible to overcome such behavior to some extent. There is a slowing of mental activity with delays in auditory and olfactory stimuli and a tendency to word-idea fixation, as is often seen in hypoxia. The resulting limitation of the power of association and perception is made especially dangerous due to the presence of overconfidence.

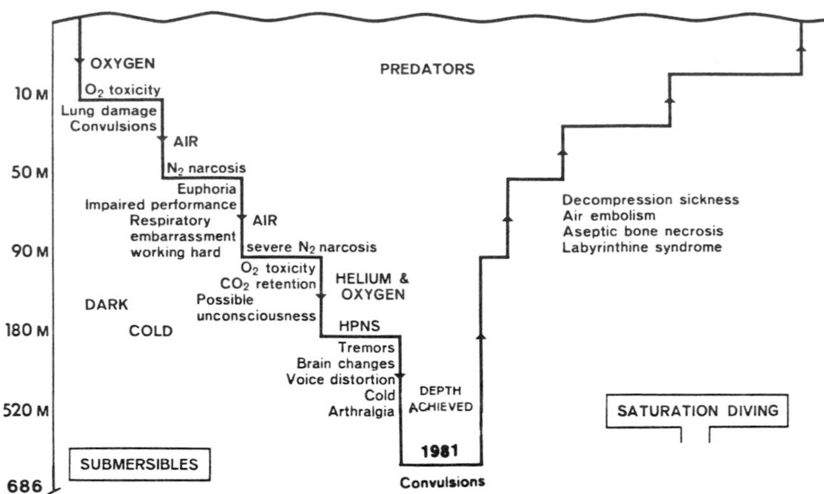

FIGURE 7–1. Physiological and medical problems of diving.

Memory will be impaired, especially short-term memory. Errors may be made in recording arithmetic data (Table 7–1). For example, 43 minutes may be confused with 48 minutes and 12:15 may be written as 15:15. Handwriting becomes increasingly larger with the severity of the narcosis. There may be a change in the sense of time. Intellectual capacities are affected more severely than psychomotor or manual abilities. However, the ability to carry out fine movements will be impaired, usually due to overexaggeration of movements. If the movements are carried out more slowly than usual, the impairment of efficiency is likely to be less severe.

There may be some numbness and tingling of the lips, legs, and feet as well as a characteristic deadpan look to the face.

At depths greater than 180 feet (6.5 ata), no trust should be placed in human performance or efficiency in breathing compressed air.

At depths greater than 300 feet (10 ata), signs and symptoms are severe, with the possibility of the diver becoming unconscious. Orders may be ignored. Intensity of vision and hearing, voice reverberation, stupor, and a sense of impending blackout and disorientation occur. Manic or depressive states can also occur, with changes in personality and a sense of levity.[16]

These signs and symptoms are very similar to those seen in alcoholic intoxication and the early stages of hypoxia and anesthesia, with an equally wide variation in susceptibility. Nitrogen narcosis is an especially important danger to the compressed air diver. The perceptual narrowing that results may permit the diver to carry out a specific task with varying degrees of competency; but, in the event of something unusual occurrring, he or she will be unable to function effectively in an emergency. Many divers who chose to ignore the narcosis problem or who believed, as with alcohol, that it is more "manly" to pretend to be unaffected by the condition have perished as a result.

TABLE 7–1. Effect of Pressure on Psychometric Tests

Pressure (feet)	0	90	100	125	150	175	200	225	250	275	300
Mean additional time to solve problems (seconds)	0.35	11.09	6.89	7.65	9.74	11.95	13.98	17.17	26.07	26.53	31.42
Mean additional errors in solving problems	0.18	0.86	0.49	0.42	0.72	0.84	1.22	0.88	2.18	2.66	3.02
Mean decrease in numbers crossed out	—	−0.59	−0.09	−2.26	−2.30	−2.49	−2.55	4.24	−5.85	−6.43	−8.74
Average reaction time (seconds)	0.214	—	—	—	0.237	—	0.242	—	0.248	—	0.257
Mean additional time to solve problems (acclimatized subjects)	1.64	2.55	3.42	3.91	4.66	8.00	11.75	15.73	16.33	17.09	24.36

From Shilling CW, Willgrube WW: Quantitative study of mental and neuromuscular reactions as influenced by increased air pressure. US Navy Med Bull 35:373–380, 1937.

The narcosis is usually more severe immediately on arrival at depth, and there may be some improvement shortly afterward followed by a relatively stable level of narcosis. This is primarily a subjective improvement as objective tests show no change.

Recovery is rapid upon decompression, although some amnesia may occur about events that occurred while narcotic. For example, a diver may have specific instructions to perform a certain task under water; he will make the dive, become narcotic, and either not perform the task or perform it badly. On return to the surface, he may report that the task had been completed satisfactorily!

Many factors potentiate the severity of the narcosis for a given depth, in addition to individual susceptibility. In particular, any increase in exogenous or endogenous carbon dioxide will synergistically potentiate the narcosis. For this reason, the narcosis is likely to be more severe in the swimming or working diver wearing breathing apparatus than in one in a pressure chamber (Table 7–2). Similarly, hard work will facilitate narcosis, as will very rapid compression, alcoholic excess or hangover, and apprehension.

Interestingly, variations in the oxygen percentage of the breathing mixture also will affect the degree of narcosis. Thus, at a constant nitrogen pressure, an increase in oxygen partial pressure will cause a greater narcosis.[17] Although a reduction of the oxygen partial pressure may reduce the narcosis if the nitrogen partial pressure is contant, this is not the case if the reduction means a concomitant increase in the nitrogen partial pressure. Albano and associates[18] noted, for example, that at 300 feet (10 ata) seven divers were more narcotic breathing a mixture of 96 per cent nitrogen and 4 per cent oxygen than breathing air (Table 7–3), a finding confirmed by Barnard and co-workers.[19]

TABLE 7–2. Mean Percentage Impairment in Ability of 14 Subjects to do an Arithmetical Test during Rest and Work on a Bicycle Ergometer (300 kg/min)

Absolute air pressures	4 atm	7 atm	10 atm	13 atm
At rest	−3.2	− 6.9	−24.6	−61.6
During exercise	−2.1	−11.6	−39.8	—

From Adolfson J: Deterioration of mental and motor functions in hyperbaric air. Scand J Psychol 6:26–31, 1965.

The novice diver may expect to be relatively seriously affected by nitrogen narcosis, but subjectively at least there will be some improvement with experience. Frequency of exposure does seem to result in some adaptation. However, adaptation to narcosis is an area about which little is known, and more research is required before any definite statements may be made.

Causes and Mechanisms of Inert Gas Narcosis

Although we have been discussing nitrogen narcosis, the more general term inert gas narcosis is more correct. Inert, in this case, refers to the inability of the respired nitrogen to interact biochemically in the body. Any mechanism of narcosis must therefore be biophysical in nature. Further, nitrogen is not alone in its ability to cause signs and symptoms of narcosis or indeed anesthesia. Behnke and associates[15] related their inference of nitrogen as the causative agent in compressed air to an old, but still very valid, hypothesis that narcotic potency is related to the affinity of an anesthetic for lipid or fat. This Meyer-Overton hypothesis[20] affirms that "all gaseous or volatile substances induce

TABLE 7–3. Arithmetic Test Results at 10 Atmospheres Absolute[18]

	FIGURES MULTIPLIED			PERCENTAGE OF ERRORS				DIFFERENCE	
Subject	(1) Ambient Pressure	(2) 10 atm air	(3) 10 atm 96% N_2–4% O_2	(4) Ambient Pressure	(5) 10 atm air	(6) 10 atm 96% N_2–4% O_2		(5)–(4)	(6)–(5)
A.G.	23	18	12	4.35	22.2	41.6		17.85	19.4
P.V.	24	19	15	4.25	79	86.6		74.75	7.6
R.S.	50	43	33	—	23	21.8		23.00	− 1.2
M.E.	40	20	14	10.00	30	42.8		20.00	12.8
S.V.	36	32	28	28.00	53.6	71.4		25.60	17.8
C.B.	27	24	20	7.4	50	60		42.60	10.0
C.U.	45	34	30		26.4	30		26.40	3.6
							M =	32.88	10.0
							t =	4.30	4.20
							p =	< 0.01	< 0.01

From Albano G, Griscuoli PM, Cirulla C: La sindrome neuropsichica di profondita. Lav Um 14:351–358, 1962.

TABLE 7–4. Correlation of Narcotic Potency of the Inert Gases, Hydrogen, Oxygen, and Carbon Dioxide with Lipid Solubility and Other Physical Characteristics

Gas	Molecular Weight	Solubility in Lipid	Molar Vol (cm^3)	Polarizability	Relative Narcotic Potency*
He	4	0.015	32.00	0.20	4.26
Ne	20	0.019	16.72	0.39	3.58
H_2	2	0.036	28.3	—	1.83
N_2	28	0.067	35.4	1.74	1
A	40	0.14	28.6	1.63	0.43
Kr	83.7	0.43	34.7	2.48	0.14
Xe	131.3	1.7	43.0	4.00	0.039 (surgical anesthesia)
O_2	32	0.11	27.9	1.58	—
CO_2	44	1.34	38.0	2.86	—

*In order from least narcotic to most narcotic.

narcosis if they penetrate the cell lipids in a definite molar concentration that is characteristic for each type of animal (or better, type of cell) and is approximately the same for all narcotics." For example, Meyer calculated this concentration as 0.07 moles/liter for mice.

In fact, the narcotic potency of inert gases may be related to many physical constants including molecular weight,[21] absorption coefficients,[22] thermodynamic "activity,"[23–25] Van der Waal's constants,[26] and the formation of clathrates.[27,28] Of these many constants, lipid solubility gives the best correlation, although polarizability and molar volume also are important in relation to the mechanism of the narcosis (Table 7–4), which involves interaction of the molecule with neuronal membranes. Thus, the size of the molecule and the degree of electrical charge upon it are important considerations.

Although nitrogen is widely recognized as the cause of compressed air intoxication, mention must be made of an alternative, but erroneous, theory that has been promoted from time to time.[29–33] This theory infers that due to the increased density of the breathing gas there is a respiratory insufficiency leading to carbon dioxide retention, and this increased carbon dioxide tension is the cause of the narcosis.

In fact, measurements of arterial carbon dioxide (Table 7–5) in humans breathing either compressed air or oxygen-helium (helium being only a very weak narcotic at most) showed that there is no increase in arterial carbon dioxide at 286 feet (9.6 ata) and at 190 feet (6.7 ata). However, nitrogen narcosis occurred when nitrogen was present, but not helium.[34] Similarly, measurements of alveolar carbon dioxide by Rashbass[35] and Cabarrou[36–37] do not support the carbon dioxide theory. Again, Hesser and colleagues[38] have shown also that the effects of raised pressures of nitrogen and carbon dioxide merely are additive and that carbon dioxide is not the cause of compressed air intoxication.

There can be no doubt that the site of action of the narcosis in the brain is at synapses or nerve junctions where there is a very small gap of 200 Å between the presynaptic terminal of one nerve and the postsynaptic terminal of another.[33–46] The mechanism therefore involves interference with the electricochemical mechanisms necessary for the transfer of the electrical potential across the synaptic gap of central synapses. Polysynaptic regions of the brain, such as the ascending reticular activating system and the cortical mantle, are likely to be the regions of the brain most affected.

TABLE 7–5. Mean Results of Human Mental Performance and Arterial Carbon Dioxide in Air and 20/80 Oxygen-Helium

	Control	20/80 He/O_2	Air 20/80 N_2/O_2
	At 286 Feet		
Arithmetic correct	16.8 ± 1.78	15.67 ± 2.08	11.0 ± 1.73
Visual analogy test	50.5 ± 5.61	51.50 ± 5.80	44.50 ± 1.21
$PaCO_2$	—	35.38 ± 4.36	34.73 ± 3.84
	At 190 Feet		
Arithmetic correct	16.8 ± 1.78	18.67 ± 1.53	15.67 ± 2.08
Visual analogy test	50.5 ± 5.61	50.00 ± 5.42	51.70 ± 4.19
$PaCO_2$	—	35.05 ± 2.56	32.68 ± 1.60

From Bennett P, Blenkarn GD: Arterial blood gases in man during inert gas narcosis. J Appl Physiol 36:45–48, 1974.

Just how the synapse is affected remains a controversial area of research. For some years considerable interest revolved around the so-called critical volume hypothesis of Miller and co-workers.[47] This hypothesis suggested that anesthesia (and thus also inert gas narcosis) occurs when the volume of a hydrophobic region is caused to expand beyond a certain critical volume. The theory also allowed an explanation for the "pressure reversal theory," which notes that increased pressure can reverse signs and symptoms of narcosis.[48] Thus, Lever and associates[49] hypothesized that a 0.4 per cent expansion of a neuronal membrane could cause narcosis, and conversely a 0.4 per cent contraction of the membrane due to pressure alone could result in the effects described in the next section as the high pressure nervous syndrome. However, the pressure reversal of different anesthetics reveals a nonlinearity that led Halsey to infer that narcosis and anesthesia may be produced by more than one site and that pressure does not necessarily act directly on the same molecular site.[50]

Further, Franks and Lieb[50a] have criticized the critical volume theory and other theories in relation to increased fluidity. They have inferred that the membrane protein may be the more likely site by exerting an effect on bilayer permeability or by interfering with normal membrane function in some other way, such as competing for the binding of some endogenous ligand (e.g., a neurotransmitter). Much current research is directed to understanding the presynaptic release and postsynaptic capture of neurotransmitters and the role of calcium ion in this mechanism.

This area remains an important area for research for solution to the mechanism of inert gas narcosis, and pressure reversal is likely to also provide the key to mechanisms of general anesthesia.

THE HIGH PRESSURE NERVOUS SYNDROME

On the basis of the lipid solubilities shown in Table 7–4, it might be expected that helium narcosis would not occur compared with that due to compressed air at 300 feet (10 ata) until about 1400 feet (43 ata). As a result helium was selected[21] as an alternative to compressed air for deep diving.

However, in 1965 during simulated dives with rapid compressions of 20 to 100 feet/minute to 600 feet and 800 feet for 1 to 4 hours, a marked decrement in performance was noted during the first hour of exposure (Tables 7–6 and 7–7), which, unlike nitrogen narcosis, was followed by a slow improvement. Further, in an opposite manner to narcosis, there was a more marked decrement in psychomotor tests, such as the ball bearing test (which required the subject to pick up ball bearings one at a time with forceps and place each in a tube of the same diameter), than in intellectual tasks such as arithmetic efficiency.[51, 52] This was due to the associated presence of a marked tremor (6 to 10 Hz) of the hands, arms, or even whole body, together with dizziness, nausea, and sometimes vomiting. This was the first report at such depths of a condition now recognized as the high pressure nervous syndrome (HPNS), which appears to reflect a general excitation of the brain compared with the decreased excitation of inert gas narcosis.

TABLE 7–6. Comparative Percentage Impairment in Psychometric Performance of Subjects Compressed to 600 Feet and 800 Feet While Breathing 5/95 Oxygen-Helium[51, 52]

	600 Ft (6) (%)	800 Ft (4) (%)
Sums correct	−18	−42
Sums attempted	− 4	− 6
No. of ball bearings	−25	−53

Similar changes were reported by Brauer and associates[53] in mice and monkeys. In such animals, HPNS appears during compression with tremors and ratchety movements. As the pressure increases, localized myoclonic jerks occur, which progress to clonic seizures. If the animal is maintained at high pressure, intermittent seizure activity will occur for as long as 12 hours. Compression beyond this point results in tonic seizures, coma, and death. Such convulsions have yet to be reported in humans.

Susceptibility to HPNS increases with increasing complexity and development of the nervous system.[54] Brauer and co-workers[55]—based on the fact that during 10 human dives at a compression rate of 24 atm/hour and, with an oxygen partial pressure of 0.5 atm and a temperature of 30°C to 33°C, the mean threshold pressure for the onset of tremors was 26.4 atm (22 to 27 atm)—calculated that convulsions should occur in humans under similar conditions at 66.3 ± 7.8 atm or 2300 feet. The onset of HPNS, however, is markedly affected by the rate of compression; slowing the rate of compression will result in the tremors and convulsions occurring at greater pressures and vice versa. Using this and other techniques, humans in fact have reached 2250 feet (686 m) without such serious HPNS.[56, 57]

TABLE 7–7. Mean Percentage Change in Performance in Subjects Breathing 95/5 Helium/Oxygen at 600 Feet for 4 Hours Compared with Performance at Atmospheric Pressure[51, 52]

Test	Surface (air)	600 ft 20 min (%)	600 ft 1½ hr (%)	600 ft 2½ hr (%)	600 ft 2½ hr (%)	600 ft 3 hr (%)	600 ft 3½ hr (%)	300 ft (decomp) (%)
Arithmetic (no. correct)	15.67	−18	+1.02	− 9.6	+ 9.6	+10.06	+ 7.4	+21.25
Arithmetic (no. attempted)	19.67	−4.2	−2.61	− 7.0	+ 4.33	+ 6.95	−0.88	+ 6.6
Ball-bearing (no. of balls)	10.67	−25	+9.37	+17.15	+26.53	+ 9.37	+15.5	+17.15

Thus, in 1968, a dive was performed at Duke University Medical Center to 1000 feet (31 ata) with a compression rate of 40 feet/hour without any tremors or other of the signs of HPNS reported during the earlier British dives in 1964-1965 to 600 and 800 feet at 100 feet/minute.[58]

However, during a further series of experiments by the French, known as Physalie,[59] with compression rates averaging about 500 feet/hour, four of the dives exceeded 1000 feet (31 ata). Tremors appeared at 21 ata (660 ft), and changes were seen in the electroencephalogram (EEG) at about 31 ata (1000 ft), with a marked increase in theta activity (4 to 6 Hz) accompanied by a depression of alpha (8 to 13 Hz). As the pressure increased, the EEG changes became worse and were accompanied by intermittent bouts of somnolence with sleep stages 1 and 2 in the EEG. If the subjects had work to do, they were able to function; but if they stopped, they lapsed into what has been termed microsleep. Due to the severity of the microsleep and EEG changes at that time, the deepest dive was aborted after only 4 minutes at 1190 feet (37 ata).

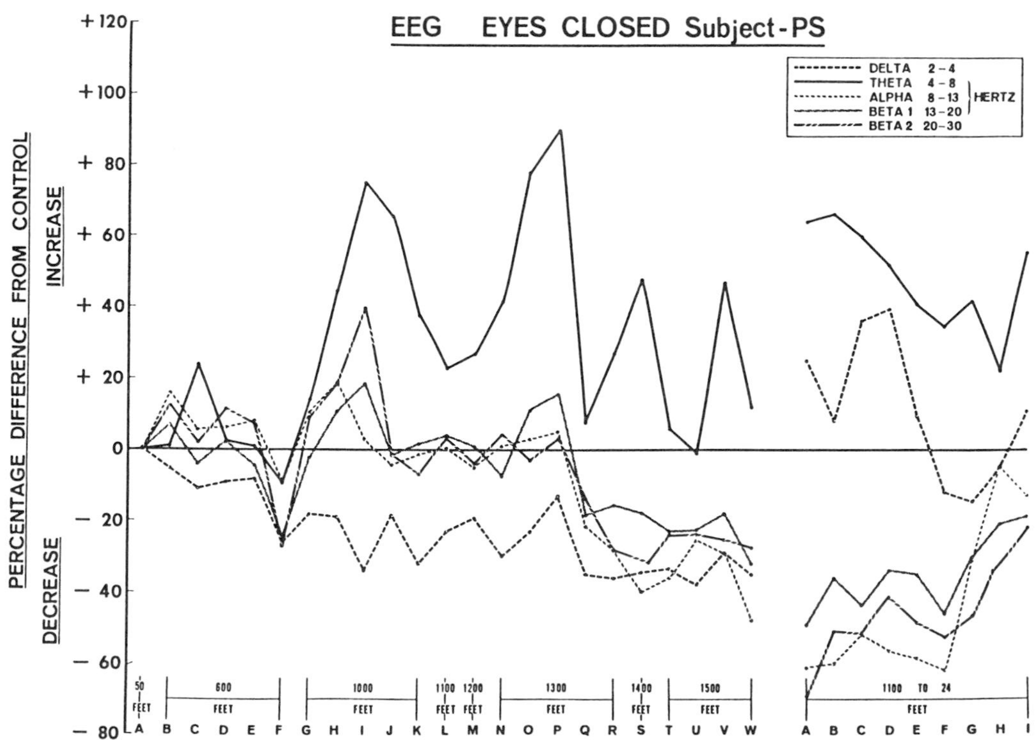

FIGURE 7–2. Spontaneous cortical electrical activity of the brain (EEG) in a subject compressed in stages to 1500 ft (46 ata) with on-line frequency analysis shows a rise in theta (4 to 8 Hz) activity with a fall in overall activity from 1300 ft (40 ata). (With permission from Bennett PB, Towse EJ: The high pressure nervous syndrome during a simulated oxygen-helium dive to 1500 ft. Electroencephalogr Clin Neurophysiol 31:383-393, 1971.)

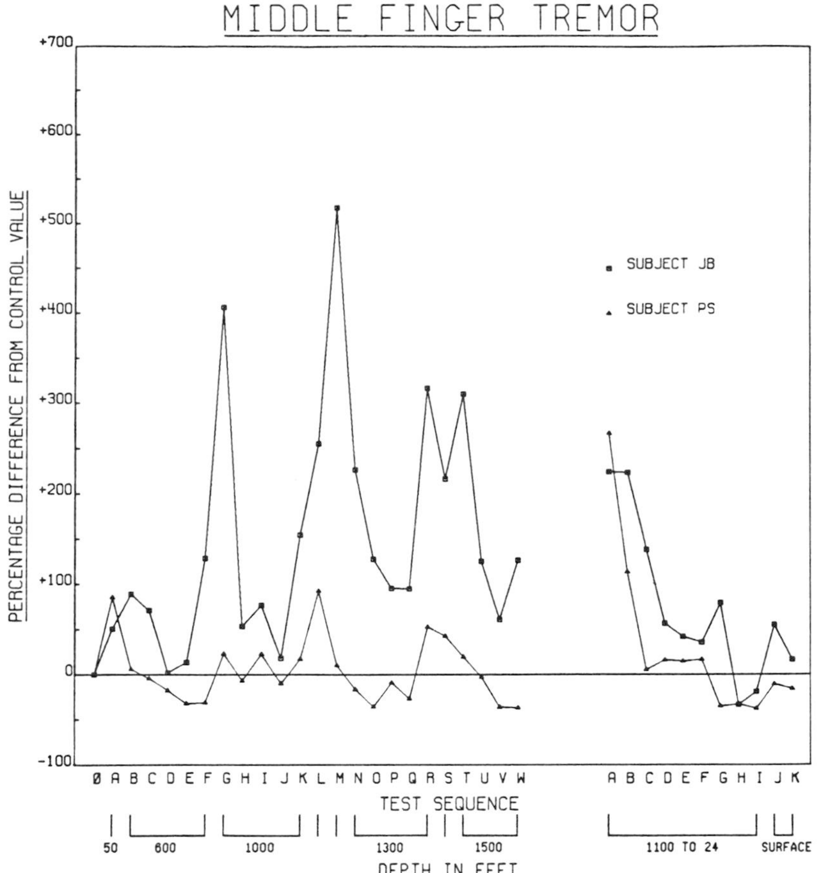

FIGURE 7–3. Percentage change in tremor of the hand measured by a transducer on the finger of men compressed to 1500 ft (46 ata) oxygen-helium. Each compression phase causes a marked increase in tremor in one subject but has little affect on the other. The tremor-sensitive subject also shows an increase in base tremor. (From Bennett PB, Towse EJ: Performance efficiency of men breathing oxygen-helium at depths between 100 ft and 1500 ft. Aerosp Med 42:1147-1156, 1971.)

Subsequently, further depth has been achieved by the use of slower rates of compression, with or without stages.

Thus, in 1970, two men were compressed for the first time to 1500 feet (46 ata), where they stayed for 10 hours. The compression rate was fast at 16 to 17 feet/minute (i.e., 100 ft/hour), but some 24 hours were spent at 600 feet, 1000 feet, and 1300 feet (19, 31, and 40 ata). During this dive, the divers were extensively monitored.[60–63]

All of the characteristics of the HPNS were seen, but the divers were able to function reasonably well. The following points were clarified by this dive.

First, in regard to the EEG, the rise in theta activity was initiated on compression, especially at pressures greater than 31 ata (1000 ft). The theta continued to rise for 6 hours, even though compression had ceased and then fell over 12 hours to lower levels (Fig. 7–2). On compression again, the cycle repeated. The rise in theta did not seem to correlate with any of the other signs of HPNS. There was interindividual susceptibility that also was apparent in the tremors. One diver showed a considerable increase in tremor, whereas the other had little response (Fig. 7–3). The occurrence of tremor in diving has been reviewed in more detail elsewhere,[4] but it should be pointed out that the tremor is in the frequency range of 8 to 12 Hz, which is normal resting tremor and not that of Parkinson's or cerebellar disease (3 to 8 Hz). Cold, alcoholism, and thyrotoxicosis also cause tremor in the 8 to 12 Hz range.

For the first time, too, it could be clearly seen that helium did not cause signs and symptoms of narcosis. Arithmetic performance was unaffected, but psychomotor tests, such as the ball bearing and peg board tests, showed a decrement mostly due to the tremors and muscular jerks.

Prevention of HPNS

Due to HPNS, diving to depths beyond 1000 feet (31 ata) impose considerable limitations on the diver, but there are a number of methods that can be used to mitigate its severity. These include choice of a suitable slow exponential rate of compression, use of long stages or holds during the compression to allow adaptation, use of nitrogen (or other narcotic) in a so-called trimix, and selection of the least susceptible divers.[2, 64, 65]

In the last 20 years well over 50 deep experimental dives have been made over 1000 feet (31 ata) in the United States, the United Kingdom, France, Germany, Norway, and Japan to study HPNS and the means for its prevention.[2, 64–66] These have involved the use of helium-oxygen, helium-oxygen plus excursions to a greater depth, nitrogen-helium-oxygen (trimix), trimix with excursions, and more recently hydrogen-helium-oxygen. These were made at a time when there seemed little operational need for diving much deeper than 1000 feet (31 ata) at most. Yet today operational diving is being done at 410 meters (1345 ft), and it seems that current interest is certainly at 450 meters (1476 ft). On this basis, it is clear that there will be a need for open ocean diving to 500 or 600 meters (1640 to 1968 ft) in the next decade. What is the best way to do such diving?

There are really only two basic methods, to compress with either helium-oxygen or trimix. The former risks incapacitating HPNS; the latter, if not used correctly, puts the diver at risk for nitrogen narcosis and some HPNS too. The protagonists and antagonists for each method divide along these issues, but in fact neither is necessarily correct.

Helium-Oxygen

During the early 1970's, studies at the British Royal Navy Physiological Laboratory (now AMTE/PL)[60–63] and by the French company Comex[67–69] showed that depths of between 1500 and 2132 feet (500 to 600 m) could be obtained by slow exponential compressions and stages. Since then there has been less interest in this type of dive. This is primarily due to the length of time involved with such compressions (e.g., 10 days to 2100 ft) which often leaves the diver still affected by varying degrees of HPNS that could be incapacitating in an ocean situation.

However, in 1976, the AMTE/PL carried out a dive to 300 meters (984 ft)[66] (AMTE/PL Dive 5)* using a *linear* compression rate of 1 meter/minute. There was nausea, unspecified epigastric sensations, intention tremor, and impending loss of consciousness. Previously in 1969 Buhlmann[70] made a much faster compression to 300 meters (984 ft) at 5 meters/minute producing only mild dizziness and an initial decrement in psychomotor tasks which was gone 2 to 3 hours later. The reasons for the differences between these two dives are not clear, but it would seem most likely to be due to personal susceptibility.

One clear characteristic of the subsequent dives with very slow compressions (AMTE/PL Dives 6, 7, and 8) is no nausea and possibly little change in the EEG. However, while very slow compressions do considerably ameliorate or even prevent HPNS in suitable subjects to 300 meters (984 ft), at 420 meters (1377 ft) even with 6 days of compression some signs of HPNS are still present, including loss of appetite, periods of unspecified epigastric sensation, and persistent intentional tremor with occasional muscle jerks. With a further depth increment of 100 meters (328 ft), these become more

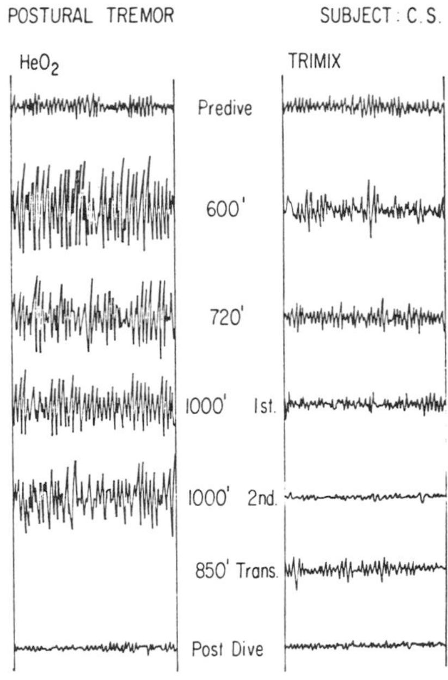

FIGURE 7–4. Postural tremor of the hand in a subject exposed either to 1000 ft (31 ata) oxygen-helium alone or trimix (He/O_2 with 18 per cent nitrogen) with the same compression time of 33 minutes. Without the nitrogen present, the classic tremor may be seen. With nitrogen added at 600 ft (19 ata) in the trimix, the tremors are suppressed. On changing back to oxygen-helium during the decompression at 850 ft, (26.6 ata), the tremor returns. (From Bennett PB, Blenkarn GD, Roby J, Youngblood D: Suppression of the high pressure nervous syndrome in human deep dives by He-N_2-O_2. Undersea Biomed Res 1:221-237, 1974 © 1974 Undersea Medical Society, Inc.)

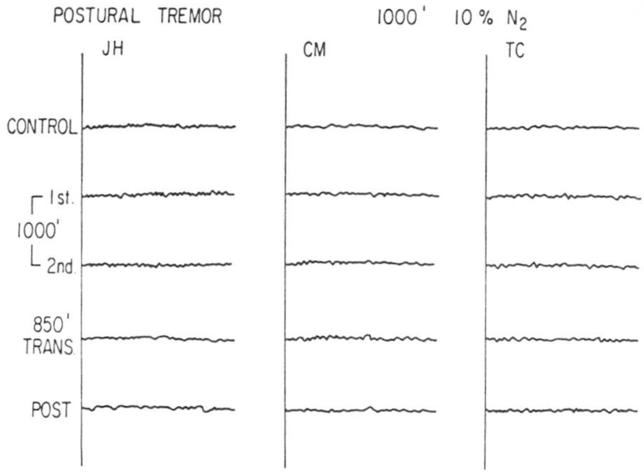

FIGURE 7–5. Tremor transducer measurements in three subjects compressed in 33 minutes to 1000 ft (31 ata) in trimix (He/O_2 with 10 per cent nitrogen). No HPNS tremors are seen. (From Bennett PB, Roby J, Simon S, Youngblood D: Optimal use of nitrogen to suppress the high pressure nervous syndrome. Aviat Space Environ Med 46:37-40, 1975.)

severe and are compounded by additional signs and symptoms severely limiting functional ability.

Thus in 1979, AMTE/PL and the USN Experimental Diving Unit carried out very similar dives. In the British dive (AMTE/PL Dive 9) to 540 meters (1771 ft) with compression at 5 meters/minute and six stages of 4 hours or more for a total of 3 days, 5 hours there was marked nausea, tremors, dizziness, vomiting, and loss of appetite. Intention tremor and epigastric sensations persisted.

The U.S. Navy dive was to 549 meters (1800 ft) with rates mostly of 30 feet/hour (9 m/hr) for a compression time of 3¾ days from 650 feet. Fatigue, dizziness, nausea, vomiting, aversion to food with 8 per cent weight loss, stomach cramps, diarrhea, myoclonic jerking, and dyspnea were present. The divers deteriorated rather than improved with time at depth, but they were able to work at 100 watts in connection with respiratory studies (Spaur, 1979, personal communication).

These experiments showed that even at comparatively slow rates of compression, the increasing hydrostatic pressure is producing severely limiting HPNS between 1400 and 1800 feet. This may in fact have been due to the rates of compression at the deeper depths being still too fast; a much more exponential rate of compression with much slower deep rates (e.g., 0.1 to 0.2 m/min) would have been more effective.

Trimix (Nitrogen-Helium-Oxygen)

In this search for some method to ameliorate or prevent HPNS in deep divers, the use of the so-called trimix (a mixture of helium and oxygen with a small percentage of nitrogen) has received special attention. This was based on the pressure reversal of narcosis theory reported in tadpoles[48] and mice.[49] Bennett and colleagues[71] noted in studies of the effects of raised pressures of the inert gases nitrogen, argon, and helium on model monolayer membranes that the first two gases caused a fall in surface tension (expansion of the monolayer), whereas the helium caused a rise (constriction) in surface tension. Inferring that the fall in tension was related to mechanisms of narcosis and the rise to an HPNS mechanism and coupled with the pressure reversal theories, Bennett suggested that adding nitrogen to helium-oxygen might well result in no change in tension and thus no narcosis or HPNS.[71–73]

The technique was first used in humans at the F.G. Hall Laboratory at Duke Medical Center in 1974 when divers were compressed with either trimix or heliox to 1000 feet in the remarkably fast time of only 33 minutes using a trimix 18 (i.e., with 18 per cent nitrogen). Although trimix did prevent HPNS compared with the heliox dive (Fig. 7–4), euphoria due to nitrogen narcosis was present in two of four divers.[72] Further studies in 1974 with five divers exponentially compressed with three brief holds or stages to 1000 feet also in 33 minutes were made with the nitrogen reduced to 10 per cent, and this indicated no performance deterioration or narcosis and no nausea, tremors, or EEG changes[73] (Fig. 7–5). Confirmation of the value of trimix later was afforded by French workers in the so-called CORAZ comparative dives, which compared the value of 9 per cent or 4.5 per cent nitrogen in a 4-hour compression to 1000 feet (305 m). The lower nitrogen appeared best for ameliorating HPNS without narcosis.[74, 75]

In 1980, Norwegian workers also made some comparative dives to 300 meters with divers

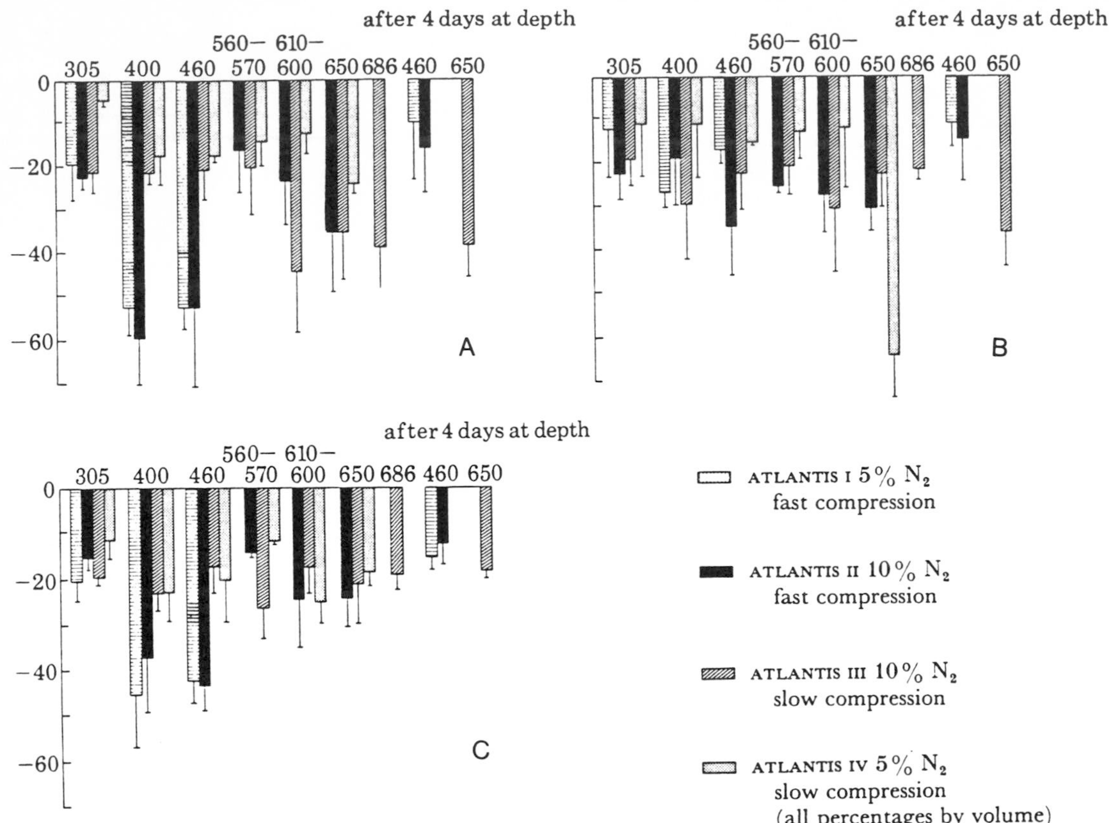

FIGURE 7–6. *A.* Comparison of the mean percentage decrement of three divers for each of the dives ATLANTIS I, II, III and IV at the addition test requiring simple arithmetic. The large decrements at 400 and 600 m for I and II owing to fast compression are evident, as is the increasing decrement for dives deeper than 500 m during II and III and the considerable improvement in ATLANTIS IV.

B. Comparison of the mean percentage decrement of three divers for each of the dives ATLANTIS, I, II, III, IV at the ball-bearing test of fine motor dexterity. There is a tendency for the tests done in less nitrogen to show less decrement, except for ATLANTIS IV when, owing to the presence of visible tremors at 650 m, the test indicates decrements of 60 per cent or more.

C. Comparison of the mean percentage decrement of three divers for each of the dives ATLANTIS I, II, III, IV at the screw plate or hand tool test of motor skills. Large decrements at 400 and 460 m due to the fast compression for I and II are not seen with the slow compressions of III and IV. Otherwise the decrements are around 20 per cent regardless of depth, rate of compression, or nitrogen percentage. (From Bennett PB, McLeod M: Probing the limits of human deep diving. Philos Trans R Soc Lond 304:105–117, 1984.)

compressed in 4 hours, 4 minutes using either trimix 10 or heliox.[76] Again while trimix successfully ameliorated much of the HPNS, there was evidence of nitrogen narcosis.[76] The next year a similar dive was made to 1640 feet (500 m) with, in one case, a heliox compression of 26 h 45 minute and the other a trimix 10 compression of 41 h 20 minute. Both groups suffered HPNS signs and symptoms, and the trimix group experienced nitrogen narcosis too. The likely reason being that the compression profiles were still too fast in critical places, and the nitrogen at 10 per cent was too high.

The Duke Atlantis IV dives from 1979 to 1982[56, 57, 77] were designed to determinutee the relationship between either 5 or 10 per cent nitrogen and either fast or slow rates of compression. Very extensive scientific studies were made which supported the view that a slow exponential compression rate with stages of about 38 to 40 hours total time to 450 meters (1476 ft) with trimix 5 (i.e., 5 per cent nitrogen in heliox) permits divers to arrive at such depths in a fit condition and able to work effectively. It was during these dives that the deepest human exposures to 686 meters (2250 ft) were made with the divers in a remarkably good condition. These tests also indicated that at depths deeper than 300 or 400 meters (984 to 1312 ft) it may not be possible to prevent some

TABLE 7–8. Duke/GUSI Compression to 600 m with Trimix 5 (N_2 5%/0.5 bar O_2 He rest)

Travel 0–180 m	= 5 m/min (36 min)
Stop at 180 m	= 2 hrs
Travel 180–240 m	= 3 m/min (20 min)
Stop at 240 m	= 6 hrs
Travel 240–300 m	= 1.5 m/min (40 min)
Stop at 300 m	= 2 hrs
Travel 300–350 m	= 0.5 m/min (1 hr 40 min)
Stop at 350 m	= 9 hrs
Travel 350–400 m	= 0.25 m/min (3 hr 20 min)
Stop at 400 m	= 2 hrs
Travel 400–430 m	= 0.125 m/min (4 hrs)
Stop at 430 m	= 2 hrs
Travel 430–460 m	= 0.125 m/min (4 hrs)
Stop at 460 m	= 12 hrs
Travel 460–490 m	= 0.100 m/min (5 hrs)
Stop at 490 m	= 2 hrs
Travel 490–520 m	= 0.100 m/min (6 hr 40 min)
Stop at 520 m	= 13 hrs
Travel 520–550 m	= 0.075 m/min (6 hr 40 min)
Stop at 550 m	= 13 hrs
Travel 550–575 m	= 0.05 m/min (8 hr 20 min)
Stop at 575 m	= 16 hrs
Travel 575–600 m	= 0.05 m/min (8 hr 20 min)

From Bennett PB, Schafstall H, Schnegelsberg W, Vann R: An analysis of fourteen successful trimix 5 deep saturation dives between 150–600 m. *In* Proceedings Ninth Symposium on Underwater Physiology and Hyperbaric Medicine. Kobe, Japan, 1986.

small (approx. 15 per cent) decrement in sensitive psychological tests (Fig. 7–6). However, the men appear fit and able to work, and this decrement was not materially worse at 686 meters compared with 300 to 400 meters.

The French company Comex initially used baboons to study the effects of trimix compressed beyond 300 meters and subsequently reached 3281 feet (1000 m) before focal seizures were seen in the EEG. They worked out a technique, tested later in human dives DRET 79/131, ENTEX V, and VIII,[80–83] which involved compression at 0.5 meter/minute to 100 meters (328 ft) followed by 0.4, 0.25 and 0.20 meter/minute for each further 100 meters and 0.14 meter/minute for the final compression to 450 meters. Nitrogen was injected at each 100 meters where the divers were held for 150 minutes.

This 40-hour compression proved very successful at ameliorating HPNS.[84] Interestingly, using the same procedures in 1983 in ENTEX IX with heliox only, there seemed little difference between the ENTEX dives with trimix or heliox. Indeed, further compression was made to 610 meters (2001 ft) for 56 hours for in-water work, although general fitness was not as good as shallower depths.

More recently a series of eight major studies involving some 14 dives between 300 and 600 meters (984 and 1968 ft) with trimix 5 were made from 1983 to 1986 at the German diving simulator GUSI at GKSS, Geesthacht near Hamburg.[85] These used modified Atlantis IV compression profiles (Table 7–8) and some 13 divers from four countries. The work involved 1298 man-days at saturation.

The results were very satisfactory with little or no HPNS on arrival, and the divers were able to carry out welding and other tasks without difficulty. At 1476 feet (450 m), two divers welded a 36-inch pipe and maintained that they felt as if they were only at 300 feet (92 m). There were no indications of nausea, visible tremors, undue fatigue, nightmares or sleep difficulty, increase in brain theta activity, or undue performance decrement certainly to 500 meters.

This work will provide, as with the French research dives, a method for compressing divers to great depths with relative comfort and safety compared with the problems seen in much earlier research and also safe decompression schedules, albeit with very slow rates of only 1 meter/hour or less.[85]

Whether man will ever dive as deep as 700 meters (2297 ft) or more must await the next period of research, but this is a formidable depth and an undoubted challenge to man's urge to overcome the limitations of his environment.

REFERENCES

1. Bennett PB: Inert gas narcosis. *In* Bennett PB, Elliott DH (eds): The Physiology and Medicine of Diving and Compressed Air Work. 3rd ed. San Pedro, CA, Best Publications, 1982.
2. Bennett PB: The high pressure nervous syndrome in man. *In* Bennett PB, Elliott DH (ed): The Physiology and Medicine of Diving and Compressed Air Work. 3rd ed. San Pedro, CA, Best Publications, 1982.
3. Hunter WL, Bennett PB: The causes, mechanisms and prevention of the high pressure nervous syndrome. Undersea Biomed Res 1:1–28, 1974.
4. Bachrach A, Bennett PB: Tremor in diving. Aerosp Med 44:613–623, 1973.
5. Lambertsen CJ (ed): Underwater Physiology: Proceedings Fourth Symposium on Underwater Physiology. New York, Academic Press, 1971.
6. Shilling CW, Beckett MW (eds): Underwater Physiology VI: Proceedings Sixth Symposium on Underwater Physiology. Washington, FASEB, 1978.
7. Bachrach AJ, Matzen MM (eds): Underwater Physiology VII: Proceedings Seventh Symposium on Underwater Physiology. Bethesda; Undersea Medical Society, 1981.
8. Bachrach AJ, Matzen MM (eds): Underwater Physiology VIII: Proceedings Eighth Symposium on Underwater Physiology. Bethesda, Undersea Medical Society, 1984.
9. Fowler B, Ackles KN, Porlier G: Effects of inert gas

narcosis on behavior—a critical review. Undersea Biomed Res 12:369–402, 1985.
10. Paton, WDM, Elliott DH, Smith EB (eds): Diving and life at high pressures. London, The Royal Society, 1984.
11. Bennett PB, Simon S, Katz Y: High pressures of inert gases and anesthetic mechanisms. *In* Fink R (ed): Molecular Mechanisms of Anesthesia. Baltimore, Williams & Wilkins, 1974.
12. Fink R (ed): Molecular Mechanisms of Anesthesia. Vol 2. New York, Raven Press, 1980.
13. Green JB: Diving With and Without Armour. Buffalo, Leavitt, 1861.
14. Hill L, Davis RH, Selby RP, et al: Deep Diving and Ordinary Diving. London, British Admiralty Report, 1933.
15. Behnke AR, Thomson RM, Motley EP: The psychologic effects from breathing air at 4 atmospheres pressure. Am J Physiol 112:554–558, 1935.
16. Adolfson J, Muren A: Air breathing at 13 atmospheres. Psychological and physiological observations. Sartryck ur Forsvars Medicin 1:31–37, 1965.
17. Frankenhaeusser M, Graff-Lonnevig V, Hesser CM: Effects of psychomotor functions of different nitrogen-oxygen gas mixtures at increased ambient pressures. Acta Physiol Scand 59:400–409, 1963.
18. Albano G, Criscuoli PM, Ciulla C: La sindrome neuropsichica di profondita. Lav Um 14:351–358, 1962.
19. Barnard EEP, Hempleman HVH, Trotter C: Mixture breathing and nitrogen narcosis. Report UPS 208, London, Medical Research Council, RN Personnel Research Committee, 1962.
20. Meyer HH: Theoris der alkoholnarkose. Arch Exp Pathol Pharmacol 42:109, 1899.
21. Behnke AR, Yarbrough OD: Respiratory resistance, oil-water solubility and mental effects of argon compared with helium and nitrogen. Am J Physiol 126:409–415, 1939.
22. Case EM, Haldane JBS: Human physiology under high pressure. J Hyg 41:225–249, 1941.
23. Ferguson J: The use of chemical potentials as indices of toxicity. Proc Roy Soc Lond B 197:387–404, 1939.
24. Fergusion J, Hawkins SW: Toxic action of some simple gases at high pressure. Nature 164:963–964, 1949.
25. Brink R, Posternak J: Thermodynamic analysis of relative effectiveness of narcotics. J Cell Physiol 32:211–233, 1948.
26. Wulf RJ, Featherstone RM: A Correlation of Van der Waal's constants with anesthetic potency. Anesthesiology 18:97–105, 1957.
27. Miller SL: A theory of gaseous anesthesia. Proc Natl Acad Sci USA 47:1515–1524, 1961.
28. Pauling L: A molecular theory of anesthesia. Science 134:15–21, 1961.
29. Bean JW: Changes in arterial pH induced by compression and decompression. Fed Proc 6:76, 1974.
30. Bean JW: Tensional changes of alveolar gas in reactions to rapid compression and decompression and question of nitrogen narcosis. Am J Physiol 161:417–425, 1950.
31. Seusing J, Drube H: The importance of hypercapnia in depth intoxication. Klin Wochenschr 38:1088–1090, 1960.
32. Buhlmann A: Deep diving. *In* Eaton B (ed): The Undersea Challenge. London, The British Sub-Aqua Club, 1963.
33. Vail EG: Hyperbaric respiratory mechanics. Aerosp Med 42:536–546, 1971.
34. Bennett P, Blenkarn GD: Arterial blood gases in man during inert gas narcosis. J Appl Physiol 36:45–48, 1974.
35. Rashbass C: The unimportance of carbon dioxide in nitrogen narcosis. Report UPS 153, London Medical Research Council, RN Personnel Research Committee, 1955.
36. Cabarrou P: L'invresse des grandes profondeurs. Presse Med 72:793–797, 1964.
37. Cabarrou P: Introduction à la physiologie de 'Homo Aquaticus.' Presse Med 74:2771–2773, 1966.
38. Hesser CM, Adolfson J, Fagraeus L: Role of CO_2 in compressed air narcosis. Aerosp Med 42:163–168, 1971.
39. Carpenter FG: Depressant action of inert gases on the central nervous system in mice. Am J Physiol 172:471–474, 1953.
40. Carpenter FG: Anesthetic action of inert and unreactive gases on intact animals and isolated tissues. Am J Physiol 178:505–509, 1954.
41. Carpenter FG: Inert gas narcosis. *In* Goff LG (ed): Proceedings First Underwater Physiology Symposium. Washington, National Research Council, National Academy of Sciences, 1955.
42. Larrabee MG, Posternak JM: Selective action of anesthetics on synapses and axons in mammalian sympathetic ganglia. J Neurophysiol 15:91–114, 1952.
43. French JD, Verzeano M, Magoun HW: A neural basis of the anesthetic state. Arch Neurol Psychiat 69:519–529, 1953.
44. Arduini A, Auduini MG: Effect of drugs and metabolic alterations on brain stem arousal mechanism. J Pharmacol 110:76–85, 1954.
45. Bennett PB: Neurophysiologic and neuropharmacologic investigations in inert gas narcosis. *In* Lambertsen CJ, Greenbaum LJ (eds): Proceedings Second Underwater Physiology Symposium. Washington, National Research Council, National Academy of Sciences, 1963.
46. Bennett PB: The effects of high pressures of inert gases on auditory evoked potentials in cat cortex and reticular formation. Electroencephalogr Clin Neurophysiol 17:388–397, 1964.
47. Miller KW, Paton WM, Smith RA, Smith EB: The pressure reversal of general anesthesia and the critical volume hypothesis. Mol Pharmacol 9:131–143, 1973.
48. Johnson FH, Flagler EA: Hydrostatic pressure reversal of narcosis in tadpoles. Science 112:91–92, 1950.
49. Lever MJ, Miller KW, Paton WM, Smith EB: Pressure reversal of anesthesia. Nature 231:368–371, 1971.
50. Halsey MJ, Wardley-Smith B, Green CJ: Pressure reversal of anesthesia—a multisite expansion hypothesis. Br J Anaesth 50:1091–1097, 1978.
50a. Franks NP, Lieb WR: Molecular mechanisms of general anesthesia. Nature 300:487–493, 1982.
51. Bennett PB: Psychometric impairment in men breathing oxygen-helium at increased pressures. Report No. 251, London, Medical Research Council, RN Personnel Research Committee, Underwater Physiology Sub-Committee, 1965.
52. Bennett PB, Dossett AN: Undesirable effects of oxygen-helium breathing at great depths. Report No. 260, London, Medical Research Council, RN Personnel Research Committee, Underwater Physiology Sub-Committee, 1967.
53. Brauer RW, Johson DO, Pessotti RL, Redding RW: Effects of hydrogen and helium at pressures to 67 atmospheres on mice and monkeys. Fed Proc 25:202, 1966.
54. Brauer RW, Way RO, Perry RA: Narcotic effects of helium and hydrogen in mice and hyperexcitability pheonomena at simulated depths of 1500 to 4000 ft

of sea water. *In* Fink BR (ed): Toxicity of Anesthetics. Baltimore, Williams & Wilkins, 1968.

55. Brauer RW, Dimov S, Fructus X, et al: Syndrome neurologique et electrographique des hautes pressions. Rev Neurol 121:264–265, 1969.
56. Bennett PB, Coggin R, McLeod M: Effect of compression rate on use of trimix to ameliorate HPNS in man to 686 m (2250 ft). Undersea Biomed Res 9:335–351, 1982.
57. Bennett PB, McLeod M: Probing the limits of human deep diving. Phil Trans R Soc Lond B 304:105–117, 1984.
58. Summit JK, Kelly JS, Herron JM, Saltzman HA: Joint US Navy–Duke University 1000 ft saturation dive. Report 3-69, Washington DC, U.S. Navy Experimental Diving Unit, 1969.
59. Fructus X, Brauer RW, Naquet R: Physiological effects observed in the course of simulated deep chamber dives to a maximum of 36.5 atm in a helium-oxygen atmosphere. *In* Lambertsen CF (ed): Proceedings Fourth Symposium on Underwater Physiology. New York, Academic Press, 1971.
60. Bennett PB, Towse EJ: Performance efficiency of men breathing oxygen-helium at depths between 100 ft and 1500 ft. Aerosp Med 42:1147–1156, 1971.
61. Bennett PB, Towse EJ: The high pressure nervous syndrome during a simulated oxygen-helium dive to 1500 ft. Electroencephalogr Clin Neurophysiol 31:383–393, 1971.
62. Bennett PB, Gray SP: Changes in human urine and blood chemistry during a simulated oxygen-helium dive to 1500 ft. Aerosp Med 42:868–874, 1971.
63. Morrison JB, Florio JT: Respiratory function during a simulated dive to 1500 ft. J Appl Physiol 30:724–732, 1971.
64. Bennett PB: A strategy for future diving. *In* Halsey MJ, Settle W, Smith EB (eds): The Strategy for Future Diving to Depths Greater than 1000 ft. 8th UMS Workshop. Report WS 6-15-75, 71-76. Bethesda, Undersea Medical Society, 1975.
65 .Bennett PB: Potential methods to prevent the HPNS in human deep diving. *In* Smith EB, Halsey NJ, Daniels S (eds): Techniques for Diving Deeper than 1500 ft. 23rd UMS Workshop Report 40 WS (DD) 6-30-80, Bethesda, Undersea Medical Society, 1980.
66. Toruk Z: Invited review: Behavior and performance in deep experimental diving with man—a review of recent work. *In* Bachrach AJ, Matzen MM (eds): Underwater Physiology VIII: Proceedings Eighth Symposium on Underwater Physiology. Bethesda, Undersea Medical Society, 1984.
67. Fructus X, Rostain JC: HPNS: A clinical study of 30 cases. *In* Shilling CJ, Beckett MW (eds): Proceedings Sixth Symposium on Underwater Physiology. Washington, FASEB, 1978, p 38.
68. Lemaire C, Murphy EL: Longitudinal study of performance after deep compressions with heliox and He-N_2-O_2. Undersea Biomed Res 3:205–216, 1976.
69. Rostain JC, Naquet R: Human neurophysiological data obtained from two simulated heliox dives to a depth of 610 m. *In* Shilling CJ, Beckett MW (eds): Proceedings Sixth Symposium on Underwater Physiology. Washington, FASEB, 1978, p 9–19.
70. Buhlmann AA, Matthys H, Overrath G, et al: Saturation exposures of 31 ats abs in an oxygen-helium atmosphere with excursions to 36 ats. Aerosp Med 41:394–402, 1970.
71. Bennett PB, Papahadjopoulos D, Bangham AD: The effect of raised pressures of inert gases on phospholipid model membranes. Life Sci 6:2527–2533, 1967.
72. Bennett PB, Blenkarn GD, Roby J, Youngblood D: Suppression of the high pressure nervous syndrome in human deep dives by He-N_2-O_2. Undersea Biomed Res 1:221–237, 1974.
73. Bennett PB, Roby J, Simon S, Youngblood D: Optimal use of nitrogen to suppress the high pressure nervous syndrome. Aviat Space Environ Med 46:37–40, 1975.
74. Charpy JP, Murphy E, Lemaire C: Performance psychometriques après compressions rapides à 300 m. Med Subaq Hyperbare 15:192–195, 1976.
75. Rostain JC: Le tremblement au cours de compressions rapides: Influence de l'azote dans le melange respiratoire. Med Sobaq Hyperbare 15:267–270, 1976.
76. Vaernes R, Bennett PB, Hammerborg D, et al: Central nervous system reactions during heliox and trimix dives to 31 ATA. Undersea Biomed Res 9:1–14, 1982.
77. Bennett PB, Coggin R, Roby J: Control of HPNS in humans during rapid compression with trimix to 650 m (2132 ft). Undersea Biomed Res 8:85–100, 1981.
78. Rostain JC, Gardette-Chauffour MC, Doucet J, Gardette B: Problems posed by compression at depths greater than 800 m in the monkey Papio papio. Undersea Biomed Res 8:15–16, 1981.
79. Lemaire C: Evaluation de la performance psychomotrice entre 10 et 450 m en ambiance helium-oxygen-azote. Med Aero Spat Med Sub Hyp 19:211–214, 1980.
80. Naquet R, Rostain JC: HPNS in man: An account of French experiments. *In* Smith EB, Halsey MJ, Daniels S (eds): Techniques for Diving Deeper than 1500 ft. Proceedings 23rd Workshop. Bethesda, Undersea Medical Society 1980, p 48–53.
81. Fructus X: Limits for both open water and chamber diving. *In* Smith E, Halsey MJ, Daniels S (eds): p 27–33, Techniques for Diving Deeper than 1500 ft. Proceedings 23rd Workshop. Bethesda, Undersea Medical Society, 1980.
82. Naquet R, Lemaire C, Rostain JC: High pressure nervous syndrome: Psychometric and clinicoelectrophysiological correlations. Phil Trans R Soc Lond B 304:95–102, 1984.
83. Rostain JC, Lemaire C, Naquet R: HPNS in man during a 12 day stay at 450 m in He/N_2/O_2. Undersea Biomed Res 9:22–23, 1982.
84. Rostain JC, Lemaire C, Garette-Chauffour MC, Naquet R: Evaluation of HPNS in 16 divers breathing He-N_2-O_2 during long stays at 45 bar. *In* Bachrach AJ, Matzen M (eds): Underwater Physiology VIII: Proceedings Eighth Symposium on Underwater Physiology. Bethesda, Undersea Medical Society, 1984, p 665–682.
85. Bennett PB, Schafstall H, Schnegelsberg W, Vann R: An analysis of fourteen successful trimix 5 deep saturation dives between 150–600 m. *In* Proceedings Ninth Symposium on Underwater Physiology and Hyperbaric Medicine. Kobe, Japan, 1986.
86. Shilling CW, Willgrube WW: Quantitative study of mental and neuromuscular reactions as influenced by increased air pressure. US Navy Med Bull 35:373–380, 1937.
87. Adolfson J: Deterioration of mental and motor functions in hyperbaric air. Scand J Psychol 6:26–31, 1965.

Chapter 8

The Toxicity of Oxygen, Carbon Monoxide, and Carbon Dioxide

STEPHEN R. THOM *and* JAMES M. CLARK

OXYGEN

Paradoxically, the same gas that is required to sustain life by preventing loss of consciousness and death from hypoxemia has toxic properties that affect all living cells at sufficiently high pressure and duration of exposure.[1–4] The rate of development of toxic effects is determined by the oxygen partial pressure (pO_2) rather than the oxygen percentage of the inspired gas. The specific manifestations of oxygen poisoning that occur in humans or animals are determined by interactions between oxygen dose, with respect to both pO_2 and duration of exposure, and relative susceptibilities of the exposed tissues. Although continued exposure to a toxic pO_2 will ultimately cause functional disruption and cellular damage in any organ system of the body, effects on the lung, brain, and eye are most prominent under practical conditions of exposure. These effects are described below.

Biochemistry of Oxygen Toxicity

Gerschman[5, 6] and Gilbert[7, 8] first proposed that oxygen toxicity is caused by the production of free radical intermediates in excessive concentrations during exposure to increased oxygen pressures. The initial involvement of these agents is now well established, and several excellent reviews summarizing what is known about the biochemistry of oxygen free radicals are available.[9–13] Although exact mechanisms are not yet known, free radical intermediates including superoxide anions, hydrogen peroxide, hydroperoxy and hydroxyl radicals, and singlet oxygen are potentially toxic to cell membranes, enzymes, nucleic acids, and other constituents. Along with better understanding of oxygen free radicals has come a greater awareness of the universal dependence of vital biological processes on cellular antioxidant defenses such as superoxide dismutase, catalase, and the glutathione system. It is now thought that the same oxygen pressures required to sustain life would cause lethal oxygen poisoning in the absence of these defenses.

Pulmonary Oxygen Toxicity

Studies in the monkey[14–17] have shown that the pathological response of the lung to oxygen toxicity can be differentiated into two overlapping phases of progressive deterioration. The first is an acute exudative phase consisting of interstitial and alveolar edema, intra-alveolar hemorrhage, fibrinous exudate, hyaline membranes, swelling and destruction of capillary endothelial cells, and destruction of type I alveolar epithelial cells. The exudative phase merges into a subacute proliferative phase that is characterized by interstitial fibrosis, fibroblastic proliferation, hyperplasia of type II alveolar epithelial cells, and partial resolution of earlier acute changes. The relative prominence of individual components in each phase is influenced by interactions of external variables, such as level of inspired pO_2 and exposure duration, with internal factors such as species differences in pulmonary tissue reactivity and susceptibility to hyperoxic exposure.

Pathological changes that are similar or identical to those caused by pulmonary oxygen toxicity in experimental animals are also found in the lungs of human patients who die after prolonged oxygen therapy.[18–21] Although such alterations are not specific for pulmonary oxygen poisoning, the clinical course of these patients in conjunction with the known susceptibility of humans to oxygen toxicity leave no reason to doubt that the observed pathological changes are in fact caused by pulmonary oxygen toxicity. In experimental animals and presumably also in humans, recovery from pulmonary oxygen intoxication is accompanied by complete resolution of changes typical of the acute exudative phase of pathology. When exposure to hyperoxia is sufficiently prolonged for the development of prominent proliferative changes, however, recovery from these pathological effects is greatly delayed and incomplete resolution may leave permanent residual scarring of the lung.

Symptoms of pulmonary oxygen poisoning begin insidiously as a mild substernal irritation that becomes progressively more intense and widespread in parallel with increasing frequency of cough. When extreme in degree, symptoms that appear to originate in the trachea and major bronchi are characterized by a constant burning sensation, which is exacerbated by inspiration and is associated with uncontrollable coughing. The most severe symptoms are associated with dyspnea on exertion or even at rest. Onset of symptoms is variable among different individuals but usually occurs after about 12 to 16 hours of exposure at 1.0 ata,[22] 8 to 14 hours at 1.5 ata,[23, 24] and 3 to 6 hours at 2.0 ata.[25, 26]

Changes in pulmonary function which have been measured in humans during and after prolonged exposures to oxygen pressures of 1.0 ata or higher include decrements in inspiratory and expiratory lung volumes and flow rates, carbon monoxide diffusing capacity, and lung compliance.[2, 4, 22–30] Arterial oxygenation was maintained at rest during early reversible stages of pulmonary intoxication[26, 29, 30] but was detectably impaired during exercise after exposure for 48 to 60 hours at 1.0 ata[29] or for 16 to 19 hours at 1.5 ata.[23, 30] In normal humans exposed continuously to oxygen pressures ranging from 1.0 to 3.0 ata, pulmonary mechanical function is impaired earlier and more severely than gas exchange function.[24, 30]

Although it is not possible to identify with certainty a level of hyperoxia which can be tolerated indefinitely with no pulmonary effects, normal humans have been exposed for periods ranging from 7 days at 0.55 ata[31] to 30 days at 0.3 ata[32, 33] with no detectable manifestations of pulmonary intoxication. However, exposure for 24 hours at 0.75 ata causes pulmonary symptoms in association with a significant decrease in vital capacity,[22] and the rate of pulmonary intoxication increases progressively at higher oxygen pressures.[24–26, 30] Nevertheless, the great majority of current applications of hyperoxia in therapy and diving do not cause pulmonary symptoms or functional deficits.[34]

Administration of hyperbaric oxygenation causes pulmonary symptoms in patients only when used very aggressively for serious conditions, such as severe decompression sickness or arterial gas embolism. Some degree of substernal discomfort is also frequently experienced by commercial divers who use intermittent hyperoxia to hasten inert gas elimination after unusually long or deep dives. When hyperbaric oxygenation is combined with saturation exposure in the treatment of refractory decompression sickness, it is not uncommon for the attendants and the patient to experience pulmonary symptoms. In all of these situations, irreversible pulmonary intoxication can be avoided by careful monitoring of symptoms and appropriate alternation of hyperoxic and normoxic exposure periods.

Central Nervous System Oxygen Toxicity

Overt manifestations of CNS oxygen poisoning include the diverse symptoms and signs listed in Table 8–1. These observations were made in divers who breathed oxygen at pressures of 3.0 ata or higher until they experienced neurological effects. The studies were designed to develop reliable methods for detecting the onset of CNS oxygen poisoning prior to the occurrence of convulsions.

Extensive investigation in hundreds of divers failed to identify a consistent preconvulsive index of CNS oxygen poisoning. Minor symptoms did not always precede the onset of convulsions, and even when a preconvulsive aura did occur, it was often followed so quickly by seizures that it had little practical value. Electroencephalography also proved to be a poor

TABLE 8–1. Signs and Symptoms of CNS Oxygen Poisoning in Normal Men

Facial pallor	Respiratory changes
Sweating	Hiccoughs
Bradycardia	Air hunger
Palpitations	Inspiratory predominance
Depression	
Apprehension	Diaphragmatic spasms
Visual symptoms	Nausea
Dazzle	Spasmodic vomiting
Constriction of visual field	Fibrillation of lips
	Lip twitching
Tinnitus and auditory hallucinations	Twitching of cheek, nose, eyelids
Vertigo	Syncope
	Convulsions

Adapted from Donald KW: Oxygen poisoning in man. Br Med J 1:667–672, 712–717, 1947.

index of incipient CNS intoxication, because brain electrical activity was not altered consistently prior to seizure onset. More recent studies have confirmed that EEG alterations in humans occur only upon initiation of the actual seizure.[35]

Although mechanisms are not known, it is well established that exercise and underwater immersion, independently or together, accelerate the onset of oxygen convulsions and can precipitate their occurrence at oxygen pressures as low as 1.6 ata.[36–39] Oxygen convulsions are also accelerated by the presence of acute hypercapnia, whether it be induced by elevation of inspired pCO_2, increased breathing resistance, or narcotic depression of ventilation.[3] The adverse effects of acute hypercapnia are mediated by cerebral vasodilation and delivery of a higher oxygen dose to the brain.[40]

Extensive investigation in animals and in humans[1, 3, 4, 35, 37] has established that oxygen convulsions are not inherently harmful. However, the condition under which they occur may make them extremely hazardous. For example, the occurrence of convulsions in an unattended diver can lead to death by drowning. Similarly, convulsions are especially hazardous in patients with fractures, osseous nonunion, head injury, cardiac abnormality, or recent surgery.

CNS oxygen toxicity in association with hyperbaric oxygen therapy is rare. The reported incidence of convulsions is approximately 0.01 per cent when care is taken to screen against factors that are known to increase risk of intoxication.[34, 41]

Visual Effects of Oxygen Toxicity

Visual manifestations of oxygen poisoning are influenced by many variables in addition to oxygen dose.[3, 42] These additional influences include the age of the exposed individual, the method of oxygen administration, and the presence of underlying conditions that may modify susceptibility to oxygen poisoning.

Retrolental Fibroplasia

Retrolental fibroplasia is a unique condition that may be induced by exposure of the premature infant to any elevation of arterial pO_2 above the normal range.[3, 42] Risk factors include gestational age less than 30 weeks, birthweight less than 1500 grams, and concurrent problems such as sepsis and intraventricular hemorrhage.[43, 44] Initial constriction of the developing retinal vessels is followed by endothelial cell destruction and arrest of the retinal circulation at an incomplete stage of development.[3, 42, 43] The remaining endothelial cells later undergo a disorganized and profuse proliferation to produce a fibrous mass of vascular tissue that ultimately causes irreversible retinal detachment and permanent blindness. Vitamin E therapy is apparently effective in reducing the severity of retrolental fibroplasia.[44]

Irreversible Effects on Visual Function

Animal studies involving extremely prolonged oxygen exposures have demonstrated severe pathological effects, such as visual cell death, retinal detachment, and cytoid body formation.[42] In guinea pigs exposed to oxygen at 3.0 ata, histopathological changes found in the corneal endothelium and lens epithelium, as well as in the retinal plexiform and inner nuclear layers, indicate that pathological effects may be more severe when the entire eye is exposed to oxygen than when hyperoxygenation occurs only by the arterial circulation.[45]

Histological studies of oxygen-induced ocular pathology have not been performed in humans. However, one patient who was exposed to 80 per cent oxygen at 1.0 ata for five months as therapy for myasthenia gravis developed nearly total blindness in association with marked constriction and "silver-wire" formation of the retinal arterioles.[46]

Reversible Loss of Peripheral Vision in Humans

Behnke and co-workers[47] first reported nearly complete, bilateral loss of peripheral vision, leaving only small islands of central vision, in a man who breathed oxygen at 3.0 ata for 3.5

hours. Recovery was essentially complete within 50 minutes postexposure. Other investigators[35, 48] also observed reversible losses of peripheral vision in subjects exposed to similar conditions.

This phenomenon was recently studied more intensively with repeated measurements of visual fields and acuity in 18 subjects exposed to oxygen at 3.0 ata for up to 3.5 hours.[35] Loss of peripheral vision started at 2.5 to 3.0 hours of exposure and progressed to involve about 50 per cent of the visual field area on average, with individual losses as great as 90 per cent at 3.5 hours of exposure. Central visual acuity was not significantly altered. Recovery of peripheral vision was essentially complete within 30 to 45 minutes after exposure termination. Mechanisms for the progressive loss of peripheral vision and its rapid recovery are not known at present.

Individual Predisposition to Oxygen Effects

An apparently increased susceptibility to visual loss during hyperoxic exposure was found in an individual who had recovered many years previously from retrobulbar neuritis in one eye.[49] While serving as a volunteer for an oxygen exposure at 2.0 ata, this subject experienced a progressive loss of vision in the previously affected eye over the last 2 hours of a 6-hour exposure. The visual field gradually expanded over the first 4 hours of recovery, but two paracentral scotomas remained and gradually cleared over a period of about 3 weeks. The observed visual disturbances appeared to involve two separate processes. One consisted of visual field constriction followed by relatively rapid reversal, while the other appeared to represent recurrence of unilateral retrobulbar neuritis with a much slower recovery.

Progressive Myopia

Approximately one third of the patients who receive daily hyperbaric oxygen treatment for a variety of chronic disease states develop some degree of myopia which usually starts after 2 to 4 weeks of therapy and is progressive thereafter.[50, 51] If the individual is initially hyperopic, the refractive error is normalized. After the series of hyperbaric oxygen therapies has ended, reversal of the myopia is nearly always complete over a period of 3 to 6 weeks. Occasionally, complete reversal of myopia can require as long as 6 to 12 months.[51] Although the basis for the myopia has not been determined, elimination of other possible causes implicates a reversible change in lens shape or metabolism.[52]

In a series of 25 patients who received a total of 150 to 850 one-hour exposures at 2.0 to 2.5 ata over a period of 2 to 19 months for refractory leg ulcers, 7 of 15 patients who had clear lens nuclei at the start of therapy developed cataracts. These persisted in five individuals and were only partially reversible in two others after termination of the therapy series.[53] The lens changes were associated with myopia that also was only partially reversible. Fortunately, most clinical conditions that respond favorably to hyperbaric oxygenation do not require such long cumulative periods of oxygen exposure.

Modification of Oxygen Tolerance

The rate of development of oxygen poisoning in intact animals and humans can be influenced by a variety of conditions, procedures, and drugs (Table 8–2). Factors that hasten the onset or increase the severity of toxic effects are listed on the left side of Table 8–2. Although none of these factors should be considered to be an absolute contraindication to the application of hyperbaric oxygenation, the presence of one or more of the listed influences as part of a disease process or its therapy should be regarded as an indication for caution.

Factors listed on the right side of Table 8–2 have been found to delay the onset or decrease the severity of overt manifestations of oxygen poisoning. Some are potentially useful as protective agents under appropriate conditions of O_2 exposure. Unfortunately, most have side

TABLE 8–2. Factors that Modify Rate of Development of Oxygen Poisoning

HASTEN ONSET OR INCREASE SEVERITY	DELAY ONSET OR DECREASE SEVERITY
Adrenocortical hormones	Acclimatization to hypoxia
CO_2 inhalation	Adrenergic blocking drugs
Dextroamphetamine	Antioxidants
Epinephrine	Chlorpromazine
Hyperthermia	Gamma-aminobutyric acid
Insulin	Ganglionic blocking drugs
Norepinephrine	Glutathione
Paraquat	Hypothyroidism
Hyperthyroidism	Reserpine
Vitamin E deficiency	Starvation
	Succinate
	Trisaminomethane
	Intermittent exposure*
	Disulfiram*
	Hypothermia*
	Vitamin E*

*Potentially useful as protective agents.

Adapted from Clark JM, Lambertsen CJ: Pulmonary oxygen toxicity: A review. Pharmacol Rev 23:37–133, 1971.

effects or other limitations that preclude their practical use in humans. Furthermore, effective protection against the multiple and diverse effects of O_2 toxicity requires wide distribution of the protective agent throughout all body tissues, as well as effective opposition to toxic effects of O_2 on a variety of enzymatic targets. The same agent may delay some effects of O_2 toxicity while hastening the onset of others. For example, administration of disulfiram delays the onset of convulsions in animals exposed to O_2 at 4.0 ata,[54, 55] but it enhances the progression of pulmonary intoxication at 1.0[56] or 2.0 ata.[57]

At the present time, the most effective and practical means for extension of oxygen tolerance in humans is the systematic alternation of oxygen exposure intervals with relatively brief normoxic intervals.[3, 4] Initially observed by Soulie,[58] the practical applications of this procedure were first elaborated by Lambertsen,[59] and its efficacy has been demonstrated in animals[60, 61] and in humans.[62] Intermittent O_2 exposure delays the onset of toxic effects in all organs and tissues, and it has none of the limitations that are associated with pharmacological protective agents. The basis for the inherent superiority of this procedure as a means for extension of O_2 tolerance resides in its dependence upon the periodic, sequential elevation and reduction of O_2 tension rather than the passage of a chemical agent across cellular membrane barriers.

CARBON MONOXIDE

Carbon monoxide (CO) is produced by the incomplete combustion of carbonaceous material. The sources of CO are plentiful and with the exception of carbon dioxide (CO_2), CO is the most abundant pollutant present in the lower atmosphere.[63] With a diver, the typical source of poisoning is contaminated air from improperly directed compressor engine exhaust, so that CO can be taken up in the air intake system. In addition to environmental sources, CO is also produced endogenously. It is a byproduct of heme catabolism and may account for perhaps 0.5 per cent saturation of hemoglobin in venous blood.[64–66] This section will focus on exogenous sources of CO and on the clinical impact of this exposure.

The toxic effects of CO result from its binding to hemoglobin and, possibly, other cellular proteins. Clinical consequences seem to be determined by a complex interaction that involves both the extent of CO binding and the physiological alterations associated with exposure. That is to say, the pathophysiology of CO is mediated by both the hypoxia associated with hemoglobin binding, as well as cardiovascular dysfunction giving rise to an ischemic insult.

Uptake

Inhaled CO rapidly diffuses across the alveoli and binds to hemoglobin. The relative affinity of CO for hemoglobin is some 200-fold greater than that of O_2, with some variation within the population.[67, 68] CO uptake follows an exponential function.[69] The rate of uptake is dependent on the percentage of inspired CO and O_2, on the ventilatory rate, and on the duration of exposure to CO.[68, 70]

Elimination

CO elimination also follows an exponential relationship.[70–73] The kinetics in any particular instance, however, is complex and appears to depend on the rate of ventilation, inspired O_2 partial pressure, and possibly the pattern of CO exposure (e.g., brief or prolonged, continuous or discontinuous).[69–76] Thus, in a clinical setting, attempts to estimate a maximum carboxyhemoglobin (COHgb) level by extrapolation using an approximate COHgb half-life (see Table 8–1) is fraught with uncertainty. Recent experience would also suggest that this is unnecessary, as the mortality and morbidity risks have not been found to correlate with the COHgb level.[76, 77]

Mechanism of CO Toxicity

There is a competition between CO and O_2 for binding to hemoproteins. The relative affinity of CO to hemoglobin ranges from 220- to 290-fold greater than that of O_2.[67, 68, 78] Hence, despite a relatively high O_2 partial pressure in the vasculature, CO binds to hemoglobin, which will reduce O_2 carrying capacity.[79, 80] Carboxyhemoglobin increases the affinity of unbound hemoglobin for O_2, thus causing a leftward shift and a more hyperbolic shape in the oxyhemoglobin dissociation curve.[81] These later effects cause a lower tissue and intracellular pO_2 than would otherwise be expected for any given blood O_2 content.

Coburn[82] has estimated that at any given time perhaps 10 to 15 per cent of the total body burden of CO is bound to extravascular proteins. There are a rather large number of proteins that bind CO, but only myoglobin, cytochrome *c* oxidase, and cytochrome P_{450}-linked enzymes have been studied with consideration to probable in vivo effects.[83–88] Even at ambient arterial O_2 tensions, CO can bind to myoglobin, which would interfere with O_2 utilization by muscle cells.[89, 80] There is no strong evidence that CO may alter in a significant fashion in vivo cytochrome P_{450}-linked enzyme activity.[91–94] Chance and co-workers[95] demonstrated that CO can bind to cytochrome *c* oxidase and emphasized that this effect was particularly enhanced during a change from anoxia to normoxia. Hence, CO binding might be expected at a time when there is a transiently high pCO to pO_2 ratio. There is uncertainty regarding the pO_2 in the vicinity of cellular mitochondria; however, even conservative estimates suggest that the tissue pCO in severe CO poisonings is only one tenth that necessary to cause 50 per cent enzyme inhibition.[96, 97] Recent data does suggest that there may be a mild compromise in mitochondrial respiratory function.[98]

As the carboxyhemoglobin level increases during CO poisoning, there is an increasing hypoxia. As pCO/pO_2 ratios increase, CO binding to proteins would be expected to increase. This has been shown with myoglobin when arterial oxygenation is reduced to below 40 mm Hg.[89, 90] A similar phenomenon may occur with cytochrome oxidase. Thus, the pathophysiology of CO may be altered, and binding at extravascular sites may take on increased importance as the carboxyhemoglobin level rises.

Animal studies involving carbohydrate metabolism and respiration have failed to identify any difference between hypoxic hypoxia and CO-mediated hypoxia, thus arguing against a cellular component to CO poisoning.[99–101] When cellular functions and not metabolism are assayed, however, animal studies have suggested that CO-mediated impairment of hemoglobin function cannot solely explain the degree of impairment observed.[102–104] Observations on the effects of very low carboxyhemoglobin levels (~4 to 5 per cent), which should have only negligible effects on tissue pO_2, also suggest that a separate, cellular-level lesion may be present.[105–107]

Pathophysiology

As carboxyhemoglobin levels rise, cerebral vessels dilate,[108] and both coronary blood flow and capillary density increase.[109–111] These are acute, compensatory reactions to CO poisoning. As CO exposure continues, central respiratory depression arises, possibly due to cerebral hypoxia.[112] Animal and human reports have described cardiac effects including a myriad of dysrhythmias, as well as pathological changes that include myocardial hemorrhages, degeneration of muscle fibers, leukocyte infiltration, mural thrombi, and multifocal myocardial necrosis.[113–116]

Acute mortality from CO may be mediated through cerebral hypoxia, either from respiratory depression or from direct, progressive pulmonary shunting and ventilation perfusion imbalance, causing a lowering of arterial O_2 tension.[80, 110, 117] Animal studies suggest that acute mortality may be principally caused by cardiac dysrhythmias, and thus death is from an ischemic insult.[118] There are indications that myocardial impairment may begin at the relatively low carboxyhemoglobin level of approximately 20 per cent. Animals that do not die acutely, but instead show neurological deterioration over the days subsequent to poisoning, appear to have a combined hypoxic and ischemic insult during acute exposure. That is, they have acutely high carboxyhemoglobin levels, and during this hypoxic stress, the normal vascular compensatory reactions are thwarted by a period of hypotension perhaps mediated through CO cardiac toxicity.[82, 118, 120, 121]

Clinical Findings

Among the earliest complaints associated with the rising carboxyhemoglobin level are frontal headache and nausea.[122] Of limited clinical value, but perhaps of value experimentally to suggest a tissue-level CO insult, are findings of diminished visual evoked responses,[122–124] visual brightness discrimination,[125] and subtle auditory dysfunction[126] with carboxyhemoglobin levels less than 10 per cent. It is extremely important to emphasize that while carboxyhemoglobin levels can perhaps be loosely associated with symptomatology, there is no direct correlation between a carboxyhemoglobin level and the severity of symptoms. This has been borne out in the authors' experience treating over 200 cases of acute CO poisoning, as well as in experience reported by others.[76, 77, 127, 128] Grossly speaking, at carboxyhemoglobin levels greater than 20 per cent, patients may experience severe headache, palpitation, confusion, weakness, syncope, and seizures. Objectively, in addition to alterations in neurological status, tachycardia and tachypnea may be noted. Notable in its absence, it is extraordinarily rare to observe "cherry red" coloration of skin except among those who have died.[129–131]

Morbidity and mortality risks appear to be

TABLE 8–3. Delayed Neurological Sequelae of CO Poisoning

Choreoathetosis	Hemiplegia
Cortical blindness	Hysteria
Dementia	Mutism
Depression	Parkinsonism
Disorientation	Peripheral neuropathy
Epilepsy	Personality changes
Gait disturbances	Speech disturbances
Hearing impairment	Urinary/fecal incontinence

greater among patients with prior cardiovascular disease and with age greater than 60 years and among those who have suffered an interval of unconsciousness during CO exposure.[127] The duration of coma portends greater risk, but it appears that any history of loss of consciousness places the patient at greater risk of CO-mediated morbidity. Approximately 30 to 40 per cent of CO victims die prior to hospitalization.[76, 131] Of those hospitalized, approximately 2 per cent die, 10 per cent make a partial recovery, and 10 per cent or more suffer what are described as delayed neurological deteriorations.[116, 131, 132]

Delayed neurological deterioration subsequent to CO poisoning was first reported by Grinker.[133] Since then several reports have described the clinical features of this disorder (Table 8–3).[127, 134–138] As might be expected, there are not uniform pathological correlations with these varied signs and symptoms. The lesions are often associated with patchy white matter damage and commonly are referred to as myelinopathy or leukoencephalopathy[132, 134–141] Among the reports of gray matter damage, the frequency of involvement of the basal ganglia is striking.[140, 141] Pathological changes similar to these may arise subsequent to any form of ischemic-hypoxic brain insult.[137, 142] There appears, however, to be a markedly greater risk among CO victims. In a large retrospective survey, Shillito and colleagues reported an incidence of delayed neurological sequelae of 0.8 per cent.[143] Meigs and Hughes observed this phenomenon in 9 of 105 cases.[116] More recent studies involving rigorous and quantitative estimations of neurological function have indicated that the incidence may be 10 to 40 per cent among patients admitted to a hospital for CO poisoning.[77, 131] Some recent opinions that reflect a small experience downplay the patient's risk.[144] Others, however, have emphasized the alarming onset of these changes in patients who seem to have recovered.[145, 146]

Treatment

In addition to general supportive care, supplemental O_2 inhalation is a cornerstone in the treatment of CO poisoning. Carboxyhemoglobin dissociation is hastened by an elevation in the O_2 partial pressure of inspired gas. Hyperbaric O_2 hastens dissociation beyond a rate achievable by breathing pure O_2 at sea-level pressure.[71, 75, 147] Due to this fact, hyperbaric O_2 has been used to treat severe CO poisoning for more than 25 years. Numerous reports attest to the efficacy of hyperbaric O_2 in reversing severe neurological and cardiovascular depression in CO poisoning.[148–153] Experience has demonstrated that hyperbaric O_2 may reverse CO-mediated neurological depression even after the carboxyhemoglobin level has fallen.[152, 154, 155] In a large retrospective study, Goulon and coworkers demonstrated that prompt administration of hyperbaric O_2 may dramatically reduce mortality.[151]

A recent separate issue regarding therapy has involved interest in treating patients with an increased risk for developing delayed neurological sequelae, even if they do not necessarily manifest evidence of serious poisoning. Several reports have indicated that prompt administration of hyperbaric O_2 may reduce the incidence of delayed neurological sequelae.[156–158] Assessment of the mechanism for hyperbaric O_2-mediated reduction in neurological sequelae is obviously hampered by a poor understanding of the mechanism behind the clinical disorder itself. Among the hypothesized mechanisms, lipid peroxidation within the central nervous system secondary to the hypoxic-ischemic insult has been suggested.[159] Brain lipid peroxidation was recently identified in an animal model, and hyperbaric O_2 was shown to block this process.[160] The underlying biochemistry responsible for this effect is not as yet fully elucidated.

Based on the body of information currently available, it is generally recommended that patients who manifest signs of serious intoxication should be referred for hyperbaric treatment. Clinical data support the administration of hyperbaric O_2 to any patient who has suffered an interval of unconsciousness, as they are at greater risk of suffering delayed neurological sequelae.[76, 77] The determination of subtle central nervous system involvement can be difficult. Utilization of a modified psychometric screening battery has been found to be useful in identifying compromised patients.[161] The body of clinical data available suggests that functional testing, rather than a carboxyhemoglobin level, may be a more sensitive method for determining the appropriate treatment among less severely symptomatic patients.

CARBON DIOXIDE

Carbon dioxide is a product of oxidative metabolism and hence is not a toxin in the most traditional sense. Intoxication results either from exposure to respiratory gases containing high concentrations of CO_2 or from retention of autogenous CO_2 due to inadequate ventilatory equipment or pathological states (e.g., emphysema). In diving medicine, acute CO_2 intoxication can be caused by inadequate CO_2 elimination from closed spaces (e.g., diving bells, submersibles, underwater habitats, recompression chambers) or from closed or semi-closed underwater breathing equipment.[162, 163]

Any physiological or toxic action of CO_2 must be referable to an increased partial pressure of molecular CO_2 and/or to an increased hydrogen ion concentration.[163] Since molecular CO_2 freely crosses cell membranes to penetrate intracellular as well as extracellular fluid compartments, these two potential agents are inseparable. In a similar manner, any toxic effects of CO_2 are superimposed upon and, to some extent, inseparable from fundamental physiological influences that include the following: (1) stimulant actions of CO_2 on central and peripheral chemoreceptors provide an important link in the regulation of internal, acid-base homeostasis; (2) relaxant effects of CO_2 on vascular smooth muscle are involved in the regulation of brain circulation; (3) excessive CO_2 partial pressures can depress the same neural structures that are stimulated by lower levels of pCO_2; and (4) CO_2-induced acidosis has nearly simultaneous influences on a wide range of biochemical reactions on both sides of membrane and vascular barriers.[162, 163]

Acute Exposure to Hypercapnia

Acute exposure to CO_2 at concentrations ranging from 0 to more than 20 per cent at normal atmospheric pressure produces effects that range from barely detectable stimulation of ventilation to loss of consciousness and convulsions, depending on the level inspired[162, 163] (Table 8–4). The ventilatory response to CO_2 administration is nearly linear over minute volumes of about 12 to 65 liters/minute for inspired levels of 4 to 10 per cent and gradually levels off to approach 90 liters/minute for 30 per cent inspired CO_2.[162] The curve for cerebral blood flow has a similar configuration in the monkey and presumably also in humans, with a nearly linear increase over the arterial pCO_2 range of about 30 to 80 mm Hg.[164]

TABLE 8–4. Signs and Symptoms of Acute Hypercapnia in Normal Men

Percent CO_2* (sea-level equivalent)	Effect
0–4	No CNS derangement
4–6	Dyspnea, anxiety
6–10	Impaired mental capabilities
10–15	Severely impaired mental function
15–20	Loss of consciousness
> 20	Uncoordinated muscular twitching, convulsions

*Biological activity of a gas is determined by its partial pressure rather than its concentration. Hence, at depth the effect of an inspired gas becomes greater.

Exposure of humans to inspired CO_2 concentrations of 15 to 20 per cent causes an abrupt and violent onset of respiratory distress that is accompanied by rapid loss of consciousness and spasms of neuromuscular twitching.[162, 163] Therapeutic exposures to inspired CO_2 levels of 20 to 30 per cent in oxygen cause convulsions within 1 to 3 minutes.[162, 163] Any accidental exposure to such a high CO_2 concentration would be extremely dangerous, because even one breath causes the onset of mental incapacitation.[162] Electrocardiographic responses to similar levels of hypercapnia include tachycardia, nodal and ventricular premature contractions, inverted P-waves, and increased amplitude of T-waves.[165, 166] In monkeys and dogs exposed to CO_2 concentrations of 30 to 40 per cent, cardiac activity was sustained for many hours and remained stable when inspired pCO_2 was gradually reduced to zero.[167, 168] However, when the dogs were moved abruptly to room air, most of the animals experienced ventricular fibrillation and death.[168] Presumably, the terminal arrhythmias were caused by failure to allow sufficient time for restoration of normal cardiac excitability by reversal of ionic shifts induced by prolonged and extreme hypercapnia.[163]

Elevation of inspired pCO_2 during exercise interferes with the elimination of metabolically produced CO_2.[163] Under these conditions, a balance between the rates of CO_2 elimination and its production is restored by concurrent increments in arterial pCO_2 and the rate of pulmonary ventilation.[169–172] Physically fit young men are able to achieve maximum levels of oxygen uptake ($\dot{V}O_2$) during exposure to inspired pCO_2 levels up to 21 mm Hg[169, 171] and can tolerate working at 80 per cent of maximum $\dot{V}O_2$ at an inspired pCO_2 of 40 mm Hg.[172]

Chronic Exposure to Hypercapnia

Chronic pCO_2 elevations in all body fluids can occur in patients with pulmonary insufficiency[173] or in normal individuals who are exposed to increased inspired pCO_2 levels for experimental purposes[170, 174] or as a potential consequence of inadequate CO_2 removal from a closed-system aerospace or undersea habitat.[163] Compensatory responses to sustained hypercapnia include renal,[175] acid-base,[176–178] respiratory,[173, 174] and circulatory[179] adaptations. The kidney responds initially by increasing the tubular reabsorption of bicarbonate and later complements this with increased ammonia production to enhance excretion of hydrogen ions.[175] Together, these processes augment both extracellular and intracellular concentrations of bicarbonate and other bases to return hydrogen ion concentrations toward normal levels.[176–178] The acid-base alterations are associated with respiratory adjustments that are manifested in normal humans by a shift of the pulmonary ventilation-arterial pCO_2 response curve to higher pCO_2 levels with no change in the slope of the curve.[174] Studies in monkeys show that cerebral blood flow responses to arterial pCO_2 elevation are also attenuated during exposure to chronic hypercapnia as manifested, in this case, by reduction in the slope of the curve with no apparent change in the initial response threshold.[180]

Normal humans have been exposed to inspired pCO_2 levels of 30 mm Hg for up to 11 days and 21 mm Hg for 30 days with no pathological or residual effects.[170, 174] Ventilatory and acid-base adjustments that occurred during the first day of chronic hypercapnia were promptly reversed upon resumption of air breathing. The ability to perform heavy exercise while breathing an inspired pCO_2 level of 21 mm Hg is not impaired by 30 days of chronic exposure.[170]

REFERENCES

1. Bean JW: Effects of oxygen at increased pressure. Physiol Rev 25:1–147, 1945.
2. Clark JM, Lambertsen CJ: Pulmonary oxygen toxicity: A review. Pharmacol Rev 23:37–133, 1971.
3. Lambertsen CJ: Effects of hyperoxia on organs and their tissues. *In* Robin ED (ed): Extrapulmonary Manifestations of Respiratory Disease. Lung Biology in Health and Disease. Vol. 8. New York, Marcel Dekker, 1978, pp 239–303.
4. Clark JM: Oxygen toxicity. *In* Bennett PB, Elliott DH (eds): The Physiology and Medicine of Diving and Compressed Air Work. London, Balliere-Tindall, 1983; pp 200–238.
5. Gerschman R: Biological effects of oxygen. *In* Dickens F, Neil E (eds): Oxygen in the Animal Organism. New York, Macmillan, 1964, pp 475–494.
6. Gerschman R, Gilbert DL, Nye SW, et al: Oxygen poisoning and x-irradiation: A mechanism in common. Science 119:623–626, 1954.
7. Gilbert DL: The role of pro-oxidants and anti-oxidants in oxygen toxicity. Radiat Res Suppl 3:44–53, 1963.
8. Gilbert DL: Atmosphere and evolution. *In* Dickens F, Neil E (eds): Oxygen in the Animal Organism. New York, Macmillan, 1964, pp 641–654.
9. Fridovich I: The biology of oxygen radicals. Science 201:875–880, 1978.
10. Fisher AB, Bassett DJP, Forman JH: Oxygen toxicity of the lung: Biochemical aspects. *In* Fishman AP, Renkin EM (eds): Pulmonary Edema. Bethesda, American Physiological Society, 1979, pp 207–216.
11. Pryor WA (ed): Free Radicals in Biology. New York, Academic Press, 1976 (Vols 1 & 2), 1977 (Vol 3), 1980 (Vol 4).
12. Halliwell B, Gutteridge JMC: Oxygen toxicity, oxygen radicals, transition metals and disease. Biochem J 219:1–14, 1984.
13. Fisher AB, Forman HJ: Oxygen utilization and toxicity in the lungs. *In* Fishman AP, Fisher AB (eds): Handbook of Physiology. Vol. 1, Sect. 3. Bethesda, American Physiological Society, 1985, pp 231–254.
14. Kaplan HP, Robinson FR, Kapanci Y, Weibel ER: Pathogenesis and reversibility of the pulmonary lesions of oxygen toxicity in monkeys. I. Clinical and light microscopic studies. Lab Invest 20:94–100, 1969.
15. Kapanci Y, Weibel ER, Kaplan HP, Robinson FR: Pathogenesis and reversibility of the pulmonary lesions of oxygen toxicity in monkeys. II. Ultrastructural and morphometric studies. Lab Invest 20:101–118, 1969.
16. Robinson FR, Harper DT Jr, Thomas AA, Kaplan HP: Proliferative pulmonary lesions in monkeys exposed to high concentrations of oxygen. Aerosp Med 38:481–486, 1967.
17. Robinson FR, Sopher RL, Witchett CE: Pathology of normobaric oxygen toxicity in primates. Aerosp Med 40:879–884, 1969.
18. Nash G, Blennerhassett JB, Pontoppidan H: Pulmonary lesions associated with oxygen therapy and artificial ventilation. N Engl J Med 276:368–374, 1967.
19. Brewis RA: Oxygen toxicity during artificial ventilation. Thorax 24:656–666, 1969.
20. Hyde RW, Rawson AJ: Unintentional iatrogenic oxygen pneumonitis—response to therapy. Ann Intern Med 71:517–531, 1969.
21. Kapanci Y, Tosco R, Eggermann J, Gould VE: Oxygen pneumonitis in man. Light and electron-microscopic morphometric studies. Chest 62:162–169, 1972.
22. Comroe JH Jr, Dripps RD, Dumke PR, Deming M: Oxygen toxicity: The effect of inhalation of high concentrations of oxygen for twenty-four hours on normal men at sea level and at a simulated altitude of 18,000 feet. JAMA 128:710–717, 1945.
23. Clark JM, Gelfand R, Flores ND, et al: Pulmonary mechanics and gas exchange in man during and after oxygen exposure at 1.5 ata for 16 to 19 hours. Am Rev Resp Dis 133(4, pt 2):A31, 1986.
24. Clark JM, Gelfand R, Flores ND, et al: Pulmonary tolerance in man to continuous oxygen exposure at 3.0, 2.5, 2.0, and 1.5 ata in predictive studies V. *In* Bove AA, Bachrach AJ, Greenbaum LJ (eds):

Underwater and Hyperbaric Physiology IX. Bethesda, Undersea and Hyperbaric Medical Society, 1987, pp 737–749.

25. Clark JM, Lambertsen CJ: Pulmonary oxygen tolerance and the rate of development of pulmonary oxygen toxicity in man at two atmospheres inspired oxygen tension. *In* Lambertsen CJ (ed): Proceedings of the Third Symposium on Underwater Physiology. Baltimore, Williams & Wilkins, 1967, pp 439–457.
26. Clark JM, Lambertsen CJ: Rate of development of pulmonary O_2 toxicity in man during O_2 breathing at 2.0 atm abs. J Appl Physiol 30:739–752, 1971.
27. Fisher AB, Hyde RW, Puy RJM, et al: Effect of oxygen at 2 atmospheres on the pulmonary mechanics of normal man. J Appl Physiol 24:529–536, 1968.
28. Puy RJM, Hyde RW, Fisher AB, et al: Alterations in the pulmonary capillary bed during early O_2 toxicity in man. J Appl Physiol 24:537–543, 1968.
29. Caldwell PRB, Lee WL Jr, Schildkraut HS, Archibald ER: Changes in lung volume, diffusing capacity, and blood gases in men breathing oxygen. J Appl Physiol 21:1477–1483, 1966.
30. Clark JM: Pulmonary limits of oxygen tolerance in man. Exp Lung Res 14:897–910, 1988.
31. Michel EL, Langevin RW, Gell CF: Effect of continuous human exposure to oxygen tension of 418 mm Hg for 168 hours. Aerosp Med 31:138–144, 1960.
32. Herlocher JE, Quigley DG, Behar VS, et al: Physiologic response to increased oxygen partial pressure. I. Clinical observations. Aerosp Med 35:613–618, 1964.
33. Robertson WG, Hargreaves JJ, Herlocher JE, Welch BE: Physiologic response to increased oxygen partial pressure. II. Respiratory studies. Aerosp Med 35:618–622, 1964.
34. Davis JC, Dunn JM, Heimbach RD: Hyperbaric medicine: Patient selection, treatment procedures, and side-effects. *In* Davis JC, Hunt TK (eds): Problem Wounds: The Role of Oxygen. New York, Elsevier, 1988, pp 225–235.
35. Lambertsen CJ, Clark JM, Gelfand R, et al: Definition of tolerance to continuous hyperoxia in man. An abstract report of Predictive Studies V. *In* Bove AA, Bachrach AJ, Greenbaum LJ (eds): Underwater and Hyperbaric Physiology IX. Bethesda, Undersea and Hyperbaric Medical Society, 1987, pp 717–735.
36. Donald KW: Oxygen poisoning in man. Br Med J 1:667–672, 712–717, 1947.
37. Yarbrough OD, Welham W, Brinton EJ, Behnke AR: Symptoms of oxygen poisoning and limits of tolerance at rest and at work. Nav Exp Diving Unit Rep 01-47, 1947.
38. Butler FK, Thalmann ED: CNS oxygen toxicity in closed-circuit scuba divers. *In* Bachrach AJ, Matzen MM (eds): Underwater Physiology VIII. Proceedings of the Eighth Symposium on Underwater Physiology. Bethesda, Undersea Medical Society, 1984, pp 15–30.
39. Butler FK, Thalmann ED: Central nervous system oxygen toxicity in closed circuit scuba divers II. Undersea Biomed Res 13:193–223, 1986.
40. Lambertsen CJ, Ewing JH, Kough RH, et al: Oxygen toxicity. Arterial and internal jugular blood gas composition in man during inhalation of air, 100% O_2 and 2% CO_2 in O_2 at 3.5 atmospheres ambient pressure. J Appl Physiol 8:255–263, 1955.
41. Hart GB, Strauss MB: Central nervous system oxygen toxicity in a clinical setting. *In* Bove AA, Bachrach AJ, Greenbaum LJ (eds): Undersea and Hyperbaric Physiology IX. Bethesda, Undersea and Hyperbaric Medical Society, 1987, pp 695–699.
42. Nichols CW, Lambertsen CJ: Effects of high oxygen pressures on the eye. N Engl J Med 281:25–30, 1969.
43. Terry TL: Extreme prematurity and fibroblastic overgrowth of persistent vascular sheath behind each crystalline lens. Am J Ophthalmol 25:203–204, 1942.
44. Hittner HM, Godio LB, Rudolph AJ, et al: Retrolental fibroplasia: Efficacy of vitamin E in a double-blind clinical study of preterm infants. N Engl J Med 305:1365–1371, 1981.
45. Nichols CW, Yanoff M, Hall DA, Lambertsen CJ: Histologic alterations produced in the eye by oxygen at high pressure. Arch Ophthalmol 87:417–421, 1972.
46. Kobayashi T, Murakami S: Blindness of an adult caused by oxygen. JAMA 219:741–742, 1972.
47. Behnke AR, Forbes HS, Motley EP: Circulatory and visual effects of oxygen at 3 atmospheres pressure. Am J Physiol 114:436–442, 1936.
48. Rosenberg E, Shibata HR, MacLean LD: Blood gas and neurological responses to inhalation of oxygen at 3 atmospheres. Proc Soc Exp Biol Med 122:313–317, 1966.
49. Nichols CW, Lambertsen CJ, Clark JM: Transient unilateral loss of vision associated with oxygen at high pressure. Arch Ophthalmol 81:548–552, 1969.
50. Anderson B Jr, Farmer JC Jr: Hyperoxic myopia. Trans Am Ophthalmol Soc 76:116–124, 1978.
51. Lyne AJ: Ocular effects of hyperbaric oxygen. Trans Ophthalmol Soc UK 98:66–68, 1978.
52. Anderson B Jr, Shelton DL: Axial length in hyperoxic myopia. *In* Bove AA, Bachrach AJ, Greenbaum LJ (eds): Underwater and Hyperbaric Physiology IX. Bethesda, Undersea and Hyperbaric Medical Society, 1987, pp 607–611.
53. Palmquist BM, Philipson B, Barr PO: Nuclear cataract and myopia during hyperbaric oxygen therapy. Br J Ophthalmol 68:113–117, 1984.
54. Faiman MD, Mehl RG, Oehme FW: Protection with disulfiram from central and pulmonary oxygen toxicity. Biochem Pharmacol 20:3059–3067, 1971.
55. Faiman MD, Nolan RJ, Oehme FW: Effect of disulfiram on oxygen toxicity in beagle dogs. Aerosp Med 45:29–32, 1974.
56. Deneke SM, Bernstein SP, Fanburg BL: Enhancement by disulfiram (Antabuse) of toxic effects of 95 to 97% oxygen on the rat lung. J Pharmacol Exp Ther 208:377–380, 1979.
57. Forman HJ, York JL, Fisher AB: Mechanism for the potentiation of oxygen toxicity by disulfiram. J Pharmacol Exp Ther 212:452–455, 1980.
58. Soulie P: Modifications expèrimentales de la rèsistance individuelle de certains animaux à l'action toxique de l'oxygène. CR Sèances Soc Biol 130:541–542, 1939.
59. Lambertsen CJ: Respiratory and circulatory actions of high oxygen pressure. *In* Goff LG (ed): Proceedings of the Underwater Physiology Symposium. Washington, DC, National Academy of Sciences, National Research Council, Publ 377, 1955, pp 25–38.
60. Penrod KE: Effect of intermittent nitrogen exposures on tolerance to oxygen at high pressure. Am J Physiol 186:149–151, 1956.
61. Hall DA: The influence of the systematic fluctuation of P_{O_2} upon the nature and rate of development of oxygen toxicity in guinea pigs. Masters Degree Thesis, University of Pennsylvania, 1967.

62. Hendricks PL, Hall DA, Hunter WL Jr, Haley PJ: Extension of pulmonary oxygen tolerance in man at 2 ata by intermittent oxygen exposure. J Appl Physiol 42:593–599, 1977.
63. Jaffe LS: Sources, characteristics and fate of atmospheric carbon monoxide. Ann NY Acad Sci 174:76–88, 1970.
64. Coburn RF, Blakemore WS, Forster RE: Endogenous carbon monoxide production in man. J Clin Invest 42:1172–1178, 1983.
65. Coburn RF, Williams WH, Forster RE: Effect of erythrocyte destruction on carbon monoxide production in man. J Clin Invest 43:1098–1103, 1964.
66. Coburn RF, Williams WJ, White P, Kohn SB: The production of carbon monoxide from hemoglobin in vivo. J Clin Invest 46:346–351, 1967.
67. Rodkey FL, O'Neal JD, Collison HA, Uddin DE: Relative affinity of hemoglobin S and hemoglobin A for carbon monoxide and oxygen. Clin Chem 20:83–84, 1974.
68. Roughton FJW, Darling RC: The effect of carbon monoxide on the oxyhemoglobin dissociation curve. Am J Physiol 141:17–31, 1944.
69. Coburn RF, Forster RE, Kane PB: Considerations of the physiological variables that determine the blood carboxyhemoglobin concentration in man. J Clin Invest 44:1899–1910, 1965.
70. Forbes WH, Sargent F, Roughton FJW: The rate of carbon monoxide uptake in normal men. Am J Physiol 143:594–608, 1945.
71. Pace N, Strajman E, Walken EL: Acceleration of carbon monoxide elimination in man by high pressure oxygen. Science 111:652–654, 1950.
72. Peterson JE, Steward RD: Absorption and elimination of carbon monoxide by inactive young men. Arch Environ Health 21:165–171, 1970.
73. Rood WS: Carbon monoxide. *In* Fenn WD, Rahn H (eds): Handbook of Physiology. Vol II, Sect 3. Washington, D.C., American Physiological Society, 1965.
74. Wagner JA, Howath SM, Dahms JE: Carbon monoxide elimination. Respirat Physiol 23:41–47, 1975.
75. Britton JS, Myers RAM: Effects of hyperbaric treatment on carbon monoxide elimination in humans. Undersea Biomed Res 12:431–438, 1985.
76. Garland H, Pearce J: Neurological complications of carbon monoxide poisoning. Q J Med 144:445–455, 1967.
77. Choi IJ: Delayed neurologic sequelae in carbon monoxide intoxication. Arch Neurol 40:433–435, 1983.
78. Killick EM: Carbon monoxide anoxemia. Physiol Rev 20:313–318, 1940.
79. Douglas CG, Haddane JS, Haldane JBS: The laws of combination of hemoglobin with carbon monoxide and oxygen. J Physiol 44:275–304, 1912.
80. Haldane J, Smith JL: The absorption of oxygen in the lungs. J Physiol 22:231–258, 1897.
81. Fenn WO, Cobb DM: The burning of carbon monoxide by heart and skeletal muscle. Am J Physiol 102:393–401, 1932.
82. Coburn RF: The carbon monoxide body stores. Ann NY Acad Sci 174:11–22, 1970.
83. Wohlrab H, Orunmala GB: Carbon monoxide binding studies of cytochrome a[3] heme in intact rat liver mitochondria. Biochemistry 10:1103–1106, 1971.
84. Taniguchi S, Hoshita N, Okuda K: Enzymatic characteristics of CO sensitive 26 hydroxylase system for 5B cholestane 3, 7, 12 triol in rat liver mitochondria and its mitochondrial localization. Eur J Biochem 40:607–617, 1973.
85. Fisher AB, Itakura N, Dodia C, Thurman RG: Relationship between alveolar P_{O_2} and the rate of p-nitroanisole O-demethylation by the cytochrome P450 pathway in isolated rabbit lungs. J Clin Invest 64:770–774, 1979.
86. Cooper DY, Levin S, Narasimhulu S, et al: Photochemical action spectrum of the terminal oxidase of mixed function oxidase systems. Science 147:400–402, 1965.
87. Lotlikan PD, Zaleski K: Inhibitory effect of carbon monoxide in the N- and ring hydroxylation of 2 acetamidofluorene by hamster hepatic microsomal preparations. Biochem J 144:427–430, 1974.
88. Antonini E: Interrelationship between structure and function in hemoglobin and myoglobin. Physiol Rev 45:123–170, 1965.
89. Coburn RF, Mayers LB: Myoglobin O_2 tension determined from measurements of carboxymyoglobin in skeletal muscle. Am J Physiol 220:66–74, 1971.
90. Coburn RF, Ploegmakers F, Gondrie P, Abboud R: Myocardial myoglobin oxygen tension. Am J Physiol 224:870–876, 1973.
91. Montgomery MR, Rubin RJ: Oxygenation during inhibition of drug metabolism by carbon monoxide or hypoxic hypoxia. J Appl Physiol 35:505–509, 1973.
92. Montgomery MR, Rubin RJ: Adaptation to the inhibitory effect of carbon monoxide inhalation on drug metabolism. J Appl Physiol 35:601–607, 1973.
93. Roth RA, Rubin RJ: Comparison of the effect of carbon monoxide and of hypoxic hypoxia. II. Hexobarbital metabolism in the isolated, perfused rat liver. J Pharmacol Exp Ther 199:61–66, 1976.
94. Roth RA, Rubin AJ: Role of blood flow in carbon monoxide and hypoxic hypoxia induced alterations in hexobarbital metabolism in rats. Drug Metab Dispos 4:460–467, 1976.
95. Chance B, Erecinska M, Wagner M: Mitochondrial responses to carbon monoxide toxicity. Ann NY Acad Sci 174:193–204, 1970.
96. Ball EG, Strittwather CF, Cooper D: The reaction of cytochrome oxidase with carbon monoxide. J Biol Chem 193:635–647, 1951.
97. Rosenthal M, LaMauna JC, Jobsis FF, et al: Effects of respiratory gases on cytochrome a an intact cerebral cortex: Is there a critical P_{O_2}? Brain Res 108:143–154, 1976.
98. Walum E, Varnbo I, Peterson A: Effects of dissolved carbon monoxide on the respiratory activity of perfused neuronal and muscle cell cultures. Clin Toxicol 23:299–308, 1985.
99. MacMillan V: Cerebral carbohydrate metabolism during acute carbon monoxide intoxication. Brain Res 121:271–286, 1977.
100. Winston JM, Roberts RJ: Glucose catabolism following carbon monoxide or hypoxic hypoxia exposure. Biochem Pharmacol 27:377–380, 1978.
101. Halebian P, Robinson N, Bave P, et al: Whole body oxygen utilization during acute carbon monoxide poisoning and isocapneic nitrogen hypoxia. J Trauma 26:110–117, 1986.
102. Raybourn MS, Cork C, Schimmerling W, Tobins CA: An in vitro electrophysiological assessment of the direct cellular toxicity of carbon monoxide. Toxicol Appl Pharmacol 46:769–779, 1978.
103. Ingenito AJ, Durlacher L: Effects of carbon monoxide on the b wave of the cat electroretinogram: Comparisons with nitrogen hypoxia, epinephrine, vasodilator drugs and changes in respiratory tidal volume. J Pharmacol Exp Ther 211:638–646, 1979.
104. Savolainen H, Kurppa K, Tenhunen R, Kivisto H:

Biochemical effects of carbon monoxide poisoning in rat brain with special reference to blood carboxyhemoglobin and cerebral cytochrome oxidase activity. Neurosci Lett 19:319–323, 1980.
105. Coburn RF, Forman HJ: Carbon monoxide toxicity. *In* Fishman AP, Farhi LE, Geiger SR (eds): Handbook of Physiology. Baltimore, Williams & Wilkins, 1987, pp 439–456.
106. Laties V: Carbon monoxide and behavior. Arch Neurol 167:68–126, 1980.
107. Longo LD: The biological effects of carbon monoxide on the pregnant woman, fetus and newborn infant. Am J Obstet Gynecol 12:69–103, 1977.
108. Traystman RJ, Fitzgerald RS, Losutoff SC: Cerebral circulatory responses to arterial hypoxia in normal and chemodenervated dogs. Circ Res 42:649–657, 1978.
109. Adams JD, Erickson HH, Stone HL: Myocardial metabolism during exposure to carbon monoxide in the unconscious dog. J Appl Physiol 34:238–242, 1973.
110. Ayres SM, Giannelli S, Meuller H: Myocardial and systemic responses to carboxyhemoglobin. Ann NY Acad Sci 174:268–293, 1970.
111. Kleinert HD, Scales JL, Weiss HP: Effects of carbon monoxide or low oxygen gas mixture inhalation on regional oxygenation, blood flow, and small vessel blood content of the rabbit heart. Pfleugers Arch 383:105–111, 1980.
112. Korner PI, Uther JB, White SW: Central nervous integration of the circulatory and respiratory responses to arterial hypoxia in the rabbit. Circ Res 24:757–776, 1969.
113. Anderson RF, Allensworth DC, DeGroot WJ: Myocardial toxicity from carbon monoxide poisoning. Ann Intern Med 67:1172–1182, 1967.
114. Cosby RS, Bergeron M: Electrocardiographic changes in carbon monoxide poisoning. Am J Cardiol 11:93–96, 1963.
115. Ehrich WE, Bellet S, Lewey FH: Cardiac changes from CO poisoning. Am J Med Sci 208:511–523, 1944.
116. Meigs JW, Hughes JPW: Acute carbon monoxide poisoning. An analysis of one hundred five cases. Arch Ind Hyg Occup Med 6:344–346, 1952.
117. Brouillard RP, Conrad ME, Bensinger TA: Effect of blood in the gut on measurements of endogenous carbon monoxide production. Blood 45:67–69, 1975.
118. Ginsberg MD, Myers RE, McDonagh BF: Experimental carbon monoxide encephalopathy in the primate. Arch Neurol 30:209–216, 1974.
119. Cramlet SH, Erickson HH, Gorman HA: Ventricular function following carbon monoxide exposure. J Appl Physiol 39:482–486, 1975.
120. Okeda R, Funata N, Takano T, et al: The pathogenesis of carbon monoxide encephalopathy in the acute phase—physiological and morphological condition. Acta Neuropathol 54:1–10, 1981.
121. Okeda AR, Funata N, Song JJ, et al: Comparative study on pathogenesis of selective cerebral lesions in carbon monoxide poisoning and nitrogen hypoxia in cats. Acta Neuropathol 56:265–272, 1982.
122. Stewart RD, Peterson JE, Baretta ED, et al: Experimental human exposure to carbon monoxide. Arch Environ Health 21:154–164, 1970.
123. Lilieuthal JL, Fugitt CH: The effect of low carbon monoxide concentrations on the altitude tolerance of man. Am J Physiol 145:359–364, 1946.
124. Vollmer ED: The effects of carbon monoxide on three types of performance at simulated altitudes of 10,000 and 15,000 feet. J Exp Psychol 36:244–251, 1946.
125. McFarland RA, Roughton FJW, Halperin MH: The effects of carbon monoxide and altitude on visual thresholds. J Aviat Med 15:381–384, 1944.
126. Beard RR, Wertheim GA: Behavioral impairment associated with small doses of carbon monoxide. Am J Public Health 57:2012–2022, 1967.
127. Min SK: A brain syndrome associated with delayed neuropsychiatric sequelae following acute carbon monoxide intoxication. Acta Psychiatr Scand 73:80–86, 1986.
128. Winter PM, Miller JN: Carbon monoxide poisoning. JAMA 236:1502–1504, 1976.
129. Matthew H: Acute poisoning: Some myths and misconceptions. Br Med J 1:519–522, 1971.
130. Norman JN, Ledingham I McA: Carbon monoxide poisoning: Investigations and treatment. Prog Brain Res 24:101–122, 1967.
131. Smith JS, Brandon S: Acute carbon monoxide poisoning—3 years experience in a defined population. Postgrad Med J 46:65–70, 1970.
132. Richardson JC, Chambers RA, Heyward PM: Encephalopathies of anoxia and hypoglycemia. Arch Neurol 1:178–182, 1959.
133. Grinker RR: Parkinsonism following carbon monoxide poisoning. J Nerv Ment Dis 64:18–28, 1926.
134. Courville CB: The process of demyelination in the central nervous system. IV. Demyelination as delayed residual of carbon monoxide asphyxia. J Nerv Ment Dis 125:534–546, 1957.
135. Gordan EB: Carbon monoxide encephalopathy. Br Med J 1:1232, 1965.
136. Hsu YK, Ch'eng YL: Cerebral subcortical myelinopathy in carbon monoxide poisoning. Brain 61:384–392, 1938.
137. Plum F, Posner JB, Hain RF: Delayed neurological deterioration after anoxia. Arch Intern Med 110:18–25, 1962.
138. Schwedenberg JH: Leukoencephalopathy following carbon monoxide asphyxia. J Neuropath Exp Neurol 18:597–608, 1959.
140. LaPresele J Fardeau, M: The central nervous system and carbon monoxide poisoning. II. Anatomical study of brain lesions following intoxication with carbon monoxide (22 cases). Prog Brain Res 24:31–74, 1967.
141. Ginsberg MD: Delayed neurological deterioration following hypoxia. *In* Faha S, Davis JN, Rowland LP (eds): Cerebral Hypoxia and its Consequences, Advances in Neurology. Vol 21. New York, Raven Press, 1976, p 21.
142. Ginsberg MD, Hedley-Whyte T, Richardson EP: Hypoxic-ischemic leukoencephalopathy in man. Arch Neurol 33:5–14, 1976.
143. Shillito FH, Drinker CK, Shaughnessy TJ: The problem of nervous and mental sequelae in carbon monoxide poisoning. JAMA 106:669–674, 1936.
144. Strahl KP, Feldman NT, Saunders RA, O'Connor N: Carbon monoxide poisoning in fire victims: A reappraisal of prognosis. J Trauma 20:78–80, 1980.
145. Larkin JM, Brahos GJ, Moylan JA: Treatment of carbon monoxide poisoning: Prognostic factors. J Trauma 16:111–114, 1976.
146. Boutros AR, Hoyt JL: Management of carbon monoxide poisoning in the absence of hyperbaric oxygen chamber. Crit Care Med 4:144–147, 1976.
147. End E, Long CW: Oxygen under pressure in carbon monoxide poisoning. J Ind Hyg Toxicol 24:302–306, 1942.

148. Smith GI, Sharp GR: Treatment of carbon monoxide poisoning with oxygen under pressure. Lancet 1:905–906, 1960.
149. Kindwall EP: Carbon monoxide poisoning treated with hyperbaric oxygen. Respir Ther 5:29–33, 1975.
150. Dostal J, Tulachova Z, Buryska J: Effect of hyperbaroxia in the recovery of metabolic acidosis in severe carbon monoxide intoxications. Roxhl Chir 53:740–744, 1974.
151. Goulon M, Barios A, Rapin M, et al: Intoxication oxycarbonee et anoxic aique par inhalation de gaz de charbon et d'hydrocarbures. Ann Med Intern 120:335–349, 1969. English translation: J Hyperbaric Med 1:23–41, 1986.
152. Myers RAM, Snyder S, Linberg S, Cowley RA: Delayed hyperbaric oxygen in suspected carbon monoxide poisoning. JAMA 246:2478–2480, 1981.
153. Onji Y, Sugimoto T, Ogawa M, Okada Y: Clinical study on carbon monoxide poisoning with special reference to hyperbaric oxygen. *In* Trapp WG, Davidson EW, Davidson AJ, Trapp PA (eds): Proceedings of the Fifth International Hyperbaric Congress. Burnaby, Canada, Simar Frasar University Press, 1973, pp 511–516.
154. Ziser A, Shnpak A, Halpern P, et al: Delayed hyperbaric oxygen treatment for acute carbon monoxide poisoning. Br Med J 289:960, 1984.
155. Yee LM, Brandon GK: Successful reversal of presumed carbon monoxide poisoning. Ann Emerg Med 14:1163–1167, 1985.
156. Myers RAM, Snyder SK, Emhoff TA: Subacute sequelae of carbon monoxide poisoning. Ann Emerg Med 14:1163–1167, 1985.
157. Mathieu D, Nolf M, Durocher A, Saulnier F: Acute carbon monoxide poisoning risk of late sequelae and treatment by hyperbaric oxygen. Clin Toxicol 23:315–324, 1985.
158. Norkool DM, Kirkpatrick JN: Treatment of acute carbon monoxide poisoning with hyperbaric oxygen: A review of 115 cases. Ann Emerg Med 14:1168–1171, 1985.
159. Marklund SL: Oxygen toxicity and protective systems. Clin Toxicol 23:289–298, 1985.
160. Thom SR: Experimental carbon monoxide-mediated brain lipid peroxidation and the effects of oxygen therapy. Ann Emerg Med 17:403, 1988.
161. Myers RAM, Messer LD, Jones DW, Cowley RA: New directions in the research and treatment of carbon monoxide exposure. Am J Emerg Med 2:226–230, 1983.
162. Lambertsen CJ: Therapeutic gases: Oxygen, carbon dioxide, and helium. *In* DiPalma JR (ed): Drill's Pharmacology in Medicine. 4th ed. New York, McGraw-Hill, 1971, pp 1145–1179.
163. Lambertsen CJ: Effects of excessive pressures of oxygen, nitrogen, helium, carbon dioxide, and carbon monoxide: Implications in aerospace, undersea, and industrial environments. *In* Mountcastle VB (ed): Medical Physiology. 14th ed. Vol 2. St. Louis, CV Mosby Company, 1980, pp 1901–1944.
164. Reivich M: Arterial P_{CO_2} and cerebral hemodynamics. Am J Physiol 206:25–35, 1964.
165. Sechzer PH, Egbert LD, Linde HW, et al: Effect of carbon dioxide inhalation on arterial pressure, electrocardiogram and plasma concentration of catecholamines and 17-OH corticosteroids in normal man. J Appl Physiol 15:454–458, 1960.
166. MacDonald FM, Simonson E: Human electrocardiogram during and after inhalation of 30% CO_2. J Appl Physiol 6:304–310, 1953.
167. Mattsson JL, Stinson JM: Tolerance of rhesus monkeys to PCO_2 of 195 mm Hg at 0.5 atmosphere total pressure. Aerosp Med 41:1051–1054, 1970.
168. Brown EB, Miller F: Ventricular fibrillation following a rapid fall in alveolar carbon dioxide concentration. Am J Physiol 169:56–60, 1952.
169. Menn SJ, Sinclair RD, Welch BE: Effect of inspired P_{CO2} up to 30 mm Hg on response of normal man to exercise. J Appl Physiol 28:663–671, 1970.
170. Sinclair RD, Clark JM, Welch BE: Comparison of physiological responses of normal man to exercise in air and in acute and chronic hypercapnia. *In* Lambertsen CJ (ed): Underwater Physiology. Proceedings of the Fourth Symposium on Underwater Physiology. New York, Academic Press, 1971, pp 409–417.
171. Luft UC, Finkelstein S, Elliott JC: Respiratory gas exchange, acid-base balance, and electrolytes during and after maximal work breathing 15 mm Hg P_{ICO_2}. *In* Nahas G, Schaefer KE (eds): Carbon Dioxide and Metabolic Regulations. New York, Springer-Verlag, 1974, pp 282–293.
172. Clark JM, Sinclair RD, Lenox JB: Chemical and nonchemical components of ventilation during hypercapnic exercise in man. J Appl Physiol 48:1065–1076, 1980.
173. Alexander JK, West JR, Wood JA, Richards DW: Analysis of the respiratory response to carbon dioxide inhalation in varying clinical states of hypercapnia, anoxia, and acid-base derangement. J Clin Invest 34:511–532, 1955.
174. Clark JM, Sinclair RD, Welch BE: Rate of acclimatization to chronic hypercapnia in man. *In* Lambertsen CJ (ed): Underwater Physiology. Proceedings of the Fourth Symposium on Underwater Physiology. New York, Academic Press, 1971, pp 399–408.
175. Kennedy TJ: The effect of carbon dioxide on the kidney. Anesthesiology 21:704–716, 1960.
176. Van Ypersele de Strihou C, Brasseur L, De Coninck J: The "carbon dioxide response curve" for chronic hypercapnia in man. N Engl J Med 275:117–122, 1966.
177. Engel K, Dell RB, Rahill WJ, et al: Quantitative displacement of acid-base equilibrium in chronic respiratory acidosis. J Appl Physiol 24:288–295, 1968.
178. Brackett NC Jr, Wingo CF, Muren O, Solano JT: Acid-base response to chronic hypercapnia in man. N Engl J Med 280:124–130, 1969.
179. Price HL: Effects of carbon dioxide on the cardiovascular system. Anesthesiology 21:652–663, 1960.
180. Raichle ME, Stone HL: Cerebral blood flow autoregulation and graded hypercapnia. Eur Neurol 6:1–5, 1971/72.

Chapter 9

Hypothermia

G. YANCEY MEBANE

Now King David was old and stricken in years; and they covered him with clothes, but he got no heat. Wherefore his servants said unto him, Let there be sought for my lord the king a young virgin: and let her stand before the king, and let her cherish him, and let her lie in thy bosom, that my lord the king may get heat.

I Kings 1:1–2

Hypothermia has always been a major factor in ocean catastrophies or cold exposure under dry conditions. It is also important to the diver, as serious hypothermia may lead to increasing inability to maintain oneself in the water, and mild hypothermia will produce fatigue and impaired cognition. Hypothermia may occur slowly under mild exposure or may be the result of a sudden exposure to severe conditions.

Hypothermia may be a significant factor in the victim of a near-drowning episode and may complicate any of the problems facing the diver, such as decompression sickness, air embolism, and nitrogen narcosis. Near drowning and hypothermia often occur simultaneously, as much of the surface water in the United States is below the 70°F (21°C) threshold year round. Even in the Sun Belt surface water temperatures will fall below 70°F during the winter. In addition, the water temperature below the first thermocline in deeper water is frequently well below 70° F. Consequently, any diver or other individual who develops a problem while in the water should be considered a possible victim of hypothermia in addition to more obvious problems. The management of near drowning and other diving accidents is covered in detail in other chapters.

Controlled hypothermia as used in surgical procedures has an excellent safety record, while accidental hypothermia has a very high mortality rate.

Man attempts to maintain a steady temperature state by controlling heat loss and production. A downward variation is hypothermia; an upward variation is hyperthermia. To aid in understanding temperature regulation, the body can be considered as a central core containing the central nervous system and the thoracic, abdominal, and pelvic viscera. A peripheral shell consists of the limbs, subcutaneous tissues, and skin. A constant core temperature is defended by the body with great vigor, while the peripheral shell temperature is subject to variation. Consequently, there is a temperature gradient from the core to the body surface.

The temperature of the core can be maintained in many ways. The insulating layers of the body cannot be changed suddenly, but the blood flow through it can be changed in volume and vascular routing.

The hypothalamus contains heat-regulating centers sensitive to minute changes in temperature of perfusing blood, and it integrates messages from the peripheral cutaneous sensors with those from within the hypothalamus to stimulate the various effector organs to correct for heat loss or gain. The systems involved in counteracting the heat loss are the somatic and autonomic nervous systems and the endocrine system. Direct constriction of arterioles and venules in the periphery occurs with lowered skin temperatures mediated through the sympathetic nervous system by the release of epinephrine. A rapid rise in peripheral vascular resistance follows, causing arteriovenous shunts to open and direct blood back to the core, while superficial veins shunt warm blood to the deeper veins. As the large central veins containing cooled blood are in close contact with a companion artery, heat is transferred to the returning blood, and the arterial blood is cooled before returning to the extremities. With vasoconstriction, the skin temperature falls and the temperature differential between the skin and water becomes less, so that heat transfer also becomes less. This is a major response to cold exposure resulting in heat conservation.

Heat production in humans can increase only as a result of muscular activity or shivering. Unfortunately, this activity may lead to increased heat loss as will be shown later.

MILD TO MODERATE HYPOTHERMIA

The individual with a core temperature of 95° to 98.6°F (35° to 37°C) may be considered mildly hypothermic and will be awake, can answer questions intelligently, and complains of cold. Moderate hypothermia can be considered to occur in the core temperature range from 90° to 95°F (32° to 35°C). At that temperature there will be apathy, mild confusion, slurred speech, and poor cooperation. The individual may also exhibit incoordination, stumbling gait, shivering, and paradoxical undressing due to a false sense of being too warm. He will have a grey bloodless appearance with a slow pulse and decreased blood pressure. Amnesia will be present.

SEVERE HYPOTHERMIA

A core temperature below 90°F (32°C) constitutes severe hypothermia; the individual will be in coma, possibly cardiopulmonary arrest, and may appear clinically dead. The victim will be stiff with dilated pupils and will be hypotensive and hyporeflexic. A cold-induced diuresis will have occurred due to suppression of antidiuretic hormone and later due to depressed tubular function in the cold kidney. The oxyhemoglobin dissociation curve shifts to the left which increases oxygen affinity. Therefore, hemoglobin does not release its oxygen to cold tissues until the partial pressure of oxygen in the tissues falls to very low levels.

All three stages of hypothermia are emergencies requiring prompt attention. However, hypothermia is an emergency in slow motion so that the rescuer has time to think before acting. Caution is indicated, for mortality may increase wtih rough handling, chest compressions, airway manipulations, and attempts at rewarming in the field.

COLD EXPOSURE

Exposure to cold results in body chilling at a rate dependent on many factors. As cold exposure occurs the body begins to lose heat at a rate that depends on the initial thermal state (body heat "storage") and on the body shape. The areas of the body showing the highest heat loss are the head, groin, and the chest wall in the midaxillary line. The rate of loss also depends on whether the individual is wet or dry and protected or unprotected. For example, the unprotected individual exposed to water at 92°F (32°C) will remain stable with no gain or loss for an indefinite period. However, unprotected exposure to water at 80°F (27°C) is equivalent to the same exposure in air at 42°F (6°C). The temperature range at which heat loss and heat production are approximately equal is the comfort zone and is 91.4° to 95°F (33° to 35°C).

MAINTENANCE OF CORE TEMPERATURE

The heat used by the body to maintain the core temperature results from the basal metabolic rate (BMR) plus the heat produced by physical exercise. Normally, exercise in dry conditions will increase heat production and body temperature. However, exercise in cold water will reduce body temperature because of increased blood flow to the limbs and increased water movement about the body. Shivering in cold water will have the same result. The increase in heat production requires increased oxygen consumption, which requires increased minute ventilation with changes in respiratory rate and chest movement. As muscle activity continues in response to the demand for heat, lactic acid accumulates contributing to metabolic acidosis and fatigue.

HEAT TRANSFER

Heat transfer occurs by physical means whenever there is a temperature gradient and always moves from the system with the higher temperature to the system with the lower temperature. The means of transfer are as follows: (1) *radiation*—emission of infra-red energy; (2) *conduction*—direct contact between surfaces; (3) *convection*—air movement (windchill) or water movement (waterchill). The cooler air comes into contact with warmer air and heat is transferred by conduction then transported elsewhere; (4) *evaporation*—the conversion of a liquid to vapor without changing temperature. This occurs on the skin and in the lungs (where there is also heat loss by convection).

Heat Loss with Immersion

With immersion the heat loss by radiation is not significant compared with that lost by conduction and convection. The water acts as an infinite heat sink and has a thermal conductivity 32 times that of air. Convection also plays a role due to the movement of water about the body resulting from muscular activity as well as water currents. Passive sweating occurs and transfers some heat, although evaporation does not take place. During a long dive there will be loss of heat from urine.

Respiratory heat loss becomes very significant in deep dives, especially if the inert gas breathed is helium because of its high thermal coefficient. It is important to be aware that none of the thermoregulatory responses affects respiratory heat loss. The heat loss is from the core, and convection is the dominant component. It is believed that the cold gas can penetrate further into the tracheobronchial tree under pressure and adds to the heat loss problem.

The direct heat loss from the body in water is largely limited by the body (core-to-skin) tissue insulation and not by the skin-to-water transfer coefficient. That is, the limiting factor in the flow of heat from the body to the surrounding environment is limited by the rate of movement of heat from the core to the skin surface in the absence of thermal protection at the skin-water interface. The thermal comfort zone varies inversely with the subcutaneous fat thickness and is the temperature range at which heat loss and heat production are approximately equal. The range is about 91.4° to 95°F (33° to 35°C) in water.

Since body cooling is inversely related to the mean subcutaneous fat thickness, transfer of heat to the water depends on the amount of insulation at the skin surface. This insulation may take the form of clothing or air or water trapped at the skin by a dry or wet suit.

Immersion Response: Unprotected

If an individual is suddenly exposed to cold water with no thermal protection, immediate disabling effects occur. With immersion there is a sudden inspiration or "gasping response," which may lead to aspiration if the victim is face down. This response continues for 1 to 2 minutes with a ventilation volume that may reach 50 to 60 liter/min for one or two minutes. The increased respiratory rate results in a drop in pCO_2, producing respiratory alkalosis, relative hypocalcemia with muscle cramps, decreased cerebral blood flow, and decreased level of consciousness. The individual has no control over the increased respiratory rate and tidal volume. There is also a sharp rise in venous and arterial pressure, accompanied by increased cardiac output. As time progresses there is decrease in muscle strength accompanied by pain and mental disorganization, with fear and panic reaction developing.

Immersion Response: Partial Protection

If there is a sudden exposure to cold water with some thermal protection, the immediate disabling effects may be blunted, but there will be vasoconstriction temporarily preventing heat loss. Vasodilatation soon occurs allowing blood to flow to the cold extremities. If vigorous exercise is undertaken or shivering develops, there is an increase in metabolic heat production. However, the agitation of water by the activity increases heat loss in excess of production, and the result is a loss of body heat and a drop in core temperature. Exercise has an adverse effect on body temperature in cold water because it increases the heat loss much more at low than at high water temperatures. Exercise always increases the rate of body heat loss regardless of subcutaneous fat thickness. It is futile to attempt to stay warm by exercise, and caution should be observed in attempts at self-rescue by swimming.

PROGRESSION OF HYPOTHERMIA

The signs and symptoms of progressive hypothermia are predictable and loosely correspond to different core temperatures (Fig. 9–1), outlined briefly below:

95° to 98.6°F (35° to 37°C): sensation of cold, shivering, increased heart rate, urge to urinate, slight incoordination in hand movements.

90° to 95°F (32.2° to 35°C): increasing muscular incoordination, stumbling gait, shivering slows or stops, weakness, apathy, drowsiness, confusion, slurred speech.

85° to 90°F (29.4° to 32.2°C): shivering stops, inability to walk or follow commands, paradoxical undressing, complaints of loss of vision, and confusion progressing to coma.

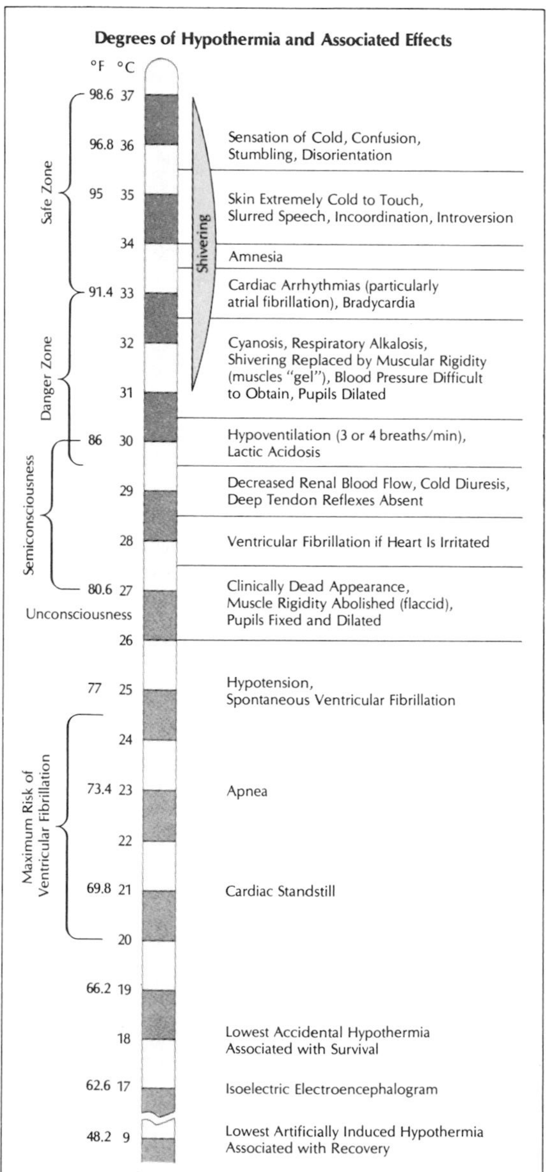

FIGURE 9–1. Degrees of hypothermia and associated effects. (From Matz R: Hypothermia: Mechanisms and countermeasures. Hosp Pract 21:45–71, 1986.)

85°F (29.4°C) or lower: muscle rigidity, decreased blood pressure, heart rate, and respirations, dilated pupils, appearance of death.

65°F (25°C): begin to take on the temperature of the environment.

WARM WATER HYPOTHERMIA

The effects of hypothermia have also been observed in relatively warm or even tropical waters. Fatigue and impaired cognition have been recognized in scientific divers as a result of slow body cooling while the diver is preoccupied with a task at hand. The diver may not recognize the problem, but it is usually expressed as a reluctance to dive. Very little is known about the effects of long, slow body cooling and the development of "undetected hypothermia." Long, slow body cooling could be encountered in individuals with no protection in 82° to 91°F (28° to 33°C) water or in those wearing a wet suit in 59°F (15°C) water. The mean skin temperature remains close to the comfort zone at 91°F (33°C), and the insidious heat drain from the body by water is scarcely noticed until core temperature drops enough to induce shivering. In some cases shivering does not occur, as the core temperature drop is not enough to induce defense mechanisms. Sports divers may encounter this phenomenon during repeated dives in warm water with no thermal protection and may suddenly find themselves very tired with no desire to continue with vacation diving plans.

CARDIOVASCULAR RESPONSE TO HYPOTHERMIA

The treatment of exposure hypothermia requires some understanding of the cardiovascular effects of a decrease in core temperature. It has been mentioned that mild hypothermia causes a sympathetic stimulation producing increased heart rate and cardiac output. There is intense vasoconstriction resulting in a shift of blood from the periphery to the core. The body interprets this fluid shift as overhydration and shuts off the production of antidiuretic hormone resulting in diuresis.

Generally, the cardiovascular system is stable in mild hypothermia. However, when the temperature falls out of the mild range and hypothermia becomes more severe, a wide spectrum of cardiac dysrhythmias may occur. At a core temperature of approximately 86°F (30°C) or above, there is a decline in heart rate, cardiac output, BMR, and oxygen consumption, although cardiovascular stability persists. Below 86°F (30°C) dysrhythmias appear initially with sinus bradycardia, then atrial fibrillation with a slow ventricular response. Ventricular fibrillation may occur spontaneously, and below 82°F (28°C) asystole is frequently encountered. The pulse and blood pressure may not be detectable, although there may exist an undetectable perfusing nonarrested rhythm.

If an arrested rhythm is present, the prognosis with asystole may be good with rapid rewarming. Ventricular fibrillation is usually refractory until the core temperature has been elevated. An arrested rhythm requires cardiopulmonary resuscitation while rewarming takes place. As the core temperature of a hypothermic victim with asystole increases, the first rhythm that appears will be ventricular fibrillation. At a core temperature below 82°F (28°C), ventricular fibrillation is refractory to cardioversion and is the usual cause of death. It is very important to be aware of the factors that may cause ventricular fibrillation in the hypothermic patient with a nonarrested rhythm. At core temperatures below 82°F (28°C), ventricular fibrillation may occur spontaneously as that is the fibrillatory threshold for the induction of ventricular fibrillation by cardiac stimulation or irritation. The very slow sinus bradycardia characteristic of such low core temperatures degenerates readily into ventricular fibrillation. The likelihood for this to take place increases with the decline in core temperature below 82°F (28°C). Mechanical factors that might induce ventricular fibrillation in such an irritable heart include airway manipulations, tracheal and nasogastric intubation, intracardiac catheters, and external chest compressions. However, external chest compressions are effective in the profoundly hypothermic heart and should not be withheld with an arrested rhythm. There are data indicating alkalosis has the potential to induce ventricular fibrillation and therefore should be avoided. Alkalosis also causes cerebral vasoconstriction and shifts the oxyhemoglobin dissociation curve to the left, resulting in decreased oxygen availability to the tissues.

MANAGEMENT IN THE FIELD

Suspecting the existence of hypothermia in an individual is the first step in management. It is crucial to avoid refractory ventricular fibrillation induced by attempts at resuscitation. As unmonitored CPR might produce such a problem, it is important to have a portable monitor available. If a portable monitor will not be quickly available and there is no indication of motor activity, the decision to proceed with CPR should be made with a realization that it may be risky and that adequate oxygenation without respiratory alkalosis can be achieved by low ventilation rates. The low tissue metabolic needs as a result of the hypothermia may indicate that the frequency of chest compressions can be reduced, but little definite information exists.

The rescuer has the responsibility to transport and rewarm without precipitating ventricular fibrillation. Rewarming is of extreme importance, of course, but should not be attempted unless proper core warming technique is available. As the cold heart is especially susceptible to ventricular fibrillation, many patients alive when found develop this complication when handled roughly during initial evaluation and transportation. If the victim is breathing spontaneously, he should be supplied with warmed oxygen by mask. The airway should be controlled by head tilt–chin lift maneuver, and oro- or nasopharyngeal airways should be avoided if possible. The apneic patient will require a higher degree of management of the airway, and skillful endotracheal intubation can be done if available. However, proper position and nasopharyngeal airway may be sufficient to allow the administration of warmed oxygen by mask. Remember! (1) Hypothermia itself may not be harmful unless cardiopulmonary arrest occurs. (2) Cold is protective to the heart and brain. (3) Spontaneous respiration if present may be slow but will be adequate.

Afterdrop

Attempts at rewarming in the field by the external application of heat may produce a phenomenon termed "afterdrop." Afterdrop is a further drop in core temperature after initiation of rewarming. This phenomenon has been explained as a result of the mixing of cold peripheral blood with the blood in the central core. Recent studies have been aimed at directly testing the circulatory explanation of afterdrop. The results have been to challenge this circulatory explanation because of the failure to demonstrate an increase in peripheral circulation at the time afterdrop occurs in the esophagus or heart. The occurrence of afterdrop may be explained as a result of heat transfer by physical means and need not involve the circulatory system. A temperature gradient will always result in heat transfer from the warmer system to the cooler one. A victim of hypothermia has transferred heat from the core to the superficial tissues and the environment. If heat is applied to the superficial tissues, the direction of heat flow will not reverse immediately. Heat will continue to flow outward from warm core areas to cooler outer regions. The resulting afterdrop may produce a significant temperature drop in the heart and may induce ventricular fibrillation. Avoiding afterdrop requires that the core organs be heated first as by venoarterial bypass or peritoneal lavage. Ideally one should have a low-reading thermometer, a monitor/defibrillator, and a portable oxygen heater/humidifier before attempting to rewarm a victim outside the hospital.

However, it sometimes becomes necessary to deal with rewarming a hypothermic victim in an area far from medical care. In this situation the first attempts should use passive methods. These would include protection against further heat loss by removing wet clothing and covering in layers, not forgetting to provide layers between the victim and the ground or deck, and to cover the head, which is a major source of heat loss. If the victim is awake, he should not be exercised, as muscular activity will bring cold blood from the periphery to the core. Active rewarming is not without hazard, and the safest method is via the airway with heated oxygen, which eliminates respiratory heat loss and provides a small amount of heat directly to the core via the lungs. More detail about this method will be found in the section on Emergency Department Management.

Immersion of the victim in a hot bath has been thought to be risky unless limited to the trunk only with the extremities left out. Similarly, body-to-body contact has been limited to bare skin in the truncal area only. If current research conclusions regarding the mechanism of afterdrop are correct, then the victim will not have increased cooling of the heart on immersion, limbs and all, in a hot bath. Heated fluids can be encouraged in the fully conscious victim only. The amount of heat energy delivered will be minimal, but the inevitable volume contraction will be helped. Coffee, tea, caffeine drinks or other diuretics, and alcohol should be strictly avoided. If intravenous fluids are available and used, they should be warmed, although the amount of heat delivered will be insignificant. Oral fluids may include balanced electrolyte solutions such as Gatorade, Gastrolyte, or Infalyte, which are also available in powder form.

The flow chart in Figure 9–2 simplifies the principles of hypothermia management in the field.

EMERGENCY DEPARTMENT MANAGEMENT

After initial stabilization in the field and rapid transport to an appropriate emergency department has been accomplished, it is still of critical importance to be gentle with the victim. The risk of inducing dysrhythmias is still present, and there is a high incidence of other traumatic injuries, especially those involving the cervical spine.

There should be continuous monitoring of cardiac rhythm and rectal core temperature. Central venous access should be obtained via catheter. Medications that might be given if indicated include glucose, naloxone, thiamine, and intravenous normal saline. Lactate should be avoided as the cold liver is unable to metabolize it. Arterial blood gas measurements that have been corrected for core temperature should be determined frequently. (Add 0.15 pH units to the measured pH for each degree Celsius that the core temperature is below 37°C.)

As rewarming occurs, oxygen consumption will rise by a factor of 2.5–3 for each 10°C increase in core body temperature. If the core temperature is determined to be less than 82°F (28°C) and a bradycardia or atrial dysrhythmia is present, there should be no chest compressions. If asystole or ventricular fibrillation is present, then compressions should be started immediately. Conversion to a more suitable rhythm will probably not be possible until the heart has been rewarmed. Medications such as Bretylium may be considered with persistent ventricular fibrillation, but caution is indicated because of the multiple variables brought about by the low temperatures. Medications exhibit a prolonged half-life and a reduced end-organ effect under such conditions. Catecholamines should be avoided as low blood pressure corresponds with low body temperature.

Appropriate rewarming methods should be instituted as quickly as possible. The most rapidly available method of core rewarming is the administration of heated, humidified oxygen. Adding hot water to the cascade humidifier on the ventilation machine warms and humidifies

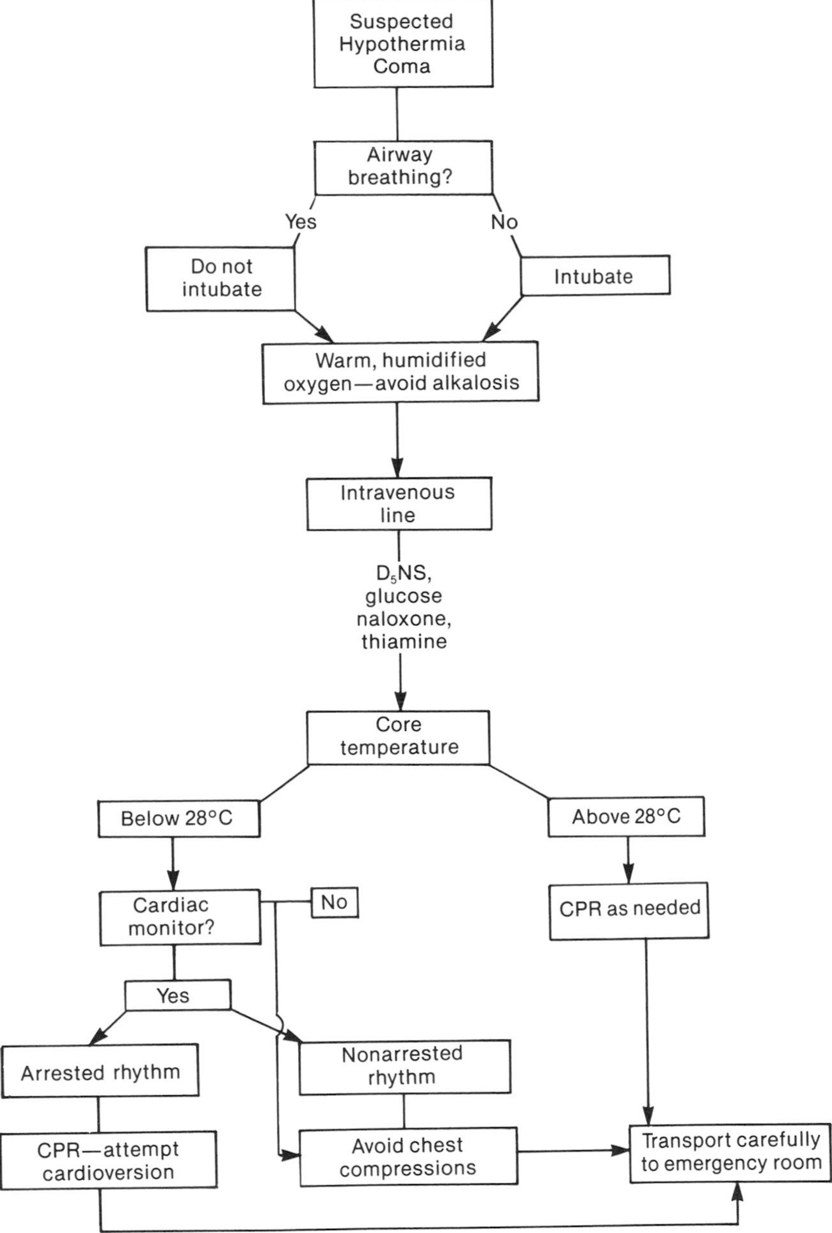

FIGURE 9–2. Management of suspected hypothermia coma in the field. (Adapted from Zell SC, Kurtz KJ: Severe exposure hypothermia. Ann Emerg Med 14:339–345, 1985.)

oxygen before it reaches the patient. Because the lungs jacket the heart, heat is delivered directly to the myocardium by convection and conduction. The effect on the core temperature will be slight, but the heart itself will be warmed fairly rapidly so that control of dysrhythmias becomes possible. Most of the inhaled heat is carried by the water vapor, whose thermal energy comes from the 540 cal/gm latent heat of vaporization of water. The water vapor must be delivered to the lung and condensed there in order to deliver significant heat.

Critical Care

If the patient has a core temperature above 82°F (28°C) with stable blood pressure, pulse, and respiration, then he may be supplied by heated, humidified oxygen while being rewarmed passively and actively under extreme caution. If the vital signs are altered, the patient is in critical condition and requires intensive measures to restore heat and protect cardiac function.

Peritoneal lavage may be used to supply heat to the core when the situation is critical. The technique is relatively simple and is available in almost any hospital, regardless of size. Proper equipment should be used. Plastic catheters designed for intravenous fluids have only one hole that may become plugged. The technique is described in the *Manual of Emergency and Outpatient Techniques* by Klippel and Anderson (Little, Brown & Co.). The lavage fluid is Ringer's lactate warmed to 105° to 110°F, rapidly instilled and immediately removed for six or seven 2-liter exchanges. The acidic pH of isotonic saline may induce some peritoneal irritation and should be avoided if possible.

The use of emergency venoarterial bypass through the femoral vessels by means of a pump-oxygenator is an excellent method of assisting the circulation for a few hours. The femoral artery–femoral vein (F-F) bypass using the cardiac pump has the advantage of very rapid rewarming with less likelihood of intracardiac temperature gradients, while supporting circulation in the absence of effective cardiac activity. A flow of 3000 ml/min is possible. F-F bypass should be continued until the patient is stable. When a core temperature of 30° to 32°C has been reached, conventional defibrillation has a chance, and the nonarrested patient is past the fibrillatory threshold.

Resuscitation should be continued until the patient is "warm and dead."

HOSPITAL MANAGEMENT

Following emergency department resuscitation and stabilization, the patient will need continued hospital care. He should receive ventilatory and circulatory support as conditions require, with continuous monitoring of vital signs. Volume assessment and control will require clinical judgment based on information received by central venous pressure and arterial catheters as well as urine output. Urine output may not be reliable because of the possibility of cold-induced diuresis or oliguria secondary to acute tubular necrosis. A central venous catheter allows venous access for fluid and medication and for assessment of volume status and does not enter or touch the irritable heart. An arterial catheter allows for frequent collection of blood samples and continuous monitoring of blood pressure. Fluid replenishment should be 5 per cent dextrose in normal saline. Potassium should be avoided in initial stages of therapy, and lactate may not be metabolized by the cold liver. The insertion of a Swan-Ganz catheter should await the restoration of core temperature above the ventricular fibrillation threshold. A Swan-Ganz may be needed for monitoring adult respiratory distress syndrome, which often occurs.

PREVENTION

The prevention of hypothermia in divers requires training, judgment, and experience. The diver must understand the use of external insulation to conserve body heat and control loss. Sports divers sometimes encounter very cold conditions in ice or winter diving in deep quarries, and they nearly always dive in water below body temperature. The commercial or scientific diver is more likely to dive under adverse temperature conditions and may need specialized systems not generally used by the sports diver. Wet suits provide some degree of thermal protection depending on the style, material, and thickness, but wet suits become compressed with increasing depth and lose much of their insulating properties. A commonly used piece of equipment by both sports and other divers is the "wooly bear" or open cell undergarment used with a dry suit. This device is quite effective under many dive conditions but does have some deficiencies. Its volume compresses 70 to 80 per cent when under a suit squeeze differential of 2 psi, and it loses insulation value if the suit is filled with helium. Should the suit become wet, as in cases of flooding, its insulation value is reduced to 5 per cent or less. Under that circumstance, the dive would have to be terminated.

Commercial divers have available to them a wet suit that is supplied with hot water from a heater on the dive vessel. The suit is constantly flooded with warm water that escapes around the wrists and ankles. The flow can be regulated by the diver. Obviously this is an expensive system limited to commercial applications, but it also has its limitations. If the water supply fails, the suit will fill with cold water in about two minutes unless there are neck, leg, and arm seals as well as a non-return valve to hold hot water in the suit. An insulated volume tank between the heater and diver helps to avoid this problem to some extent. Serious hypothermia may develop rapidly with a system failure.

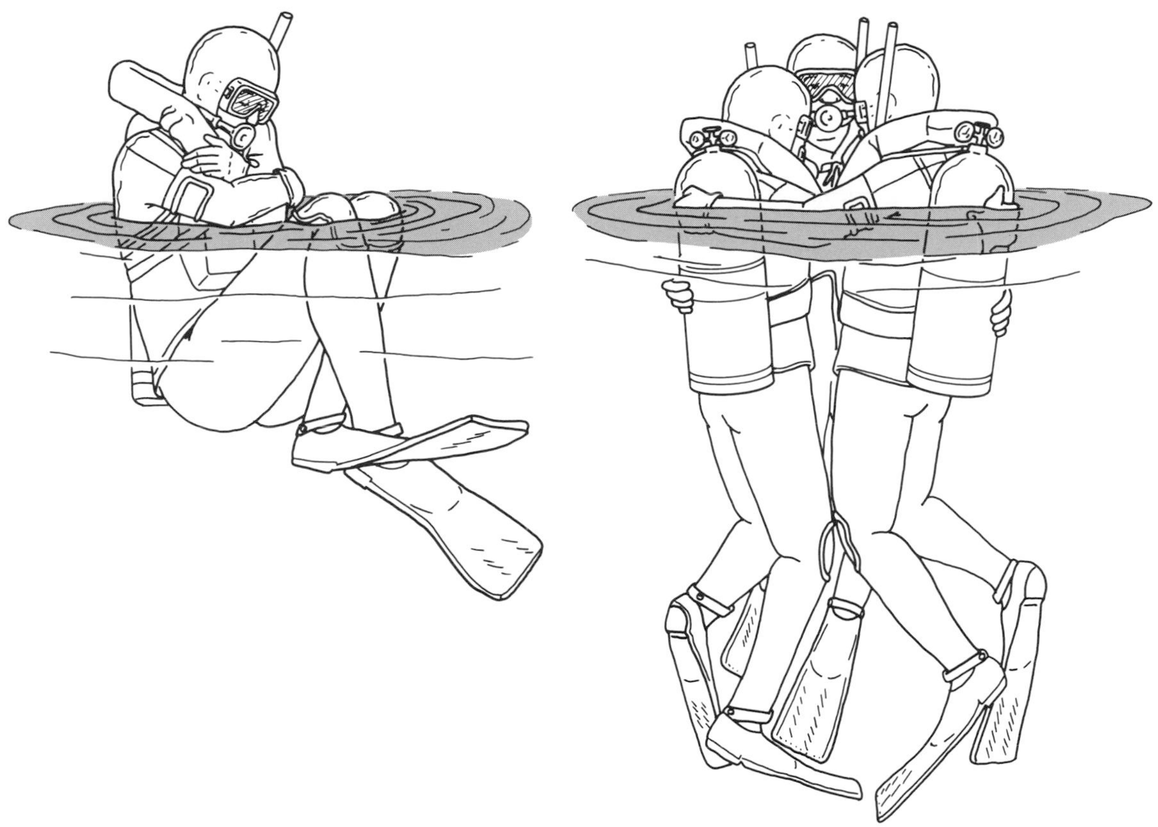

FIGURE 9–3. A diver wearing a flotation device can minimize heat loss and increase chances of survival by assuming the Heat Escape Lessening Position (H-E-L-P) (left), in which the knees are pulled up to the chest and the arms are crossed. Groups of three or more divers can conserve heat by wrapping their arms around one another and pulling into a tight circle (right).

Electrically heated suits still have a reliability and safety problem to overcome.

Prevention of hypothermia also includes preparation for unexpected immersion. Divers traveling by boat to the dive site should have a flotation device available other than their diving equipment. The personal flotation device (PFD) should be designed to keep the wearer afloat with no effort on his part, to keep the head out of the water, and to be self-righting. The diver should practice using his PFD in order to be familiar with its use. Seat cushions or flotation devices that require the victim to hold on are not satisfactory in cold water, as hypothermia will soon cause the loss of muscle power and the victim will lose his grip. The diver should be prepared for actions to be taken once in water. These would include efforts to minimize heat loss such as remaining still and assuming the H-E-L-P position (heat escape lessening position). This position is assumed by drawing the knees up to the chest and holding with crossed arms (Fig. 9–3). The position is unstable and is not easy to achieve without practice as one tends to roll forward or backward. Consequently, it is well to practice the position from time to time. The huddle position with other persons is surprisingly effective in conserving heat. Everyone wraps arms around one another and pulls into a tight circle, afterward remaining as still as possible.

The psychological preparedness of knowing what to expect if suddenly immersed in cold water, how to use flotation, and how to stay put and wait for rescue will significantly increase the chances for survival.

REFERENCES

Auerbach P: Medicine for the Outdoors. Boston, Little Brown, 1986.

Bennett PB, Elliott D: The Physiology and Medicine of Diving. San Pedro, Best Publishing, 1982.

Blackman JR: Caught in cold water. Emer Med January, 69–83, 1985.

Edmonds C, Lowry C, Pennefather J: Diving and Subaquatic Medicine. San Pedro, Best Publishing, 1983.

Klippel AP, Anderson CB: Manual of Outpatient and Emergency Surgical Techniques. Boston, Little, Brown, 1979.

Matz R: Hypothermia: Mechanisms and countermeasures. Hosp Pract 21:45–71, 1986.

Shilling CW, Carlston CB, Mathias RA: The Physicians Guide to Diving Medicine. New York, Plenum Press, 1984.

Strauss RH: Diving Medicine. New York, Grune & Stratton, 1976.

Webb P: Afterdrop of body temperature during rewarming. J Appl Physiol 60:385–390, 1986.

Zell SC, Kurtz KJ: Severe exposure hypothermia. Ann Emerg Med 14:339–345, 1985.

Chapter 10

Near Drowning

TOM S. NEUMAN

In the approximately 100 to 150 scuba fatalities in the United States each year, drowning is the leading cause of death.[1–10] Additionally, near drowning is frequently a complicating factor in nonfatal scuba accidents. More importantly, drowning is responsible for approximately 7000 deaths in the United States each year, and there are approximately 90,000 near drownings as well.[11–12] Until recently, drowning was considered to be, after motor vehicle accidents, the chief cause of death among children 4 to 14 years of age[13]; however, with the advent of effective automobile child restraint laws, drowning has become the leading cause of death in some states.[14, 15] Thus, although scuba and diving accidents are a small percentage of the total number of drowning and near-drowning incidents, the physician who either is interested in diving medicine, is frequently in or around aquatic environments, or deals with emergencies must be thoroughly familiar with the management of these patients.

Drowning and near-drowning incidents can occur in a variety of ways. About 1500 of the total yearly drowning fatalities are related to boating accidents, and approximately 500 are victims who die trapped in submerged motor vehicles.[16] Most drownings occur in fresh water (swimming pools, ponds, lakes, and streams), but this may be due to less supervision—since approximately 80 per cent of drownings occur at places other than those designated for swimming,[17–21]—in contrast to the smaller inherent danger of ocean swimming on supervised beaches.

The major location of drowning incidents in the toddler group is the residential pool, generally because of inadequate safety measures in the home.[22–25] In the United States, drownings in males are approximately five times more common than in females, and blacks drown approximately twice as often as whites.[19] As with fatal automobile accidents, the single most important factor in drowning incidents involving adults is alcohol. Multiple studies done in widely different geographical areas, such as the United States,[11, 19] New Zealand,[26] Africa,[27] and Australia,[28–29] reveal that in well over half of the adults who drown, alcohol is a significant contributing factor.

With scuba-related drownings or near-drowning incidents, the most comon factor is the diver running out of air at depth or in a cave.[1–10] The second most common cause of death in divers is arterial gas embolism (AGE), and this entity, when not fatal, is frequently complicated by near drowning as well.

Although not generally reported in the diving fatality statistics, there is strong evidence that intentional hyperventilation prior to breath-hold diving is associated with both drowning and near-drowning episodes.[30–32] Hyperventilation reduces the partial pressure of arterial carbon dioxide (Pa_{CO_2}) such that the breath-hold break point is prolonged sufficiently for hypoxemia to occur before the individual is forced to breathe. The hypoxemia in turn causes the individual to lose consciousness, and the submersion incident then occurs (See "Shallow Water Black-out" in Chapter 6).

Hypothermia leading to drowning and near-drowning incidents has been reported frequently; however, in diving fatalities this is an unusual occurrence. It is important to remember that hypothermia per se is rarely the cause of death for people immersed in water. Rather, hypothermia gradually reduces a person's ability to function, until the point of unconsciousness is reached. At that time, the victim's head falls into the water, resulting in drowning or near drowning. Perhaps the most famous historical example of this is the sinking of the *Titanic*. When that tragedy occurred, the sea was perfectly calm and help was but a few hours away. There were no fatalities among those in life rafts, and there were no survivors among those in the water.[33] More recently, the *Lakonia* sank resulting in 200 passengers immersed in 16°C water. In less than three hours, 113 died.[34] All victims succumbed to the combined effects of hypothermia and drowning. However, as discussed in the next section, hypothermia can have a tremendous protective effect on the near-drowning victim. There are several documented occurrences of individuals being submerged for extended periods and of having complete recoveries.[35–38]

Hypothermia is only one of many conditions that can precipitate drowning by causing unconsciousness. In the case of scuba diving incidents, physicians must be aware of the possibility that contamination of the diver's air supply with any number of toxic gases may have occurred. Carbon monoxide is by far the most likely contaminant to produce unconsciousness rapidly under water leading to a fatal episode.[10] The treatment of carbon monoxide poisoning is beyond the scope of this chapter; however, it is a condition that may have to be treated at the same time as near drowning.

Other forms of gas toxicity producing unconsciousness under water can also occur (O_2-induced seizures, CO_2 poisoning); however, no specific therapy is required other than removing the victim from the exposure. Other medical conditions that can produce unconsciousness (i.e., generalized seizures[19, 39]) in or under the water have been implicated in a number of nondiving fatalities, although within the recent past neither seizure disorders nor diabetes (unconsciousness induced by hypoglycemia) has been implicated as an underlying cause of a scuba fatality in the United States (whether or not associated with drowning).

Finally, it must be mentioned that near drowning can complicate traumatic injury as well. Obviously, scuba divers can be struck by boats and suffer closed head injury or any of a variety of propeller injuries.[10] In addition, the diver can sustain a neck fracture while going through the surf zone. Although neck fractures are common in surfers and even more common in individuals diving into shallow pools or ponds,[40–42] occult neck fracture should always be considered in the near-drowning victim. Although not a "diving" accident per se, more than half of the 7000 spinal cord injuries associated with aquatic accidents result in permanent paralysis, and "stick in the mud" accidents (spinal cord injuries due to diving) are caused more frequently by water sports than by all other sporting activities combined.[43]

PATHOPHYSIOLOGY

Within the past 20 years, a considerable amount of experimental evidence has been collected which in large part explains the pathophysiology of drowning and near drowning. Without question, the major pathophysiological event is hypoxemia, with or without aspiration, secondary to immersion in any fluid medium. Most of the demonstrable pathology leading to long-term morbidity found in near-drowning victims can be explained by hypoxemia.[44–48]

Approximately 10 to 15 per cent of near-drowning victims do not aspirate any fluid during the period of immersion.[49,50] It has been hypothesized that reflex laryngospasm persists until reflex ventilatory activity ceases and, as a result, aspiration does not occur. In these victims, the period of hypoxemia is generally only as long as the immersion incident itself, and if ventilation can be re-established prior to the development of injury secondary to hypoxemia, recovery is generally rapid and uneventful.

When aspiration occurs, the pathophysiological processes are markedly different, although in the majority of cases the underlying primary process remains hypoxemia. Unlike the victim without aspiration, the individual who does aspirate remains hypoxemic, even after being removed from the fluid medium and even after ventilation is re-established. As a result, in this latter group the period of hypoxemia is potentially much longer, and secondary damage due to the hypoxemia is more likely to occur. The continuing hypoxemia is due to direct lung injury from the aspirated fluid, which causes areas of low ventilation perfusion ($\dot{V}_A/\dot{Q}$) ratio to develop.

The mechanisms by which hypoxemia develops have not been completely elucidated. With salt water aspiration, it is believed that the hyperosmotic fluid causes transudation of fluid into alveoli, and the aspiration of debris (sand, diatoms, algae, and so forth) causes a reactive exudate. As a result, alveoli become filled and are not ventilated, and hypoxemia occurs. In fresh water aspiration, it is believed that surfactant is washed out of the lungs, causing areas of focal alveolar collapse, leading to areas of shunt and low $\dot{V}_A/\dot{Q}$ ratio, again resulting in hypoxemia. These abnormalities then persist until the lung damage resolves or until surfactant can be regenerated. As victims often swallow large amounts of fluid during the near-drowning episode, further decreases in ventilatory function can occur as a result of elevation of the diaphragm from gastric distention. Regardless of the cause, hypoxemia and decreased alveolar ventilation can produce a number of consequences. Elevations of arterial carbon dioxide tension (P_aCO_2) and decreases in pH occur quickly. The former, of course, is due to decreased alveolar ventilation ($\dot{V}_A$) and increased CO_2 production; the latter is due to the combined effects of increased P_aCO_2 and decreased oxygen delivery to the tissues, resulting in increased lactic acid generation. This metabolic component can be extremely significant as the victim often struggles violently during the near-drowning episode. Finally, cardiovascular collapse can occur resulting in cardiac arrest. If hypoxemia and decreased cardiac output persist long enough, anoxic cerebral damage can ensue.[35, 51–57]

In the past, it was believed that a significant portion of the physiological changes associated with near drowning were a result of serum electrolyte changes that occurred with aspiration of salt or fresh water. These misconceptions were based on a series of carefully controlled experiments in which intubated dogs had increasing quantities of salt or fresh water instilled into their endotracheal tubes. When sea water was instilled beginning at a dose of 1 ml/lb, hypernatremia, hyperchloremia, and hyperkalemia (average K^+ concentration of sea water is approximately 11 mEq/liter[58]) quickly occurred producing what appeared to be lethal electrolyte changes. When fresh water was instilled, hyponatremia, hypochloremia, and hyperkalemia (presumably from hypo-osmolar red cell lysis) quickly occurred resulting in ventricular fibrillation and death.[59–61] Yet repeated observations in human near-drowning victims conclusively demonstrate that clinically significant abnormalities in serum electrolytes rarely occur.[46, 48, 53, 62–66] Although there are minor changes in serum Na^+ and Cl^- in the direction expected from the type of aspirated fluid (hypernatremia in salt water aspiration and hyponatremia in fresh water aspiration), significant changes in serum potassium have not been reported. Indeed, the hyperkalemia seen in the original dog studies, which was allegedly due to red cell lysis, cannot be explained in that fashion, as the major intracellular cation in the dog erythrocyte is sodium rather than potassium.[47] This is not meant to imply that red cell lysis does not occur with fresh water aspiration, but rather to emphasize that the clinical significance of this occurrence has perhaps been overemphasized.

In all probability, significant electrolyte changes do not occur in the human near-drowning victim because the quantity of aspirated water is simply not large enough to produce such changes (Table 10–1).[46, 48, 53, 62–67] This appears to be true for the drowning victim as well, for in the limited circumstances where it has been investigated, major electrolyte changes were not noted in fatal incidents either.[68] The exception to this situation appears to be submersion victims in the Dead Sea where electrolyte concentrations are greater than those in usual sea water. Victims of near drowning in that unique environment do have major electrolyte abnormalities, and it is believed that these disturbances are responsible for the fatal arrhythmias that have occurred in that group.[58, 69]

The remaining specific consequence of aspiration is pneumonia, which can occur in near-drowning victims. This is occasionally a cause of long-term morbidity and mortality.[70, 71] Although hemoglobinuria,[72] diffuse intravascular coagulation,[73] and renal failure[74, 75] have been reported in near-drowning victims, they are probably nonspecific responses to the hypoxemia, acidosis, and hypotension previously described.

It should be apparent that hypothermia as previously described can be protective for the cold-water victim. Since cardiac arrest is secondary to hypoxemia in near drowning, it presumably takes a significant amount of time to occur. If during this time the fluid in which the victim is immersed is cold enough, if the surface area to mass ratio of the victim is large enough, and if the victim swallows enough water, the individual's core temperature may decrease enough that oxygen demands are markedly decreased, protecting the victim from the effects of the hypoxemia.

CLINICAL PRESENTATION

From the previous discussion of the pathophysiology of near drowning, it should be apparent that the clinical presentation of the near-drowning victim can vary considerably. Additionally, the patient's appearance at the scene of the incident (the prehospital setting) may differ from that at the hospital. The patient who is unconscious at the scene without vital signs may be hemodynamically stable and neu-

TABLE 10–1. Serum Electrolytes in Human Near-Drowning Victims

	Na⁻ (mEq/Liter)			Cl⁻ (mEq/Liter)			K⁺ (mEq/Liter)		
	#	Mean	Range	#	Mean	Range	#	Mean	Range
Fresh water victims	22	137	126–146	25	101	88–116	21	4.4	3.0–6.3
Sea water victims	26	147	132–160	28	111	96–127	25	4.2	3.2–5.4

From Modell JH: Blood gas and acid base changes. *In* The Pathophysiology and Treatment of Drowning and Near Drowning. Springfield, IL, CC Thomas, 1971, pp 44–45.

rologically intact in the emergency room (ER), whereas the victim initially hemodynamically stable at the scene might deteriorate significantly before arrival at the hospital independent of the emergency care rendered. As the clinical presentation can be so varied, it is easiest to describe the clinical status of the cardiovascular, pulmonary, and neurological systems individually.

Cardiovascular System

All too frequently, victims of significant near drownings suffer cardiac arrest. Frequently, the cardiac arrest responds to resuscitative measures in the field, but it is not uncommon for a victim to be brought to the ER still requiring cardiopulmonary resuscitation (CPR). If the patient responds to CPR with a stable rhythm or if the patient never suffers a cardiac arrest, supraventricular tachycardias (SVT) are commonly seen. If the patient presents with a viable rhythm, it too will most likely be an SVT secondary to hypoxemia and acidosis.[76, 77] Usually the patient is hemodynamically intact (i.e., adequate blood pressure and pulse with a presumably adequate cardiac output); on occasion, patients will be in shock and will require cardiovascular support. The treatment for the hemodynamically unstable patient will be covered in the next section.

Pulmonary System

Patients with water aspiration may present with little or no respiratory complaints or with severe pulmonary edema.[78] This is due to direct lung injury and is not cardiogenic in origin. Patients who have aspirated any significant quantity of water will have a widened alveolar-arterial (A-a) oxygen gradient and anything from mild to severe hypoxemia. P_aCO_2 can be low or elevated depending upon the alveolar ventilation (Table 10–2). Chest x-rays can show patchy infiltrates (Fig. 10–1) (most commonly peripherally or in medial basal regions) or frank pulmonary edema (Fig. 10–2).[79–82] The pulmonary edema is, as stated, noncardiogenic and is a form of the adult respiratory distress syndrome (ARDS).[79]

Neurological Status

The neurological status of patients can also be quite varied. In order to compare results among different groups, a classification scheme has been devised to describe these patients.[83, 84] In this classification system, patients are placed into category A, B, or C based upon their initial neurological status. Category A patients are *a*wake; category B patients are *b*lunted; and category C patients are *c*omatose. Within category C, patients are further classified as C_1, C_2, or C_3, depending upon their best motor response. The C_1 comatose patient has a decorticate response, the C_2 patient has a decerebrate response, and the C_3 patient has no motor response at all. Treatment for these groups is potentially different and will be discussed in the following section.

TREATMENT

The near-drowning patient who presents in cardiac arrest should be treated vigorously, since salvage with normal neurological function has been described even after prolonged cardiac arrest.[35–38] As cardiac arrest in this setting is invariably due to hypoxemia and acidosis, the first goal must be to establish a reliable airway and to supply as high a fractional inspired oxygen concentration (F_IO_2) as possible. Until the results of arterial blood gas (ABG) determinations are available, 100 per cent oxygen should be used. Furthermore, as aspiration of stomach contents is a constant threat in the comatose patient, bag-valve-mask oxygenation has no place in the advanced care of these patients. The preferred method of establishing an airway is endotracheal intubation. This must be accomplished, however, keeping in mind the possibility of a concomitant unstable neck injury.

It should also be remembered that patients with cardiac arrest secondary to near drowning

TABLE 10–2. Arterial Blood Gas and pH Values Found on Admission to the Hospital After Near Drowning

pH	P_aCO_2 (torr)	Base Excess (mEq/liter)	P_aO_2 (torr)	F_IO_2
In Fresh Water:				
6.95	64	−19	245	1.0
7.01	38	−22	28	0.2
7.05	59	−16	40	1.0 R
7.13	30	−19	67	0.2
7.14	45	−14	68	0.2
7.18	33	−15	110	1.0
7.19	29	−16	108	±0.8 R
7.21	37	−13	175	1.0
7.22	54	−7	123	1.0 R
7.28	54	−3	35	0.4
7.33	41	−4	127	1.0
7.40	32	−4	103	0.2
7.44	32	−2	76	0.2
7.45	35	1	84	0.2
In Sea Water:				
7.03	36	−21	58	1.0
7.08	58	−14	21	1.0 R
7.20	46	−10	27	0.2
7.29	49	−4	364	1.0 R
7.31	35	−8	85	0.8 R
7.35	47	−1	45	0.2
7.46	25	−5	71	0.2
7.47	26	−3	82	0.4

R = Mechanical ventilation.
From Modell JH: Blood gas and acid base changes. *In* The Pathophysiology and Treatment of Drowning and Near Drowning. Springfield, IL, CC Thomas, 1971, pp 17–18.

can have a profound metabolic acidosis and that the doses of bicarbonate necessary to reverse such an acidosis may be far larger than the blind doses recommended for patients suffering cardiac arrest from primary heart disease.[85] Generally, in immersion incidents, the cardiac arrest is secondary to hypoxemia and acidosis, while in cardiac arrest secondary to primary heart disease, acidosis and hypoxemia are secondary to the cardiac arrest itself. As a result, ABG determinations are necessary to determine exact bicarbonate dosing. Concurrent with the above resuscitative measures, a nasogastric tube should be inserted to decompress the stomach, and measurement of body temperature should be obtained to rule out hypothermia. In the presence of a significantly lowered body temperature, a patient should not be declared dead and aggressive rewarming measures must be instituted (see Chapter 9).

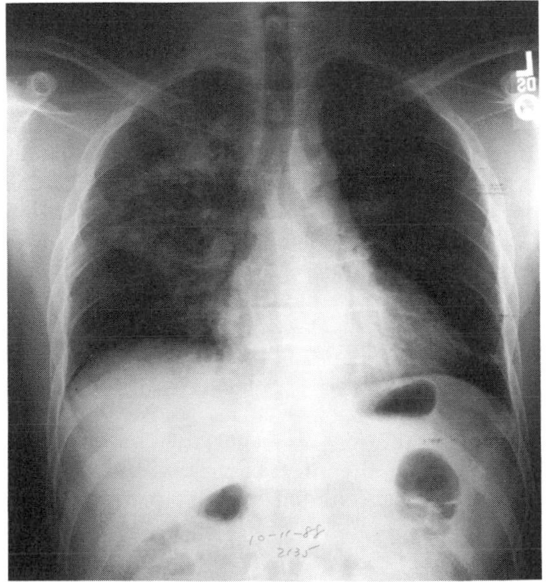

FIGURE 10–1. Localized, patchy infiltrates in right lung of a near drowning victim.

Once an adequate airway has been obtained and spontaneous cardiac activity achieved, attention must be directed to ensuring adequate oxygen delivery to the tissues by obtaining an adequate P_aO_2. Generally, in the near-drowning victim, hemodynamic stability is relatively easy to achieve; however, on rare occasion, patients will have marked decreases in blood pressure and associated decreases in cardiac output. The initial therapy for hypotension of most etiologies is a trial of fluids, yet for a near-drowning victim with pulmonary edema, this may not be appropriate. As a result, this group of patients is best managed with invasive hemodynamic monitoring. With knowledge of pulmonary artery wedge (PAW) pressure and cardiac output, more rational decisions concerning the need for fluids or pressors can then be made.[78, 86] It is important to realize that with noncardiac pulmonary edema of any cause, isolated measurement of the central venous pressure (CVP) is generally not an accurate method of judging intravascular fluid volume. In addition, changes in CVP, whether up or down, do not necessarily correspond to changes of the PAW pressure or left ventricular filling pressures. As a result, the use of CVP measurements in the management of the near-drowning victim is extremely limited; direct measurement of PAW and cardiac output may need to be obtained in addition to the ABG in patients with hypotension and evidence of pulmonary edema.

Positive end expiratory pressure (PEEP) has been shown, both experimentally and clinically, to be extremely effective in reversing the abnormal $\dot{V}_A/\dot{Q}$ relationships leading to hypoxemia.[87–91] Usually only modest amounts of PEEP will be necessary to achieve adequate oxygenation, and the improvement in pulmonary function can be quite dramatic (Figs. 10–2 and 10–3). PEEP apparently does not alter the course of the underlying pulmonary injury but rather allows for adequate oxygenation while the lung is recovering. PEEP also allows this recovery to take place at a level of inspired oxygen that is not in itself toxic to the lung.[92] Usually the pulmonary injury resolves over a period of 48 to 72 hours. As a result, ventilatory support in most circumstances is relatively brief unless infections develop.[87]

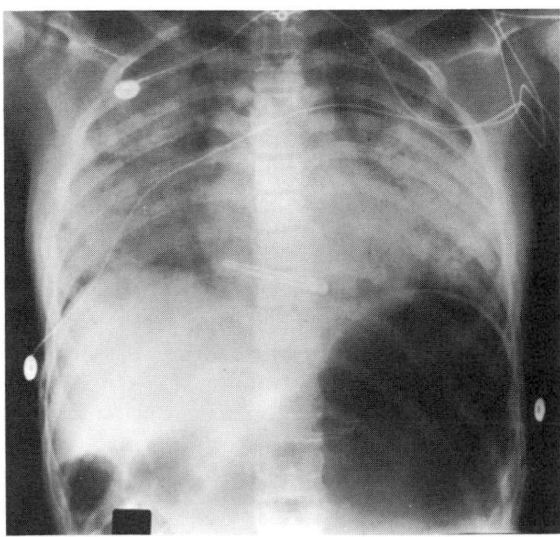

FIGURE 10–2. Diffuse pulmonary edema pattern in a near drowning victim. Note gastric distention.

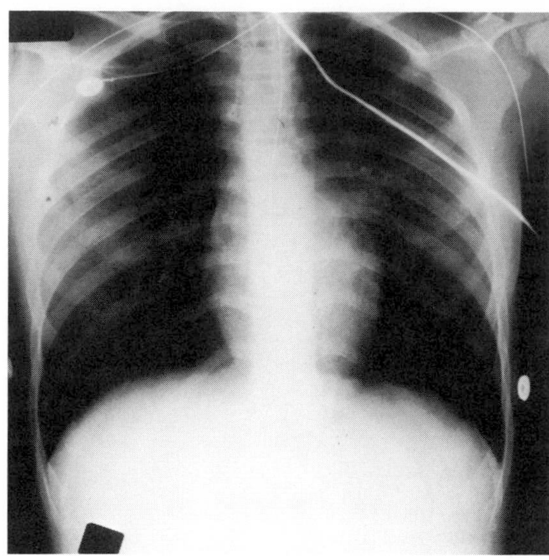

FIGURE 10–3. Same subject as in Figure 10–2 following therapy with PEEP.

The use of antibiotics in the near-drowning victim who aspirates ocean water or swimming pool water is usually restricted to those individuals who become febrile, develop new pulmonary infiltrates, and/or develop purulent secretions.[93] Prophylactic antibiotics do not seem to improve mortality or decrease morbidity.[45, 94] Since most pulmonary infections in the near-drowning victim appear to be hospital acquired, prophylactic antibiotics seem to select for more resistant organisms.[62] In addition to clinical experience, experimental evidence also suggests that the use of prophylactic antibiotics is not indicated. If the victim aspirates heavily contaminated water with a known or suspected organism, the use of prophylactic antibiotics may be appropriate.[95]

Adrenocortical steroids used to treat the lung injury associated with near drowning are also probably unwarranted. Experimental evidence in this form of aspiration as well as others strongly suggests that steroids do not improve the long-term outcome or short-term morbidity.[96, 97] Their is, however, one uncontrolled series of four cases which suggests that high-dose steroids may be beneficial in near-drowning victims who present with pulmonary edema.[98]

The final area of treatment that must be addressed at the time of hospital admission is "cerebral resuscitation." A detailed analysis of the management of the brain-injured individual is beyond the scope of this chapter; however, a brief synopsis may be useful for those who may have to treat a near-drowning victim.

Historically, it has been extremely difficult to estimate the incidence of long-term neurological dysfunction following near-drowning episodes. Various different studies have different entrance criteria and different degrees of follow-up. Estimates in large series range from zero to approximately 10 per cent.[25, 62, 63, 76, 99, 100] In the late 1970's after a small experience of near-drowning incidents with a high incidence of long-term neurological sequelae, it was suggested that the incidence of neurological dysfunction following near-drowning episodes could be lowered by aggressive attempts at cerebral salvage.[101] This so-called *hyper* therapy included barbiturate coma, controlled hyperventilation, diuretics, paralysis, intentional hypothermia, and adrenocortical steroids. The rationale for this therapy was to lower intracranial pressure (ICP), reduce cerebral edema, and lower cerebral oxygen demand. All of these measures were to prevent further secondary damage to the neurological system. This mode of therapy presumes that further damage—after the initial anoxic insult—does occur and that it can be prevented by these measures.

Unfortunately, after approximately a decade of experience with this mode of therapy, it is not clear that morbidity and mortality have appreciably improved. The largest study performed by the group that originally advocated *hyper* therapy reports an incidence of neurological morbidity of 7 per cent.[102] This is not appreciably different from multiple studies performed prior to the advent of this therapy.[25, 62, 63, 76, 99, 100] Additionally, other studies have suggested that, although very high ICPs are associated with a poor outcome,[103] normal ICPs do not ensure neurological recovery,[104] and this therapy does not necessarily prevent elevations of ICP. Indeed, it appears that elevations of ICP are the result of brain injury rather than the cause of it.[105] Certainly most authorities agree that if this therapy is indicated at all,[106] it should be reserved for the most severely affected and then only in the setting of an ICU staffed, equipped and experienced in handling this type of patient.[84, 107] Even in such a setting, the portions of this therapy that are associated with significant morbidity should be reserved for victims whose ICP cannot be controlled by any other more conventional means (i.e., hyperventilation, head elevation, osmotic diuretics).

The decision to admit the near-drowning victim is usually straightforward. Any victim who has lost consciousness, has respiratory tract symptoms, an abnormal chest x-ray, or abnormal arterial blood gases should be admitted to the hospital, since pulmonary damage may not be clinically manifest for several hours after the incident.[45, 108]

TABLE 10–3. Treatment of the Near-Drowning Victim

1. Ensure patient airway. If necessary:
   a. Clear secretions and debris in airway and suction. (It is not necessary to try to "empty" lungs of water.)
   b. Intubate.
2. Ventilate with as high a percentage of oxygen that can be delivered.
3. If cardiac arrest has occurred, resuscitate according to American Heart Association recommendations.
4. Assess circulation and administer a gentle trial of volume infusion for hypotension.

If patient is a diver or has been breathing compressed air, consider the diagnosis of arterial gas embolism and arrange transfer to a hyperbaric chamber, if needed.

5. Obtain arterial blood gases, chest x-ray (and C-spine films, if indicated), complete blood count, urinalysis, electrocardiogram, prothrombin time, and serum electrolytes.
6. Insert nasogastric tube and Foley catheter, if necessary.
7. Apply PEEP as necessary to maintain adequate P_aO_2 and to allow reduction of F_IO_2.
8. For continued hemodynamic instability, consider placement of a Swan-Ganz catheter and measurements of PAW pressure, PA pressure, and cardiac output.
9. For a deeply comatose victim, consider ICP monitoring. Use hyperventilation, bed positioning, and diuretics to improve cerebral perfusion pressure. If the above measures fail to control the ICP, consider more aggressive measures (paralysis, barbiturate coma, hypothermia).
10. Treat complications (i.e., pneumonia, seizures, DIC, renal failure) supportively.

The previous discussion has dealt entirely with a victim of near drowning; however, in the setting of a diving accident, an unconscious victim may have sustained an air embolism as well. Whenever doubt exists, both conditions should be treated simultaneously if possible (Table 10–3).

PROGNOSIS

The prognosis in the near-drowning victim is entirely dependent upon the duration of immersion, length of the anoxic period, and the degree of damage secondary to the anoxic episode. Patients who arrive at the hospital neurologically intact have an excellent prognosis and should survive neurologically unimpaired. Additionally, the occurrence of a cardiac arrest does not in itself suggest a poor outcome. If the cardiac arrest responds to first aid at the scene of the accident, the outcome may be excellent. Cardiac arrest that persists through the period of initial first aid and transport to the hospital is a poor prognostic sign,[76] but the presence of spontaneous respirations upon presentation to the ER following cardiac arrest in the field is a good prognostic sign.[109] The duration of immersion correlates with the degree of damage secondary to the anoxic episode and therefore with the outcome. For example, if parents estimate that a child is "missing" or has been immersed for more than five minutes, this is associated with a poor outcome.[99]

Finally, it should be emphasized that any prediction concerning eventual outcome cannot be made in the presence of a hypothermic victim.

REFERENCES

1. Schench HV, McAniff JJ: United States underwater fatality statistics, 1972. U.S. Department of Commerce, NOAA. U.S. Government Printing Office Report No. URI-73-8, December, 1973.
2. Schench HV, McAniff JJ: United States underwater fatality statistics, 1973. U.S. Department of Commerce, NOAA. U.S. Government Printing Office Report No. URI-SSR-75-9, May, 1975.
3. Schench HV, McAniff JJ: United States underwater fatality statistics, 1974. U.S. Department of Commerce, NOAA. U.S. Government Printing Office Report No. URI-SSR-75-10, April, 1976.
4. Schench HV, McAniff JJ: United States underwater fatality statistics, 1975. U.S. Department of Commerce, NOAA. U.S. Government Printing Office Report No. URI-SSR-77-11, March, 1977.
5. Schench HV, McAniff JJ: United States underwater fatality statistics, 1976. U.S. Department of Commerce, NOAA. U.S. Government Printing Office Report No. URI-SSR-78-12, December, 1978.
6. McAniff JJ: United States underwater fatality statistics, 1970–78. National Underwater Accident Data Center, University of Rhode Island. Report No. URI-SSR-80-13, September, 1980.
7. McAniff JJ: United States underwater fatality statistics, 1970–79. National Underwater Accident Data Center, University of Rhode Island. Report No. URI-SSR-80-14, August 1981.
8. McAniff JJ: United States underwater fatality statistics, 1970–80, including a preliminary assessment of 1981 fatalities. National Underwater Accident Data Center, University of Rhode Island. Report No. URI-SSR-82-15, December, 1982.
9. McAniff JJ: United States underwater fatality statistics, 1970-81, including a preliminary assessment of 1982 fatalities. National Underwater Accident Data Center, University of Rhode Island. Report No. URI-SSR-83-16, 1983.
10. McAniff JJ: United States underwater fatality statistics, 1970-82, including a preliminary assessment of 1983 fatalities. National Underwater Accident Data Center, University of Rhode Island. Report No. URI-SSR-84-17, 1984.
11. Aquatic deaths and injuries: United States. MMWR 31:417–412, 1982.
12. Schuman SH, Rowe JR, Glazer HM: Risk of drowning: An iceberg phenomenon. JACEP 6:139-172, 1977.
13. Editorial: Immersion and drowning in children. Br Med J 2:146–147,1977.
14. United Press International. San Diego *Union*, May, 1985.
15. Decker MD, Dewey MJ, Hutchison RH, Schaffner W: The use and efficacy of child restraint devices: The Tennessee experience, 1982 and 1983. JAMA 252:2571–2575, 1984.
16. Spyker DA: Submersion injury: Epidemiology, prevention, management. Pediatr Clin North Am 32:113–125, 1985.
17. Press E, Walker J, Crawford I: An interstate drowning study. Am J Public Health 12:2275–2289, 1968.
18. Virginia Department of Health, Bureau of Vital Records and Health Statistics: Vital Statistics Monthly Report. Richmond, 1978.
19. Dietz PE, Baker SP: Drowning: Epidemiology and prevention. Am J Public Health 64:303–312, 1974.
20. Baker SP, O'Neill B, Karpf RS: The Injury Fact Book. Lexington, MA, Lexington Books, 1984.
21. National Safety Council: Accident Facts, 1984. Chicago, National Safety Council, 1984.
22. Pearn J, Hsia EY: Swimming pool drownings and near drownings involving children: A total population study from Hawaii. Milit Med 190:15–18, 1980.
23. Pearn J, Nixon J: Prevention of childhood drowning accidents. Med J Aust 1:616–618, 1977.
24. Rowe MI, Arango A, Allington G: Profile of pediatric drowning victims in a water-oriented society. J Trauma 17:587–591, 1977.
25. Pearn JH, Wong RY, Brown J, et al: Drowning and near drowning involving children: A five-year total population study from the City and County of Honolulu. Am J Public Health 69:450–453, 1979.
26. Cairns FJ, Koelmeyer TD, Smeeton WM: Deaths from drowning. NZ Med J 97:65–67, 1984.
27. Davis S, Smith LS: Alcohol and drowning in Cape Town. S Afr Med J 62:931–933, 1982.
28. Plueckhahn VD: The aetiology of 134 deaths due to "drowning" in Geelong during the years 1957–1971. Med J Aust 2:1183–1187, 1972.
29. Plueckhahn VD: Alcohol and accidental drowning. Med J Aust 2:22–25, 1984.
30. Craig AB: Underwater swimming and loss of consciousness. JAMA 176:255–258,1961.
31. Craig AB: Causes of loss of consciousness during underwater swimming. J Appl Physiol 16:583–586, 1961.
32. Snively WD, Thuerbach J: Voluntary hyperventilation as a cause of needless drowning. W Va Med J 68:153–157, 1972.
33. Mersey, Lord (Wreck Commissioner): Report of a formal investivation into the circumstances attending the foundering on 15th April 1912 of the British Steamship Titanic of Liverpool after striking ice in or near latitude 41° 46′ N, longitude 50° 14′ W, North Atlantic Ocean, whereby loss of life ensued. His Majesty's Stationery Office, London, 1912.
34. Martin TG: Near drowning and cold water immersion. Ann Emerg Med 13:263–273, 1984.
35. Sekar TS, McDonnell KF, Namsirikul P, et al: Survival after prolonged immersion in cold water without neurologic sequelae. Arch Intern Med 140:775–779, 1980.
36. Siebke H, Breivik H, Rod T, et al: Survival after 40 minutes submersion without cerebral sequelae. Lancet 1:1275–1277, 1975.
37. Wolford JP: Cold water near-drowning response. JEMS, Spring, 1984.
38. Young RSK, Zaineraitis ED, Dooling EO: Neurologic

outcome in cold-water drowning. JAMA 244:1233–1235, 1980.
39. Walker D: New Zealand diving-related fatalities. SPUMS 14:12–16, 1984.
40. Burke DC: Spinal cord injuries from water sports. Med J Aust 2:1190–1194, 1972.
41. Green BA, Gabrielsen A, Hall WT, et al: Analysis of swimming pool accidents resulting in spinal cord injury. Paraplegia 18:94–100, 1980.
42. Kewalramani LS, Kraus JF: Acute spinal cord lesions from diving: Epidemiological and clinical features. West J Med 126:353–361, 1977.
43. Perspectives in disease prevention and health promotion. MMWR 31:417–419, 1982.
44. Modell JH: Blood gas and acid base changes. *In* The Pathophysiology and Treatment of Drowning and Near Drowning. Springfield IL, CC Thomas, 1970, pp 13–15.
45. Hoff BH: Multisystem failure: A review with special reference to drowning. Crit Care Med 7:310–317, 1979.
46. Modell JH, Davis JH, Giammona ST, et al: Blood gas and electrolyte changes in human near-drowning victims. JAMA 203:337–343, 1968.
47. Rivers JF, Orr G, Lee HA: Drowning: Its clinical sequelae and management. Br Med J 2:157–161, 1970.
48. Segarra F, Redding RA: Modern concepts about drowning. CMA 110:1057–1062, 1974.
49. Modell JH: Biology of drowning. Annu Rev Med 29:1–8, 1978.
50. Cot C: Asphyxia from drowning: Treatment based on experimental findings. Bull Acad Natl Med (Paris) 105:758, 1931.
51. Halmagyi DF, Colebatch HJ: Ventilation and circulation after fluid aspiration. J Appl Physiol 16:35–40, 1961.
52. Colebatch HJ, Halmagyi DF: Lung mechanics and resuscitation after fluid aspiration. J Appl Physiol 16:684–696, 1961.
53. Haglund P, Favarel-Garrigues J, Nicod J, Lobera A: Biological disturbances during drowning in sea water. Resuscitation 3:121–127, 1974.
54. Modell JH, Moya F, Newby EJ, et al: The effects of fluid volume in sea water drowning. Ann Intern Med 67:68–80, 1967.
55. Modell JH, Moya F: Effects of volume of aspirated fluid during chlorinated fresh-water drowning. Anesthesiology 27:662–672, 1966.
56. Giammona ST, Modell JH: Drowning by total immersion: Effects on pulmonary surfactant of distilled water, isotonic saline and sea water. Am J Dis Child 114:612–616, 1967.
57. Greenberg MI, Baskin SI, Kaplan AM, et al: Effects of endotracheally administered distilled water and normal saline on arterial blood gases of dogs. Ann Emerg Med 11:600–604, 1982.
58. Yagil Y, Stalnikowicz R, Michaeli J, Mogle P: Near drowning in the Dead Sea: Electrolyte imbalances and therapeutic implications. Arch Intern Med 145:50–53, 1985.
59. Swann HG, Brucer M, Moore C, et al: Fresh-water and sea-water drowning: A study of the terminal cardiac and biochemical events. Texas Rep Biol Med 5:423–438, 1947.
60. Swann HG, Brucer M: The cardiorespiratory and biochemical events during rapid anoxic death. VI. Fresh-water and sea-water drowning. Texas Rep Biol Med 7:604–618, 1949.
61. Swann HG, Spafford NR: Body salt and water changes during fresh and sea-water drowning. Texas Rep Biol Med 9:356–382, 1951.
62. Modell JH, Graves SA, Ketover A: Clinical course of 91 consecutive near-drowning victims. Chest 70:231–238, 1976.
63. Fandel I, Bancalari E: Near drowning in children: Clinical aspects. Pediatrics 58:573–579, 1976.
64. Barrett O, Martin CM: Drowning and near drowning: A review of 10 years experience in a large Army hospital. Milit Med 136:439–443, 1971.
65. Modell JH, Weibley TC, Ruiz BC: Serum electrolyte concentrations after fresh-water aspiration. Anesthesiology 30:421–425, 1969.
66. Hasan S, Avery WG, Fabian C, Sackner M: Near drowning in humans: A report of 36 patients. Chest 59:191–197, 1971.
67. Wong LL, McNamara JJ: Salt-water drowning. Hawaii Med J 43:208–210, 1984.
68. Modell JH, Davis JH: Electrolyte changes in human drowning victims. Anesthesiology 30:414–420, 1969.
69. Alkan ML, Gaszes T, Kotev S, et al: Near drowning in the Dead Sea. Isr J Med Sci 13:290–294, 1977.
70. Vieira DF, Van Saene HKF, Miranda DR: Invasive pulmonary aspergillosis after near drowning. Intensive Care Med 10:203–204, 1984.
71. Rosenthal S, Zuger JH, Apollo E: Respiratory colonization with *Pseudomonas putrefaciens* after near drowning in salt water. Am J Clin Pathol 64:382–384, 1975.
72. Munroe WD: Hemoglobinuria from near drowning. J Pediatr 64:57–62, 1964.
73. Ports TA, Deuel TF: Intravascular coagulation in fresh-water submersion. Ann Intern Med 87:60–61, 1977.
74. Neale TJ, Dewar JM, Kimber J, et al: Acute renal failure following near drowning in salt water. NZ Med J 97:319–322, 1984.
75. Grausz H, Amend WJC, Earley LE: Acute renal failure complicating submersion in sea water. JAMA 217:207–209, 1971.
76. Peterson B: Morbidity of childhood near drowning. Pediatrics 59:364–370, 1977.
77. Kaukinen L: Clinical course and prognostic signs in near-drowned patients. Ann Chir Gynaecol 73:34–39, 1984.
78. Lheureux P, Vincent JL, Brimioulle S: Fulminant pulmonary edema after near drowning: Remarkably high colloid osmotic pressure in tracheal fluid. Intensive Care Med 10:205–207, 1984.
79. Fine NL, Myerson DA, Myerson PJ, Pagliaro JJ: Near drowning presenting as the adult respiratory distress syndrome. Chest 65:347–349, 1974.
80. Hunter TB, Whitehouse WM: Fresh-water near drowning: Radiological aspects. Radiology 112:51–56, 1974.
81. Rosenbaum HT, Thompson WL, Fuller RH: Radiographic pulmonary changes in near drowning. Radiology 83:306–312, 1964.
82. Neuman TS: Near Drowning. *In* Moser KM, Spragg RS (eds): Respiratory Emergencies. 2nd ed. St. Louis, CV Mosby Company, 1982, pp 282–284.
83. Conn AW, Montes JE, Barker GA, Edmonds JF: Cerebral salvage in near drowning following neurological classification by triage. Can Anaesth Soc J 27:201–210, 1980.
84. Modell JH, Graves SA, Kuck EJ: Near drowning: Correlation of level of consciousness and survival. Can Anaesth Soc J 27:211–215, 1980.
85. Standards and guidelines for cardiopulmonary resus-

citation (CPR) and emergency cardiac care (ECC). JAMA 255:2905–2984, 1986.

86. Tabeling BB, Modell JH: Fluid administration increases oxygen delivery during continuous positive-pressure ventilation after fresh-water near drowning. Crit Care Med 11:693–696, 1983.
87. Modell JH, Calderwood HW, Ruiz BC, et al: Effects of ventilatory patterns on arterial oxygenation after near drowning in sea water. Anesthesiology 46:376–384, 1974.
88. Van Haeringen JR, Blokzijl EJ, van Dyl W, et al: Treatment of the respiratory distress syndrome following nondirect pulmonary trauma with positive end expiratory pressure with special emphasis on near drowning. Chest 66(Suppl):30S–34S, 1974.
89. Bergquist RE, Vogelhut MM, Modell JH, et al: Comparison of ventilatory patterns in the treatment of fresh-water near drowning in dogs. Anesthesiology 52:142–148, 1980.
90. Oaks DD, Sherck JP, Maloney JR, Charters AC: Prognosis and management of victims of near drowning. J Trauma 22:544–549, 1982.
91. Rutledge RR, Flor RJ: The use of mechanical ventilation with positive end expiratory pressure in the treatment of near drowning. Anesthesiology 38:194–196, 1973.
92. Lindner KH, Dick W, Lotz P: The delayed use of positive end expiratory pressure (PEEP) during respiratory resuscitation following near drowning with fresh or salt water. Resuscitation 10:197–211, 1983.
93. Kizer KW: Resuscitation of submersion casualties. Emerg Med Clin North Am 1:643–652, 1983.
94. Hughs JA: Drowning—An overveiw. JACEP 6:172, 1977.
95. Wynne JW, Modell JH: Respiratory aspiration of stomach contents. Ann Intern Med 87:466–476, 1977.
96. Calderwood HW, Modell JH, Ruiz BC: The ineffectiveness of steroid therapy for treatment of fresh-water near drowning. Anesthesiology 43:642–650, 1975.
97. Downs JB, Chapman RL, Modell JH, Ian Hood C: An evaluation of steroid therapy in aspiration pneumonitis. Anesthesiology 40:129–135, 1974.
98. Sladen A, Zauder HL: Methyl prednisolone therapy for pulmonary edema following near drowning. JAMA 215:1793–1795, 1971.
99. Orlowski J: Prognostic factors in pediatric cases of drowning and near drowning. JACEP 8:176–179, 1979.
100. Pearn J: Neurologic and psychometric studies in children surviving fresh-water immersion incidents. Lancet 1:7–9, 1977.
101. Conn AW, Edmonds JF, Barker GA: Cerebral resuscitation in near drowning. Pediatr Clin North Am 26:691–701, 1979.
102. Conn AW, Barker GA: Fresh-water drowning and near drowning: An update. Can Anaesth Soc J 31:538–544, 1984.
103. Dean JM, McComb JG: Intracranial pressure monitoring in severe pediatric near drowning. Neurosurgery 9:627–630, 1981.
104. Nussbaum E, Galant SP: Intracranial pressure monitoring as a guide to prognosis in the nearly drowned, severely comatose child. J Pediatr 102:215–218, 1983.
105. Sarnaik AP, Preston G, Lieh-Lai M, Eisenbrey AB: Intracranial pressure and cerebral perfusion pressure in near drowning. Crit Care Med 13:224–227, 1985.
106. Rogers MC: Near drowning: Cold water on a hot topic? J Pediatr 106:603–604, 1985.
107. Frewen TC, Sumabat WO, Han VK, et al: Cerebral resuscitation therapy in pediatric near drowning. J Pediatr 106:615–617, 1985.
108. Putman CE: Drowning: Another plunge. Am J Roentg Radium Ther Nucl Med 125:543–549, 1975.
109. Jacobsen WK, Mason LJ, Briggs BA, et al: Correlation of spontaneous respiration and neurologic damage in near drowning. Crit Care Med 11:487–489, 1983.

Chapter 11

Marine Animal Injuries

CARL EDMONDS

Serious injury from a marine animal attack is not very common. Nevertheless, there are over 1000 marine vertebrates that are believed to be either venomous or poisonous. The invertebrates are even more numerous and less well documented.

The first group of marine animals referred to in this chapter are those that bite. Lacking the malevolent weapons designed by humans, this group of animals has the capability to revert to this primitive method of defense. In most such cases, the provocation lies with the human who threatens the animal's domain. Often the human has entered the territory with a clear intent to destroy, for example, fishermen, divers carrying spear guns, or underwater construction workers. In other cases, a wader, swimmer, or diver intrudes by accident or by choice into the territorial area of the marine animal.

The incidence of serious attacks from biting marine animals is very small, although speculation and folklore among marine enthusiasts have given them a high profile. The types of animal incriminated include killer whales, seals, sea lions (Fig. 11–1), grouper, barracuda, eels, and many types of fish. Two marine animals—sharks and crocodiles—do cause a genuine concern as they have been responsible for verified fatalities and are the source of much public interest. They will be discussed in more detail.

The second group of marine animals inflicts pain or causes incapacity by stinging victims in order to obtain food or to protect against predators. These stinging marine animals possess a venom that must be injected by fangs, spines, stinging tentacles, and so forth. Some animals hide the venom delivery system until threatened or attacked. Others highlight or display the lethal-looking appendages, relying on prevention of the attack more than on counterattack. Some species deliver an electric current instead of a venom.

Such animals selected for discussion in this chapter include sea snakes; stonefish, stingray, and other fish; sea wasp, *Physalia*, and other coelenterates; cone shells, blue-ringed octopus, sea urchins, electric rays, and coral.

There are many others that could have been included, but these are too numerous to cover

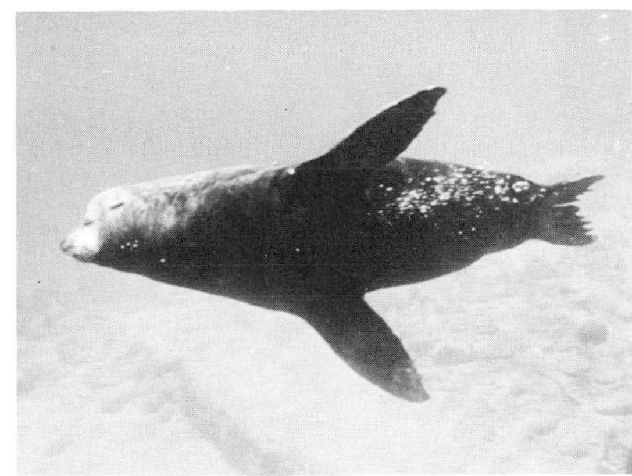

FIGURE 11–1. Bull sea lion found in the Sea of Cortez. Normally rather docile, the male can become aggressive during mating season. (Photo by Bonnie J. Cardone, used with permission from Peterson Publishing Company, Los Angeles, CA)

This chapter contains material that is reproduced with permission from *Dangerous Marine Creatures*, by Carl Edmonds, and from *Diving and Subaquatic Medicine*, 2nd Edition, by Edmonds, Lowry, and Pennefather.

in one chapter. The references are chosen to provide a recommended reading list.

As a final pièce de résistance, which works well for species survival but which sacrifices the individual, is the poisonous fish. Here a predator succeeds in killing and ingesting the marine animal but suffers or dies from the effects. Survivors of the predator species thus learn to respect and avoid these poisonous species.

SHARK ATTACK

General

Our knowledge of sharks has been based more on fiction than on fact. Earlier this century they were regarded by Europeans as scavengers and cowards, and it was seriously argued whether they did, in fact, attack humans. The subsequent controversy resulted in a mass of accumulated data that left no doubt.

Sharks comprise a very efficient and successful evolutionary group of animals. Many of the present day sharks and rays are of the same genera as those that swam in the Cretaceous seas over 100 million years ago. The majority of the 250 species of sharks are marine inhabitants; many will enter estuaries, some will travel far up rivers, and a few are fresh-water species. Most live in the relatively shallow waters off the major continents or around islands and inhabit the temperate or tropical zones (Fig. 11–2).

The shark is perhaps the most successful of all predators. It has roamed the seas since the very dawn of history, and islanders and seafaring people have incorporated this creature into the center of their folklore. The shark is variously feared, respected, worshipped, idolized, and exploited. Mariners, fishermen, and divers, who are not renowned for their strict observance of factual reporting, have perpetuated shark obsessions. Rescue and first-aid groups may have ulterior motives in sometimes exaggerating the risk of shark attack.

Shark attack remains a genuine but unlikely danger to seafaring people. Although rare, the attack is often terrifying in intensity, and the degree of mutilation produced has a strong emotive effect on civilized man. In the marine environment, without the protection afforded by a superior civilization, sophisticated technology, or the terrestrial senses, man is a weak and vulnerable creature.

There has been a detectable change in attitude since the advent of scuba diving. Initially, divers engaged in an orgy of destruction against sharks, using spears, powerheads, and carbon dioxide darts. More recently, as divers have observed and then admired the beauty of these animals, attitudes have changed. As in other areas, the camera has replaced the gun. We now look on the sea and its inhabitants as an equally vulnerable and limited resource.

Once a shark attack has occurred, most of those involved would consider the species identification as somewhat academic. This is not necessarily so. Different species have different characteristics, and only 30 of the 250 species have been reported as attacking humans. Also, preventative measures must be based on an understanding of shark behavior.

The Isuridae form the most notorious of the shark families. They have a fusiform shape, tapered from the pointed snout, with an equally

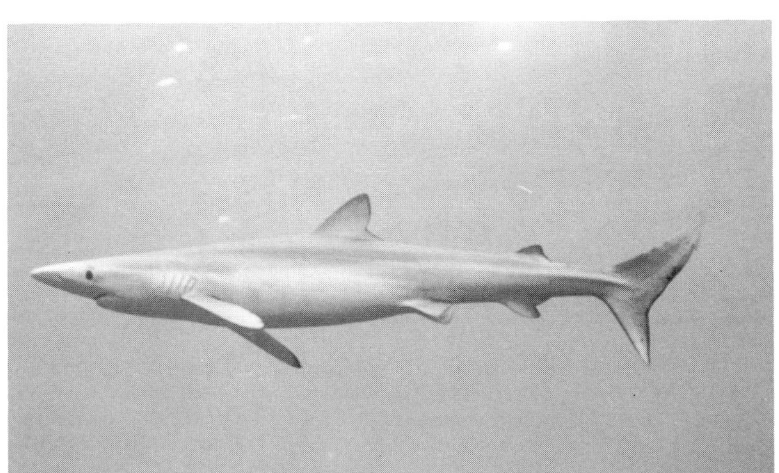

FIGURE 11–2. Blue shark *(Prionace glauca)*. (Photo by Bonnie J. Cardone)

lobed muscular tail. They are capable of fast but stiff-bodied swimming, with short rapid strokes. The large dark eyes testify to the deep water habits of the porbeagle and the mako; the great white is a more shallow inhabitant.

The great white is the epitome of a man-eating shark. The larger specimens (usually female) weigh between one and two tons and measure up to 21 feet long. The teeth are triangular, serrated, and disproportionately large—sometimes over two inches long. Great whites are especially found in cold waters with large seal and sea lion populations and therefore are found in shallower areas than the other Isuridae, who feed on deep sea fishes. The west and northeastern coasts of North America, southern Australia, and south Africa are well-documented areas of habitation and are also favored by surfers and abalone divers.

San Francisco, because of the 120 miles of coast between Tomales Point and Bodega Bay to the north and Santa Cruz and Monterey Bay to the south, is known as the white shark attack capital of the world. The adult females give birth in late summer or early fall in shallow waters south of Point Conception, with the pups remaining inshore and feeding on the prolific fish life. As they grow older, they travel north and offshore to the pinniped (seal, sea lions) breeding areas, around islands.

Over the last few decades there has been an increased number of shark attacks along the west coast of the United States on both abalone divers and surfboard riders. Almost four out of every five such attacks are unequivocally due to the great white. It is believed that the attacks are of a feeding type, whereby the surface swimmer or surf craft is mistaken for a seal or sea lion.

Carcharhinids, requiem, or gray sharks are among the largest and most aggressive, with varied and confusing nomenclature. They range from 3 to 12 feet long, usually with the second dorsal fin much smaller than the first and the upper lobe of the tail much longer than the lower.

Examples include the tiger shark and the oceanic white tip. The tiger shark is so named because the young are born with stripes. Cousteau described the oceanic whitetip as the most dangerous of all sharks. It is certainly one of the most abundant and congregates rapidly at midocean disasters, such as shipwrecks and airplane accidents.

Hammerheads are easily identified by the T-shaped head with eyes and nostrils widely separated, giving the shark a wide area of perusal as it slowly swings its head from side to side. It may grow to a 20-foot length and is often gregarious, having been observed in packs of 10 to 20 sharks.

Shark Attack Patterns

There are different types of attack, and these may be identified by the behavior of the animals and the subsequent nature of the injury. Three of these types represent different degrees of a feeding attack, and the fourth and fifth represent a territorial intrusion.

The feeding response seems to be related more to the presence of specific stimuli than to the nutritional requirements of the animal. The presence of physical and chemical stimuli, such as that released from injured or freshly killed animals, can attract sharks and may result in a feeding response. Sharks in a feeding pattern tend to circle the victim, gradually increasing their swimming speed. As the circles begin to tighten, the sharks may commence a criss-cross pattern going across the circle. At this stage, they may produce the first type of injury by contact, when they bump or brush against the prey. The shark's very sharp skin can cause extensive injuries, and it is thought that the information obtained by the animal at this time may influence the likelihood of progression of the feeding pattern.

The shark bite is usually performed with the animal in a horizontal or slightly upward direction, with the head swung backward and the upper teeth projecting in a forward direction. This results in a great increase in the mouth size and a display of the razor sharp teeth.

Once the animal has a grip on its prey, if the feeding pattern continues, the mouthful will usually be torn out sideways or the area will be totally severed. If other sharks are in the vicinity, they may reflexly respond to the stimuli created by the attack and commence the third type of feeding pattern behavior—a feeding frenzy.

It has been noted that sharks may swim together in an orderly and smooth manner, but when abnormal vibrations are set up (e.g., by one of the animals being shot or hooked), then the abnormal activity of that animal may trigger feeding responses in the others, and this may progressively increase into a feeding frenzy. In this instance, the sharks are likely to attack both the original prey and the predator or any other moving object. During this feeding frenzy, cannibalism has been observed, and the subsequent carnage can be extensive. This sequence of circling/bumping/biting may not always be followed, especially in the case of the great white, which has the size and strength to attack without warning behavior. The first bite on a large animal may be to wound or kill, more than to eat. Thus, the prey may be bitten and released, to die from blood loss. The shark can then feed without risk of retaliation from its victim.

Once a potential human victim separates from others, he appears more likely to be attacked. Staying within a group offers some protection. Even going to the aid of a victim rarely results in the rescuer being attacked, although there are at least two cases where this did happen. At least four people have been attacked on more than one occasion, and one had his artificial leg bitten.

The fourth type of attack is agonistic and involves an animal having its territorial rights infringed on by an intruder—either a swimmer or a diver. It may also happen if the shark is angry, frightened, or engaged in dominance behavior. It is quite unlike the feeding pattern, and the shark tends to swim in a far more awkward manner, shaking its head with a lateral motion, snout upturned with mouth slightly opened, spine arched, and pectoral fins angled downwards. In this position, it appears to be more rigid and awkward in its movements than the feeding animal. It has been described, both in appearance and motivation, as an animal adopting a defensive and snapping position. If the intruding diver vacates the area, confrontation will be avoided and an attack prevented.

Probably most of the attacks from territorial sharks are of this type. If the intruder does not vacate the area, the shark may snap or rake the victim with the teeth of its upper jaw. This may result in slashing wounds.

Another territorial type of attack may be precipitated by a person entering the water suddenly, onto or near an unsuspected shark. This happens from falling, jumping, or diving into the water, with the shark responding by snapping at the intruder.

Prevention of Shark Attack

Prevention of shark attack depends very much on the marine locality. The following procedures will be relevant in different situations.

Heavily Populated Beaches

The most effective method of reducing the incidence of shark attack is by net enclosures or meshing. Total bay enclosures are effective in sheltered areas, if consistent surveillance is carried out to ensure the integrity of the net. Only small areas are suitable for this technique, and at least one shark attack has occurred within a netted area.

Areas exposed to adverse weather or surf are best protected by meshing. This was introduced to the heavily populated beaches around Sydney, Australia, which had an awesome reputation for shark attack. In 1937 intermittent meshing was introduced along the metropolitan beaches. No shark attacks have been recorded on meshed beaches, since its introduction at Sydney or its surrounding cities.

Meshing involves the intermittent use of a heavy-gauge net, which is submerged from buoys to the seaward side of the breaking waves. It may be left overnight or for 24 hours and then retrieved. The net wraps around the animal and interferes with its gill function. As the shark is unable to retreat, it will struggle and attempt to push itself forward through the mesh. This results in the shark being further immobilized and thus produces death by suffocation.

The South Africans extended the Australian experience, both by increasing the extent of meshing and conducting high quality research into shark morphology and behavior. The Natal Anti-Shark Measures Board is an impressive monument of the importance of this work.

Survival Situation

The entry of an airplane into the water and sometimes the noises associated with a ship sinking are very effective in attracting sharks to an area. Thus, the survivors of such accidents may become victims of shark attack. The most effective way to prevent this is to use life rafts and have the survivors move into them as quickly as possible. As an alternative, the Johnson shark screen is very effective.

The shark screen is a bag of thin, tough plastic with a collar consisting of three inflatable rings. The survivor partially inflates one of the rings by mouth and then climbs into the bag. He fills it with water by dipping the edges, and it presents to any shark as a large, solid-looking black object. The other rings can be inflated at leisure. The bag retains fluid and excreta that may stimulate shark attack.

Swimmers

Swimmers are advised not to urinate in the water or to swim with abrasions or bleeding wounds. They are also advised to move gently and not to thrash around on the surface. They should stay with a group or at least with a buddy. This is cynically claimed to reduce the chance of shark attack by 50 per cent, but, in fact, it probably reduces it far more. Swimmers are also advised not to swim in water with low visibility, near drop-offs or deep channels, or toward late afternoon or night when sharks tend to be involved in feeding.

It is sometimes claimed that women should not dive or swim while menstruating. There is no evidence to support the belief that decomposing blood will attract sharks; in fact, both experimental and statistical evidence points to the opposite.

Divers

The incidence of shark attacks on scuba divers appears to be progressively increasing and now comprises one third of all shark attacks. Wet suits offer no protection and may well increase the likelihood of shark attack despite popular hopes to the contrary. Divers are advised in the same way as swimmers but with added precautions. Underwater explosives tend to attract sharks. Shark attacks are more likely at increased depth and can be provoked by playing with or killing other sharks. It is preferable to dive in areas where spear fishing is not performed. Divers are also advised not to tether fish or abalone near their bodies.

Powerheads, carbon dioxide darts, and the drogue dart (this has a small parachute attached which disrupts the shark's orientation and swimming efficiency) are all specialized pieces of equipment which may be appropriate in certain diving situations.

Experimentation was performed on the use of Kevlar incorporated into wet suits as a shark-bite–resistant material. It is currently being used as bulletproof vest material and is able to stop a .45 caliber bullet. However, it does not stop penetration of teeth from a relatively mild dusky shark.

Steel-meshed diving suits definitely discourage an attack but are dangerous unless extra precautions are taken to ensure buoyancy.

If one is diving in shark-infested waters, the use of a shark billy can be effective. The shark billy is of greatest value to experienced divers who often encounter sharks. It is a sturdy stick, with a nail stuck into it; the billy is used to push away any curious or interested shark.

Action to Take if Shark Attack is Threatened

Although the shark may do the unexpected, more often the behavior is predictable. If sharks are encountered, it is best to descend to the seabed or to the protection of rocks, cliff face, or some other obstacle so as to interfere with the normal attack patterns described earlier. If the shark retreats, slowly move along the shelter or head for the beach or boat when the shark is at its greatest distance. Always stay in a group, both under and on the surface.

If the shark is involved in feeding behavior, separate yourself from the probable source of the stimulus. Abandon any caught fish. If you are producing the stimulus, such as by overhand swimming, kicking, or prying abalone off rocks, then desist in the activity. As calmly as possible, and without heading into open water, leave the area. Continue to face the shark.

If the attack is agonistic in nature, with the typical posturing described previously, remain motionless for a few seconds while you appraise your situation. Face the shark, be prepared to fend it off with anything at your disposal, and calmly vacate the area, swimming backwards.

If the shark comes within a meter or two, any action may disrupt the feeding or agonistic pattern, so that yelling, blowing bubbles, or sudden body actions may be of value. Kicking or striking the shark in a sensitive area—eyes, snout, gills—with a knife, snorkel, or other instrument may terminate the attack.

Deterrents of Historical Interest

A vast number of experiments have been carried out to demonstrate ways of preventing shark attack. The less attention given to the repeated failures with chemical, electrical, sound, and bubble deterrents, the better.

CROCODILES, CAIMANS, AND ALLIGATORS

General

These reptiles, survivors of the dinosaur age, are found in the tropics and subtropics of the Americas, Australia, Indo-Pacific islands, Asia, and Africa. Crocodiles, despite their unlovable appearance, live a highly developed social life. They are very territorial and communicate under water by a variety of deep throated sounds and higher pitched oral noises. They display emotions by specific body postures and become more aggressive during breeding times. The young are hatched from eggs and are protected by both parents.

The species considered as man eaters are the saltwater crocodile and the Nile crocodile, which grow to 8 meters in length, and the American crocodile and American alligator, which grow to 3.5 meters. South American caimans are of the same family as alligators. The Indian mugger crocodile may attack humans if provoked while nesting. All crocodilians are carnivorous. They grow from one to 10 meters long, and the larger specimens are the ones potentially dangerous to humans. The largest grow up to a ton in weight.

South American caimans can grow up to 5 meters long, although most are much less. As one moves north to the Gulf of Mexico, the southern United States, and the Caribbean, crocodiles are more numerous. The crocodiles of Florida were nearly wiped out by hunting in the Everglades and during land development of the Keys. Conservation attempts over the last decade have resulted in a rise of some crocodilian populations, but this also has consequences that are diffcult to reconcile. As the animals grow older and larger, conflicts with humans emerge. They are often believed to be responsible for damage to fishermen's nets, and they may prey on both domestic animals and humans.

Alligators are slower moving and generally less dangerous to humans. Crocodiles have narrower snouts than alligators, and the fourth tooth on each side of the lower jaw is usually visible when the mouth is closed.

The fact that the animal is found in fresh water may signify that it has swum inland from the estuary, not that it is necessarily a freshwater crocodile. The latter are found in lakes and rivers that have no connection with the sea, and in some countries these crocodiles may be large and dangerous. For reptiles, they have very complex brains and are intelligent enough to stalk a human, strong enough to destroy a water buffalo, and gentle enough to release its own young from the eggs with its teeth. It even carries the newly hatched babies in its massive jaws.

Crocodiles tear their food off the carcass, twisting and turning in the water to achieve this. They then swallow it whole. Stones are also swallowed, and these increase the animal's specific gravity so as to be neutrally buoyant in water.

The animal often lies along the banks of rivers, with only the nostrils protruding above water to breath. Prey, especially land animals, that come to the river bank may be suddenly grabbed in the crocodile's immensely strong jaws and twisted off its feet. Once the prey is in the water and does not have the traction usually produced by its feet, it is more vulnerable to panic and drowning. Crocodiles can also move fast on land and can attack there or while free swimming—as has been demonstrated by recent attacks.

On land, attacks occur especially at night when the animal commonly stalks for food. They move surprisingly fast (faster than most humans), issue a hissing sound, and sometimes attack by sweeping the victim with its powerful tail.

SEA SNAKES

General

These air breathing reptiles number some 50 species. They are usually found in tropical or temperate zones and are most frequent in the Indo-Pacific area. Sea snakes can be subdivided into two major types according to their feeding habits. The bottom feeders have the capability of diving to considerable depths, perhaps even to 200 meters to locate and devour their prey (eels, fish, and so forth). The Laticauda, or banded sea snakes, are characteristic of this type. They are necessarily restricted to coastal and relatively shallow waters, often breed and lay their eggs onshore in crevices or caves, and are capable of existing for long times out of water.

The second group is the pelagic "blue water" type, exemplified by the yellow-bellied sea snake, *Pelamis platurus*. These snakes are surface feeders that drift with the warm tides. Mating takes place at sea, and the snake is viviparous. It may be found in packs far out to sea, but if it is washed up on beaches or land, it is unable to survive. This snake does not tolerate extremes of temperature and is rarely found when the average sea temperature drops below 20°C. The lethal limit for the snake's body temperature is 33° to 36°C, and the snake avoids high temperatures in tropical regions by diving into the cool waters away from the surface. It is for this reason they are more frequently found on the surface during rain or on cloudy days.

The sea snake has adapted to the hypertonic saline environment by developing salt-excreting glands under the tongue. It has also developed a flattened paddle-shaped tail and a laterally compressed body that make it an efficient swimmer. It is capable of remaining submerged for two hours, perhaps by decreasing its metabolic rate and developing an increased tolerance for hypoxia. The lung is greatly enlarged, extending all the way to the base of the tail. Parts of this lung may function as a hydrostatic organ, regulating the snake's buoyancy. Sea snakes are inquisitive and are sometimes aggressive, especially if handled or trodden upon. They appear to be attracted by fast-moving objects (e.g., divers being towed by a boat), and under these circumstances they can congregate and become troublesome. They are also caught in trawling nets, especially in the tropics.

Land snakes may also take to the water, sometimes causing difficulty with identification. The identification of a sea snake is confirmed by the observation of a paddle-shaped tail. No land snake has this flattened tail. Sea snake venom is approximately 2 to 10 times as toxic as that of the cobra, but they tend to deliver less of it, and only about one quarter of those bitten by sea snakes ever show signs of poisoning. It appears that there is some reluctance to inject venom even when they do bite. Nevertheless, the venom of one fresh adult sea snake of some species is enough to kill three men.

In most species the apparatus for delivering the venom is poorly developed even though the mouth can open widely; in other species the mouth is small and the snake has difficulty in biting wide enough to pierce the diver's clothing or any other protective material. Sea snake venom is a heat stable, nonenzymatic protein that appears to block neuromuscular transmission by acting on the postsynaptic membrane and possibly affecting the motor nerve terminals. It has a specific action in blocking the effects of acetylcholine. Autopsy findings include patchy and selective necrosis of skeletal muscles and tubular damage in the kidneys if the illness lasts longer than 48 hours.

Clinical Features

An initial puncture when bitten is usually noted. Fang and teeth marks vary from 1 to 20, but usually there are 4, and the teeth may remain in the wound. After a latent period without symptoms, and this may vary from 10 minutes to several hours, generalized features will be noted in approximately one quarter of the cases.

Mild symptoms include a psychological reaction, such as euphoria, anxiety, or restlessness. The tongue may feel thick. Thirst, dry throat, nausea, and vomiting occasionally develop. Generalized stiffness and aching may then supervene. If weakness does progress into paralysis, then it is usually of the ascending Guillain-Barré type, with the legs involved an hour or so before the trunk, then the arms and neck. Another manifestation of paralysis extends centrally from the area of the bite, e.g., from the bite on the hand to the forearm, arm, other arm, body, and legs. Usually the proximal muscle groups are the more affected, and trismus and ptosis are characteristic. Muscular twitchings, writhings, and spasms may be seen, and the patient may develop difficulty with speech and swallowing as the paralysis extends to the bulbar areas. Facial and ocular palsies then develop. Respiratory distress due to involvement of the diaphragm may result in dyspnea, cyanosis, and finally death in a small number. Cardiac failure, convulsions, and coma may be seen terminally.

Myoglobinuria may develop. When this is seen, one must consider the other possible effects of myonecrosis, namely, acute renal failure, with electrolyte and potassium changes, uremia, aggravation of the muscular paralysis, and weakness. The myonecrotic syndrome with renal failure usually supervenes on the other muscular paralysis and may thus prolong and aggravate this state. When recovery occurs it is usually rapid and complete.

Treatment

First Aid

It was originally thought that a venous ligature above the site, together with removal of the surface venom, was indicated. The current tendency is to apply pressure bandages, using a wide strap and about the same tension as for a sprained ankle and wrapping around the area of the bite and proximal to it. This is thought to reduce both venous and lymphatic drainage of the area.

It is essential to give reassurance and to keep exertion to a minimum. The affected limb or body area should be immobilized. If possible, the snake should be retained for identification because, although it may be harmless, the treatment certainly is not.

In the event of severe manifestations, mouth-to-mouth respiration may be required.

Medical Treatment

Apart from the above first-aid procedures, full cardiopulmonary resuscitation may be required. Fluid and electrolyte balance must be corrected, and acute renal failure is usually obvious from the oliguria, raised blood urea, and electrolyte changes. Hemodialysis may result in a dramatic improvement in the muscular paralysis and in the general clinical condition. The acute renal tubular necrosis and the myonecrosis are considered temporary if life can be maintained.

Treatment may be necessary for the cardiovascular shock and convulsions, and often respiration does require assistance or even complete control. Sea snake antivenom can be used cautiously in serious cases. It contains 200 micrograms per ampule. Care must be taken to administer it strictly in accordance with the directions in the brochure. The antivenom can be dangerous to allergic patients. Emergency precautions for anaphylactic shock are required. Polyvalent land snake antivenom can be used if the sea snake antivenom is unavailable, although with both the value has yet to be absolutely proven.

The sea snake antivenom is comprised of three antivenoms, each with a very specific action. Unfortunately, although it does counter the three most common venoms, there are some that are not affected. If it is necessary to use land snake antivenom, then probably the Tiger snake type is preferred. Patients with sea snake bite should be hospitalized for 24 hours because of the delay in symptoms developing. Sedatives may be required, and it is reasonable to administer diazepam (Valium) 5 mg as required. This will assist in sedating the patient, without interfering significantly with respiration.

FISH STINGS

General

Many fish have spines and a venom apparatus, usually for protection and occasionally for incapacitating their prey. Spines may be concealed, only becoming obvious when in use (e.g., stonefish), or the spines may be highlighted as an apparent warning to predators (e.g., butterfly cod, or firefish).

Some fish envenomations have resulted in death, especially by the stonefish and stingray. These will be described separately. Others, such as the infamous scorpionfish and firefish (family Scorpaenidae), catfish (family Plotosidae and Ariidae), and stargazers (family Uranoscopidae), have also been responsible for occasional deaths in humans. Weeverfish (family Trachinidae), toadfish (family Batrachoididae), rabbitfish (family Siganidae), and some species of leatherbacks (family Caragindae) are also believed to have a potentially serious venom apparatus. As a general rule, fish that have been damaged—such as those in fishing nets—cause less problems clinically, probably because some of the envenomation system may have been previously used.

Wounds that bleed profusely are less likely to be associated with intense symptoms. Some spines are inexplicably not associated with venom sacs and therefore produce few symptoms.

Other fish may produce injury by knife-like spines that may or may not result in envenomation, e.g., old wife fish (family Enoplosidae), surgeonfish and unicornfish (family Acanthuridae), ratfish (family Chimaeridae). In many cases the slime that exists on the spines may contribute to the symptomatology and to subsequent infections as much as the possible venom.

Identification of the species of fish responsible for a wound is not always possible. Fortunately, the symptomatology does not greatly vary.

Clinical Features

The first symptom is usually an immediate local pain that increases in intensity over the following few minutes. It may become excruciating, but pain from an average sting usually lessens after a few hours (more rapidly with a minor sting and longer with a major sting). Maritime folklore attempted to reassure victims with the adage that the pain will lessen "with the turn of the tide."

The puncture wound is anesthetized, but the surrounding area is hypersensitive. Pain and tenderness in the regional lymph glands may extend even more centrally. Locally the appearance shows one or more puncture wounds, with an inflamed and sometimes cyanotic zone. Surrounding the cyanotic zone is an area that is pale and swollen, with pitting edema.

Generalized symptoms are sometimes severe. The patient is often very distressed by the degree of pain, which is disproportionate to the clinical signs. This distress can merge into a delirious state. Malaise, nausea, vomiting, and sweating may be associated with temperature elevation and leukocytosis.

Occasionally a cardiovascular shock state may supervene and lead to death. Respiratory distress may develop in severe cases.

Treatment

First Aid

The patient should be laid down and reassured. The affected area should be rested in an elevated position. Since these fish toxins are usually heat labile, arrangements can then be made to immerse the wound in hot (up to 50°C), water for 30 to 90 minutes or until the pain no longer recurs. Unaffected skin as well as the wound should be immersed to avoid scalding. If the area cannot be immersed, as on the head or body, hot packs may be applied.

As an alternative, if other methods are not available and if the therapist is prepared to risk any legal repercussions, a small incision can be made across the wound and parallel to the long axis of the limb to encourage mild bleeding and to relieve pain. A ligature or tourniquet is not indicated. Local vasoconstriction is already a hazard to tissue vascularity without aggravating it by further circulatory restriction.

The duration of the hot water immersion depends on the symptoms. If the site of injury is removed and the pain recurs, it should be reimmersed. The wound should be washed and cleaned after the treatment is no longer required.

Medical Treatment

This includes first aid as above. Local anesthetic, e.g., 5 to 10 mg lidocaine 2% without adrenaline (epinephrine), if injected through the puncture wound, will give considerable relief. Local or regional anesthetic blocks may also be of value. Emetine, 0.5 to 1.0 ml at a concentration of 50 mg/ml, injected into wound site is of great value but is hard to obtain.

Treatment may be needed for generalized symptoms of cardiogenic shock or respiratory depression. Systemic analgesics or narcotics are rarely needed, although they may be of value in severe cases.

Local cleansing of the wound, with removal of any broken spines or their integuments, is best followed by the application of a local antibiotic such as neomycin or bacitracin. Tetanus prophylaxis may be indicated if there is necrotic tissue or if the wound has been contaminated.

If the stings are severe, they can mimic the lesions described under the headings of stonefish or stingray. The treatment sections of these injuries should be referred to, since the principles (other than the use of antivenom) have general application to all fish stings.

STONEFISH

General

Perhaps the most venomous fish known, stonefish (Fig. 11–3) inhabit the whole tropical Indo-Pacific region. Many species similar to *Synanceja verrucosa* and *S. trachynis* are found in other tropical areas. Some of the Scorpenidae, such as the spotted scorpionfish of the Caribbean, probably have comparable toxicity.

This fish grows to about 30 cm in length. It lies dormant in shallow waters, buried in mud, coral, or rocks, and is practically indistinguishable from the surroundings. It can catch a small passing fish by sucking it into its gaping mouth.

The 13 dorsal spines, capable of piercing sneakers and skin, become erect when the fish is disturbed. Apart from the tip of the spine, the fish is covered by loose skin or integument. When pressure is applied, two venom glands discharge along ducts on each spine into the penetrated wound. The fish may live for many hours out of the water.

The venom is an unstable protein, with a pH of 6.0 and a molecular weight of 150,000. It produces an intense vasoconstriction and therefore tends to localize itself. It is destroyed by heat (2 min at 50°C), alkalis and acids (pH greater than 9 or less than 4), potassium permanganate, and congo red. The toxin is a myotoxin that acts on skeletal, involuntary, and cardiac muscles, blocking conduction in these tissues. This results in a muscular paralysis, respiratory depression, peripheral vasodilation, shock, and cardiac arrest. It is also capable of producing cardiac arrhythmias.

Each spine has 5 to 10 mg of venom and is said to be neutralized by 1 ml of antivenom produced by the Australian Commonwealth Serum Laboratories. Occasionally a stonefish spine may have no venom associated with it. It

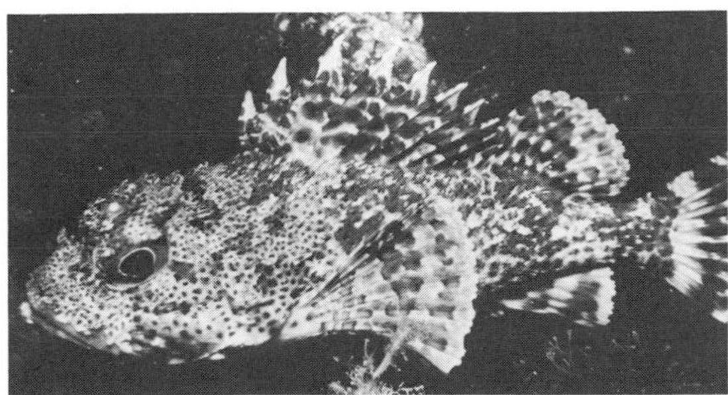

FIGURE 11–3. ***Scorpaena guttata*, cousin of the stonefish. Both species have venomous spines. (Photo by Bonnie J. Cardone, used with permission from Peterson Publishing Company, Los Angeles, CA)**

is thought that the venom is regenerated very slowly, if at all.

Clinical Features

Whether local or general symptoms predominate seems to depend on many factors, such as the geographical locality, the number of spines involved, depth of spine penetration, protective covering, previous sting, first aid treatment, and so forth.

Local

Immediate pain is noted. This will increase in severity over the ensuing 10 minutes or more. The pain, which is excruciating, may be sufficient in some cases to cause unconsciousness and thus drowning. Sometimes the pain comes in waves, a few minutes apart.

Ischemia of the area is followed by cyanosis, which is probably due to local circulatory stasis. The area becomes swollen and edematous, often hot, with numbness in the center and extreme tenderness around the periphery. The edema and swelling may become gross, extending up the limb. Paralysis of the adjacent muscles is said to immobilize the limb, as may pain.

The pain is likely to spread proximally to the regional lymph glands, e.g., in the axilla or groin. Both the pain and the other signs of inflammation may last for many days; delayed healing, necrosis, and ulceration may persist for many months. Swelling can likewise continue, although in a gradually lessening degree for many months. The long-term sequelae are not as common in patients treated correctly in the first few days with antitoxin, debridement, cleansing, and local antisepsis.

General

Signs of mild cardiovascular collapse are not uncommon. Pallor, gross sweating, hypotension, and syncope on standing may be present. Respiratory failure may be due to pulmonary edema, depression of the respiratory center, cardiac failure, and/or paralysis of the respiratory musculature. Bradycardia, cardiac arrhythmias, and arrest are also possible. Malaise, exhaustion, fever, and shivering may progress to delirium, incoordination, generalized paralysis, convulsions, and death. Convalescence may take many months and may be characterized by periods of malaise and nausea.

Treatment

First Aid

Rescue the patient from the water and provide the necessary reassurance. Immobilize the victim and keep the affected limb in an elevated position. Immerse the limb in hot water (up to 50°C) for 30 minutes. This may produce rapid relief especially if given early. Adjacent unaffected skin should also be immersed to ensure that scalding does not occur. The local application of a weak solution of potassium permanganate may relieve pain.

If there is loss of consciousness, apply external cardiac massage and mouth-to-mouth respiration as indicated. Do not cease these measures unless death is confirmed. Resuscitation may be required for many hours.

Medical Treatment

Medical treatment will depend on the site and severity of the symptoms.

Local

Local anesthetic agent without adrenaline, infiltrated into and around the wound, is the treatment of choice, especially if administered early. It may also remove the pain in the regional lymphatic area. A repeat injection will probably be needed. Local injection into the site with either hyoscine *N*-butyl bromide (scopolamine) or emetine (pH of 3.4) is a conventional remedy that gives relief if injected within the first 15 minutes. Emetine may be given in a dose of 25 mg in 0.5 ml.

Systemic analgesics and narcotics are seldom indicated or useful, although intravenous narcotics are sometimes used. Elevate the affected limb to reduce pain and swelling and apply local antibiotics to prevent secondary infection. After the initial resuscitation and analgesia have been effected, debridement of necrotic tissue must be considered if there is any significant damage and necrosis from the spine. Otherwise both local and generalized symptoms can continue for many months. Even when treatment has been inadequate or delayed, surgical excision of the damaged area may be necessary to reduce symptomatology and hasten recovery.

General

Stonefish antivenom may be administered with 1 ml neutralizing 10 mg of venom (i.e., the venom from one spine). Initially, 2 ml of antivenom is given intramuscularly, although in severe cases the intravenous route can be used.

Further doses can be given if required, but it should never be given to those with horse serum allergy. It should be stored between 0°C and 5°C but not frozen, protected from light, and used immediately on opening. Tetanus prophylaxis is sometimes needed, and systemic antibiotics may be used as secondary infection is likely.

Appropriate resuscitation techniques may have to be applied. These include external cardiac massage and defibrillation and endotracheal intubation with controlled respiration. Monitoring procedures should include records of clinical state (pulse, respiration), blood pressure, central venous or pulmonary pressure, electrocardiogram, arterial pO_2, pCO_2, and pH. Clinical complications of bulbar paralysis should be treated as they arise.

Prevention

Wear thick sole shoes when in danger areas. Be particularly careful on coral reefs and while entering or leaving boats. A stonefish sting is said to confer some degree of immunity for future episodes.

STINGRAYS

General

Stingrays (Fig. 11–4) are found extensively from the tropics to the temperate regions. They are bottom dwellers; their flat bodies are often submerged in sand and only detectable by a protruding eye or two, a piece of tail, or the spiracles showing above an elevated disc of sand or mud.

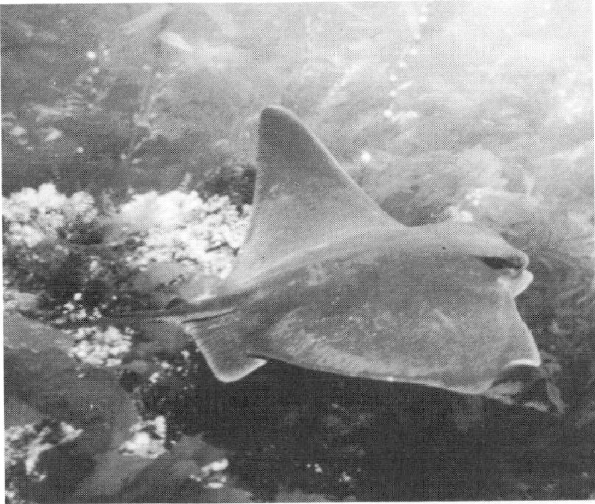

FIGURE 11–4. Stingray or bat ray *(Myliobatis)*. Barb at base of tail can be directed by rapid flexion of the tail. (Photo by Bonnie J. Cardone, used with permission from Peterson Publishing Company, Los Angeles, CA)

Damage from the spine may cause death either from physical trauma, such as the penetration of the body cavities (pleural, pericardial, or peritoneal) or from the venom of the spine. In Australia deaths tend to be from the former, whereas in the United States death is more likely from the venom effects. There are said to be 1500 injuries per year from stingrays in the United States.

The stingray is unaggressive but is capable of protecting itself against intruders. It buries itself in sea or riverbeds; an unwary wading victim may step on its dorsal surface or a diver may descend over it. The stingray swings its tail upward and forward, either producing sword-like lacerations or driving the spine into the limb (especially the ankle) or body of the victim. An integument over the serrated spine is ruptured. Venom escapes and passes along ventrolateral grooves into the perforated wound. Extraction of the saw-shaped spine results in further tissue damage due to the serrations and retropointed barbs and may leave spine or sheath within the wound.

The venom is a protein (molecular weight greater than 100,000) that is heat labile, water soluble, and with an intravenous LD 50 of 28 mg/kg body weight. Low concentrations cause increased P-R interval associated with bradycardia. A first degree atrioventricular block may occur with mild hypotension. Larger doses produce vasoconstriction, second and third degree atrioventricular blocks, and signs of cardiac ischemia. Most cardiac changes are reversible within 24 hours. Some degree of respiratory depression is noted with greater amounts of venom. This is probably secondary to the neurotoxic effect of the venom on the medullary centers. Convulsions may also occur.

Clinical Features

Local

Pain is usually immediate and is the predominant symptom, increasing over 1 to 2 hours and easing after 6 to 10 hours. However, it may persist for some days.

The area is swollen and pale, with a bluish rim. It is several centimeters in width and spreads around the wound after an hour or two. The pain may be constant, pulsating, or lancinating. Bleeding may be profuse and may relieve the pain. A mucoid secretion may follow. Integument from the spine may be visible in the wound, which may gape and extend for a few centimeters in length. Aggravation of pain within days may be due to secondary infection. Local necrosis, ulceration, and/or secondary infection are common and, if unchecked, may cause incapacity for many months. In earlier years even amputation resulted. Osteomyelitis in the underlying bone has been reported.

General

The following manifestations have been noted: anorexia, nausea, vomiting, diarrhea, frequent micturition, and salivation. Pain extends to the area of lymphatic drainage. Muscular cramps, tremors, and tonic paralysis may occur in the affected limb or may be more generalized. Fainting, palpitation, hypotension, cardiac irregularities (conduction abnormalities, blocks), and ischemia are possible.

Respiratory depression may occur, with difficulty in breathing, cough, and pain on inspiration. Other features include nocturnal fever with copious sweating, nervousness, confusion, or delirium.

Fatalities are possible, especially if the stingray's spine perforates the pericardial, peritoneal, or pleural cavities. The initial symptoms last from hours to days but may recur or persist for weeks or months after the injury, even though the wound may have closed over. These include a dull ache over the area and a swelling that may develop under the influence of gravity. Thus, an ankle may become painful and swollen after standing or walking. It may be alleviated by resting with the foot elevated. An X-ray should be performed to exclude a foreign body (stingray spine) in the soft tissues. Usually a fibrotic nodule can be removed if the area is surgically explored, and rapid recovery follows this minor surgery. The nodule may be due to a tissue reaction from a piece of spine or sheath. Antibiotics do not help at this stage.

Treatment

First Aid

The patient should be laid down, and the affected area should be placed in an elevated position. Surface venom is removed by washing or irrigating the area with water. If the spine or integument is still present, it should be gently extracted. If bleeding has not occurred naturally, it may be encouraged by a small incision. The area is immersed in hot water, up to 50°C, until pain has stopped (usually in 30 to 90 min). Adjacent unaffected skin should also be immersed to prevent scalding. Following pain relief, the limb should be immobilized in an elevated position and covered with a clean dressing, for example, an unused newspaper. The patient's state may become far more serious than it first appears.

Medical Treatment

Local anesthetic without adrenaline (epinephrine) infiltrated into and around the wound, or by regional block, will relieve the pain. Systemic analgesia may be required. A tourniquet is rarely if ever indicated and only if the medical practitioner is very seriously worried about generalized symptoms, with care being taken to avoid aggravating the already ischemic tissues.

X-ray will demonstrate foreign bodies and bone injury. The basic physiological signs (TPR, BP, CVP, urine output, and so forth), serum electrolytes, electroencephalogram, and electrocardiogram are monitored as indicated. Broad spectrum antibiotics, e.g., tetracycline 250 mg qid and local application of neomycin, are used at an early stage. Debridement, cleansing, and suturing, if required, are performed as early as permitted by the patient's general state. Symptomatic treatment is given for the clinical features. Tetanus prophylaxis is indicated if wounds are necrotic or contaminated.

Prevention

Divers, swimmers, and waders are advised to shuffle their feet when walking in the water. This gives the ray time to remove itself, which it cannot do if a foot is on its dorsum. Although wearing rubber boots decreases the severity of the sting, the spine will penetrate most protective material. Care is needed when handling fishing nets.

COELENTERATES

General

This phylum of 9000 species contains jellyfish, sea anemones, fire coral, stinging hydroids, and so on. It constitutes one of the lowest orders of the animal kingdom and has members that are grossly dissimilar in general appearance and mobility. Although many appear flowerlike, all are carnivorous animals.

The common factor among the coelenterates is the development of nematocysts or stinging capsules. They are like coiled springs held within an envelope whose shape varies with the species. The tentacles that carry the nematocysts adhere to the victim by either sticky mucus or specialized nematocysts with penetrating spines. The triggering mechanisms that is responsible for the firing of the nematocyst is thought to be initiated by many factors (e.g., trauma or the absorption of water into the nematocyst capsule causing it to swell).

The function of the nematocysts is to incapacitate and retain prey, which is then used as food by the coelenterate. The nematocysts of different types of coelenterate may be identifiable and are therefore of value in the differential diagnosis of marine stings. There may also be a characteristic pattern of nematocyst stings, depending on their aggregation on the tentacle of the coelenterate and on the morphology of the tentacles. Thus, the Portuguese man o'war usually produces a single long strap with small blisters along it, whereas the sea wasp has multiple long red lines often with the tentacle adherent. Stinging hydroids (Fig. 11–5) and fire coral, being nonmobile, sting only when touched by the diver.

Clinical Features

Clinical factors may vary from a mild itch locally to severe systemic reactions. The local symptoms vary from a prickly or stinging sensation developing immediately on contact to a burning or throbbing pain. The intensity increases over 10 minutes or so, and the red inflamed area may develop blisters or even necrotic ulcers in severe cases. The pain may spread centrally, with lymphadenopathy, and may be associated with abdominal pain and chest pain.

Generalized symptoms include fever, increased secretions, gastrointestinal disorders, cardiovascular failure, respiratory distress, and signs of a toxiconfusional state.

The intensity of both local and generalized manifestations of coelenterate stinging may vary according to the following: (1) the species involved (the sea wasp is often lethal, whereas many jellyfish can be handled with impunity); (2) the extent of the area involved; (3) the maturity of the animal; (4) the body weight of the subject, with the generalized symptoms being more severe in children than adults; (5) the thickness of the skin in contact; and (6) individual idiosyncracies such as allergic reac-

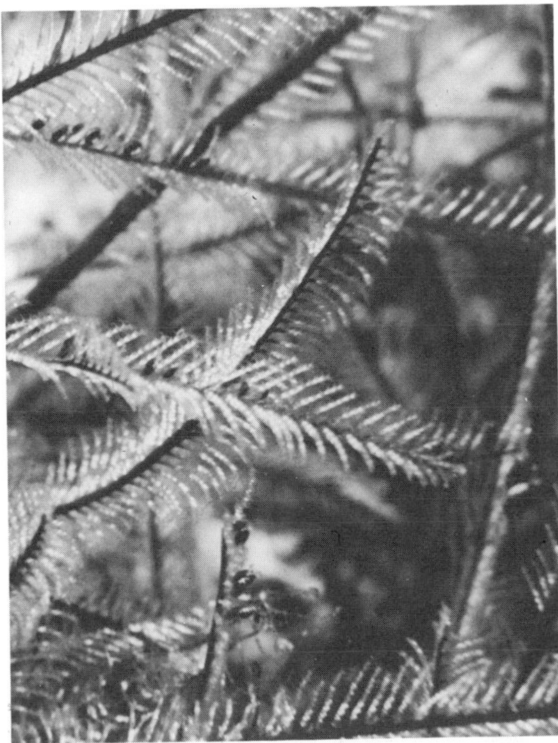

FIGURE 11–5. Stinging hydroids from the Sea of Cortez. Fine fronds contain hundreds of nematocysts. (Photo by Bonnie J. Cardone, used with permission from Peterson Publishing Company, Los Angeles, CA)

tions, pre-existing cardiorespiratory disease, and so forth.

As the most dangerous, coelenterates of the Cubomedusae family (sea wasp or box jellyfish) are dealt with in detail. *Physalia*, or Portuguese man o'war, is so widespread that it is also dealt with in detail.

CUBOMEDUSAE (Sea Wasp, Box Jellyfish)

General

These species are restricted to the warm waters of the Indo-Pacific region, with the 70 or more documented fatalities most numerous in the waters off northern Australia, from November to April. Other species are found in equatorial waters, such as Tamoya from the Gulf of Oman.

The sea wasp is said to be the most venomous animal known. It is especially dangerous to children and patients with cardiorespiratory disorders (e.g., asthmatics). Its box-shaped body can measure 20 cm along each side and has up to 15 tentacles measuring up to three meters in length on each side of its four pedalia.

The severity of the sting increases with the size of the animal, the extent of contact with the victim, and the delicacy of the victim's skin. Deaths have occurred with as little contact as 6 to 7 cm of tentacle. Adjacent swimmers may also be affected to a variable degree. The tentacles tend to adhere with a sticky jelly-like substance but these can usually be removed by bystanders, due to the protection afforded by the thick skin on the palms of the hands. This protection is not always complete, and stinging can occur even through surgical gloves.

The venom is made up of at least two different fractions, one with a molecular weight of approximately 75,000 and one of 150,000. The lethal dermatonecrotic and hemolytic fractions are specific antigens for each species, and cross immunity does not develop. The effects on the cardiovascular system include an initial rise in arterial pressure, which is followed by hypotensive/hypertensive oscillations. This is probably due to interference with vasomotor reflex feedback systems. The hypotensive states are related to bradycardia; cardiac irregularities (especially delay in atrioventricular conduction) are due to cardiotoxicity, baroreceptor stimulation, and/or brain state depression. Ventricular fibrillation or asystole will precede cerebral death.

Clinical Features

The patient usually screams as a result of the excruciating pain occurring immediately on contact and increasing in intensity, often coming in waves. He then claws at the adherent tentacles (whitish strings surrounded by transparent jelly). He may become confused, act irrationally, or lose consciousness and may drown because of this.

Local

Multiple interlacing whiplash lines—red, purple, or brown, 0.5 cm wide—develop within seconds. The markings are in a beaded or ladder pattern and are quite characteristic. These acute changes will last for some hours. They are also described as transverse weals. If death occurs, the skin markings then fade. If the patient survives, the red, swollen skin may develop large weals, and, after 7 to 10 days, necrosis and ulceration develop over the area of contact. The skin lesions may take many months to heal if deep ulceration occurs. Itching may also be troublesome and recurrent. Pigmentation and scarring at the site of these lesions may be permanent.

General

Excruciating pain dominates the clinical picture, while impairment of the conscious state may proceed to coma and death. The pain diminishes in 4 to 12 hours. Amnesia occurs for most of the incident following the sting. If death occurs, it usually does so within the first 10 minutes; survival is likely after the first hour.

Cardiovascular effects dominate the generalized manifestations. The patient may develop cardiac shock, with a disturbance of consciousness. Hypotension, tachycardia, and a raised venous pressure may also occur. It is also possible that the clinical state may oscillate within minutes from episodes of hypertension, tachycardia, rapid respirations, and normal venous pressure of those of hypotension, bradycardia, apnea, and elevated venous pressure. The oscillation may give a false impression of improvement just prior to the patient's death.

Respiratory distress, pulmonary congestion, edema, and cyanosis may be due to the cardiac effects or to a direct midbrain depression. Paralysis and abdominal pains may occur. Malaise and restlessness may persist, with physical convalescence requiring up to a week. Irritability and difficulty with psychological adjustment may take weeks or months to disappear. Immunity to the sting is said to occur following repeated and recent contacts, although it is likely that the cross immunity between the species is incomplete or absent.

Treatment

First Aid

Prevent drowning. Apply vinegar or mild denaturing agents to reduce the likelihood of discharge of the nematocysts. The tentacles should be removed as rapidly and gently as possible. Cardiopulmonary resuscitation may be needed and may need to be repeated on a number of occasions.

Medical Treatment

First aid as above. Local applications include lidocaine or other local anesthetic ointment. Local steroid applications may also be of value. These may assist even after the first few minutes, during which time the traditional vinegar is believed to have some prophylactic value. Analgesics include morphine (15 mg) or Demerol (100 mg) administered intravenously; these may also protect against shock. Pentazocine has also been used with good results.

Hydrocortisone 100 mg is administered intravenously every two hours if needed. Local steroid preparations are valuable for treating local manifestations such as swelling, pain, itching, and so forth. Intermittent positive pressure respiration, possibly with oxygen, replaces mouth-to-mouth artificial respiration, if needed. This will require constant attention because of the varying degree of respiratory depression. General anesthesia with endotracheal intubation and controlled respiration are needed if analgesia cannot otherwise be obtained.

Chlorpromazine 100 mg intramuscularly, diazepam 10 mg intravenously, or other sedatives may be of value after the immediate resuscitation, as they will assist in sedating and tranquillizing the patient without causing significant respiratory depression. Other drugs may be used but are unproven in this clinical disorder. They include noradrenaline (Levophed) or isoproterenol (Isuprel) drips. Electrocardiogram monitoring is indicated as are pulse rate, blood pressure, central venous or pulmonary pressure, respiratory rate, arterial gases, and pH levels. External cardiac massage and defibrillation are given if required. Verapamil has been investigated as has calcium gluconate.

Sea wasp antivenom has been developed by the Australian Commonwealth Serum Laboratories and is derived from the serum of hyperimmunized sheep. Twenty thousand units may be sufficient to control the effects of a moderate sting on adults. This may need to be increased to 100,000 U for a child with massive injury. Local steroid ointment may relieve the severe itching that may follow the acute skin lesion.

Prevention

This includes the wearing of adequate protective clothing (overalls, wetsuits, body stockings, and so forth). Swimming or wading should be restricted to the safe months of the year. Care is especially needed on cloudy days toward the end of the hot season. Dragging a section of a beach with a 2.5 cm mesh has been used, not very successfully, to clear the area for bathing.

PHYSALIA (Portuguese Man O'War)

General

There was one reported death in Florida from *Physalia*, but the animal was not convincingly identified. The animal has a pneumatophore (a gas-filled transparent sac, usually blue colored), which can reach 20 cm in length and which allows it to drift at an angle to the wind. It floats on the surface of the water and trails many short frilled tentacles and one or more long "fishing" tentacles. The latter may extend for 10 meters and is responsible for most of the stings.

One toxin of *Physalia* is termed hypnotoxin and is a peptide or protein material. This is denatured by heating to 60°C for 15 minutes or by adding either alcohol or acetone. It causes neurological depression, affecting motor and sensory areas, and also has edema-producing properties. Respiratory depression occurs in envenomated animals and has been described in human victims.

Clinical Features

Local

Initially there is a sharp sting. This may be aggravated by pulling on the tentacle, rubbing the area, or applying fresh water. The sting rapidly increases to an intense ache that spreads to involve surrounding joints and then moves centrally. The axilla or groin may be affected, and the associated draining lymph glands become tender. The duration of the severe pain may range from a few minutes to many hours. It is superseded by a dull ache that lasts a similar period.

The affected area develops a red line with small white punctate (pinpoint) lesions often in a ladder-like pattern, and in severe cases a central weal or blister appears after the erythema. The weals only last a few hours looking like a string of beads, and the erythema clears within 24 hours. Rarely, there is ulceration, discoloration, and scarring.

General

General signs are not uncommon but rarely last longer than one day. The patient may be slightly shocked and may develop syncope, with a rapid pulse and hypotension. Generalized chills and muscle cramps may develop. Abdominal symptoms include nausea, pain, and vomiting.

Neurological signs have been noted, with the patient showing irritability and confusion. Death is possible if the patient develops respiratory depression.

Treatment

First Aid

This includes rescuing the victim from the water, laying him down, and giving reassurance. Vinegar is partially effective in preventing further nematocyst discharge, and subsequent injury. Many household substances used against burns have been of value, but alcohol can aggravate the condition. By far the best application for relief of pain is a local anesthetic agent (e.g., lidocaine 5%). The tentacle should be removed as gently as possible to reduce the likelihood of further nematocyst discharge.

Medical Treatment

Local anesthetic (topical) is excellent as a pain reliever and is usually far superior to other applications. In a series of stingings performed on volunteers, both immediately and following a 10-minute delay, the following results were obtained. Lidocaine 5% ointment was superior to both Ultralan 0.5% and lidocaine gel, and both of these were far better than Benadryl cream. Methylated spirits was the least effective of all. Commercial preparations were effective for only a short time.

If the eye is affected, it would be logical to apply a nonaqueous local anesthetic solution (e.g., cocaine eye drops or ointment) followed by a steroid ointment. Aqueous drops should be avoided. Homatropine 1% and cocaine drops may be instilled later, although some tend to use a steroid antibiotic eye ointment combination, e.g., Hydrophenical or Sofradex. Antibiotic is used to ensure that the corneal ulcers do not become infected.

Despite the paucity of verified deaths, it would be wise to monitor severely affected cases as one does with *Chironex* stings and to give cardiovascular and respiratory assistance if needed. Tranquilizers and muscle relaxants (e.g., diazepam 10 mg IV) may be indicated in distressed patients.

It is possible that allergy-prone patients are more susceptible to the *Physalia* and other coelenterates. The use of hydrocortisone may be indicated in these patients (100 mg IV repeated as needed). Severe itching may develop within a few days, but this responds to steroid ointments such as Ultralan.

CONE SHELLS

General

Highly favored by shell collectors of the tropics and warm temperate regions, these attractive univalve mollusks (Fig. 11–6) have a proboscis that extends from the narrow end but which is able to reach most of the shell. Holding the shell even by the "big end" may not be entirely safe and may court a sting with a resultant 25 per cent mortality. The cone shell inhabits shallow waters, reefs, ponds, and rubble.

It is usually up to 10 cm in size. It has a siphon, sometimes ringed with orange, that

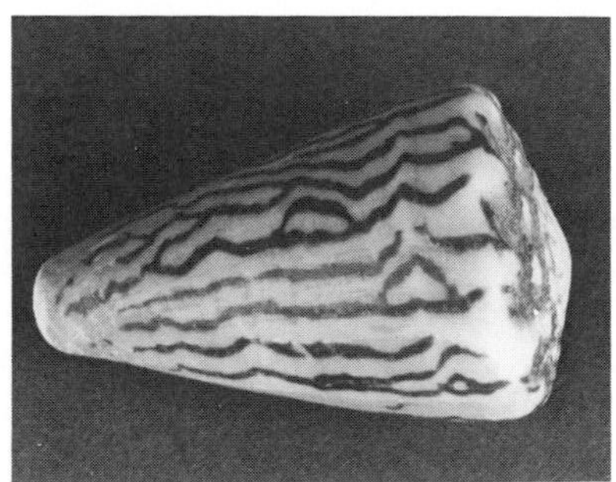

FIGURE 11–6. Cone shell *(Conus princeps)*. The proboscis can reach almost to the large end of the shell. (Photo by Bonnie J. Cardone, used with permission from Peterson Publishing Company, Los Angeles, CA)

detects its prey and may be the only part visible if the cone burrows under the sand. The proboscis, which delivers the coup de grâce, carries 1 to 20 radular teeth that penetrate and inject venom into its prey, thus immobilizing the victim.

Probably only the fish-eating cones are dangerous to humans, but as these are difficult to distinguish at first sight, discretion on the part of shell collectors is recommended. The venom is composed of two or more substances. One interferes with neuromuscular activity and elicits a sustained muscular contracture; the other abolishes nerve fiber excitability and summates with tubocurarine but is uninfluenced by eserine. The major effect appears to be directly on skeletal muscular activity. Children are very vulnerable.

Clinical Features

Local

The initial puncture effects may vary from no pain to extreme agony and may be aggravated by salt water. The wound may become inflamed and swollen, sometimes white and ischemic, with a cyanotic area surrounding it, and it may be numb to touch.

General

Numbness and tingling may ascend from the sting to involve the whole body and especially the mouth and lips. This may take about 10 minutes to develop. Skeletal muscular paralysis may spread from the site of injury and may result in anything from mild weariness to complete flaccid paralysis. Difficulty with swallowing and speech may occur prior to total paralysis. Visual disturbances may include double and blurred vision (paralysis of voluntary muscles and pupillary reactions). These changes may take place within 10 to 30 minutes of the sting. Respiratory paralysis may dominate the clinical picture. This results in shallow rapid breathing and a cyanotic appearance, proceeding to apnea, unconsciousness, and death. Other cases are said to result in cardiac failure, although this is probably secondary to the respiratory paralysis. The extent of neurotoxic damage is variable. If the patient survives, he is active and mobile within 24 hours. The sequelae and especially the local reaction may last a few weeks.

Treatment

First Aid

The following recommendations are made.

1. *Without paralysis.* The patient should be rested and constantly reassured. The limb must be immobilized, and if there is little inflammation a pressure bandage may delay venom absorption.
2. *With paralysis.* Mouth-to-mouth respiration may be needed. This may have to be continued for hours or until medical facilities are obtained. This artificial respiration is the major contribution to saving the patient's life. External cardiac massage as well as mouth-to-mouth are needed if the patient has neither pulse nor respiration. The patient may be able to hear but not to communicate and thus requires reassurance. If he is in shock, place him in a prone position with his feet elevated.

Medical Treatment

With respiratory paralysis, administer artificial respiration with intermittent positive pressure adequate to maintain normal pO_2, pCO_2, and pH levels of arterial blood. Endotracheal intubation prevents aspiration of vomitus and facilitates tracheobronchial toilet, when indicated. With total paralysis, the following regime is needed: intravenous nutrition (nothing by mouth), eye toilet and protection, and attention to pressure areas. External cardiac massage, defibrillation, vasopressors, and so forth may be indicated by the clinical state and electrocardiogram monitor. Local anesthetic can be injected into the wound. Respiratory depressants, respiratory stimulants, and drugs used against neuromuscular blockade are not indicated.

BLUE-RINGED OCTOPUS (Octopus maculosa or Hapalochaena maculosa)

General

This animal usually weighs from 10 to 100 grams and is currently found only in the Australasian and Central Indo-Pacific region. Its span, with tentacles extended, is from 2 to 20 cm but is usually less than 10 cm. It is found in rock pools at low tide. The color is yellowish brown with ringed markings on the tentacles and striations on the body. These markings change to a vivid iridescent blue when the animal is feeding or becomes angry, excited, disturbed, or hypoxic. The heavier specimens are more dangerous, and handling these attractive creatures has resulted in death within a few minutes. Many such incidents have probably escaped detection by the coroner. Autopsy features are nonspecific and the bite fades after death.

The toxin (maculotoxin) is more potent than that of any land animal. Analysis of posterior-salivary extracts demonstrates a hyaluronidase and cephalotoxins of low molecular weight (probably less than 500). These have similar effects to tetrodotoxin, and recent work has suggested that the octopus toxin may be identical to this.

Clinical Features

Local

Initially the bite is usually painless and may thus go unnoticed.

General

A few minutes after the bite, a rapid, painless paralysis dominates the clinical picture, which progresses in the following order: abnormal sensations around mouth, neck, and head; nausea and/or vomiting; dyspnea with rapid, shallow, and stertorous respirations leading to apnea, asphyxia, and cyanosis; visual disturbance (involvement of the extraocular eye muscles results in double vision, blurred vision, and ptosis, whereas intraocular paralysis results in a fixed dilated pupil); difficulty in speech and swallowing; generalized weakness and incoordination progressing to complete paralysis. The duration of paralysis is between 4 and 12 hours, but the weakness and incoordination may persist for another day. The patient's conscious state is initially normal, even though he may not be able to open his eyes or respond to his environment. The respiratory paralysis (causing hypoxia and hypercapnia) finally results in unconsciousness and then death, often within minutes of the commencement of symptoms unless resuscitation is continued. Cardiovascular effects of hypotension and bradycardia are noted in severe cases.

There may be a cessation at any stage of the above clinical sequence—that is, the effects may cease with the local reaction or with a partial paralysis or may proceed to a complete paralysis and death. Less severe bites may result in generalized and local muscular contractions, which may continue intermittently for six hours or more. This occurs with a subparalytic dose. Other symptoms noted in mild cases include a lightheaded feeling, depersonalization, paresthesia, weakness, and exhaustion.

Treatment

First Aid

The following recommendations are made:

1. *Before paralysis.* Immobilize the limb and apply a pressure bandage to reduce the absorption of venom. Rest the patient, preferably on his side in case of vomiting, and do not leave him unattended. Obtain medical assistance and give reassurance.

2. *With paralysis.* Apply mouth-to-mouth respiration to ensure that the patient does not become cyanotic. Attention must be paid to cleaning the airway of vomitus, tongue obstruction, dentures, and so forth. If any airway is available, this should be inserted—but it is not essential. Artificial respiration may have to be continued for hours, until the patient reaches a hospital. If delay has occurred, then external cardiac massage may also be required. Reassure the patient, who can hear but not communicate, that he will be all right and that you understand his condition. Enlist medical aid but never leave him unattended.

Medical Treatment

For respiratory paralysis, artificial respiration with intermittent positive pressure respiration is necessary to maintain normal pO_2, pCO_2, and pH levels of arterial blood. Endotracheal intubation also prevents aspiration of vomitus and facilitates tracheobronchial toilet, when indicated. Oral foods or fluids are contraindicated. Eye toilets and protection are needed. Respiratory stimulant may be of some value in the recovery phase.

SEA URCHINS

General

Of the 600 species of sea urchins (Fig. 11–7), approximately 80 are thought to be venomous or poisonous to humans. They belong to the phylum Echinodermata, named after the hedgehog (Echinos) because of its many-spined appearance. In some, such as *Diadema setosum*, the long spined or black sea urchin, the damage is mainly done by the breaking off of the sharp

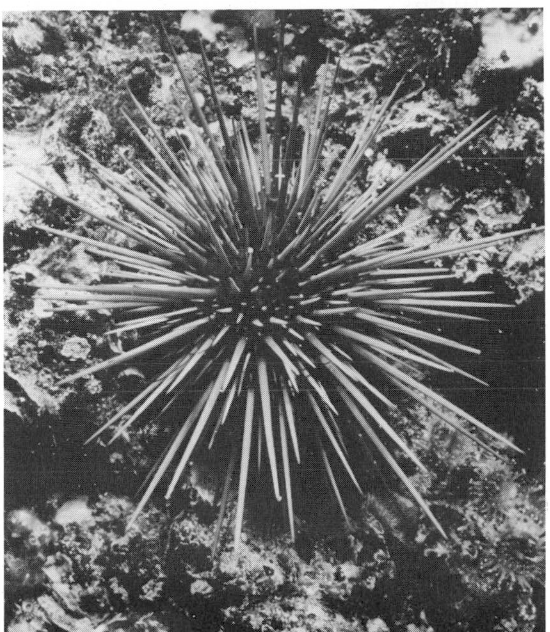

FIGURE 11–7. Red sea urchin *(Strongylocentrotus franciscanus)*. The long spines break off readily in the skin when contacted. (Photo by Bonnie J. Cardone, used with permission from Peterson Publishing Company, Los Angeles, CA)

brittle spines after they have penetrated the diver's skin. Sometimes the spines will disappear within a few days, but in other cases they become encrusted and may remain for many months to emerge at sites distant from the original wound. The spines are covered by a black pigment, which can then be mistaken for the actual spine during its removal.

The most potent sea urchins are the Toxopneustidae, which have short thick spines poking through an array of flower-like pedicellariae. Deaths have been reported from this, and the venom is thought to be a dialyzable acetylcholine-like substance.

The starfish *Acanthaster Planci* (crown-of-thorns) can also cause damage by the spines piercing the skin, but these seem to have a far more inflammatory action suggestive of a venom. Injuries from the crown-of-thorns have been more commonly reported since divers attempted to eradicate them from reefs. A characteristic general symptom is nausea or vomiting. It was proclaimed that the crown-of-thorns destroyed reefs at a rate of 5 km per month. It is not likely to be a natural phenomenon.

Treatment

The long spines tend to break easily and therefore need to be removed vertically without any horizontal movement. A local anesthetic may be required if surgical extraction is contemplated. Drawing pastes such as magnesium sulfate have been used. Some find relief with the use of the heat, and others have removed the spines by the use of a snake-bite suction cup.

One technique that would be described as barbaric, had it not been for the fact that it seems to work, is to apply extra trauma and movement to the area in order to break up the spines within the tissue. It does seem as if, in this case, activity is more beneficial than rest and immobilization. With the latter, the limb tends to swell and become more painful. Since the spines are proteinaceous, they are usually absorbed. Attempts at surgical removal are sometimes necessary if symptoms persist.

The use of hot water baths and local anesthetic as treatment of the crown-of-thorns sting seems to be of some value in early stages. Treatment of the Toxopneustidae must be based on general medical principles.

ELECTRIC RAYS

Electric rays (Fig. 11–8) are found in temperate and tropical oceans, as is the other marine fish that produces electric discharge, the stargazer. The rays are commonly encountered by divers, as they are found in relatively shallow depths and can be submerged in mud or sand.

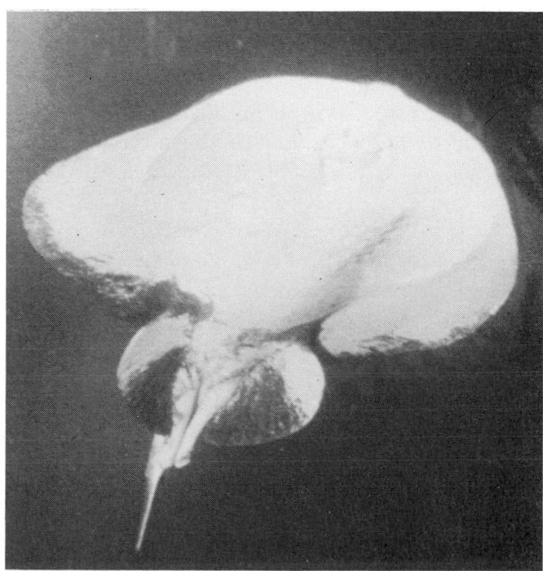

FIGURE 11–8. Electric ray (torpedo ray). Electric discharge up to 200 volts can briefly paralyze a diver. (Photo by Bonnie J. Cardone, used with permission from Peterson Publishing Company, Los Angeles, CA)

The electrical discharge varies from 8 to 220 volts and is passed between the electrically negative ventral side of the ray to the positive dorsal side. The thick electric organs are usually discernible on each side. Activation of an electric discharge is a reflex action, the result of tactile stimulation. The ray can deliver a successive series of discharges, but these are of lessening intensity. There is a latent period in which the fish recuperates its electric potentials. It is not necessary to actually touch the ray to get a shock.

The electric shock may have a serious effect in disabling a man temporarily and presumably could be more hazardous to a child. Subsequent danger may come from drowning or aspiration. There are usually no local manifestations visible on the affected skin. Recovery is uneventful, and treatment is not usually required.

SPONGES

General

These sedentary animals require some defense from mobile predators, and they have developed a skeleton of calcareous and siliceous spicules. They also have a toxin that is not well understood. About a dozen sponges from the 5000 or so known species have been incriminated as toxic, and these are found mainly in the temperate or tropic zones. Skin lesions have developed from sponges that have been deep frozen or dried for many years.

Clinical Features

One group of symptoms relates to the contact dermatitis associated with the areas of sponge contact. After a variable time, between 5 minutes and 2 hours, the dermal irritation is felt. It may be precipitated by wetting or rubbing the area. It may progress over the next day or so and feel as if ground glass has been abraded into the skin. Hyperesthesia and paresthesia may be noted. The symptoms can persist for a week or more with inflammatory and painful reactions around the area. The degree of severity is not related to the clinical signs, and some patients may be incapacitated by the symptoms without any objective manifestations.

The dermal reaction may appear as an erythema, with or without papule and vesicle development. There is sometimes a desquamation of the skin in the second or third week, but in other cases the skin lesions have recurred over many months.

Treatment

The only adequate treatment is prevention, using gloves when handling sponges and not touching anything that has been in contact with the sponge. The use of alcohol, lotions, or hot water will usually aggravate the condition. Local application of a cooling lotion, such as calamine, may be of some value, but in general the skin lesion is treated with the conventional dermatological preparations—with very limited success.

CORAL CUTS

General

Because of their sharp edges and man's awkwardness in the sea environment, corals (Fig. 11–9) often cause lacerations. The sequelae of this may well equal the intensity of the more impressive marine animal injuries. Not only is the coral covered by infected slime, but also pieces of coral or other foreign bodies will often remain in the laceration. It is possible that some of the manifestations, especially initially, are due to the presence of discharging nematocysts. There have also been occasional patients who have been affected by the marine organism *Erysipelothrix*.

Certain vibrio may be present in the marine environment which can cause serious infection. These must be cultured in a saline media if identification is to be made.

Clinical Features

A small, often clean-looking laceration is usual on the hand or foot. It causes little incon-

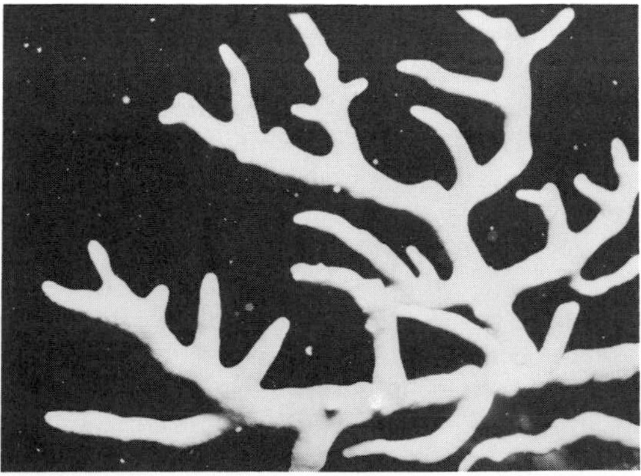

FIGURE 11–9. Fire coral (*Millepoia* sp.) found in the Caribbean. All stinging marine animals have microscopic capsules called nematocysts that contain a small dart with a toxin. (Photo by Bonnie J. Cardone, used with permission from Peterson Publishing Company, Los Angeles, CA)

venience at the time of injury and may well go unnoticed. A few hours later there may be a "smarting" sensation, especially during washing. At that stage, there is a mild inflammatory reaction around the cut. Within the next day or two, the inflammation becomes more widespread with local swelling, discoloration, and tenderness. In severe cases there may be abscess formation developing with chronic ulceration and even osteomyelitis.

After healing there may be a small numb area of skin with a fibrous nodule beneath it, a keloid reaction to the foreign body (coral).

Treatment

This involves thorough cleansing of the area, removal of the foreign material, and application of an antibiotic powder or ointment such as neomycin.

One sequelae of coral cuts is sometimes a very unpleasant pruritus that can be troublesome for many weeks. It responds to the use of a local steroid preparation such as Ultralan 0.5%.

FISH POISONING

There are many species of fish and other marine animals which inflict harm by poisoning those who eat them. Fish poisoning is becoming more prevalent because of the increase in fish consumption resulting from the health benefits of fish in reducing risk for atherosclerosis. Of the many types of poisoning, four stand out because of their relatively high incidence or severity. These are ciguatera poisoning, paralytic shellfish poisoning (PSP), scombroid poisoning, and tetrodotoxin poisoning.

Ciguatera Poisoning

Ciguatera poisoning is caused by ingesting many of the common fish found in tropical waters. The toxin, an ichthyosarcotoxin,[1] is a heat-stable, lipid-soluble compound that originates from a dinoflagellate. The toxin passes through the food chain and is concentrated in fish such as red snapper, amberjack, barracuda, and surgeonfish. Ingestion of the affected fish, whether cooked or raw, can produce poisoning.

The victim usually notices symptoms within 12 hours of ingesting the affected fish; often they appear within minutes. Presentation may vary from minor symptoms to coma and death. Paresthesia or dysesthesia, arthralgia, and myalgia are common. Abdominal cramps, diarrhea, nausea, and vomiting are less common. Paresis, hypotension, and shock may occur. The active disease is most severe for 6 to 10 (average 8.5) days,[2] but many victims complain of symptoms for prolonged periods that may extend to a year or more. Some victims have recurrence of symptoms when any fish or fish product is ingested.

There are no diagnostic laboratory tests, although in some areas there is a specific immunoassay for the toxin in suspected fish products. Because the disease is endemic to certain locations in the tropical latitudes, it is important to seek advice from natives before eating any fish from local waters. Some areas of the world have a custom of feeding suspected fish to a pet cat or kitten (most sensitive). If the animal becomes sick, then the fish is not eaten by humans.

Treatment of ciguatera poisoning is nonspecific and primarily supportive.[3] A variety of treatments has been suggested. These include calcium gluconate, corticosteroids, atropine, vitamin B complex, pyridoxine, amitriptyline, and others.[4] Palafox and colleagues listed the clinical features of 24 patients with ciguatera (Table 11–1) and suggested that mannitol may be helpful in comatose patients to treat cerebral edema.[5]

Paralytic Shellfish Poisoning

This poisoning occurs in humans after ingestion of shellfish that are contaminated by toxins of planktonic organisms known as dinoflagellates. These plankton are found to "bloom" in the open sea and bays under certain conditions of temperature and organic material concentrations. They often become concentrated enough to color the waters. The Red and Yellow Tides

TABLE 11–1. Clinical Features of Ciguatera Poisoning in 24 Patients

SIGN OR SYMPTOM	%
Circumoral or facial paresthesia	96
Paresthesias in extremities	96
Cold to hot reversal	79
Paresis	17
Coma	8
Abdominal pain	42
Diarrhea	38
Nausea	33
Vomiting	33
Muscle pain in extremities	75
Arthralgia	75
Hypotension	12

Data from Palafox NA, Jain LG, Pinano AZ, et al: Successful treatment of ciguatera fish poisoning with intravenous mannitol. JAMA 259:2740–2742, 1988.

that occur periodically throughout the world are due to proliferation of these plankton. The high concentration may deplete the sea of oxygen and cause death of fishes, but mollusks can filter these organisms and concentrate the toxin in their muscles. Contamination may be found in mussels, beach and surf clams, razor clams, and butter clams, among others.[6]

Shellfish poisoning may take on different manifestations. A gastrointestinal form is related with nausea, vomiting, diarrhea, and abdominal pain. Symptoms may appear hours or days after eating the shellfish. The paralytic type begins by immediate sensations of tingling in the mouth and lips after eating a contaminated shellfish. The sensation spreads to the rest of the body, numbness may follow the tingling, and ultimately paralysis develops. Dizziness, increased salivation, thirst, dysphagia, and respiratory paralysis may occur.

In some subjects the symptoms are typical of an acute allergic reaction, with bronchospasm and oral mucosal edema.

There is no specific treatment for this disease. If oral sensations are perceived, the food should not be eaten. When systemic symptoms are found, the food should be removed from the stomach by gastric lavage. Vomiting should be induced if a gastric tube is not available. When muscle paralysis is present, careful monitoring for respiratory insufficiency should be done, and respiratory support should be provided if necessary.

Scombroid Poisoning

This form of poisoning originates in the scombroid fishes, which include tuna, mackerel, skipjack, bonito, and albacore.[6] Epidemics have been described related to canned tuna. The disease occurs when the fish, which are usually safe to eat, are left for several hours at room temperature or outside in a warm climate. When at room temperature for several hours, histidine in the muscle tissues is converted to saurine by bacteria. This is one instance in which bacteria have a role in producing the toxin. The toxin, however, is not a bacterial toxin.

Clinical Presentation

The fish may have a spicy or peppery taste. Within 30 to 60 minutes, a histamine-like intoxication develops. The subject experiences headache, flushing, dizziness, throbbing of blood vessels, palpitations, and tachycardia. Hypotension may result. In addition, bronchospasm, urticaria, and anaphylactic shock may occur. Gastrointestinal symptoms include nausea, vomiting, diarrhea, abdominal pain, thirst, and dysphagia.

Treatment includes gastric lavage and circulatory and respiratory support. Antihistamines are considered to be of value.

Tetrodotoxin Poisoning

This type of poisoning is typified by the well-known fugu poisoning in Japan. Fugu poisoning occurs from ingestion of puffer fish, which contains lethal amounts of the poison in the gonads and the liver. The toxin inhibits sodium transport across cell membranes and affects neuronal transmission in motor and sensory peripheral nerves and in the central nervous system. Cardiac conduction and contractility are also affected.

Clinical Presentation

The severity depends on the amount of toxin ingested. In Japan, specially trained fugu chefs are considered expert if they leave small amounts of the toxin in the fish to provide a mild tingling sensation in the mouth. Mortality from a large dose of toxin can reach 60 per cent.

Neurological involvement often begins with muscular fasciculations and twitching and may progress to total flaccid paralysis. Speech and respiration may be compromised, and ocular paralysis may occur. A curare-like state will ensue in which the patient is totally immobile but conscious and aware of all that is going on around. Treatment for early poisoning includes gastric lavage and support of respiration. When paralysis occurs, respiratory support is required for 24 hours or more. The toxic effects usually remit spontaneously if the patient is otherwise supported. Sedation should be given to the totally paralyzed patient as consciousness is retained. No specific treatment has proven to be effective.

REFERENCES AND RECOMMENDED READING

1. Morris JG: Ciguatera fish poisoning. JAMA 244:273–274, 1980.
2. Chretein JH, Fermaglich J, Garagusi VF: Ciguatera poisoning: Presentation as a neurologic disorder. Arch Neurol 38:783, 1981.
3. Hughes JM, Merson MH: Fish and shellfish poisoning. N Engl J Med 295:117–1120, 1976.

4. Hokama Y, Abad MA, Kimura LH: A rapid enzyme-immunoassay for the detection of ciguatoxin in contaminated fish tissues. Toxicon 21:817–821, 1983.
5. Palafox NA, Jain LG, Pinano AZ, et al: Successful treatment of ciguatera fish poisoning with intravenous mannitol. JAMA 259:2740–2742, 1988.
6. Halstead BW: Dangerous Marine Animals. Centreville, MD, Cornell Maritime Press, 1980, pp 142–160.
7. Halstead BW: Dangerous Marine Animals. Centreville, MD, Cornell Maritime Press, 1980, pp 161–183.
8. Edmonds C, Lowry C, Pennefather J: Diving and Subaquatic Medicine. Sydney, Australia, Diving Medical Center, 1981, pp 316–352.

Sharks and Shark Attack

Coppleson VM: Shark Attack. Sydney, Angus and Robertson, 1958.

Davies DH: About Sharks and Shark Attack. Pietermaritzburg, Shuter and Shooter, 1964.

Ellis R: The Book of Sharks. New York, Grosset and Dunlap, 1975.

Johnson RH: Sharks of Tropical and Temperate Seas. Singapore, Les Editions Du Pacifique, 1978.

Wallet T: Shark Attack in Southern African Waters. Cape Town, Struik, 1983.

Venomous Marine Animals

Bulletin, Supplement of the Post Graduate Committee in Medicine (Gilbert P. Whitley 4.05, Vol 18, No. 3). University of Sydney, 1963.

Cleland JB, Southcott RB: Injuries to Man from Marine Invertebrates in the Australian Region. Canberra, Austalian Government Printing Office, 1965.

Edmonds C: Marine Animal Injuries to Man. Melbourne, Wedneil Publishers, 1984.

Edmonds C, Lowry C, Pennefather J: Diving and Subaquatic Medicine. 2nd ed. Sydney, Diving Medical Centre, 1981.

Halstead BW: Dangerous Marine Animals. Centreville, MO, Cornell Maritime Press, 1980.

Sutherland SK: Australian Animal Toxins. Melbourne, Oxford University Press, 1983.

Chapter 12

Human Performance Under Water

ARTHUR J. BACHRACH
and GLEN H. EGSTROM

Human performance under water occurs when, for example, a commercial diver inspects a pipeline, a sports diver engages in underwater photography, or a Navy diver repairs a propeller. For many years the emphasis in diving medicine has been on physiological problems such as decompression, largely a matter of getting the diver safely to the worksite and back without untoward physical problems. However, as Bennett observed in 1965,[1] while this emphasis is "of vital necessity, it should not be forgotten that this consititutes wasted effort if man, working under pressure, is not in perfect physical and mental condition."

In recent years the emphasis has shifted, in large measure, to an understanding of those factors that have an effect on the diver's ability to perform effectively and safely under water. With this shift, the physician's role has also changed from one concentrating almost exclusively on physiological factors to one involving an awareness of those elements of human performance that are crucial to the diver's safety and efficacy. The physician's understanding of physiological effects has had to expand to include the impact of such factors as cold water, decompression, breathing gas mixtures, and emotional elements (anxiety, panic) on the diver's performance. Thus, the normal physiological orientation of the physician is extended to include the psychophysiological realm, and the functions of screening and treating divers take on new dimensions.

The problem has been compounded to some degree by a blurring of the distinctions that once differentiated commercial and military divers from the sports diving community. In recent years increasing numbers of sports (or recreational) divers have entered diving activities that involve decompression. What was originally an activity involving breath-hold diving or relatively shallow, no-decompression dive profiles, has taken on new requirements when pursuits such as wreck diving necessitated divers staying longer at greater depths to perform tasks. In addition, some cave divers have developed dive profiles for cave dives that go as deep as 700 feet and require the use of helium/oxygen breathing mixtures. Developments in enriched air (nitrox) breathing mixes have also been of interest to divers because they allow extensive bottom time. While wreck diving and cave diving represent diving activities that require profiles and, perhaps, breathing mixes that differ from standard scuba and skin-diving procedures, divers still refer to such activities as "sports" or "recreational" diving. It is our position that once a diver enters a decompression schedule dive or uses a mix that is not a standard compressed air mixture (and the two are often related), the dive should no longer be considered recreational. The planning and operation of a decompression dive, the use of breathing mixes such as nitrox or heliox, and need for different equipment make such dives *working* dives. Even if the purpose of the dive is adventure and recreation, the character of the dive has changed and the diver is now a working diver, subject to all the subsequent demands of needing to know more about operations and equipment than the shallow, "no-decompression" warm-water diver has even considered.

This position does not suggest that divers should reject activities such as wreck diving or cave diving as recreational pursuits; all we ask is that a diver entering such endeavors recognize that the demands are more severe and that the requirements for sound physical and emotional conditions, as well as training and diving skills, are dramatically increased. The demands placed upon the diving physician who evaluates candidates for diving programs are likewise increased.

THE ELEMENTS OF PERFORMANCE

In the examples of diving activities noted, once again the central feature of a diver performing a task under water becomes our main focus. Our goal in this chapter is to examine the principal factors involved in an evaluation of human performance under water.

All too often performance is described in general and abstract terms—for example, saying that a diver "inspects" or "repairs" an object under water. In the planning of a dive operation, more than a general description of an overall task is needed; more valuable is specifying the particular behaviors that make up the entire performance in a complex task. Such specificity is also valuable to the scientist or physician who wishes to evaluate the ability of the diver to work at a performance task. For example, for some time there was a question as to whether a diver working in dark waters needed to have perfect color vision. The divemaster planning an operation might not be concerned if a diver working under turbid conditions lacked optimal color vision but might well be concerned if this same diver were acting as a gas manifold or hyperbaric chamber operator for whom color coding plays a role. Even here, the experienced operator can learn the placement of certain valves and, perhaps, can overcome a lack of color discrimination. By knowing the requirements of the performance task and the faculties of the individual who is to perform the task, a more effective decision as to assignment of divers to jobs can be made, thus ensuring better efficacy and safety.

Generally, psychologists in performance research agree upon three elements that constitute an overal performance sequence:

1. *Perception*: sensing the stimulus event (visual, tactile, auditory)
2. *Information processing*: cognitive or mediational processing by which the information perceived is evaluated and a course of action (motor) is selected
3. *Motor response*: the actual motor activity directed toward completing the task.

In various analyses of these factors, behavioral components have been further delineated.

One classification of these variables which attempts to provide greater specificity of performance elements was reported by Christensen and Mills[2] and was later modified by Berliner, Angell, and Sherarer[3] and by Bachrach.[4] In this system the performance elements include:

1. *Perceptual processes*
   a. Searching for and receiving information: the performing individual (operator) detects, inspects, observes, reads, surveys
   b. Identifying objects, actions, and events: the operator discriminates, identifies, locates
2. *Mediational processes* (cognitive)
   a. Information processing: the operator categorizes, calculates, codes, computes, itemizes
   b. Problem solving and decision making: the operator analyzes, calculates, computes, compares, estimates, plans, selects course of action
3. *Motor processes*
   a. Simple/discrete: the operator activates, closes, connects, disconnects, sets
   b. Complex/continuous: the operator adjusts, aligns, tracks, regulates, synchronizes

With this type of model, an assessment of which elements are most affected by external events can be accomplished. For example, in a review of the effects of alcohol on driving behavior, Moskowitz and Austin[5] concluded that the primary effects of alcohol in the performance of skills are on *mediational* processes—information processing and response-selection—rather than on the sensory/perceptual inputs or on the motor response. In other words, the driver under the influence of alcohol may have the capacity to detect the red light (sensation/perception) and complete the motor response needed to activate the brake pedal, but the information processing needed to interpret the significance or meaning of the signal light and to make a decision based upon this input is adversely affected. In a similar manner, when Bradley[6] suggests that cold is a major factor in commercial diving fatalities in the North Sea, owing in large measure to the loss of judgment by the diver, he is stating that an external event (cold) affects information processing in the form of judgment and decision making.

In the classification of performance elements discussed above, the original authors (Christensen and Mills[2]) added the element of *communication processes,* very important in task completion. In communication processes, the operator advises, answers, reports, transmits, requests, answers, and/or instructs. Communication is another function that may be adversely affected as a part of the operator's performance if, for example, cold has distracted the diver's attention so that inputs from topside are not perceived, or, as seen in Bradley's study, a loss of judgment resulting from cold exposure interferes with information processing. Problems in communication were also significant as disruptions of perception and information processing in the studies reported by Moskowitz and Austin[5] on alcohol effects.

With this classification of the key elements in human performance as a model, we may proceed to evaluate the factors that make human performance under water a special field of research and practice.

The primary factors to be considered in this chapter as they relate to performance are *environment, diver training, diver condition* (including emotional factors, principally panic), and the *type of work* performed. Other chapters in this volume will deal in depth with the all important performance factor of *equipment* (see Chapter 3) as well as the effects of hypothermia (see Chapter 9) and drugs in diving.

Environment

Among the environmental factors of primary interest in underwater human performance are the *water medium* itself, *temperature,* and *visibility.*

The impact of the water medium on diver performance is significant, for the water necessarily alters performance. Movements in a viscous medium are patently different from those performed in air. In a study conducted at UCLA, Weltman and colleagues[7] compared the learning of an underwater assembly task (UCLA pipe puzzle) in two groups of divers; the first group was trained to do the task on dry land, while the second group learned to perform the task under water. The dry land group had the obvious advantage of direct contact with the training staff as well as immediate corrective feedback on their performance. Nevertheless, the water-trained group experienced a 25 per cent faster mean completion time on the task, suggesting that not only are the movements different in water but also that performance itself (and accordingly performance assessment) must be different from water to dry land. Many performance assessments are accomplished using dry land baselines. The studies by Weltman and his colleagues suggest a more fitting comparison might be how well a task can be performed under *optimal* diving conditions (clear, comfortable, low-current water, with a minimum of protective gear), so that the assessment could compare performance under given diving conditions with ideal conditions, not against dry land or hyperbaric chamber baselines, which cannot duplicate underwater characteristics.

The water environment degrades performance in many ways. Relative weightlessness in a tractionless milieu is a major problem. The condition markedly affects the use of tools; there is the problem of recoil and the difficulty in maintaining a stable posture. This problem is greatly compounded under conditions of high current, when swiftly flowing or surging water moves the diver, making it difficult to maintain stability and control over tools and equipment.

Low visibility is another environmental factor that degrades performance. Turbidity and other obscuring elements in the water make observing and performing a task more difficult. The diver often has to resort to tactile sensory inputs almost exclusively when faced with visibility loss, but this is a problem when the turbid water is also cold, necessitating the use of protective gloves, which markedly diminish feeling. Changing technologies of acoustic imaging offer great promise as an aid to "seeing" in dark waters.

The most disruptive of all environmental conditions is temperature; cold exposure represents the most severe stress in diving. Not only does cold itself adversely affect performance, but also, as noted, the diver's work is further affected by the impact of protective gear such as gloves and the impediment of other forms of clothing, all of which diminish mobility and manual performance.

Cold Stress and Effects on Performance

Webb[8] observed that "cold is a serously limiting factor in many diving operations" and is likely to be a causative or contributing factor in commercial diving accidents; however, "because cold exposure is routine in diving, it is accepted and its potential for harm is discounted."

In one report, Padbury and co-workers[9] offer a similar comment: "the diving industry is skeptical whether undetected hypothermia is a real enough danger to warrant monitoring, let alone development of equipment or procedures to prevent it." The term "undetected hypothermia" is used by research workers and field personnel (along with synonyms of "insidious," "silent," and "progressive" hypothermia) to describe the slow effects of cold exposure on the diver. The process is a slow cooling that occurs often without perception of change on the part of the diver.

Progressive hypothermia suggests that the critical factor is the *rate of cooling*. Kuehn[10] comments upon this variable, noting that rapid heat loss results in a greater drop in rectal temperature accompanied by more shivering, whereas the identical loss of heat over a longer period of time results in little temperature drop (when compared with rapid cooling), less shivering, and fewer complaints about cold discomfort. The concern about slow cooling is that the diver may not be aware of progressive changes, which are not as profound as those associated with rapid cooling, creating a potential for hazard. Bradley's study[6] implicates such cold exposure as a causative or contributing factor in 11 per cent of North Sea commercial diving fatalities; in another 15 per cent, loss of judgment (a cognitive decrement resulting from cold stress) appeared to be a crucial element in the accident and its unfortunate consequences.

Among the principal physical symptoms associated with progressive hypothermia are muscle stiffness, numbness, weakness, and loss of muscle strength, all of which reduce the diver's ability to respond effectively and markedly affect performance in such critical motor areas as manual dexterity. This degradation of physical capacity, coupled with loss of judgment and decision-making competence, places the diver in a vulnerable position as far as safety and performance are concerned.

Some problems encountered by the diver working in a cold environment are caused by distraction. The diver's concentration on the task requirements at hand may well mask the perception of the physiological changes that are occurring with slow cooling. Another form of distraction is a feeling of discomfort from cold exposure, which can interfere with optimal performance of the task requirements and can lead to serious consequences. As Childs[11] observed, "distraction due to discomfort may cause the diver to ignore threats to his safety underwater and, finally, realizing he is in danger, he may be in further difficulty because of a loss of power and dexterity in his hands." Distraction was considered to be a major factor in problems in performance reported by Vaughan,[12] who found that Navy divers showed impaired performance in reaction time and target detection early into cold water exposures. Similar findings were reported by Davis, Baddeley, and Hancock,[13] who recorded significant decrements in tasks of simple arithmetic, logical reasoning, word recall and recognition (all cognitive tasks), as well as manual dexterity in divers exposed to 5°C water temperatures.

Another study suggesting that distraction from cold exposure may be a factor in degraded performance is the one by Padbury and colleagues[9] in which divers were locked out of a 450-meter chamber dive in cold water. The divers were wearing open-circuit hot-water suits for warming but showed uneven temperatures. In one diver, undetected hypothermia appeared when rectal temperature fell from 37.8°C to 36.3°C in a 66-minute lockout, but he had no complaints of cold or discomfort. It should be remembered that a core temperature drop of 1° to 1.5°C moves the diver from the "comfort" range of ±1°C on 37°C into the "tolerable" range of ±2° to 2.5°C. The drop recorded in this diver over a 66-minute lockout was not severe but was approaching the discomfort level. Among the results of this study were the findings that no performance decrements occurred in manual perforance as measured by finger dexterity or arm/wrist speed. However, vigilance (a cognitive task), as measured by arithmetic speed and visual reaction time, was degraded on the first cold exposures but improved with later trials. The assumption that distraction from cold exposure adversely affects early performance while later trials show improvement appears valid if one considers adaptation to the novel stimulus of cold exposure over time. Other factors need to be taken into account as well. Over a number of exposures, humans can adapt and tolerance levels can change by ± ½°C. Perhaps of greater importance is the difference between a chamber dive in a wet pot and an open sea exposure. Even with temperature and pressure controlled, an open sea dive represents conditions of danger not present in a controlled environment.

A neurophysiological basis for changes in performance is provided by preliminary studies reported by Reeves, Winsborough, and Bachrach,[14] who placed subjects in swim trunks in a cold immersion tank, which effectively produced colonic temperature reductions to an average of 35.5°C. The cold exposures were either 60 to 90 minutes or up to a core temperature reduction of 1.5°C below baseline, whichever occurred first. The techniques used included electrophysiological evaluation of central nervous system (CNS) activity and employment of visual and auditory event-related potentials to measure the effects of cold immersion on nerve conduction. Related performance measures such as tapping and grip stength were used to determine behavioral factors in nerve conduction velocity. The authors concluded that multineuronal conduction velocity in both the central and peripheral nervous systems can be reliably slowed as a result of reducing core temperatures by an average of 1.5°C. Increased latency in nerve conduction was associated with degraded cognitive performance. Reduction in nerve conduction velocity was significantly correlated with tapping rate (the number of times a subject could finger tap within a set time), while no correlation was found between nerve conduction velocity and grip strength. These data suggest that tapping as a performance task involves intermittent neuromuscular activity, whereas grip strength is a static and steady effort less susceptible to interference from changes in nerve conduction. The study also lends support to the need for specifying performance tasks with precision so that a better evaluation of responses can be made. The authors suggest that further work in "sham" immersion in cold water is needed, in which subjects would be placed in cold water sufficient to be noxious but not to induce reductions in core temperature. The authors believe that this could contribute to an understanding of the effects found in the study, whether the increased latency is associated with cold, discomfort-induced distraction, or, as seems probable, a combination of both elements.

Another critical performance element in divers affected by cold exposure is that of *memory*. Coleshaw and colleagues[15] reported that memory registration was impaired as core temperatures fell below 36.7°C in subject divers during a cold chamber diver. Results revealed a 70 per cent loss of memory for data at core temperatures of 34° to 35°C. A significant feature of this study was the assessment of recall of facts memorized during hypothermic exposures under warm water conditions following the cold immersion. The subjects were comfortable, although still slightly hypothermic, but showed marked impairment in reasoning ability as well as in memory for facts learned under cold exposure. The 70 per cent loss agrees with the measured loss of 75 per cent of material learned in an underwater task when recalled on the surface post-dive, as reported by Jim Stewart of the Scripps Institution of Oceanography.[16]

From the above review of selected studies on the effects of cold exposure on diver performance, it is clear that the major effect appears to be in the mediation of information—the cognitive, information-processing element so crucial in task completion under water.

Diver Training

A specific and precise analysis of performance elements serves in the development of more effective programs in diver training. In recent years the emphasis has shifted, particularly in industry and in the military, from a concentration on selection for a particular job, followed by training and field performance, to the reverse. It is now understood that the first step in performance is a task analysis that defines the requirements of the performance and the specific behaviors needed to accomplish it. First, the tasks and the behaviors associated with them are specified, then the most effective training procedures to perfect the needed skills are developed, and finally those individuals whose aptitudes and backgrounds seem most appropriate for the training designed to lead to optimal performance are screened and selected.

An important part of training also involves responses that are designed not to accomplish a task but to avoid or eliminate events that might interfere with the performance. For example, Egstrom[17] found that divers surveyed indicated that an important skill required in the field was the ability to escape from entanglement. The group surveyed was composed of commercial divers who had gone through formal training but who had not been trained in escape from entanglement in lines or debris under water. Such feedback is important in assessing elements of performance and which procedures might be added to standard teaching programs. In a similar fashion, a knowledge of emergency procedures is crucial for all divers, recreational as well as military and commercial. The inclusion of skill training in handling emergencies should be a part of all training programs; unfortunately, little formal emphasis has been placed on emergency procedures, and virtually no standardization of such procedures exists.

One of the most controversial of all emergency procedures has been the emergency ascent. When a diver runs out of air, or some untoward event occurs, it is desirable to return to the surface rapidly, but carefully, so that the risk of an air embolism is not encountered. Emergency ascent training has been controversial because many diving trainers and physicians believe that the risks involved in teaching the emergency ascent outweigh the possible benefits to be derived from the low-frequency occurrence of a real emergency. In 1977 the Undersea Medical Society convened a group of 35 diving authorities from all areas of diving to resolve the question of the value of emergency ascent training. The consensus, reflected in a workshop report,[18] was that a controlled emergency ascent was desirable, if feasible, as an independent action on the part of the diver in difficulty. If such independent action were not possible for one reason or another, a dependent action such as buddy breathing was recommended. The experts agreed that training was essential to the success of these emergency procedures and that there was a need for improved standardization of emergency ascent training and the use of equipment. More than a decade has passed since that important workshop, and there is still no significant progress in the standardization of emergency procedures. This reflects in large measure a failure of the training agencies to agree and the proliferation of techniques available for an out-of-air emergency. For example, the "Octopus" is used as an additional second-stage regulator without any standardization of the placement of the second stage, creating a hazardous uncertainty during a time of emergency.[19]

There is also, unfortunately, a lack of standardization in training programs for commercial and recreational divers; divers have no means of knowing precisely what kinds of skills and experience a fellow diver brings to the dive. The variety of courses offered to potential recreational divers ranges from essentially a few hours' training to a thorough grounding in diving practice. Cooperation among the training agencies to develop ideal levels of training would solve many of the problems currently encountered.

It is our opinion that one of the major problems in diver training today is the emphasis on an increased reliance on equipment. When diver training began formally in the United States in the 1950's, there was a requirement on individual, personal skills in handling oneself in the water and being in good physical condition. The diver learned proper weighting techniques so that the weight belt became a means of controlling buoyancy; the ability to use the weight belt (and jettisoning it when necessary) was a personal skill that, for example, also taught the diver about his or her own physical characteristics of buoyancy. This personal skill has been replaced by training in the use of a buoyancy compensator, which is, undoubtedly, a useful tool but not a substitute for individual self-reliance in case of an emergency. The increasing reliance on equipment rather than on personal skills also seems to include the belief, in some quarters, that one need not be able to swim in order to become a diver. Consequently, earlier requirements for demonstrating watermanship skills have all but disappeared.

We have referred to emergencies frequently in the above discussion. The reasons are simple. If nothing goes wrong on a dive, the level of training and the experience of the diver may not be crucial, and, despite a lack of skill, a dive can proceed safely. When a physician or diving instructor evaluates a diving candidate, the possibility of an emergency and the need for a coping response should be kept in mind. The candidate can then be evaluated in terms of needed skill training and, equally important, in terms of physical and emotional condition.

Diver Condition

Perhaps the most important single factor in underwater human performance is the condition of the diver. Given optimal diving conditions, properly planned diving operations, and well-engineered equipment, the physical and psychological state of the diver remains the critical element in performance. The diver in good physical condition is more likely to be able to perform successfully and to cope readily with problems encountered in the underwater environment. This means that the diver should have sufficient endurance and strength to withstand the stresses of the underwater environment and the ability to handle the equipment, perform the task, and cope with emergencies that may arise. Behaviorally, it means that the diver in good condition must have a confidence in his or her own skills (in very large measure a function of adequate training) and thus sufficient competence to cope with impending problems. A combination of effective training and good physical condition appears to be a critical requisite of coping behavior in divers.

With regard to strength and endurance, the level of work in sport diving should be kept well within aerobic limits. Divers should be trained to recognize the signs of overexertion and to use them as alarms to trigger behavior designed to reduce the work load until respiration rate and pulse rate are back to a comfortable level.

One further comment about the diver's physical condition: about a decade ago, Eldridge[20] reported on a number of deaths in scuba divers, all in cold water and all involving males in an age range of 35 to 55 years. She referred to these deaths as a "sudden unexplained death syndrome" and suggested cardiovascular mechanisms in older males as a possible causative factor. In a discussion of this report, Bachrach[21] suggests the possibility of vagotonic changes in older males as one factor to be considered. There have been recent reports of "sudden death" occurring in divers, reviving an interest in the phenomenon among diving personnel. When evaluating the diver's physical condition, especially in older males, the diving physician should give careful consideration to factors such as vasovagal state, factors that also involve behavioral elements. As Engel[22] notes, "vasodepressor syncope occurs in our machismo culture more commonly among men than women, especially in settings in which the man feels the ambience to be one of strong social disapproval of any display of weakness," a description of what has come to be known as Type A behavior.

The Problem of Panic

Of all the factors that interfere with effective performance under water and, in many cases, lead to serious consequences such as death, the problem of panic is clearly paramount. The lack of confidence and competence and less than adequate physical condition can lead to a loss of control, which appears to be a factor in most diving fatalities. In a study of sports diving fatalities, Sand[23] implicated panic as the major factor leading to a casualty in a diving accident in 80 per cent of the cases studied. Most diving researchers would agree that panic, with the diver losing control, is indeed the leading cause of fatalities. The problem of panic and loss of control has been addressed by several authors in recent years.[19, 24–28] As Bachrach and Egstrom[25] observed, a certain amount of apprehension may be expected in a diver experiencing a novel situation, such as entering a kelp bed for the first time. It is not possible for a training program to cover every conceivable hazard a diver may eventually encounter, although, as we have noted, a good training program teaches emergency coping procedures and self-confidence in handling novel situations. The diver performing adequately obtains as much information as possible about the particular dive—the conditions, the dive plan, the necessary equipment, and the potential problems—thus reducing apprehension by information gathering. The positive aspects of the dive, the beautiful sights to be encountered, the opportunity to perform exciting tasks such as underwater photography, and the pleasure of being under water should be emphasized as keys to pleasant anticipation as well as apprehension reduction.

Although apprehension may be brought under control by proper planning, adequate knowledge, good role modeling, and reassurance by the divemaster, panic is a loss-of-control state wherein a diver perceives that he or she is losing control but cannot extricate himself or herself from the dangerous situation.

In virtually all the fatalities reported, there has been no indication of equipment failure. Rather, from the condition of the victims the inference is that human error was at fault. The victim usually has air left in the tank, the weight belt is still in place, and the buoyancy compensator is uninflated—all suggestions of a human error resulting from a lack of problem-solving behavior leading to panic.

An early sign common to most panic situations is *rapid breathing*. A change in breathing rate and pattern is the first sign in virtually any type of stress—heat, cold, altitude, diving—and is readily observable. The change in breathing rate and pattern in the apprehensive diver goes from smooth and regular to rapid, irregular, and shallow. The latter is a type of respiration that produces an inefficient exchange of oxygen and carbon dioxide, leading to a sensation of air hunger which may further exacerbate feelings of panic. It is frequently reported that a diver in a panic condition on the surface is seen struggling with arms and legs to keep the head above water; the struggle results in the head being higher, but it increases the work load on the body and also increases pulse and respiration rates. The struggling diver supporting the weight of the head (approximately 17 pounds) can only sustain this work load for a matter of seconds; if shoulders are raised out of the water, the weight to be supported could easily be 30 to 36 pounds. The problem is compounded by exhaustion from the work of struggling. Divers have been reported to sink in a matter of seconds or, at the most, in a minute or so. Implications for cardiac consequences of the panic and struggle have been assumed, including the sudden death syndrome mentioned earlier.

Another early sign of panic is *agitation*, which is associated with the change in breathing rate and pattern discussed above or with erratic movement. A diver in control moves along smoothly, with respiration and swimming movements controlled and regular. An apprehensive diver's movements are likely to be jerky and irregular. Bevan[26] comments upon a movement seen in a diver on the verge of panic, noting that such a diver is apt to bring the knees forward and swim with short, jerky strokes rather than with smooth movements using the thighs and legs for propulsion.

Another sign of agitation concerns *orientation*. A controlled diver is oriented toward the water ahead, toward the bottom to observe sights and events, or toward the diving partner to maintain contact. The apprehensive diver, who may be approaching panic, is oriented toward the surface, often checking orientation toward the presumed safety of the surface and the dive boat. A diver in control will make frequent equipment checks to make certain that there is enough remaining air in the tank for a safe ascent and that the bottom time is carefully monitored; the apprehensive diver checks equipment too often, manifesting discomfort and preoccupation with gauges.

Preventing panic is largely a function of good physical condition and adequate training so that a diver develops competence and confidence. Skill acquisition is of great importance so that appropriate coping responses can be brought to bear in a problem situation. It is not uncommon to witness a diver venturing into an unfamiliar surf condition who fails not only to evoke the appropriate behavior but also to respond to pertinent directions given by the dive partner. Often such behavior leads to failure to take simple precautions such as holding on to the face mask when the surf is about to break on the diver. The subsequent loss of the face mask caused by the surge of the water creates additional stress and results in the onset of panic in what should be a minor emergency.

In the training of the diver, effective program sequences of diver training are crucial so that actual experience with required skills is built into the diving program. A necessary skill in the water for the apprehensive diver is being able to properly gain positive buoyancy, a first priority for a fatigued or anxious diver. The diver who still has a snorkel or regulator in the mouth should be trained to back float with the mouthpiece removed for greater air passage.[28] Floating on one's back, with the buoyancy compensator sufficiently inflated, can provide a diver with rest and a diminution of struggling, which lessens exhaustion and possible submergence.

Although the prediction of behavior is not an exact science, there are some behavioral patterns that have been identified[19] which may help the diving physician and diving instructor look for potential problem individuals. The diving candidate most vulnerable to panic appears to have three characteristics:

1. The individual has a high level of generalized anxiety and is more likely to respond with anxiety to a wider range of situations viewed as stressful. This general, behavioral type of anxiety is referred to by psychologists as *trait* anxiety,[29] as opposed to *state* anxiety, which is more situational.
2. The vulnerable individual has a low sense of self-confidence and competence and is unsure of an ability to cope (has a sense of helplessness[19]) in facing potential stress situations.
3. The individual has a low level of social support, an inability to work well with other people, and an inability to provide or receive support from others. In some cases this represents a "macho" type of behavior, a need to excel and exceed on one's own. The lone diver is a myth; every diver is involved in a social net—from the diving partner of the recreational diver to the topside personnel of a working dive.

A proper screening of divers should identify characteristics that need attention by diving instructors and diving partners. Good training programs can develop skills and self-confidence, along with a recognition of the importance of the social support that can help to ameliorate anxious tendencies.

Drugs and Diving

The drugs considered here are not the medications divers may take, such as antihistamines, but, rather, controlled substances, marijuana, and cocaine. The behavioral effects of such compounds are similar in many ways to those of alcohol ingestion, with profound effects on information processing, decision making, and judgment. Marijuana, for example, is known to affect the individual's sense of timing.[19] The awareness of the passage of time is a critical variable in dive planning, information necessary to monitor air consumption and decompression limits. Tzimoulis[30] comments on the problem of sleepiness as a result of marijuana intoxication. The information-processing impairment resulting from marijuana may not be a problem in an uneventful dive, but if an emergency arises, the diver's ability to bring adaptive reserves to bear in coping behavior is severely diminished. Physiologically, marijuana has another effect that can be serious for the diver: it can cause hypothermia. Studies by Pertwee[31] have shown that tetrahydrocannabinol (THC), the active ingredient in marijuana, lowers body temperature by acting centrally (primarily in the anterior hypothalamus) to reduce heat production in response to cold.

Cocaine is reported to be "the most commonly abused central nervous system stimulant."[32] Cocaine drastically affects information-processing abilities, placing the diver at risk. Physiologically, the risks are major ones. Cocaine, as a stimulant, produces a hypermetabolic state that "may place the diver at risk of subsequent fatigue, mental depression, acidosis and an inability to respond to life-threatening emergencies."[32]

A crucial physiological effect of cocaine is that of cardiac alteration. Isner and colleagues,[33] in a report of cardiac consequences of the use of cocaine, showed serious, often fatal, effects including ventricular arrhythmias and sudden cardiac death. These consequences have been sadly demonstrated in recent years in young, otherwise fit athletes.

Type of Work: Changing Technologies

When evaluating human performance under water, one must recognize that in recent years the role of the diver has changed significantly. In place of the "mud diver," who performed alone in a hardhat with simple tools, the demands of an ever-expanding diving technology have required more sophisticated working divers trained in the use of new diving techniques and procedures. From the working diver in a surface-supplied hardhat diving mode, to the saturation diver performing at greater depths for longer durations freed from stringent decompression obligations, the changes in technology and resulting physiological stresses have been profound. With saturation diving the necessity for mixed-gas breathing, such as helium/oxygen, to replace air at depth in itself created problems in heat loss and speech intelligibility as well as neurological effects, such as the high pressure nervous syndrome. Differences in performance effects between shallow and deep diving were discussed by Biersner,[34] who noted that neuromuscular performance is most affected by deep dives and cognitive, information-processing processes are less affected. The opposite appears to be true for shallow dives using compressed air rather than heliox as a breathing mix, as intellectual functions are degraded more than motor responses.

The concerns about neurological effects of deep diving, particularly possible long-term effects on divers, were in part responsible for an increased emphasis on diving technology and the development of diving techniques such as 1-ata diving systems (JIM and WASP, for example) and the remotely operated vehicles (ROVs), which are now a standard part of diving procedures in deep exploration and work. The utility of ROVs is demonstrated in such outstanding deep dives as the discovery of the *Titanic* and, in tandem with 1 ata systems such as the WASP, in the work on the deep archeological dive on the wreck of the *HMS Breadalbane*.

Busby[35] observes that "there seems to be no stopping the ROV now. The concept of sending a human being into the cold, dark high-pressure environment of the deep sea has had its day." He supports this view by referring to performance tasks accomplished using the ROV SCARAB in recovering the voice and data recorder from the downed Air India Flight #182 in 1985 at a depth of 6601 feet off the coast of Ireland. He notes that this was a task that could not have possibly been performed by a human diver, just as the work on the *Titanic* at 2½ miles down could not have been accomplished with human operators. Busby sums up his position by noting that the human diver has obviously not been replaced by the ROV in all circumstances but that "the ROV has demonstrated that the human diver need not be subjected to potentially hazardous situations and that it is frequently not economical to do so." In a real sense, this parallels developments in the space program in which, as Busby observes, "the romantic aspects of human involvement have given way to the practical and economic aspects of getting the job done."

The human diver is not going to be replaced by a machine in all circumstances, and the need for human performance will continue. If, as seems likely, the human operator at great depths is no longer a practical alternative to mechanical means of performing work, owing to both physiological and economic reasons, what does this mean for the study of human performance under water? We believe that the emphasis has necessarily shifted from concerns about the physiology of deep diving to the development of improved training techniques, more effective decompression schedules for working dives, and better equipment such as improved tools, diving suits, and other protective gear, as well as aids to the diver in performing tasks. The last item includes the previously mentioned development of acoustic imaging techniques to help the diver "see" in turbid waters. The use of the operator in the 1-ata diving system WASP in tandem with an ROV on the wreck of the *HMS Breadalbane* was a breakthrough in diving technology, for the human operator in the 1 ata system was able to communicate with topside personnel to send the ROV with a camera to any position on the wreck.

The future of human performance under water depends in large measure on the effective use of technology and human skill.

REFERENCES

1. Bennett PB: Narcosis due to helium and air at pressure between 2 and 15.2 ata and the effects of such gases on oxygen toxicity. *In* Proceedings of the Symposium on Human Performance Capabilities in Undersea Operations. Panama City, Florida, 1965 (unpublished).
2. Christensen JM, Mills RG: What does the operator do in complex systems? Human Factors 9:329–340, 1967.
3. Berliner C, Angell D, Shearer JW: Behaviors, measures and instruments of performance evaluation in simulated environments. Presented at the Symposium and Workshop on the Quantification of Human Performance, Albuquerque, New Mexico, 1964.
4. Bachrach AJ: Underwater performance. *In* Bennett PB, Elliott DH (eds): The Physiology and Medicine of Diving and Compressed Air Work. 2nd ed. London, Bailliere Tindall, 1975, pp 264–284.
5. Moskowitz H, Austin G: A critical review of the drug/performance literature. 2. A review of selected research studies from the last decade on the effects of alcohol on human skills performance. Final Report to U.S. Army Medical Research and Development Command. Washington, DC, Associate Consultants, 1979.
6. Bradley ME: An epidemiological study of fatal diving accidents in two commercial diving populations. *In* Bachrach AJ, Matzen MM (eds): Underwater Physiology VII: Proceedings of the Seventh Symposium on Underwater Physiology. Bethesda, Undersea Medical Society, 1981, pp 869–876.
7. Weltman G, Egstrom GH, Willis MA, Cuccaro W: Underwater Work Measurement Techniques: Final Report, UCLA ENG-7140. BioTechnology Laboratory, UCLA, 1971.
8. Webb P: Impaired performance from prolonged mild body cooling. *In* Bachrach AJ, Matzen MM (eds): Underwater Physiology VIII: Proceedings of the Eighth Symposium on Underwater Physiology. Bethesda, Undersea Medical Society, 1984, pp 391–400.
9. Padbury EH, Ronnestad I, Hope A, et al: Undetected hypothermia: Further indications. *In* Bove AA, Bachrach AJ, Greenbaum LJ (eds): Underwater and Hyperbaric Physiology IX: Proceedings of the Ninth International Symposium on Underwater and Hyperbaric Physiology. Bethesda, Undersea and Hyperbaric Medical Society, 1987, pp 153–161.
10. Kuehn LA: Thermal effects of the hyperbaric environment. *In* Bachrach AJ, Matzen MM (eds): Underwater Physiology VIII: Proceedings of the Eighth Symposium on Underwater Physiology. Bethesda, Undersea Medical Society, 1984, pp 413–439.
11. Childs CM: Loss of consciousness in divers—a survey and review. *In* Proceedings: Medical Aspects of Diving Accidents Congress. Luxembourg, 1978, pp 3–23.
12. Vaughan WS: Distraction effects of cold water performance of higher-order tasks. Undersea Biomed Res 4:113–116, 1977.
13. Davis FM, Baddeley AD, Hancock TR: Diver performance: The effect of cold. Undersea Biomed Res 2:77–88, 1975.
14. Reeves DL, Winsborough MM, Bachrach AJ: Neurophysiological and behavioral correlates of cold water immersion. *In* Bove AA, Bachrach AJ, Greenbaum LJ (eds): Underwater and Hyperbaric Physiology IX: Proceedings of the Ninth International Symposium on Underwater and Hyperbaric Physiology. Bethesda, Undersea and Hyperbaric Medical Society, 1987, pp 589–598.
15. Coleshaw SRK, van Someren RNM, Wolff AH, et al: Impairment of memory registration and speed of reasoning caused by mild depression of body core temperature. J Appl Physiol 55:27–31, 1983.
16. Stewart JR: Personal communication.
17. Egstrom GH: UCLA-ENG Diving safety research project. NDAA-4-6 158-44021.
18. Egstrom GH: Emergency ascents. *In* Kent M (ed): Emergency Ascent Training. Fifteenth Undersea Medical Society Workshop. Bethesda, Undersea Medical Society, 1979.
19. Bachrach AJ, Egstrom GH: Stress and Performance in Diving. San Pedro, Best Publishing, 1987.
20. Eldridge L: Sudden unexplained death syndrome in cold water scuba diving. Annual Scientific Meeting, Undersea Medical Society, 1979. Supplement to Undersea Biomedical Research, 6:41, 1979.
21. Bachrach AJ: Psychophysiological factors in diving. *In* Davis J (ed): Hyperbaric and Undersea Medicine. San Antonio, Medical Seminars, 1981.
22. Engel GL: Psychological stress, vasodepressor (vasovagal) syncope, and sudden death. Ann Intern Med 89:403–412, 1978.
23. Sand R: Diving fatalities in Puget Sound 1970–1974. *In* Man-in-the-Sea Symposium, Seattle, Washington, 1975 (Underwater Association Newsletter, May, 1975).
24. Bachrach AJ: Diving behavior. *In* Human Performance and Scuba Diving: Proceedings of the Symposium on Underwater Physiology. La Jolla, California,

Scripps Institution of Oceanography, 1970. Chicago, Athletic Institute, 1970, pp 119–138.

25. Bachrach AJ, Egstrom GH: Apprehension and panic. *In* British SubAqua Club Diving Manual, 10th ed. London, British SubAqua Club, 1977, pp 40–45.
26. Bevan J: Diver panic—how to beat it. Triton 18:311–312, 1973.
27. Egstrom GH, Bachrach AJ: Diver panic. Skin Diver Magazine 20:11–36, 1971.
28. Strauss MB: A program for panic prevention. Skin Diver Magazine 23:50–51, 1973.
29. Spielberger CD: Anxiety—state-trait process. *In* Spielberger CD, Sarason IG (eds): Stress and Anxiety, Vol 1. New York, John Wiley, 1975.
30. Tzimoulis P: Divers don't do drugs. Skin Diver Magazine 32:4, 1982.
31. Pertwee RG: Effects of cannabis on thermal regulation. Marijuana '84: 9th International Congress of Pharmacology, 3rd Satellite Symposium on Cannabis, 1984 (abstract).
32. Walsh JM, Ginzburg HM: Use of drugs and related substances under diving conditions. *In* Shilling CW, Carlston CB, Mathias RA (eds): The Physician's Guide to Diving Medicine. New York, Plenum Press, 1984, pp 445–459.
33. Isner JM, Estes N, Thompson PD, et al: Cardiac consequences of cocaine: Premature myocardial infarction, ventricular tachyarrhythmias, myocarditis and sudden death. American Heart Association, 58th Scientific Sessions, 1985.
34. Biersner R: Human performance at great depths. *In* Lambertsen CJ (ed): Underwater Physiology: Proceedings of the Fourth Symposium on Underwater Physiology. New York, Academic Press, 1971, pp 479–485.
35. Busby F: Remotely operated vehicles. *In* Bachrach AJ, Desiderati BM, Matzen MM (eds): A Pictorial History of Diving. San Pedro, Best Publishing, 1988. Presented by the Undersea and Hyperbaric Medical Society, pp 138–149.

Chapter 13

Women and Diving

MAIDA BETH TAYLOR

Although women now participate in all types of competition and amateur sports, in prior years sports and exercise for women were confined to low intensity activities. In spite of these early restrictions, many women established world-recognized reputations in sports prior to the 1950's.

With the acceptance of women in most sport activities, and the evident capability for high-quality performance of female athletes, many women have directed their interest to sport, commercial, and military diving. Like their male counterparts, female divers may develop medical problems from diving, and, therefore, they require attention to medical status, therapy of diving disorders, and education in health and safety. Of note, the oldest and largest population of commercial divers–the Ama of Japan—are, for the most part, women. This chapter is devoted to the particular problems encountered in women divers.

The first section of the chapter offers a brief review of cardiopulmonary and skeletal differences in women and the effects of these on sports performance. Next there is discussion of the effects of heavy exercise on female developmental, endocrine, and reproductive functions. The ultimate direction of this chapter will be to provide background and substance to answer a common query: should the pregnant woman dive?[1] Special focus on pregnancy and exercise, fetal effects of maternal exercise, and effects of pressurized gases on the maternal-fetal unit will explain both the obvious and hidden risks to mother and fetus.

ANATOMICAL AND PHYSIOLOGICAL SEX DIFFERENCES AFFECTING SPORTS PERFORMANCE

Although the differences may not be universal, owing to great genetic and individual variation and overlap, women typically have a lower threshold for peak performance than men, by virtue of smaller cardiovascular, pulmonary, and skeletal systems. Smaller bones with smaller articular surfaces carry less weight. Leg length is shorter and represents 51 per cent of total height in women compared with 56 per cent in men. The shoulder width is narrower while the hip is wider, with an attendant increased valgus angulation of the knee inward and a greater varus angulation at the hip outward. These skeletal modifications, in conjunction with a lower center of gravity, provide women with a narrower stance for balance.

Physiologically, women hold less potential for power, speed, work capacity, and stamina than do men. At a specified height, a woman has a smaller heart than a man. Coupled with a smaller lung and smaller thorax and smaller stroke volume, women cannot functionally achieve the maximal oxygen consumption capacity that a man can reach. Despite training, women have a higher percentage of body fat. For example, sedentary college-age women have approximately 25 per cent body fat, while trained athletic women reach 10 to 15 per cent. Trained males, however, average 7 to 10 per cent body fat. Of total body mass, trained males have relatively more muscle (40 per cent), while comparably fit women have only 23 per cent muscle.[2]

Women possess other physical differences with seemingly more positive aspects. Females conserve energy by a number of mechanisms better than do males. Increased body fat provides better insulation from heat loss and, incidentally, increased buoyancy. The sudorific response (sweating) occurs at a higher core temperature, again conserving energy but making women perhaps more susceptible to heat stress. The basal metabolic rate is lower in women, once more lowering basic caloric needs. Women also demonstrate more tendon laxity and flexibility, allowing for greater range of motion but also predisposing to torsion and dislocation injuries.

The functional anatomy of women predispose them to certain injuries in sports. The increased angulation of the knee and hip joints causes lateral malposition of the patella. Coupled with overuse, women are prone to a set of abnormalities known as a patellofemoral stress syndrome, a "catchall" term that includes patella subluxation, chondromalacia patella, lateral patella compression syndrome, and patella tendonitis. All variations of the disorder are usually treated with a combination of rest for acute symptoms and exercise aimed at strengthening the vastus medialis to help stabilize lateral slip of the patella. In severe cases in competitive athletes, surgical stabilization of the patella may be required.

Women are also at increased risk for shoulder injuries, including anterior subluxation, shoulder impingement, and thoracic outlet syndrome. This group of injuries often occurs in swimmers, as tendon and muscle hypertrophy puts stress on points of insertion and articulation. Neck injuries, particularly ballistic trauma such as whiplash, also are more common. Cranial size, volume, and weight are only slightly smaller in woman, while the bones and muscles of the neck are significantly reduced in size. When the head accelerates or decelerates suddenly, the force generated may be similar to that in a man, but the supporting structures are gmuch smaller and more vulnerable to injury. This type of injury is not common in the surface swimmer, but platform and springboard divers are at risk.

EXERCISE, DEVELOPMENT, AND REPRODUCTIVE ENDOCRINOLOGY

Pubertal Development

In the industrialized world during the past 100 years, the secular age of menarche has fallen from 17 to 12. Generally, one can say that girls are reaching their terminal height at an earlier age and soon thereafter reach the critical body mass necessary for initiation of cyclic ovarian hormone production and, eventually, ovulation. Puberty is a vague term assigned to the triad of developmental landmarks—thelarche, pubarche, and menarche. These events are linked temporally and physiologically, with breast and pubic hair development starting between ages 8.5 and 13. Although a great deal of variability occurs in the onset of these developmental landmarks, in the rapidity of their progression, and in their interrelationships, in general, breast development starts first in 66 per cent of girls, followed by growth of pubic hair, then an accelerated rate of linear growth in height before menstrual function starts. The most constant predictor of menses is the decrease in the rate of growth—the deceleration phase of the peak height velocity. The decline of the rate of growth heralds the onset of menarche usually within six months.

Pubertal development is mediated and altered by many factors including weight, height, heredity, nutrition, environment, and climate. Because of its effects on weight, body fat, and calorie requirements, exercise can profoundly alter developmental landmarks. Most of the research in this area has been done by Michelle Warren and Rose Frisch[3–7] studying developmental delay in young ballet dancers, but their findings also apply to other young, competitive athletes who run, swim, or bike. First, menarche is delayed often by two to four years. Bone age is also consistently two to four years behind chronological age in premenarcheal athletes. Menstrual cycles, once initiated, are often infrequent or irregular. The high incidence of observed oligomenorrhea and irregular cycles continues into young adult life if high levels of activity persist.

Athletes reach their terminal height at a later age than do controls, owing to later closure of epiphyses, but the final height does not appear to be altered. Similarly, breast development is delayed. Young athletes gain weight at puberty more slowly, gain less, and stop gaining sooner than sedentary controls. During periods of inactivity, such as during summers when intramural competitions cease or during times of injury, young athletes may experience rapid developmental progression, implying that rest allows energy to be directed to development rather than to sports activity.

Interestingly, both Marcus and Warren[8, 9] have reported increased orthopedic problems in young female athletes who are amenorrheic. Warren found an increased incidence of scoliosis in amenorrheic dancers and also found that the incidence correlates with duration of amenorrhea. Similarly, Frisch noted an increased incidence of stress fractures in teen-age and young adult runners, again the injury rate increasing with the duration of amenorrhea.

Girls who continue their athletic endeavors

into young adult life and women who undertake intensive athletic training during their reproductive years are likely to have continued impaired reproductive function. The incidence of amenorrhea in top female athletes is reported to range from 3.4 to 66 per cent, compared with 2 to 10 per cent in the general population. Vigorous exercise induces a progressive impairment of gynecological endocrinology.

Initially, the luteal phase of the menstrual cycle shortens from the normative 14 days to 8 to 10 days. This aberration can be detected by both a lower peak and a shortened duration of the rise in basal body temperature. Serum progesterone levels parallel the temperature changes, with lower hormone levels in the luteal phase in athletes. Progesterone levels persist for a shortened duration, reflecting the impaired function of the corpus luteum. As the endocrine abnormality progresses, anovulatory cycles ensue, with loss of the luteinizing hormone (LH) surge at mid cycle, no ovulation, no corpus luteum formation, and cessation of progesterone secretion.[10–14] Uterine bleeding may continue to occur as scant, irregular bleeding or as light menstrual-like flow at intermittent, long intervals. The disorder then progresses to a state of euestrogenemic amenorrhea, with serum estrogen levels high enough to maintain secondary sex characteristics and bone density, but not high enough to cause endometrial proliferation.

Further progression of endocrine dysfunction leads to hypoestrogenemic amenorrhea. At this stage, profound disruption of the regulatory mechanisms in reproduction occurs. Endocrine tests reveal prepubertal hypothalamic function with low tonic level of LH and follicle stimulating hormone (FSH), decreased pulse frequency of LH secretion, and an LH/FSH ratio of less than one.[15, 16] Prolonged, continued impairment of the hypothalamus offers little ovarian stimulation, and serum estrogen levels—most notably the level of estradiol, the potent estrogen of the reproductive age—fall. If low levels of estradiol persist, regression of secondary sex characteristics, particularly breast development, can occur.

Bone Development

More important from the vantage point of the coach, trainer, or physician is the role estradiol plays in maintenance of bone. The skeleton is composed of two types of bone, which are structurally and metabolically different. Cortical bone comprises the shafts of the long bones and is traditionally measured at the junction of the lower and middle third of the radius. Trabecular bone comprises the vertebral bodies, pelvis, flat bones, and the ends of the long bones. Measures of trabecular bone are done on the vertebral column or on the wrist or distal radius. Vertebral measures, though more important clinically in determining bone density, are less sensitive and less reproducible than measures of the wrist or radius. Cortical bone is less metabolically active than trabecular bone. Cortical bone remodels at a rate of 10 per cent per year, while trabecular bone turns over at 40 per cent per year. Thus, trabecular bone is more vulnerable to agents or events impairing bone metabolism.

Bone mineralization reaches a maximum rate in early adult life and continues through age 35. One might think of the early adult years as a time for making deposits in a "bone bank" account. This prepares a woman for the withering of bone later in life when estrogen levels fall. Prior to menopause, cortical bone is lost at a rate of 0.3 to 0.5 per cent per year. In early menopause this rate of loss increases to 2 to 3 per cent. Being more metabolically active, trabecular bone is lost at a rate of 1.2 to 2.4 per cent per year prior to menopause. The rate accelerates to 6 per cent per year for the first two years after the climacteric. Thus, 25 per cent of cortical and 32 per cent of trabecular bone will be lost between ages 50 and 80.[17]

Amenorrheic athletes develop osteoporosis; their rates of bone loss approximate the accelerated rates of bone loss seen in menopause.[18–21] The losses can be stopped and reversed by exogenous hormone administration or by the resumption of normal cycles.[25] New data, however, suggest that the losses may not be completely reversible, and that amenorrheic athletes will never recover normal bone density. This makes eminent sense when one remembers that these women are losing bone at a profound rate at a time when they should in fact be building bone, a form of double jeopardy. Osteoporosis is also exacerbated by low dietary levels of calcium. In weight loss or in calorie-restricted diets, the kind of diet often undertaken by young women athletes, dairy products with their generally high fat levels are often left out. By limiting the substrate needed for bone mineralization, another level of risk is imposed on these women. Therefore, in dieting or training when dairy intake is limited, calcium supplementation is imperative. Poor protein intake also reduces bone mineralization. Smoking, alcohol, and thyroid disease add to the risk of osteoporosis.

Gravity and weight-bearing exercise positively affect bone density. Working against gravity is the best means of promoting bone mineralization. Standing, walking, and running in the presence of normal estrogen levels all lead to heavier, denser bones. But weight-bearing exercise cannot correct for a lack of estrogen. Women runners who are cyclic have denser bones than sedentary women, and postmenopausal runners have 40 per cent more bone than controls.[22] Amenorrheic runners have less bone than cyclic runners, and though bone mass is greater with greater distance, the mass is still well below the levels of cyclic runners. Note here that swimming and other non–weight-bearing exercises do not increase bone density and do nothing to counter hypoestrogenemic osteoporosis. Swimming can be regarded as a safe, alternative form of aerobic activity for the osteoporitic or injured athlete.

A long career in commercial diving may damage the microcirculation of bone, with osteonecrosis now a well-recognized outcome. No evidence exists that osteonecrosis occurs in sport diving, but female commercial divers are likely to incur the same risk for dysbaric osteonecrosis as their male counterparts. Superimposed on the risk for osteoporosis, women divers may be at risk for more profound disability than their male counterparts.

Exercise-Induced Amenorrhea

Several predisposing factors have been proposed and confirmed for exercise-induced amenorrhea. The most important measurable cause of amenorrhea in athletes is weight loss coupled with loss of body fat. As more weight loss occurs in training, the incidence of amenorrhea increases. Amenorrhea correlates with low body weight at the start of training, actual weight loss, and percentage of body fat lost. The age of onset of training also correlates with incidence of athletic amenorrhea. Women who start training prior to the initiation of regular menstrual cycles are more likely to be amenorrheic than women who start training after their cycles are established. In a similar mode, women who have had prior pregnancy, evidencing maturity and stability of the reproductive axis, are less likely to become amenorrheic when they undertake strenuous training.

If the hypothalamic axis is inherently unstable, a rather modest level of exercise can cause disruption of cycles. Some women with highly erratic cycles may become amenorrheic by running only nine miles per week. This translates into a three-mile run three times per week, a level of aerobic activity equal to the lower end of the recommended scale for cardiovascular conditioning. Stated another way, some women possess an inherently fragile reproductive balance and may suffer significant reproductive impairment at very low levels of training.

Both Prior and Shangold[10, 23] report that even women with stable reproductive function will develop menstrual irregularity if training is intense. The degree of irregularity and the incidence of dysfunction increase directly with intensity of training. Shangold found that as college runners increase their mileage, menstrual irregularity increases. Prior demonstrated similar events in runners, swimmers, and cyclists, though the latter two groups showed less severe aberrations at equivalent levels of energy expenditure. Interval, sprint, and other forms of speed work tend to disturb cycles more than steady aerobic demand. Periods of intensive training, during which the individual is trying to increase levels of performance and fitness, lead to more abnormalities than continued maintenance of a stable level of activity.

Several other poorly defined factors in athletic amenorrhea have been proposed. Stress of training is not easily quantified or studied. Amenorrheic runners often feel that training is more stressful than do eumenorrheic runners. This may reflect an inherent difference in the personality of these women. Individuals who perceive training as pleasurable or satisfying may feel less stressed by the high demand of their endeavor. Perhaps more competitive individuals find training more stressful. The differences in perceived level of stress may reflect differences in inherent athletic ability. Persons with natural talent and ability may not have to "work" as hard to reach a level of performance, and therefore will experience training as less physiologically demanding and less psychologically stressful.

Although not clearly elucidated, menstrual dysfunction in female athletes results from the complex interaction of neurotransmitters, hormone-releasing factors, and peripheral sex steroids. Several acute hormonal changes occur in response to exercise, but they are generally mild and short lived. These include a decline in LH and increases in prolactin, estradiol, and progesterone. The level of FSH is unaltered. Intensive exercise ultimately results in diminished LH pulse amplitude and pulse frequency, chronically lowered estradiol levels, and failure of ovulation with an absence of progesterone secretion. Researchers in this area surmise that chronic, daily changes in hormones may lead to cumulative effects on the endocrine system, especially if intense workouts are long and closely spaced. The overall effect of training may be greater than is implied by the small acute changes measured after a single training session. Amenorrheic runners also have been found to have increased levels of endorphins and enkephalins during exercise.[24] Research has implied that increased levels of these compounds lower FSH and LH, and the lowering effect can be blocked with the narcotic antagonist naloxone.

Fertility and Exercise

Athletes with exercise-induced amenorrhea are anovulatory and therefore infertile. Since estradiol levels are low, this type of infertility does not respond to clomiphene citrate, the agent most commonly used for ovulation induction. Clomiphene acts as an anti-estrogen, inducing the hypothalamus to secrete increased levels of LH to drive the ovary to produce more peripheral sex steroids. The desired response normally induces follicle growth and development. Therefore, in the hypoestrogenemic female with impaired LH metabolism, clomiphene offers no therapeutic effect. The use of more dramatic, complex, and expensive ovulation induction agents—such as gonadotropin releasing factor, FSH and LH extracts, and human chorionic gonadotropin—poses a difficult medical and ethical dilemma. If an individual is so active and hypoestrogenemic that her body cannot support ovulation, how well will she support a pregnancy? The safest therapy for exercise-induced infertility is a decrease in level of activity, increased calorie consumption, and weight gain. Ovulation may take some time to recur, since a higher percentage of body fat is needed to re-establish cycles than to initiate them.

Pregnancy and Exercise

Gestation imposes increased physiological and metabolic requirements, and the pregnant athlete superimposes the demands of training on the demands of pregnancy. Both pregnancy and exercise elicit hyperdynamic physiological responses; therefore, the pregnant athlete will have to be a "superwoman" to meet all these demands. When assessing the benefits and risks of exercise in pregnancy, the accomplishments and rewards of the gravida as athlete must be balanced with the needs of the developing fetus, which is a noncompetitor but not a nonparticipant. Sound training principles protect the athlete from injury, and even more stringent guidelines need to be observed during pregnancy to protect the fetus from inadvertent injury.[25, 26]

Aside from the obvious gross changes in the uterus as it enlarges, major physiological adaptations occur in the respiratory and cardiovascular systems to support the needs of the fetus. Although the diaphragm elevates owing to compression by the expanding uterus, total lung capacity remains unaltered since the chest wall splays laterally and the anteroposterior diameter of the chest increases. Inspiratory capacity and tidal volume increase, while there is an attendant decrease in functional residual capacity, residual volume, and end expiratory reserve volume. Although respiratory rate remains unchanged, tidal volume increases and thus minute volume increases, resulting in an increase in oxygen uptake and maximum ventilatory capacity.[27]

Cardiovascular alterations, mediated by hormonal changes, occur during the first trimester. These changes are dramatic even though the uterus remains rather small and the actual hemodynamic demands are low. Heart rate increases by 10 to 15 per cent coincident with a 20 to 40 per cent rise in stroke volume, resulting in a 30 to 50 per cent increase in cardiac output. Blood volume expands by 20 to 100 per cent (mean 50%) comprised of a 33 per cent increase in red cell mass and a 50 per cent increase in plasma volume. Therefore, hematocrit falls to 33 to 36 per cent (the so-called dilutional anemia of pregnancy), but overall oxygen-carrying capacity improves greatly. Coordinated with increased level of erythrocyte 2,3, diphosphoglycerate (2,3 DPG) causing a decrease in oxygen affinity in red cells and shifting the oxyhemoglobin dissociation curve to the left, oxygen delivery at the tissue level also improves. Mediated by progesterone and its relaxing effects on smooth muscle, peripheral vascular resistance falls, lowering systolic and, even more so, diastolic blood pressure. Thus, pronounced venous pooling occurs in the lower extremities and uterus.[28]

Also of importance in discussing exercise in pregnancy are musculoskeletal alterations, most notably the increased joint laxity and ligament loosening, again mediated by progesterone. While promoting relaxation of the pelvic floor joints and ligaments to facilitate delivery of the fetal head, these changes destabilize extremity joints and predispose the pregnant woman to joint injury, torsion accidents, and dislocations. The growing uterus imposes a passive increase in weight bearing, increasing the lordotic curve of the spine, increasing stress and compression on lower back vertebae and nerve roots, and predisposing to sacroiliac syndrome, back strain, and sciatica. The hip, knee, and ankle are also at increased risk of stress injury. As pregnancy progresses and the uterus comes out of the pelvis, becoming a true abdominal organ, the center of gravity of the gravida shifts forward. During the late second and entire third trimesters, this center changes almost constantly, producing gait and balance instability and increasing the woman's vulnerability to injury.

Acute and chronic responses to the demands of exercise are altered in pregnancy. Maximal aerobic response is reached sooner, not unlike wearing weights while exercising.[29–32] Any well-conditioned female athlete will maintain her level of fitness if she maintains her level of activity; and she will experience an increased level of fitness as pregnancy progresses, doing more work as the passive load increases with the expanding mass of the pregnancy. Even if level of activity declines slightly, conditioning will be maintained. Untrained women may train without problems using a slow paced program of aerobic activity. One study demonstrated a 15 per cent increase in level of fitness and a 33 per cent increase in maximal oxygen consumption; sedentary controls evidenced a 10 per cent decline in maximal aerobic capacity.[33]

Animal studies demonstrate that uterine blood flow decreases with exercise and that the decrease correlates with intensity and duration of activity. In sheep exercised at 70 per cent of maximal output for 40 minutes, uterine blood flow fell 24 per cent. Placental blood flow also decreased but less dramatically, and actual fetal oxygen delivery fell only 11 per cent.[34] Since the fetal oxygen delivery system holds a 50 per cent reserve, this decline is not significant in normal pregnancy. Exercise produces a number of other physiological effects that, in theory though not clearly in practice, may lower oxygen delivery to fetal tissues. Increased maternal oxygen consumption and muscle blood flow play only a small role. Increased catecholamines, particularly epinephrine, are known to decrease uterine blood flow, but sympathomimetics increase uterine blood flow. Overall, exercise increases sympathetic tone. Increased maternal temperature directly increases fetal temperature and metabolic rate. After exercise, fetal cooling lags behind maternal, but this has not been demonstrated to produce adverse effects.

Animal studies of exercise and pregnancy have not demonstrated adverse fetal effects. In 1980 Clapp[35] exercised ewes to exhaustion, and while uterine and umbilical blood flow decreased, uterine and umbilical oxygen uptake was unaltered. Maternal lactic acidemia developed with no demonstrable uteroplacental and fetal lactic acid excess. Bagnall[36] exercised rats throughout gestation and found decreased maternal weight gain but complete fetal sparing. Bell[37] also studied ewes and measured seven metabolic parameters, including glucose, lactate, insulin, and glucagon, noting rapid changes of maternal and fetal levels of all metabolites measured, but also rapid return to baseline level after activity ceased. He found that lambs of ewes that exercised regularly were larger, fatter, and had more muscle glucagon than controls. This single paper has been responsible for the notion that exercise promotes fetal well-being and enhances intrauterine growth. No other work has confirmed improved fetal growth with maternal exercise in any species. Mottola[38] found that sedentary rats have, on the average, three more pups per litter than do exercised rats, and that pups in both groups had comparable birthweights. This suggests that some fetuses were resorbed to compensate for the increased demands of exercise, but those surviving were spared any ill effects.

Studies of fetal responses to maternal exercise in human subjects fail to demonstrate any short- or long-term damage to the fetus, nor do these studies show any benefit to infants of active mothers. Most human studies have been conducted at low, submaximal levels of activity, and the results cannot be extrapolated to committed or elite athletes. Most studies have been done at 65 to 80 per cent of maximal oxygen consumption, and at worst a short-lived fetal bradycardia was observed in a few subjects, with no adverse fetal outcomes at term.[39–45] Carpenter[46] is the only researcher to report on maximal levels of output. In third-trimester women, he recorded fetal hearts in 85 submaximal observations and in 79 maximal sessions. One fetal bradycardia occurred in the submaximal group in a woman who experienced a vasovagal episode. In the maximal output group, 16 bradycardias were observed, all occurring within three minutes of the cessation and all recovering without incident. The flaw in the study is that the women went from maximal activity to rest, probably causing a profound drop in cardiac output, an increase in peripheral venous pooling, and very likely, a rapid fall in uterine blood flow. Good training principles mandate a cool down, to avoid hypotension and decreased cerebral perfusion; the uterus probably deserves the same.

Exercise has no clearly documented effects on pregnancy outcomes, fetal or maternal. No differences in birthweight, length, or Apgar scores can be confirmed. In point of fact, the notion that exercise is good for the fetus comes from one sheep study that found slightly higher birthweights in lambs of ewes that were exercised. One study demonstrates a higher one-minute Apgar in offspring of fit mothers but no significant difference in 5-minute Apgar. No study has been done on cord gases of "fit" infants. On the maternal side of the equation, no differences have been observed in need for induction, duration of gestation, length of stages of labor, anesthetic requirements, use of forceps, or need for episiotomy. One paper in 1987[47] did find a decreased rate of cesarean section in fit women, but other papers in the past contradict this claim. There is also one report of a slight decrease in the length of second stage labor, again contradicted by other reports. Subjective observations of fit women have promoted a consensus that they tolerate the physical demands of pregnancy well, have better attitudes in labor, experience less fatigue postpartum, and recover their prior level of activity sooner than their unfit counterparts. These may not be the result of exercise but rather may reflect the positive, active attitude of these women, who may be predisposed and committed to good health behaviors. Their personalities get them up and moving. In the past, our society has promoted the perception of the puerperium as a time when women are ill and should adhere to sick role behaviors. Less than 30 years ago, women were kept at bed rest for 2 to 4 weeks postpartum. Many individuals, families, and subcultures in our society still think that the parturient should be treated as ailing. Women invested in fitness clearly reject these vestiges of the past.

When the pregnant woman is high risk, exercise is generally contraindicated, particularly in disorders predisposing to impaired uteroplacental exchange or prematurity. Any recreational activity must be carefully monitored or even precluded in maternal diseases such as asthma, renal disease, hypertension, anemia, diabetes, heart disease of NYHA class II or more, and autoimmune conditions. Obstetric contraindications to exercise include but are not limited to intrauterine growth retardation, twins, uterine anomalies, prior infant under 2500 grams, incompetent cervix, myomata uteri, placenta previa, abruption, postdate pregnancy, and history of second or third trimester losses. Also considered poor risks for activity in pregnancy include women with seizure disorders and nerve root or disc disease.

Fetal Physiology and Gas Exchange

Uterine blood flow approximates 5 liters per minute or 10 per cent of cardiac output of the mother, which is equal to cerebral blood flow levels. Eighty per cent of flow distributes to the placental bed and 20 per cent perfuses the uterine musculature. Within the closed fetal circulation, umbilical blood flow reaches 270 ml per minute, 50 per cent of the total fetal cardiac output. Twenty per cent of the umbilical flow is shunted and does not participate in fetal gas exchange. Gas exchange occurs in the intravillous space and is characterized by a multivillous streaming system, maximizing the surface area for gas exchange. Gas exchange between the two circulations is passive and is limited by diffusion. The rate of exchange is affected by a long list of hematological and hemodynamic factors including intervillous blood flow, placental blood flow, oxygen tension in the maternal arterial blood, oxygen tension in fetal blood, oxygen affinity of maternal and fetal bloods, hemoglobin concentration in each system, oxygen-carrying capacity of each circulation, placental diffusion capacity, placental vascular geometry, the ratio of maternal-to-fetal blood flow in the exchange areas, shunting, and placental and uterine oxygen consumption.

The fetal environment is severely hypoxic, and Bancroft[48] has called the fetus "a maskless mountaineer atop of Everest in utero." The tissue defenses of the fetus mimic adult hypoxic protections, although the fetal responses are quantitatively different. Fetal erythropoiesis is higher, maintained by an increased, chronic level of erythropoietin. Increase in hematocrit, however, is limited by the flow dynamics of Poiseuille's law, with a dramatic increase in viscosity over 80 per cent. Fetal hematocrit averages 60 per cent. Maximum blood flow of the most oxygenated blood is directed to critical tissues—the brain, coronary arteries, and adrenals. The oxygen dissociation curve is shifted markedly to the left. This is achieved by altered molecular configuration of the fetal hemoglobin molecule. The beta chains are replaced by gamma chains, and the attendant binding of oxygen is tighter, with higher oxygen saturations at lower oxygen tensions. This altered binding is not dependent on 2,3 DPG as it is in the adult. But just as is seen in adult hemoglobin, increased temperature, increased carbon dioxide, and increased hydrogen ion concentration all cause a shift of the curve to the right and decreased oxygen affinity.

Gas transfer takes place in the intervillous space. The gradient of oxygen tensions is exactly the same as the gradient in the alveolar capillary bed, 10 mm Hg. Transit time for the red cell in the capillary also equals transit time in the lung, about 1 second. Fifteen to 20 per cent of uterine blood flow is shunted through the myometrium, and 15 to 20 per cent of umbilical flow is shunted through fetal and placental channels, with a resultant 30 per cent of flow uninvolved in gas exchange. Little reduction in the shunt is physiologically possible and there are limits on increased rates of exchange. Another limiting factor in exchange comes from the fact that placental oxygen consumption is higher than that of the lung, lung metabolic need being almost negligible.

In the placenta, maternal-to-fetal blood flow ratio ranges from 0.4 to 2 with a mean of 0.8, close to the predicted optimum of 1 to 1. Areas of high maternal-fetal flow are equivalent to areas of high ventilation-perfusion in the lung. This wasted maternal circulation or overarterialization of flow offers the fetal-maternal system a considerable reserve. Increases in the maternal or fetal flow rates do little to increase oxygen transfer. The system is at most times functioning at an ideal, maximal level. If stressed or compromised, gas exchange does not improve, but rather is maintained since the resting state holds a 50 per cent physiological reserve. Increases in inspired maternal oxygen do little to alter fetal gas delivery, even at maternal arterial oxygen concentrations of 500 to 600 mm Hg. Increases can, however, be achieved using hyperbaric states.

The Soviet medical community claims extensive experience treating both maternal and fetal hypoxic conditions with hyperbaric therapy. They also treat diseases presumed to be due to poor maternal-fetal exchange with hyperbaric oxygen. The literature cites hyperbaric oxygen treatment of cyanotic heart disease, pulmonary hypertension, anemic disorders, intrauterine growth retardation, preeclampsia, diabetes, and even habitual abortion. Statistics are poor, with almost no analysis beyond reporting of percentages of improved outcome. Treatment schedules do not approximate any of our common treatment tables. Hyperbaric oxygen is administered at 1.5 to 2 ata often for extended periods of time, with patients laboring in chambers and with delivery and even cesarean section being performed under pressure.

In acute hypoxic situations, the fetus responds by differential redistribution of flow to three classes of circulatory beds: non-negotiable, negotiable, and expendable. Blood flow is centralized to critical tissues, paralleling the diving reflex of marine mammals. Liggins,[49] working with the weddell seal, found that the fetus demonstrates a diving reflex during maternal dives, with centralization of flow and bradycardia in both carrier and carried. The human fetus "dives" during hypoxia with a reflex mediated afferently by the trigeminal-vagal nerve plexus. Hypoxia induces bradycardia and peripheral vasoconstriction. Note also that fetal adrenal secretion is dominated by norepinephrine, the dominant adrenergic mediator in diving mammals. Nelson[48] summarizes the physiology in this paraphrase of the classic tenet of genetics: "The physiologic ontogeny of the human fetus may very usefully recapitulate the phylogeny of the diving reflex.

In considering the possible effects of diving, pressure, and hyperbaric states on the fetus, one needs to know the effects that changes in concentration of inspired gases have on the fetal-maternal unit. Moderate levels of hypoxia, hypercapnia, and hypocapnia do little to alter placental gas exchange. Marked changes in inspired gases, however, cause decreases in fetal perfusion. Research from the anesthesia literature reveals that when inspired oxygen drops to 6 per cent, maternal cardiac output increases, systemic vascular resistance decreases, and uteroplacental vascular resistance increases, with concomitant decreases in uterine blood flow. The same changes occur at 12 per cent oxygen concentration, but less dramatically. When carbon dioxide increases in maternal circulation, uterine blood flow increases up to 60 mm Hg. With CO_2 over 60 mm Hg, vascular resistance increases and uterine blood flow declines. Low levels of CO_2 probably cause no great changes, but the anesthesia literature cites uteroplacental vasoconstriction with an attendant decline in uterine blood flow, fetal hypoxia, acidosis, and neonatal depression when CO_2 falls to 17 mm Hg. Fall of CO_2 in the study reviewed was achieved by mechanical hyperventilation and is thought to be due to an artifact of mechanical positive pressure ventilation.[50]

WOMEN AND DIVING

Little attention has been paid to the special anatomical, physiological, and psychological differences between men and women in the diving literature. To extract relevant information is difficult since reports are scant in number and substance. Data can be derived from sources in diving and hyperbaric medicine, anesthesia, and aerospace science.[51–53]

Because of smaller stature and smaller muscle mass, women possess different strength and energy potential during exercise. Thermal stress represents one of the major energy burdens in diving. Anatomically and physiologically, women respond to cold in subtly different ways. Surface area to volume ratio is slightly higher in women, increasing the area of conductive heat loss. It is agreed, however, that the differential is small in practical terms. More important, women possess much smaller muscle mass, with less metabolically active tissue to generate heat during activity. Although women carry more subcutaneous fat than men, the relative insulation value is poor. Women demonstrate a greater ability to vasoconstrict limb blood flow, thereby conserving heat, but again the advantage is unclear. When all variables are taken together, the conclusion is that women are more susceptible to thermal stress than are men. Of interest is work by Hong, who studied Korean Ama divers (see Chapter 6). He quantitatively demonstrated that men and women divers lost the same amount of heat when working in cold water for 60 minutes. Men worked in 27° water and cooled to a core temperature of 36.4° C. Women worked in 22.5° water and cooled to 35° C. The physiological mechanisms in response to cold stress appeared to differ between the two groups. Men seemed to produce and lose much more metabolic heat, while women did not appear to "compensate" for rapid thermal losses. The women, in fact, voluntarily tolerated a state of prolonged hypothermia. Skin-fold thickness is presented as an explanation of the differences. Although most measures and parameters put women at a disadvantage in tolerance to cold exposure, practice offers contradictory evidence. Long distance, open water swim records for distance and time in water are often held by women, such as Diane Nyad. Even if women are more vulnerable to hypothermia, thermal stress should not pose a sex-specific hazard for women divers when properly equipped.

Women possess a lower aerobic capacity than do men, with significantly lower upper body strength. During sport diving (generally not a severe aerobic endeavor), these differences should hold little influence. Most experienced divers insist that less work and exertion help to conserve air and extend bottom time. In commercial diving and when swimming in bad currents, women performing the same work load as men are likely to become exhausted sooner when cold stress and hyperventilation are superimposed. Male divers and instructors need to be aware that they must avoid pushing female divers into situations demanding overexertion.

Decompression Sickness and Air Embolism

Commonly held wisdom in diving medicine states that women are at increased risk for decompression sickness (DCS). Work by Bassett[54] in 1973 found higher rates of DCS in female flight nurses when compared with men at similar altitude exposure. Bangasser[55] published a retrospective survey of female divers in 1978. Subjects had varied diving experience; 649 subjects reported on 88,028 dives with 29 reported cases of DCS, an 0.033 per cent rate per dive. The incidence increased for basic divers to 0.043 per cent and fell for instructors to 0.023 per cent. These rates were considered excessive when compared with a 0.007 per cent incidence for male instructors. No adequate physiological explanation could be found though a number were postulated. These included increased percentage of body fat, differential body fluid dynamics, hormonal influences, differential limb perfusion, and hypothetical differences in platelet aggregation acting as a trigger for bubble formation. Later work, however, has demonstrated that when men and women with comparable levels of aerobic fitness are compared, the differences in the rates of DCS disappear. This observation offers the prescription that if women are to dive safely, they should ensure that they are in good physical condition.

The suggestion in the literature that women are at increased risk of DCS cannot be ignored, and one cannot assume that all divers are aerobically fit. Often an unfit, unathletic woman is cajoled into sport diving by an avid, active male friend or spouse, or the woman may wish to avoid being left on the beach or boat, and will engage in activities beyond her level of physical readiness.

No reports exist in the literature of an excess incidence of air embolism in women, nor is there any suggestion of differential rates of air embolism between the sexes. The incidence of patent foramen ovale is the same in men and women, and its role in decompression sickness and air embolism is not clear. Women as well as men should be advised of the dangers of shallow compressed air diving.

Considering psychological characteristics of divers, Morgan[51] states that female and male divers are more similar than different. Both men and women divers have psychometric profiles not unlike those of elite athletes. The profile is termed the "iceberg," with below-average scores on negative scales (tension, depression, fatigue, and confusion) and higher scores on the scale of physical vigor. Women are more likely to have panic reactions but are less likely to perceive themselves in life-threatening situations. These perceptions, however, do not meet statistical significance. These data were obtained from women who started diving rather early in the vogue of the sport. As more women become sport divers, perhaps women with more traditional psychological profiles will become part of the population, and pertinent differences will appear.

Diving and Menstruation

There is no evidence of increased shark attacks on menstruating female divers. The only risk of menstruation is embarrassment if spills or leaks occur.

Premenstrual syndrome (PMS) is a poorly defined psychophysiological disorder in women. Physical complaints include bloating, food cravings, mastodynia, and headaches. Psychological symptoms include irritability, anger, hostility, and moodiness. No consistent, simple, reproducible remedy exists.[56] The underlying disorder is also undefined, though recent work postulates that a neurotransmitter defect may exist in predisposed women, altering endorphin activity.[57] Women with *severe* PMS have been found to have abnormal personalities reflecting underlying mood and personality disorders. Their symptoms seem to be exacerbated in the premenstrual phase. No one should dive, male or female, who evidences depressive or antisocial tendencies.

DIVING, HYPERBARICS, AND PREGNANCY

Diving during pregnancy might provide a short, pleasurable activity for the mother. Like swimming, the perceived weightlessness of diving may give the woman temporary respite from the burden she carries on land. The short-term pleasure of diving must be balanced against the potential long-term effects on the fetus as a passive passenger at depth.

Most workers investigating DCS and fetal risk agree that the fetus is at no increased risk of bubble formation during decompression. In fact, three researchers[58–61] demonstrated that the fetus is more resistant to bubble formation than is the mother. Only Fife[62] found an increased risk in fetal lambs, but later Stock[63] repeated the experiment and asserted that the increased risk was an artifact of instrumentation. Studies of DCS have also measured rates of birth defects after induced DCS in animals. Most of the experiments have been done at pressures (6.4 to 7.1 ata) in excess of those encountered in sport diving. Despite the high pressures and high rates of DCS imposed on the study animals, only one of three studies in the literature demonstrates an increased rate of malformation after DCS. In Gilman's study, hamsters with untreated DCS had increased rates of defects, while treated animals did not.

Of more importance perhaps than birth defects is a very high rate of fetal death in utero found by animal researchers. Studies of dogs and rats show no increased rates of fetal death, but virtually all sheep studies show high fetal loss rates. The impression is that the closer to term the greater the risk. The fetal circulation depends on the large patent foramen ovale and ductus arteriosus for the delivery of the most well-oxygenated blood from the umbilical vein directly to critical tissues, bypassing the systemic and pulmonary circulation. The fetal cardiovascular system lacks an effective filter; thus any bubbles formed are likely to be directed to the brain and coronary arteries. This selective perfusion scheme probably accounts for the lethality of DCS in animals. Thus, researchers in the field concur that any bubbles in the fetus are more ominous than many bubbles in the mother.

Concern about potential fetal oxygen toxicity comes from two quarters. First, diving at depth on compressed air presents increased partial pressure of oxygen in fetal circulation. Second, diving accidents often necessitate hyperbaric therapy, exposing the fetus, sometimes repeatedly, to high levels of oxygen in utero. Miller[65] exposed rats to 100 per cent oxygen at 2 to 3 ata for six hours and found not only an increase in cardiovascular malformations, but an increased rate of fetal resorption. One hundred per cent oxygen at 1 ata and air at 3 ata caused no increased adverse outcome. Fukikura[66] treated rabbits with 100 per cent oxygen at 3.6 and 4 ata for two to three hours and found high rates of retrolental fibroplasia similar to that seen in infants treated for prematurity with high oxygen. Gilman[67] used standard U.S. Navy treatment table 6 on hamsters with no increased rate of defects in the offspring.

Human data on hyperbaric oxygen and the fetus are very limited. The Soviets, as mentioned above, have used hyperbaric oxygen repeatedly and for long durations in mothers, but at relatively low pressures. They do not report any fetal problems. Van Hoesen[68] recently reported a case of maternal carbon monoxide poisoning treated with 100 per cent oxygen at 2.4 ata for 90 minutes, with delivery five weeks later of a normal infant. Hollander[69] also published a similar successful case. A few cases of maternal air embolism have been treated with hyperbaric oxygen (see below). All fetuses died, probably owing to the magnitude of the insult, not as a consequence of therapy.

Two surveys have been conducted questioning the outcome of women who dived while pregnant. In her survey Bangasser[55] included questions on birth defects and losses in women who dived, and found no increased rates. Bolton[70] also did a retrospective questionnaire. Limiting the study to the most recent pregnancy, 109 women dived before prior to and during gestation. Sixty-nine dived before pregnancy but stopped when pregnancy was diagnosed. Although no statistical analysis was done, the survey suggests higher rates of low birthweight, birth defects, neonatal respiratory difficulties, and other problems in the dive group that continued diving perinatally. Of particular interest is the list of defects reported: multiple hemivertebrae, absence of a hand, ventricular septal defect, possible coarctation of the aorta, hypertrophic pyloric stenosis, and a birthmark. No major defects were reported in the non-dive group. The cardiac anomalies are worrisome, but the first two defects listed are rare and dramatic. They were also associated with deep diving—120 and 160 feet, respectively. Much attention should be paid to these two items, and a good measure of caution is indicated by them. The need for caution is reinforced by a distressing case reported by Turner and Unsworth,[71] excerpted below.

> We have seen a baby born with arthrogryposis and some dysgenic features whose mother had been scuba diving in early pregnancy. The mother was a 22-year-old primigravida. She and her husband went on holiday from the 40th–50th days post LMP (last mentrual period). The mother dived at least once daily to a total of twenty dives in these 15 days. Most dives were to a depth of 60 ft or less but three were to 100 ft and one to 110 ft. The ascent rate used by the mother and her husband was 60 ft/min, though this was usually estimated rather than timed. When decompression was required, a modified version of the U.S. Navy tables was used. All the dives except one were without complications. The exception involved an "equipment failure" of the husband, whom she was accompanying, at the end of a strenuous 15 min bottom time dive at 60 ft. The rate of ascent of both was described as "very rapid." She felt well but tired after this dive. No medications were used apart from oral Sudafed (pseudoephedrine) 60 mg on two or three occasions early in the holiday to aid ear cleaning.
>
> The rest of the pregnancy was uneventful. The abnormalities noted in the baby were unilateral ptosis, small tongue, micrognathia, and short neck. The penis was adherent to the scrotum. The upper limb joint movements were all normal except the hands. The fingers were fixed in flexion with some webbing between the 3rd, 4th, and 5th fingers, the thumb was digit-like but had two phalanges. The hip joints were dysplastic with reduced range of movement, and one hip was dislocated. There was fixed flexed deformity of the knees and bilateral equinovarus deformity of the feet. The head circumference was normal and motor development was appropriate for the baby's age at 3 months. Karyotype, electromyogram, and muscle biopsy were all normal.

No data, reports, or discussions of air embolism and its effects on mother and fetus in pregnancy appear in the diving literature. Fifteen cases of embolism from sex play have appeared in the obstetric journals, all in young women in the second or third trimester. The embolism occurred from air being forceably blown into the vagina. The first 12 cases reported maternal and fetal death in all instances. The next case reported was treated with hyperbaric oxygen 39 hours after the event and lived; however, she retained moderate neurological deficits. The infant was stillborn.[77] Another woman lived with no therapy and delivered a healthy, but premature, infant. The good outcome in this case has been ascribed to only a small volume of air entering the arterial circulation.[73] The most recently reported case occurred at 22 weeks of pregnancy and was treated 9 hours postinsult. The mother survived without sequelae, but the infant was stillborn three weeks later.[74] These reports demonstrate the lethality of embolism in the fetus if air evolves in the uteroplacental bed. Overpressure diving accidents with pulmonary air embolism would surely present less gas directly to the uterine bed, and the mother's circulation would act as a filter. Since the volume of gas lethal to the fetus has not been measured and is probably very small, and since bubbles would be preferentially delivered to the heart and brain, even shallow diving presents grave fetal risks.

The hazard of diving during pregnancy extends beyond DCS and air embolism. Since both of these injuries usually dictate hyperbaric oxygen therapy, the safety of treatment merits examination. The medical literature offers no evidence of adverse fetal outcomes from controlled hyperbarism. The classic paper on maternal and fetal effects of hyperbaric states by Assali[75] in 1968 detailed changes in uterine and fetal blood flow during administration of hyperbaric oxygen. On 100 per cent oxygen at 1 ata, maternal arterial pO_2 reached 500 mm Hg, but fetal umbilical vein pO_2 only increased by 10 to 15 mm Hg. When pressure was increased to 3 ata, maternal pO_2 rose to 1300 mm Hg; umbilical vein rose to 300 mm Hg, but umbilical artery levels reached only 50 mm Hg. Maternal and fetal arterial pressures did not change significantly. Placental and umbilical flow rates decreased slightly during hyperbaric oxygen administration. The major finding was alterations in fetal blood flow pattern. Ductus arteriosus flow decreased dramatically when the oxygen tension in the pulmonary blood rose. At the same time, flow increased in the ascending aorta, but effective fetal cardiac output decreased. Apparently the fetal pulmonary bed is exquisitely sensitive to oxygen tension and responds with vasodilation as oxygen tension rises. Thus, hyperbaric oxygen causes a shift from a fetal blood flow pattern to a neonatal pattern. The shift reverses when oxygen tension returns to normal. One can only speculate on the long-term effects of prolonged exposure of the fetus to high oxygen in utero due to neonatalization of the fetal circulation.

A more immediate problem, though still speculative, is concern that basic physiological changes in pregnancy may compound diving risks. Many divers experience some anxiety at the outset of a dive. Combining the increased exercise demand, cold stress, pregnancy load, and sympathomimetic reflex of anxiety, the potential for potent vasoconstriction is present; therefore, the possibility of decreased uterine blood flow may be significantly increased for the pregnant diver. Although diving is submaximal in its cardiovascular demands, occasional short, hard bursts of activity are often needed. Such episodic demands are more likely to compromise uterine blood flow than gradual increases or sustained requirements of aerobic activity. Abrupt shifts in flow dynamics may produce unrecognized, short episodes of decreased fetal perfusion. For this reason, racket sports and power weightlifting are generally less than ideal forms of exercise during pregnancy. If diving elicits erratic cardiopulmonary response, it should be avoided.

During pregnancy, maternal body fluid distribution is altered, with increased interstitial fluid and edema. These so-called third-space fluids have diminished exchange of dissolved gases in the central circulation. Though not addressed in any of the literature, maternal third-space fluid might offer a reservoir for nitrogen retention. The potential sites for nitrogen sequestration include the increased deposits of body fat found during pregnancy. On the average, women increase body fat from a normative 28 to 33 per cent to 33 to 36 per cent during pregnancy. Combining third-space and fat stores as harbors for nitrogen, off gassing time for pregnant women may not correspond to the limits established in the standard repetitive dive tables. Some of this loss of effective circulation may be counterbalanced while diving by centralization of maternal circulation during immersion, which has recently been observed.[76]

Fluid retention during pregnancy also causes nasopharyngeal swelling. Women with no prior allergic symptoms often complain of nose and ear stuffiness in pregnancy. Obviously, the risk of ear and sinus squeeze will be increased. Many pregnant women become decongestant-dependent and will incur the risk of rebound congestion when the medication wears off. If rebound occurs during diving, ascent may be slow and arduous.

During the early months of gestation, approximately two thirds of pregnant women experience some degree of gastrointestinal dysfunction, including increased nausea, vomiting, increased gastric acidity, and gastric reflux. Later in pregnancy, as the uterus enlarges, reflux increases. Gastric emptying time is delayed; obstetricians and anesthesiologists have come to regard all pregnant women as having full stomachs regardless of the timing of the last meal. If motion sickness on the dive boat adds to morning sickness, the pregnant diver is in for difficult diving. Consequently, the pregnant diver clearly is at high risk of vomiting into her regulator, an accident few sport divers are prepared to handle safely.

Pregnancy induces a state of relative vasodilation accompanied by an increased basal metabolic rate. While vasodilation may increase risk of hypothermia, a higher metabolic rate may increase risk of hyperthermia. During diving, the thermal risk will be defined by water temperature, length of dive, and quality of diving garment. Heavy activity in a heavy wet suit in warm water will lead to hyperthermia. Light activity with no protective clothing in cool water may lead to hypothermia. One paper from Finland[77] cited increased neural tube defects in women who used saunas during pregnancy. Though no other confirmatory reports exist demonstrating adverse outcomes of hyperthermia, obstetricians generally advise women to avoid hyperthermia when pregnant. Ama divers, who endure repeated cold stress, were reported to have a higher incidence of low birth-weight infants. Since these women incur exceptionally high levels of exertional demand as professional divers, and often consume fewer calories than are required to compensate for thermal debt, their smaller infant size may not be due solely to thermal stress.

Comfort during diving is not a medical issue, but pregnancy introduces problems in fit and function of dive gear. The changing size of the abdomen throughout gestation will soon stress even the most flexible wet suit. The safe location and placement of weight belts under, over, or around the gravid belly may create an unforeseen inability to ditch them during an emergency. Over the uterus, the belt will not fall free; under the uterus, the belt may be poorly positioned for quick release. Edema of hands and feet reduces gas exchange, increasing the likelihood of the bends. Balance with the fetus in front and tanks in back may pose an interesting challenge. Though obviously not a problem in water, balance instability will make leaving or entering a boat more difficult.

Any diving hazard has the potential to harm the fetus. If envenomation occurs from marine animals, undefined fetal toxic effects may follow. Specific antitoxins may also hold risks. In a litigious society such as ours, diving and pregnancy seem incompatible. The woman who wants to dive may not drink coffee in order to protect her fetus from unknown risk, although caffeine is not a teratogen. She may take vitamins and avoid paint fumes but will ask if diving is safe during pregnancy. In view of the elective nature of diving, even though pregnancy does not clearly increase maternal incidence of DCS or air embolism, the unborn may be at severe risk if a diving accident occurs. Summarizing all that has been cited and said, pregnant women should not dive.

REFERENCES

1. Williams J, Moon RE, et al: Utility of divers' alert network (DAN) non-emergency telephone information service [abstract]. Undersea Biomed Res 15(suppl):31, 1988.
2. Ellison AE (ed): Athletic Training and Sport Medicine. Chicago, American Academy of Orthosurgeons, 1984.
3. Frisch RE, McArthur JW: Menstrual cycles: Fatness as a determinant of weight for height necessary for their maintenance or onset. Science 185:949, 1974.
4. Frisch RE, Wyshak G, Vincent LV: Delayed menarche and amenorrhea in ballet dancers. N Engl J Med 30:17, 1980.
5. Frisch RE, Botz-Welbergen AV, McArthur JW, et al: Delayed menarche and amenorrhea of college athletes in relation to age of onset of training. JAMA 246:1559, 1981.
6. Warren M: The effects of exercise on pubertal progression and reproductive function in girls. J Clin Endocrinol 51:1150, 1980.
7. Scott EC, FS Johnston: Critical fat, menarche and the maintenance of cycles: A critical review. J Adol Health Care 2:2249, 1982.
8. Marcus R, Cann C, Madvig P, Minkoff J, et al: Menstrual function and bone mass in women distance runners: Endocrine and metabolic features. Am Intern Med 102:158–163, 1985.
9. Warren MP, Brooks-Gunn J, Hamilton LH, et al: Scoliosis and fractures in young ballet dancers. N Engl J Med 314:1348, 1986.
10. Prior JC, Cameron K, Ho Yuen B, et al: Menstrual cycle changes with marathon training: Anovulation and short luteal phase. Can J Appl Sports Sci 7(3):173, 1982.
11. Prior JC, Ho Yuen B, Clement P, et al: Reversible luteal phase changes and infertility associated with marathon training. Lancet 2:269, 1982.
12. Shangold M, Freeman R, Thysen B, et al: The relationship between long-distance running, plasma progesterone and luteal phase length. Fertil Steril 31:130, 1979.
13. O'Herlihy C: Jogging and suppression of ovulation. N Engl J Med 306:50, 1982.
14. Bullen BA, et al: Induction of menstrual disorders by strenuous exercise in untrained women. N Engl J Med 312:1349, 1985.
15. Cumming DC, Vickovic MM, Wall SR, et al: Defects in pulsatile LH release in normally menstruating runners. J Clin Endocrinol Metab 60:810, 1985.
16. Veldhuis JD, et al: Altered neuroendocrine regulation of gonadotropin secretion in women distance runners. J Clin Endocrinol Metab 61:557, 1985.
17. Riggs L, Melton L: Involutional osteoporosis. N Engl J Med 314:1676, 1986.
18. Jones KP, Ravnikar VA, Tulchinsky D, Schiff I: Comparison of bone density in amenorrheic women due to athletics, weight loss and premature menopause. Ob Gyn 66:5–8, 1985.
19. Drinkwater B, Nilson K, Chestnut CH, et al: Bone mineral content of amenorrheic and eumenorrheic athletes. N Engl J Med 311:277, 1984.
20. Lindberg JS: Exercise induced amenorrhea and bone density. Ann Intern Med 101:647, 1984.
21. Drinkwater BL, Nilson K, Ott S, Chestnut CH: Bone mineral density after resumption of menses in amenorrheic athletes. JAMA 256:380, 1986.
22. Lane N, et al: Long distance running, bone density and osteoarthritis. JAMA 255:1147, 1986.
23. Shangold MM, Levine HS: The effect of marathon training upon menstrual function. Am J Obstet Gynecol 143:862, 1982.
24. Carr DB, Bullen BA, Skrinar GS, et al: Physical

conditioning facilitates the exercise-induced secretion of beta-endorphin and beta-lipotropin in women. N Engl J Med 305:560, 1981.
25. American College of Ob-Gyn Technical Bulletin no. 87: Women and exercise. Washington, DC, ACOG, September, 1985.
26. American College of Ob-Gyn. Exercise during pregnancy and the post partum period. Washington, DC, ACOG, 1985.
27. Bonica JT: Obstetric analgesia and anesthesia: Basic considerations. Clin Ob-Gyn 2(3):469–495, 1975.
28. Williams AW, Lim YL: Blood volume and haemodynamics in pregnancy. Clin Ob-Gyn 2(2):301–320, 1975.
29. Edwards MJ, Metcalfe MJ, Danham MJ, Paul MS: Accelerated respiratory response to moderate exercise in late pregnancy. Resp Physiol 45:229–241, 1981.
30. Artal R, Platt LD, Sperling M, et al: Exercise in pregnancy. I. Maternal cardiovascular and metabolic responses in normal pregnancy. Am J Obstet Gynecol 140:123, 1981.
31. Lotgering GK, Gilbert RD, Longo LD: Maternal and fetal responses to exercise during pregnancy. Physiol Rev 65:1, 1985.
32. Lotgering GK, Gilbert RD, Longo LD: The interactions of exercise and pregnancy: A review. Am J Obstet Gynecol 149:560, 1984.
33. Dibblee L, Graham TE: A longitudinal study of changes in aerobic fitness, body composition and energy intake in primigravid patients. Am J Obstet Gynecol 147:908–914, 1983.
34. Lotgering FK, Gilbert RD, Longo LD: Exercise responses in pregnant sheep: Oxygen consumption, uterine blood flow, and blood volume. J Appl Physiol 55:834, 1983.
35. Clapp JF: Acute exercise stress in the pregnant ewe. Am J Obstet Gynecol 136:489, 1980.
36. Bagnall KM, Mottolo MF, McFadden KD: The effects of strenuous exercise on maternal rats and their developing fetuses. Can J Appl Sport Sci 8(4):254–259, 1983.
37. Bell AW, Bassett JM, Chandler KD, Boston RC: Fetal and maternal endocrine responses to exercise in the pregnant ewe. J Dev Physiol 5(2):129–141, 1983.
38. Mottola M, Bagnall KM, McFaffed: The effects of maternal exercise and developing rat fetuses. Br J Sports Med 17:117–121, 1983.
39. Artal R, Paul RM, Romem Y, et al: Fetal bradycardia induced by maternal exercise. Lancet 2:258, 1984.
40. Clapp JF: Fetal heart rate response to running in midpregnancy and late pregnancy. Am J Obstet Gynecol 153:251, 1985.
41. Collings C, Curet LB: Fetal heart response to maternal exercise. Am J Obstet Gynecol 151:498, 1985.
42. Collings CA, Curet LB, Mullin JP: Maternal and fetal responses to a maternal aerobic exercise program. Am J Obstet Gynecol 145:702, 1983.
43. Dale E, Mullinax KM, Bryan DH: Exercise during pregnancy: Effects on the fetus. Can J Appl Sports Sci 7:98, 1982.
44. Dressendorfer RH, Goodin RC: Fetal heart rate response to maternal exercise testing. Phys Sport Med 8(11):91, 1980.
45. Hauth JC, Gilstrap LC, Widmer K: Fetal heart rate reactivity before and after maternal jogging during the third trimester. Am J Obstet Gynecol 142:545, 1982.
46. Carpenter MW, Sady SP, et al: Fetal heart rate response to maternal exertion. JAMA 20:3006, 1988.
47. Hall DC, Kaufmann DA: Effects of aerobic and strength conditioning on pregnancy outcomes. Am J Obstet Gynecol 157(5):1199–1203, 1987.
48. Smith C, Nelson NN: The Physiology of the Newborn Infant, 4th ed. Springfield, IL, Charles C. Thomas, 1976.
49. Liggins GC, Qvist J, Hochachka PW, et al: Fetal cardiovascular and metabolic responses to simulated diving in the weddell seal. J Appl Physiol 49(3):424–430, 1980.
50. Shnider SM, Levinson G: Anesthesia for Obstetrics. Baltimore, Williams & Wilkins, 1979.
51. Morgan WP: Psychologic characteristics of the female diver. *In* Fife W (ed): Women in Diving: 35th Undersea and Hyperbaric Medical Society Workshop. NHMS publ number 71 (WS-WD):45–53, April 1987.
52. Jennings R: Women and the hazardous environment: When the pregnant patient requires hyperbaric oxygen therapy. Aviat Space Environ Med 58:370–374, 1987.
53. Newhall JF: Scuba diving during pregnancy: A brief review. Am J Obstet Gynecol 140:893–894, 1981.
54. Bassett BD: Decompression sickness in female students exposed to altitude during physiologic training. Annual Scientific Meeting of Aerospace Medical Association 1973, pp 241–242.
55. Bangasser SA: Medical profile of the woman scuba diver. *In* National Association of Underwater Instructors. Proceedings of the 10th International Conference on Underwater Education. Colton, CA, NAUI:31–40, 1978.
56. American College of Ob-Gyn: Committee opinion #66. Premenstrual syndrome. Washington, DC, ACOG, January 1989.
57. Facchinetti F, et al: Premenstrual fall of plasma. Beta-endorphin and patients with premenstrual syndrome. Fertil Steril 47(4):570–573, 1987.
58. McIver RG: Bends resistance in the fetus. *In* Preprints of scientific program. Annual Scientific Meeting. Washington, Aerospace Medical Association. 31, 1968.
59. Nemiroff MJ, Willson JR, Kirschbaum TH: Multiple hyperbaric exposure during pregnancy in sheep. Am J Obstet Gynecol 140:651, 1981.
60. Powell MR, Smith MT: Fetal and maternal bubbles detected noninvasive in sheep and goats following hyperbaric decompression. Undersea Biomed Res 12:59–69, 1985.
61. Wilson JR, Blessed WB, Blackburn PJ: Hyperbaric exposure during pregnancy in sheep: Staged and rapid decompression. Undersea Biomed Res 10:10–15, 1983.
62. Fife WP, Simmang C, Kitzman JV: Susceptibility of fetal sheep to acute decompression sickness. Undersea Biomed Res 5:287–292, 1978.
63. Stock MK, Lanphier EH, Anderson DF, et al: Responses of fetal sheep to simulated no decompression dives. J Appl Physiol 48:776–780, 1980.
64. Gilman SC, Greene KM, Bradley ME, Biersner RJ: Fetal development: Effects of simulated diving and hyperbaric oxygen treatment. Undersea Biomed Res 9:297–304, 1982.
65. Miller PD, Telford ID, Haas GR: Effect of hyperbaric oxygen on cardiogenesis in the rat. Biol Neonate 44:52, 1971.
66. Fukikara T: Retrolental fibroplasia and prematurity in newborn rabbits induced by maternal hyperoxia. Am J Obstet Gynecol 90:354–358, 1964.
67. Gilman S, Bradley M, Greene K, Fischer G: Fetal

development: Effects of decompression sickness and treatment. Aviat Space Environ Med 54:1040–1042, 1983.

68. Van Hoesen KB, Camporesi EM, et al: HBO therapy for CO poisoning during pregnancy [abstract]. Undersea Biomed Res (suppl)15:61, 1988.
69. Hollander DI, Nagey DA, Welch R, Pupkin M: HBO therapy for the treatment of acute carbon monoxide poisoning in pregnancy: A case report. J Reprod Med 32(8):615–617, 1987.
70. Bolton ME: Scuba diving and fetal well-being: A survey of 208 women. Undersea Biomed Res 7:183–189, 1980.
71. Turner G, Unsworth I: Intrauterine bends? Lancet 1:905, 1982.
72. Bray P, Myers RAM, Cowley RA: Orogenital sex as a cause of non fatal air embolism in pregnancy. Obstet Gynecol 61:653–657, 1983.
73. Fyke FE, Kazmier FJ, Harms RW: Venous air embolism: Life-threatening complication and orogenital sex during pregnancy. Am J Med 78:333–336, 1985.
74. Barnhardt TL, Goldmann RW, Thombs PA, Kindwall RP: Hyperbaric oxygen treatment of cervical air embolism from orogenital sex play during pregnancy. Crit Care Med 16:729–730, 1988.
75. Assali NS, Kirschbaum TH, Dilts PV: Effects of hyperbaric oxygen on uteroplacental and fetal circulation. Circ Res 22:573–588, 1968.
76. Katz VL, McMurray R, Berry MJ, Cefalo RC: Fetal and uterine responses to immersion and exercise. Obstet Gynecol 72(2):255–230, 1988.
77. Lipson A, et al: Sauna and birth defects [letter]. Teratology 32(1):147–148, 1985.

Chapter 14

Diving in the Elderly and the Young

ALFRED A. BOVE

DIVING IN THE ELDERLY

Although age limitations are commonly imposed on commercial and military divers, there are no formal limitations on the sport diver. Divers under the age of 10 years and over the age of 75, while not common, are known to participate in sport scuba diving. Limitations to the young and to the elderly follow different patterns, but youth and age alone should not be considered as contraindications.

Although there has been a trend toward increased physical activity in older individuals, the majority of elderly people do not exercise and indeed are often discouraged from participating in regular exercise. Good physical condition is essential for diving. Although physical capacity is known to decline with age,[1–3] it is unclear whether this loss is related to aging or to the reduction in physical activity that is common in older individuals and is to some extent caused by social factors that relegate physical activity and exercise to the younger population. Because of the continuing reduction in the amount of physical activity experienced by older individuals, there tends to be a deconditioning effect associated with age. Therefore, most elderly divers are not capable of sustaining the exercise work load of younger individuals.

The reduction in physical capacity must be accounted for when advising older divers. Several studies have examined older athletes and have found marked physiological differences in these individuals when compared with age-matched, nontrained persons.[4–6] The findings suggest that the decline in physical capacity with age can be minimized by continued physical training.[7] Thus with elderly divers, conditioning programs are essential for safe diving. Recommendations for diving in the elderly should be provided when chronic or acute illness does not preclude such activity and when physical condition is at a level that allows the diver to perform safely. This section reviews some of the changes in physiological responses known to occur with aging and, based on these concepts, provides some recommendations for diving in the elderly.

Cardiovascular Consideration

It is generally accepted that systolic and diastolic blood pressures rise with age.[2] Thus, the standard accepted range of normal blood pressures is known to increase slowly with age, so that at age 70, for example, an acceptable high limit for normal systolic blood pressure would be higher than the acceptable high level of normal in a 20- to 30-year-old individual. Individuals with hypertension should be treated before being cleared for diving. Blood pressure elevation in the elderly is due in part to alterations in the compliance or stiffness of the aorta.[8] Clinical observations[9] and experimental studies[10] suggest that reduced aortic smooth muscle tone would occur following prolonged exercise training. The finding of reduced aortic strip tension following exercise in experimental studies[10] also suggests that an exercise program might reduce peripheral vascular resistance and increase aortic compliance, thus lowering blood pressure in elderly subjects. Training of these individuals can provide some blood pressure control and should be recommended as part of a conditioning program for diving.

Peripheral vascular resistance is also known to increase with age. This increase may be caused by a reduction in skeletal muscle mass[11, 12]; however, the change is probably caused by multiple factors and is not necessarily related to long-standing hypertension. Since most of the systemic vascular resistance resides in the vasculature of skeletal muscle, it is possible that the increase in peripheral vascular resistance found in elderly individuals is a result of combined increased hormonal sensitivity[13] and reduced muscle mass, with partial loss of microvascular channels in the peripheral vascular bed. The known increase in susceptibility to decompression sickness in the elderly may be related to this loss of vasculature with subsequent changes in inert gas kinetics. Studies in hypertensive populations suggest that peripheral vascular resistance is lowered with exercise.[14, 15] A program of endurance exercise training in elderly hypertensives reduces blood pressure because of changes in peripheral vascular resistance and possibly because of changes in the vascular tone of the large distributing arteries. Blood pressure response to acute exercise in older individuals is known to be altered by training[2, 4, 16]; however, elderly individuals with apparently mild hypertension may develop marked elevation of blood pressure during exercise, including diving. If exercise produces a significant elevation of blood pressure (diastolic >110, systolic >210 mm Hg), it is necessary to provide antihypertensive treatment prior to instituting a diving program.

Cardiac Performance

Studies in experimental animals and in patients[17–20] indicate that a reduction in contractile performance of the myocardium occurs with age. This reduction is small and generally of minimal consequence, although it can be detected in studies designed specifically to examine the contractile characteristics of the myocardium.[21] Catecholamine responses in the elderly are enhanced[13, 22]; however, it is unclear whether catecholamine receptors in the elderly have the same sensitivity as receptors in a younger population.[23] Some studies[13] have demonstrated increased blood catecholamine levels in response to exercise in the elderly, suggesting that the control system that stimulates the heart during exercise requires release of greater amounts of catecholamines to obtain a cardiac response appropriate for the exercise level. The myocardium in the elderly is also known to have increased stiffness.[24, 25] Thus, diastolic ventricular relaxation in elderly subjects is impaired, and high heart rates are presumably less well tolerated in the older age groups than younger individuals. A well-known alteration in cardiac performance associated with age is the decline of maximum heart rate.[3, 7, 26] The cause for this alteration in heart rate response in the elderly is not clear; however, it is possible that changes in autonomic tone or in the state of innervation of the heart by the autonomic system are responsible.[23]

In addition to reduced maximal heart rate with aging, maximum oxygen uptake also declines with age beyond the late twenties.[1, 18, 27] Reduction in maximum oxygen uptake with age may occur rapidly or slowly depending on the state of physical condition and the continuity of endurance training over many years. Thus, the decline of maximal oxygen uptake with age described from early studies was found to be associated with a state of poor physical conditioning. A program of physical activity continuing over several decades has been found to reduce the decline of oxygen uptake originally thought to be age related.[28, 29] Lactate production with exercise may also be exaggerated in older untrained subjects.[30] This information again provides evidence that alterations in physical work capacity, oxygen uptake, and other indices of physical capacity are not only age related, but also are due to inactivity or detraining. Loss of physical strength with age may also result from detraining.[31] Because of the decline in maximal oxygen uptake with age, maximal work capacity is reduced in older individuals when compared with that of individuals in the third and fourth decades; similar changes occur in both male and female populations.[32] Reduced capability in elderly divers must be accounted for in recreational diving.

Ventilatory Performance

Data from Christensson and colleagues[33] showed an increase in unventilated lung compartments with age. These results suggest that older divers may experience more breathing difficulty than younger divers. Brischetto and co-workers[34] found a reduced ventilatory sensitivity to CO_2 production with exercise in the elderly.

Superimposition of chronic illness adds further to the decline of work performance in the elderly. It is not reasonable to expect elderly divers to perform on an equal level with younger divers. Sport diving programs should allow for differences in physical performance when considering elderly diving candidates. The elderly individual will experience a greater amount of physical stress when exercising at a given level in comparison to younger individuals, even when the state of physical training is approximately equivalent in the two individuals.

Metabolic Changes

Other contributing factors for consideration of diving in the elderly include age-related alterations in the metabolic state.[35] Older individuals may have more glucose intolerance than younger individuals.[36] Symptomatic hypoglycemia should disqualify an individual from diving. The activity of the thyroid gland may be diminished, and the elderly individual, therefore, will be less tolerant to alterations in temperature. Elderly persons are noted to have reduced basal metabolic rates when compared with younger individuals,[12] and these differences in metabolism also should be considered when evaluating older individuals for diving. Both heat and cold tolerance may be reduced in elderly divers.[37] This population may also have a reduced corticosteroid response to stress. In general, elderly persons will not be able to withstand prolonged exertion and will have a relative heat and cold intolerance. The risk of hypothermia is therefore greater in elderly divers.

Other Age-Related Alterations

In addition to known cardiovascular, endocrine, metabolic, respiratory, and nervous system changes with age, connective tissue structure also changes. As age progresses, collagen polymerizes from a relatively soluble form to a relatively insoluble form that is stiffer than the younger, nonpolymerized collagen.[38] The changes in collagen structure result in increased stiffness of tendons, ligaments, and joints. Current data suggest that alterations in collagen structure cannot be avoided in the elderly. Thus, the known increase in stiffness of joints and tendons with associated reduction in range of motion should be accounted for in elderly diving candidates.

It remains unclear whether older divers are more susceptible to decompression sickness. Hoiberg[39] showed no age effects on decompression sickness. However, this report involved only Navy divers under 50 years of age.

Another important consideration in dealing with diving in the elderly is alteration in neurological function.[22] Normally a slowing of certain central nervous system functions can be noted with age. The elderly have a lengthening of reflex time and somewhat less precise motor control compared with younger individuals. Because of these changes, it is important to document a neurological examination prior to diving for later comparison if needed.

Evaluating the Elderly Diver

When dealing with elderly normals or elderly patients who wish to dive, physical capacity must be determined. Often this evaluation will reveal that physical capacity is significantly reduced compared with individuals of younger age, although elderly individuals who have continuously exercised may have surprisingly good physical capacity. One should also consider the increased incidence of chronic disease. The elderly individual is more likely to have coronary disease, which may be undiagnosed. Pulmonary function may be reduced, there may be endocrine metabolic disorders either manifest or undiagnosed, and renal function may be impaired because of arteriosclerosis. All of the alterations that occur in the elderly as part of the aging process or as a result of chronic illness must be considered in evaluation for diving.

The reduced work capacity of older individuals requires low exertion diving programs. Older subjects can be tested for exercise capacity using a standard stress test. In exercise testing, elderly individuals in general do not achieve the same levels of exercise capacity as younger individuals, and when chronic illnesses are present, exercise tolerance may be severely limited. Severe limitations to physical capacity due to chronic illness or detraining should prohibit diving.

The known reduction in thermal tolerance (both hot and cold) also must be considered in diving programs for the elderly. In the elderly, exposure to cold may result in severe hypothermia. Careful instructions concerning reduced work capacity and altered cardiovascular responses in extremes of temperature should be provided to the individual in the training program. By considering these factors, diving programs can be provided for the elderly.

Chronic diseases known to be of higher incidence in the elderly present special problems in diving. A significant and important problem in the elderly is the high incidence of cardiovascular disease. Atherosclerosis can affect blood flow to the brain, heart, kidneys, or skeletal muscle, such as the legs. Many times these arterial obstructions are undetected, and high flow demands induced by swimming with diving gear may result in inadequate oxygen supply and abnormal function of a tissue or organ. Because these disorders are higher in frequency in the elderly, it is important to search carefully by physical examination, history, and appropriate laboratory studies to rule out the possibility of significant atherosclerosis. Of most importance is the presence of coronary atherosclerosis with coronary artery obstruction, which limits flow to the myocardium. Flow demands in the myocardium can increase substantially with diving, and in the presence of severe atherosclerosis with impaired blood flow, myocardial infarction, serious arrhythmias, or sudden death may follow. In the elderly avoidance of serious cardiac problems while diving can be achieved through appropriate screening evaluation[40] including an exercise stress test with electrocardiographic and blood pressure monitoring, which documents the physical capacity of the patient and detects coronary artery disease. The value of an exercise stress test in this population cannot be overemphasized. This test provides both diagnostic screening for coronary disease and the information needed to judge capacity for diving. A study of this type is essential in elderly individuals prior to instituting a diving program.

Consideration of diving in the elderly must also take into account alterations in bone and joint structure and strength to avoid musculoskeletal injury from diving. The osteoporosis of the elderly can be a significant problem if an elderly diver is subjected to trauma that might lead to a fracture. Poorly conditioned individuals beginning a diving program should be instructed to avoid heavy lifting or traumatic situations that might result in injury to bones, joints, or tendons, since these structures are weak compared with those of younger divers and heal more slowly. For poorly conditioned individuals who have not exercised for long periods of time, the initial training may result in a musculoskeletal injury that precludes further conditioning.

In conclusion, it is reasonable to provide clearance for some elderly subjects to undertake sport diving. Programs for the elderly require special considerations because of the reduced physical capacity and alterations in the neurological, cardiovascular, pulmonary, and endocrine systems. Diving candidates should undergo exercise testing in a controlled environment with electrocardiographic and blood pressure monitoring. With a careful evaluation, an elderly individual in good health can be given clearance for diving. Taking into account all of these variables, it is possible and desirable to provide diving programs to healthy, moderately conditioned elderly subjects. These divers, however, should not be considered to be as capable as younger divers.

DIVING IN THE YOUNG

Medical considerations for young divers are directed toward emotional maturity, ability to learn and understand the requisite physiological, physical, and environmental data needed for safe diving, and physical strength necessary for handling diving equipment. In commercial and military diving, the lower age limit is 19 years, but most commercial divers are two to three years older. Sport diving imposes no legal limit, but most diver training organizations require candidates to be 15 years old for full certification. Training is provided to younger candidates who receive conditional certification until age 15.[41] Pouliquen[42] reported on a diving program for children from 4 to 12 years old. This program provides training and supervised scuba diving and had no claimed problems in 7000 dives undertaken by children.

Questions have been raised concerning injury to developing bones. To date no evidence has been provided to support this concern. Nevertheless, young divers should use diving profiles that minimize risk for decompression sickness. Shallower, shorter dives for children will remove any concern for bone injury.

Equipment must be properly fitted to the young diver. Wetsuits, buoyancy compensators, and compressed air tanks designed for adults will be difficult to manage and may be unsafe for a child of small body habitus. Small size equipment may require custom manufacture in some cases.

Evaluating the Young Diver

A review of factors to be considered in young divers was presented by Dembert and Keith.[43] The medical guidelines presented throughout this book should be applied to all divers, including the younger diver. Physical conditioning is usually of less concern than in the elderly diver but must still be considered. Most children active in recreational or organized sports are in good physical condition. Although poor physical condition is less common in the young, those young divers who are poorly conditioned have increased risk of accident or injury. Dembert and Keith[43] suggest that the young diver weigh at least 45 kg and be 150 cm tall or greater. Medical guidelines are similar to adult guidelines.

As in the elderly, the young diver is best trained with a group of peers to avoid stress produced by keeping up with older and more physically capable divers.

In summary, there appear to be no physiological constraints to diving in children below age 15. Physical constraints should be considered in small children (< 45 kg or < 150 cm tall) because of minimum strength requirements for safe diving. Of greatest concern in the healthy child are the capability to learn and understand the physics and physiology needed for safe diving and the presence of a mature attitude toward safe diving.

REFERENCES

1. Dehn MN, Bruce RA: Longitudinal variations in maximal oxygen intake with age and activity. J Appl Physiol 33:805–807, 1972.
2. Raven PB, Mitchell J: The effect of aging on the cardiovascular response to dynamic and static exercise. *In* Weisfeldt HL (ed): The Aging Heart. New York, Raven Press, 1980, pp 269–296.
3. Bruce RA, Fisher LD, Cooper MN, Gey GO: Separation of effects of cardiovascular disease and age on ventricular function with maximal exercise. Am J Cardiol 34:757–763, 1974.
4. Ordway GA, Wekstein DR: The effect of age on selected cardiovascular responses to static (isometric) exercise. Proc Soc Exp Biol Med 161:189–192, 1979.
5. Currens JH, White PD: Half a century of running: Clinical, physiological, and autopsy findings in the case of Clarence De Mar ("Mr. Marathon"). N Engl J Med 265:988–993, 1961.
6. Cantwell JD, Watt EW: Extreme cardiopulmonary fitness in old age. Chest 65:357–359, 1974.
7. Heath GW, Hogherg JM, Ehsani AA, Holloszy JO: A physiologic comparison of young and older endurance athletes. J Appl Physiol 51:634–640, 1981.
8. Cox RH: Effects of age on the mechanical properties of rate carotid artery. Am J Physiol 233:H256–H263, 1977.
9. Pulike G, Frenkle R: Sensitivity to catecholamines and histamine in the trained and untrained human organism. Eur J Appl Physiol 34:199–204, 1975.
10. Thorp GD: The effects of exercise training on blood pressure and aortic strip tension of normal and spontaneously hypertensive rats (abstr). Fed Proc Fed Am Soc Exp Biol 35:796, 1976.
11. Sidney KH, Shephard RJ, Harrison JE: Endurance training and body composition in the elderly. Am J Clin Nutr 30:326–333, 1977.
12. Suominen H, Heinkken E, Liesen H, et al: Effects of 8 weeks' endurance training on skeletal muscle metabolism in 56–70 year old sedentary men. Eur J Appl Physiol 37:173–180, 1977.
13. Palmer GJ, Ziegler MG, Lake CR: Response of norepinephrine and blood pressure to stress increases with age. J Gerontol 33:482–487, 1978.
14. Boyer JL, Kasch FW: Exercise therapy in hypertensive men. JAMA 211:1668–1671, 1970.
15. Hansen JS, Nedde WH: Preliminary observations on physical training for hypertensive males. Circ Res 26(Suppl):49–53, 1970.
16. Montgomery DL, Ismail AH: The effect of a four month physical fitness program on high and low-fit groups matched for age. J Sports Med 17:327–333, 1977.
17. Gerstenblith G, Lakatta EG, Weisfeldt ML: Age changes in myocardial function and exercise response. Prog Cardiovasc Dis 19:1–21, 1976.
18. Becklake MR, Frank H, Dagenais GR, et al: Influence of age and sex on exercise cardiac output. J Appl Physiol 20:938–947, 1965.
19. Yin FCP, Spurgeon HA, Weisfeldt L, Lakatta EG: Mechanical properties of myocardium from hypertrophied rat hearts. Circ Res 46:292–300, 1980.
20. Dock W: How some hearts age. JAMA 195:148–150, 1966.
21. Mann DL, Mackler PT, Bove AA: Reduced left ventricular contractile reserve in aged subjects (abstr). Clin Res 29:220A, 1981.
22. Eisdorfer C: Neurotransmitters and aging: Clinical correlates. *In* Adelman RC, et al (eds): Neural Regulatory Mechanisms During Aging. New York, Alan R. Liss, 1980, pp 53–59.
23. Lakatta EG: Age related alterations in the cardiovascular response to adrenergic medicated stress. Fed Proc Fed Am Soc Exp Biol 39:3173–3177, 1980.
24. Weisfeldt M: Left ventricular function. *In* Weisfeldt ML (ed): The Aging Heart. New York, Raven Press, 1981, pp 297–316.
25. Templeton GH, Platt MR, Willerson JT, Weisfeldt ML: Influence of aging on left ventricular hemodynamics and stiffness in beagles. Circ Res 44:189–194, 1979.
26. Sidney KH, Shephard RJ: Maximal and submaximal exercise tests in men and women in the seventh, eighth, and ninth decades of life. J Appl Physiol 43:280–287, 1977.
27. Saltin B, Brimby G: Physiological analysis of middle aged and old former athletes. Circulation 38:1104–1114, 1968.
28. Montoye HJ, Block WD, Gayle R: Maximal oxygen uptake and blood lipids. J Chronic Dis 31:11–118, 1978.
29. DeVries HA: Physiologic effects of an exercise training regimen upon men aged 52–88. J Gerontol 25:325–336, 1970.
30. Seals DR, Hurley BF, Schultz J, Hagberg JM: Endurance training in older men and women. II. Blood lactate response to maximal exercise. J Appl Physiol 57:1030–1033, 1984.
31. Petrofsky JS, Burse RL, Lind AR: Aging, isometric strength and endurance, and cardiovascular responses to static effort. J Appl Physiol 38:91–95, 1975.
32. Petrofsky JS, Burse RL, Lind AR: Comparison of physiological responses of men and women to isometric exercise. J Appl Physiol 38:863–868, 1975.
33. Christensson PM, Arborelius M, Kautto R: Volume of trapped gas in lungs of healthy humans. J Appl Physiol 51:172–175, 1981.
34. Brischetto JJ, Millman RP, Peterson DD, et al: Effect of aging on ventilatory response to exercise and CO_2. J Appl Physiol 56:1143–1150, 1984.

35. Sartin J, Chaudhuri M, Obenrader M, Adelman RC: The role of hormones in changing adaptive mechanisms during aging. Fed Proc 39:3163–3167, 1980.
36. Montoye HJ, Block WD, Metzner H, Keller JB: Habitual physical activity and glucose tolerance. Diabetes 26:172–176, 1977.
37. Wagner JA, Horvath SM: Cardiovascular reactions to cold exposures differ with age and gender. J Appl Physiol 58:187–192, 1985.
38. Versar F: Aging of the collagen fiber. Int Rev Connect Tissue Res 2:243–300, 1964.
39. Hoiberg A: Consequences of U.S. Navy diving mishaps: Decompression sickness. Undersea Biomed Res 13:383–394, 1986.
40. Camm AJ, Evans KE, Ward EE, Martin A: The rhythm of the heart in active elderly subjects. Am Heart J 99:598–603, 1980.
41. Linaweaver PG: Physical standards for diving. *In* Shelling CW, Carlston CB, Mathias RA (eds): The Physicians Guide to Diving Medicine. New York, Plenum Press, 1986, p 494.
42. Pouliquen H: L'enfant et la plongee. J So Pacific Underwater Med Soc 3:3, 1982.
43. Dembert ML, Keith JF: Evaluating the potential pediatric scuba diver. Am J Dis Child 140:1135–1141, 1986.

Chapter 15

Pathophysiology of Decompression Sickness

T. J. R. FRANCIS, A. J. DUTKA, and J. M. HALLENBECK

It has been generally accepted for some years that the formation of gas bubbles within tissues is the event that precipitates the onset of decompression sickness.[1] The birth of a bubble, however, is only the first of a sequence of events that, depending upon their location, may be symptomless or may result in conditions that range in severity from pruritus to convulsions and death. Indeed, so varied are the manifestations of decompression sickness (Table 15–1), that the nascent bubble has been compared with the spirochete as "the great imitator."[2]

Faced with the bewildering variety of signs and symptoms produced by decompression sickness, the physician, nurse, or medical technician must always be alert to the possibility of this diagnosis after any hyper- or hypobaric exposure. This chapter will discuss the conditions under which decompression sickness occurs, the mechanisms involved in bubble-induced tissue injury, and the signs and symptoms of the classic "bends."

BUBBLE FORMATION

Decompression sickness cannot occur unless there is a sufficient volume of inert gas dissolved in the tissues, so that when the ambient pressure maintaining it in solution is sufficiently reduced, the gas leaves solution and forms bubbles. The body is able to safely remove the excess tissue inert gas load that results from a gradual release of ambient pressure by passively transferring the gas down a concentration gradient from the tissues to the blood stream and then to the lungs, where gas tensions in the blood equilibrate with the breathing mixture. There is, however, a finite maximum rate at which this process can proceed. If the release of ambient pressure is too rapid, tissue gas tensions may exceed the local tissue pressure sufficiently that bubbles form. This is the physiological basis for the practical observation—now over 100 years old and described first by foremen of caissson workers—that rapid ascent following a prolonged period at depth leads to the bends.

Uptake and Release of Inert Gas by the Body

When humans are suddenly exposed to an increased inert gas tension, a rapid transfer of gas occurs across the alveolar membrane, so that the arterial and atmospheric gas tensions equilibrate within a few minutes.[3] The variables that now determine the rate of gas uptake by any tissue in the body may be expressed as a mass balance equation:

$$S_t(dP_t/dt) = \dot{Q} \cdot S_b(P_a - P_v)$$

or: Net accumulation = uptake from arterial blood − removal in venous blood, where S_b and S_t are the solubilities of the gas in blood and tissue, $\dot{Q}$ is the blood flow, P_t is mean tissue gas tension, and P_a and P_v are the gas tensions in arterial and venous blood. The up-

TABLE 15–1. Frequency of Signs and Symptoms in 935 Cases of Decompression Sickness

SIGN OR SYMPTOM	NUMBER OF INSTANCES WITHIN 935 CASES	PERCENTAGE OF INSTANCES WITHIN 935 CASES	NUMBER OF INSTANCES MANIFESTED INITIALLY	PERCENTAGE OF INITIAL MANIFESTATIONS
Localized pain	858	91.8	744	76.6
Numbness or paresthesia	199	21.2	41	4.3
Muscular weakness	193	20.6	8	0.8
Skin rash	140	14.9	42	4.4
Dizziness or vertigo	80	8.5	24	2.5
Nausea or vomiting	74	7.9	8	0.8
Visual disturbances	64	6.8	14	1.4
Paralysis	57	6.1	2	0.2
Headache	37	3.9	5	0.5
Unconsciousness	26	2.7	6	0.6
Urinary disturbances	24	2.5	0	—
Dyspnea ("chokes")	19	2.0	4	0.4
Personality change	15	1.6	0	—
Agitation or restlessness	13	1.3	0	—
Fatigue	12	1.2	2	0.2
Muscular twitching	12	1.2	0	—
Convulsions	11	1.1	0	—
Incoordination	9	0.9	0	—
Equilibrium disturbances	7	0.7	0	—
Localized edema	5	0.5	0	—
Intestinal disturbance	4	0.4	0	—
Auditory disturbance	3	0.3	0	—
Cranial nerve involvement	2	0.2	0	—
Aphasia	2	0.2	0	—
Hemoptysis	2	0.2	0	—
Emphysema—subcutaneous	1	0.1	0	—

From Rivera JC: Decompression sickness amongst divers: An analysis of 935 cases. Milit Med 129:314–334, 1963.

take or release of gas by a particular tissue depends on both the rate of blood flow to the tissue and the rate of gas diffusion into the tissue from blood. For most tissues, it is not known which of these processes is the principal determinant of the rate of gas transfer. It may be seen that if the blood flow ($\dot{Q}$) to a given tissue is low, then even if all the dissolved inert gas were to leave the blood for that tissue, the rate of gas uptake would be slow. Equally, if a situation were to exist whereby a tissue had a very high blood flow but only a small proportion of the dissolved inert gas were to leave the blood stream ($P_a - P_v \cong 0$), then the rate of gas uptake would also be slow. In a situation where tissue gas uptake is entirely perfusion limited, venous gas tension will equal that of the tissue. Under these circumstances, tissue gas uptake when arterial inert gas tension is increased from some original value, P_0 to P_a can be described by the equation:

$$P_t = P_0 + (P_a - P_0) \cdot (1 - e^{-kt})$$

where k, the rate constant, $= S_b/S_t \cdot \dot{Q}$.

The mathematical modeling of diffusion-limited systems is complex and beyond the scope of this text. Interested readers may wish to refer to Hills,[3] who discusses a number of models.

Although direct data are very hard to obtain, it is generally accepted that perfusion is the rate-limiting step in tissue inert gas loading in most cases. However, it is likely that this assumption is incorrect under certain circumstances. For example, when the rate of perfusion is so high as not to be rate limiting, where intercapillary distances are large, or where there is a barrier to diffusion, it is diffusion that might be expected to be rate limiting.

Under either condition, the rate of gas uptake by a tissue can be expressed as an exponential function from which a tissue half-time can be derived ($T½ = 0.693/k$). This tissue half-time is an estimate of the time it would take the gas tension in a given tissue to reach $(P_a - P_0)/2$ if the ambient gas tension were suddenly raised from P_0 to P_a. Tissues with a short half-time are often termed "fast" and those with a long half-time, "slow." Table 15–2 shows some of the variables that influence half-times for a number of tissues that range from slow adipose tissue to fast kidney.

Inert gas elimination from tissues is, for the most part, simply the reverse of gas uptake. However, if during decompression, a tissue becomes sufficiently supersaturated that gas bubbles form, then it is likely that the rate of

TABLE 15–2. The Blood Flow, Intercapillary Distance, and Fat Content of Some Tissues

TISSUE	BLOOD FLOW (ml·min⁻¹·100 g⁻¹)	INTERCAPILLARY DISTANCE (μm)[4]	FAT CONTENT† (% dry weight)
Adipose	2.6[5]	(R) fat-rich 34 (R) fat-poor 18	84.9[6]
Spinal cord: white	10–15[7]	—	> 75.0[8]
gray	50–70[7]	—	30.0[8]
Cerebrum: white	21[9]	33	54.9[10]
gray	83[9]	18	32.7[10]
Skin	0.5*[11]	—	33.6[6]
Striated muscle: rest	3–5[12]	(D) 11, (H) 15	22.1[6]
exercise	50–75[12]		
Kidney: cortex	(R) 508[13]	8	mean 24.4[6]
medulla	(R) 96–208[13]	7	

Measurements in humans, except R = rat, D = dog, H = horse
*May vary greatly with thermoregulation
†Defined as ether extract

gas elimination will be reduced. This is because (1) gas molecules within a bubble are less available for diffusion out of the tissue than when they are in solution, and (2) the presence of bubbles within a tissue will increase the hydrostatic pressure (particularly in tissues of low compliance, such as tendon) and consequently will reduce tissue perfusion. However, the evidence for inequalities in rates of tissue saturation and desaturation is at present somewhat limited.[14–16]

Once exposed to hyperbaric conditions, body tissues continue to take up inert gas until they equilibrate with the partial pressure of that gas in the breathing mixture. This state is known as *saturation*. A significant, rapid lowering of the ambient pressure surrounding a body saturated with gas will lead to decompression sickness regardless of the pressure at which it is saturated. Aviators and astronauts, for example, saturated with nitrogen at one atmosphere may suffer serious decompression sickness if rapidly decompressed to as little as 30,000 feet.[17] The "bounce" diver, on the other hand, must worry not only about the rate of decompression but also about the amount of time spent under hyperbaric conditions.

How long can a diver continue to take on gas and still remain able to surface immediately? In some recent experiments a few subjects remained at 25 to 28 fsw (about 1.8 ata) until they were completely saturated with inert gas and returned directly to the surface without suffering harm.[18] A few cases of decompression sickness have been reported after two to three hours at 30 fsw.[19] The amount of time the diver can spend on the bottom without risk of decompression sickness upon immediate surfacing decreases progressively with depth, extending from 60 minutes at 60 fswg to less than 5 minutes at 200 fswg. These are the familiar "no decompression" limits as recommended by the U.S. Navy tables. The sport diver is usually taught to stay within these limits to avoid the necessity of ascending slowly or stopping to allow equilibration of tissue gas with an intermediate ambient pressure. It is important to remember from the diagnostic viewpoint that diving within these limits does not guarantee the absence of decompression sickness. This is especially the case if a diver has made several dives during the same day and has not completely brought his tissues to equilibrium with atmospheric pressure between dives, or if he is subjected to a lower atmospheric pressure soon after diving (flying home from vacation, for instance). Even if there have been no repetitive dives and the individual has not flown soon after diving, there are occasional cases of decompression sickness even after dives within the no decompression limits, particularly deeper dives. This may reflect the effect of factors that increase the rate at which a diver takes on gas, such as hyperventilation from exercise, cold or fear; factors that increase the amount of gas that a diver may take up, such as hypothermia; or factors that may increase the individual's susceptibility to decompression sickness, such as age and obesity.[20, 21]

Other Forces Influencing Bubble Formation

All tissues can tolerate some degree of excess gas tension without the gas necessarily bubbling out of solution. A force opposing bubble nucleation is tissue pressure. This is the sum of the ambient pressure and local pressures generated by forces such as tissue elasticity. A reduction of local elastic forces may permit the formation of bubbles. Exercise taken soon after a dive that has substantial decompression risk may increase the incidence of bends; this is possibly due to the lowering of local tissue pressure by stretching of elastic capsules, much like stretching a balloon to make it easier to inflate.[22]

There is a considerable energy cost in transforming dissolved gas into bubbles; this permits tissues to carry an excess gas load and consequently to tolerate a certain amount of supersaturation. A priori calculations of the energy cost using the physical values for pure water saturated with an ideal gas suggest that even a rapid decompression from 100 ata would be insufficient to result in the nucleation of bubbles.[23] This value depends critically on the surface tension of the dissolving liquid. Although the supersaturation pressure required to cause the nucleation of bubbles in physiological fluids is much lower than in pure water,[24] predictions based on such calculations determine that tissues should tolerate much higher levels of supersaturation than those levels that are implied by the occurrence of decompression sickness after reasonably shallow dives. This conclusion has led to the postulate that there are numerous microbubble nuclei already present in the body which will avidly take up additional gas from solution without incurring the energy cost involved in the formation of new bubbles. Evidence for the existence of microbubble nuclei has been provided by experiments showing that hamsters may be protected from bends by an initial short exposure to very deep depths, designed to drive these microbubble nuclei into solution, and by similar experiments in transparent shrimp.[25, 26]

Long experience suggests that divers can surface with a significant inert gas load and yet remain symptom-free. This observation has been interpreted as evidence that the gas remains in solution within tissues under these circumstances, but it may also mean that the body can tolerate a certain amount of bubble formation without obvious ill effects. This last possibility is supported by work suggesting that bubbles can be detected in the large vessels of asymptomatic divers after decompression.[27]

The calculation of decompression tables relies for the most part on the assumptions that the body is composed of multiple compartments and that each compartment can tolerate a certain degree of supersaturation. Initial observations in humans and goats[28] suggested that subjects could ascend up to one half the depth of the dive without developing decompression sickness. The diver could then spend some time at the new intermediate depth allowing his tissues to equilibrate and then ascend again. This remains the basis for the staged decompression used mainly by military and commercial divers. In saturation diving, which is carried out using a pressurized chamber in which the divers can be maintained in relative comfort for long periods of time while decompressing, this staged procedure is replaced by a slow continuous decompression. The original concept was that each tissue compartment could tolerate a constant ratio of dissolved gas pressure to ambient pressure, and the calculation of the time required at each intermediate depth depended on allowing the slowest compartment at that depth to "offgas." These compartments are not readily identified with a particular tissue but are approximations that more or less fit the observed incidence of bends after certain dives.[29] These mathematical assumptions are necessary because very little is really known about the rates at which various body tissues offgas. The selection of the rate of decompression is essentially an empirical process, calculated by algorithm derived from theory and proved by a record of successfully completed dives. Many profiles within most diving tables have been tested by only a few dives, and current algorithms are likely to be invalid if extended beyond the tested envelope.

CONSEQUENCES OF BUBBLE FORMATION

Tissue bubbles may invariably be present when the signs and symptoms of decompression sickness are present, but the converse of this statement is certainly not true. The occurrence of symptoms depends on the number of bubbles, their location, the presence of other associated injuries, and probably on a biological predisposition in the diver. In fact, direct evidence for bubble formation in most clinically relevant situations is lacking, due at least in part to the insensitivity of current bubble detectors. This is especially true for pain-only limb bends, which in many types of diving remains the most common form of decompression sickness. Certainly, there are situations, such as a catastrophic "blow-up" (the diver loses buoyancy control and rises suddenly to the surface), where many tissues, almost simultaneously, become supersaturated with inert gas and massive, uncontrolled bubble formation occurs with rapidly fatal consequences for the host. The detection of bubbles at postmortem presents no problem in this situation, and their effects on function are abundantly clear. Thankfully, blow-ups in divers are rare. Unfortunately, though, animal modeling of decompression sickness, particularly in small rodents, has for many years relied upon this technique in order to consistently generate decompression sickness. Thus, the extrapolation of findings from animal studies to the human experience should be treated with caution and account should be taken of the various features of each model.

The effects of bubble formation can be divided into two broad categories. An expanding bubble may produce mechanical effects, such as the distortion or tearing of tissues and the obstruction of blood flow. The mechanical effects may also include a release of the energy stored in the process of bubble formation as heat, when nascent bubbles collapse or coalesce. The presence of a gas-bubble interface is also a powerful stimulus to several systems involved in blood coagulation, the activation of leukocytes, fibrinolysis, and complement-mediated injury. These comprise the nonmechanical effects of bubbles.

Mechanical Effects of Bubbles

The formation of gas bubbles within the body is theoretically possible in a number of compartments—namely, within cells, between cells, and within blood vessels. In the latter case, bubbles could predominate in the arterial side of the circulation, acting as emboli and resulting in tissue infarction. Alternatively, gas could be released from a tissue at such a rate that the capillary bed becomes filled with bubbles and results in blood flow obstruction at that level. Finally, bubbles could accumulate in the venous side of the circulation, particularly in areas of low flow, and, combined with the effects of a blood-bubble interaction (vide infra), could provoke a sufficient obstruction to blood flow as to result in venous infarction.

Intracellular Bubble Formation

It is evident that if bubbles were to form and grow within cells, significant tissue destruction, akin to that seen after a freeze/thaw injury, would result. Such findings, however, are rare in the decompression literature. Unicellular organisms and erythrocytes have proven to be very resistant to intracellular bubble nucleation,[30, 31] and, although bubbles have been seen to form within decompressed hen's eggs,[32] such a diffusion-limited system is probably a poor model for larger organisms. Evidence for an intracellular gas phase in vertebrates is at present limited to the findings of mitochondrial membrane abnormalities[33] and of small bubbles within adipocytes of rapidly decompressed rodents.[34] The paucity of findings of intracellular gas and the rarity of hemolysis, for example, in decompression sickness make it reasonable to conclude that intracellular gas nucleation is an infrequent primary event in the pathogenesis of decompression sickness.

Intercellular Bubble Formation

The earliest description of the ill effects of decompression commented on the appearance of a bubble in the aqueous humor of a viper's eye,[35] an observation that has subsequently been repeated in the dog.[36] Bubbles have also been reported in the urine and CSF of acutely decompressed animals.[28] What role such bubbles play in decompression sickness remains unclear.

Despite the theoretical possibility for their existence, evidence for extracellular bubbles occurring within tissues has rarely been described in the literature. Two early reports claimed to demonstrate extracellular bubbles located principally in the white matter of the spinal cord of goats with decompression sickness.[28, 37] Subsequent investigation, however, has raised questions as to whether these tissue spaces were in fact evidence of intravascular gas bubbles.[38, 39] Although extracellular gas bubbles have been seen in the peripheral nerve myelin of rapidly decompressed guinea pigs,[40] whether this is a frequent occurrence within humans is unclear. The possible role in human decompression sickness of bubbles formed in spinal cord myelin and tendon is discussed below.

Intravascular Bubble Formation

Although the appearance of gas bubbles within blood vessels has been directly observed in the exteriorized cheek pouch of decompressed hamsters, accounts of their origin are conflicting. In one report, arterial bubbles appeared first,[41] and in others bubbles first appeared on the venous side.[42, 43] In these reports no nucleation of bubbles was seen within the field of vision, and bubbles were only observed subsequent to a severe decompression insult.

Most of the available evidence for the presence in vivo of gas bubbles in the blood stream following decompression is based on their detection by Doppler flowmeters. There are a number of limitations to this technique which should be borne in mind when considering the results: (1) bubbles can only be detected if they are moving, (2) the signals from small bubbles may be confused with those from blood components and other emboli such as platelet aggregations and lipid droplets, and (3) artifactual signals may arise from any movement of the transducer. The Doppler is a relatively insensitive technique for estimating bubble size, and where high intensity ultrasound is used, there is a theoretical possibility that its use may actually provoke bubble nucleation. Finally, the analysis of Doppler records is not wholly objective, particularly if the observer was not blinded to the outcome of the decompression.

Despite their limitations, numerous Doppler studies have been performed. The overwhelming evidence from both animal[44–46] and human[27, 47–49] studies is that during decompression, gas bubbles are first detected in the venous side of the circulation, that arterial bubbles are rarely observed except under conditions of severe decompression stress, but that when they are detected, their presence is accompanied by manifestations of serious decompression sickness. An important finding is that precordial Doppler monitoring for circulating gas bubbles is of limited diagnostic use. Although the detection of circulating gas is crudely correlated with decompression stress, it does not appear to correlate well with the clinical manifestation of decompression sickness.[27, 50]

The origin of arterial gas bubbles has been a matter of some controversy. It is unlikely that arterial blood is a frequent site of bubble nucleation, since there is a relatively high pressure opposing their formation and, having just passed through the lungs, the inert gas tension will have approached ambient. An alternative to gas nucleation as a mechanism for the appearance of arterial bubbles is microscopic pulmonary barotrauma, resulting in the release of showers of alveolar gas bubbles into the pulmonary veins.[51] Although there is little evidence for this as a primary mechanism for decompression sickness, there is some evidence that pulmonary barotrauma and arterial gas embolism may provoke decompression sickness in otherwise safe, no-stop dives.[52, 53]

A more probable origin of arterial bubbles is the transpulmonary passage of venous bubbles. The lung is a most efficient filter of glass beads[54] and gaseous emboli[55] in the size range of bubbles measured in the central venous blood of decompressed dogs,[56] but there is evidence that this capability may be reduced under certain circumstances. In the presence of massive intravenous bubbling, the filtering capacity of the lungs can be exceeded,[57, 58] which may be due to the opening of pulmonary arteriovenous shunts[59] or to a raised pulmonary artery pressure.[60] Other factors that may reduce the filtering capability of the lung are hypoxia,[59] oxygen toxicity,[61] and pulmonary vasodilators such as aminophylline.

Another potential source of arterial gas bubbles is the paradoxical embolism of venous bubbles through an intracardiac shunt. Actual or potential asymptomatic shunts are likely to be quite common in the diving community. The prevalence of a patent foramen ovale, for instance, varies from 6 to 35 per cent in the adult population.[62, 63] These abnormalities do not result in a significant right to left shunt under normal circumstances,[64] but transient flow quite often occurs during a Valsalva maneuver,[65] and there may be considerable shunting during the pulmonary hypertension that is associated with significant pulmonary gas embolism.[60]

Nonmechanical Effects of Bubble Formation

The ability of bubbles to distort tissue and to obstruct blood flow would be injurious even if the fluid surrounding the gas phase were bland and unreactive. However, blood is a highly reactive fluid, and the effects of a bubble are amplified by the activation of systems usually quiescent during normal intravascular flow. Tissues other than blood will also react to bubbles, but most experiments have addressed the activation of blood elements.

The interface between the gas phase and blood is a physical-chemical discontinuity, and its maintenance is associated with enormous electrochemical forces. These forces cause the denaturation of proteins, as the hydrophobic portions of the molecules will tend to have a lower free energy when surrounded by air than when surrounded by water[66] (Fig. 15–1). The denaturation of proteins can lead to the accumulation of globules of free fats and may also participate in the release of fatty acids from cell membranes, with the resultant formation of fat emboli.[67] Fat emboli have been observed in several pathological studies of decompression sickness and may contribute to the central nervous system damage.[68]

The forces that cause denaturation may also expose active sites on enzymes in the blood

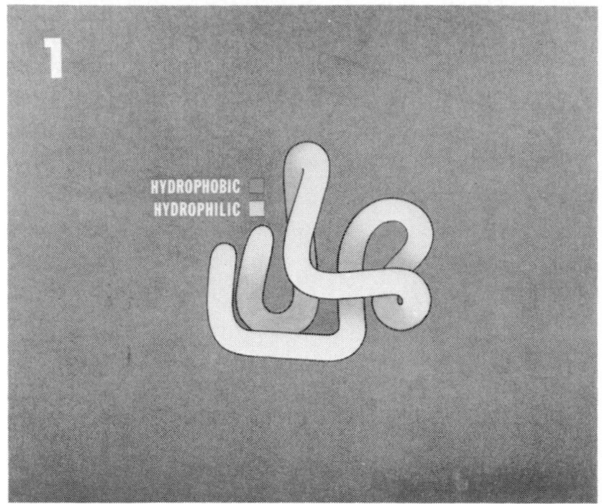

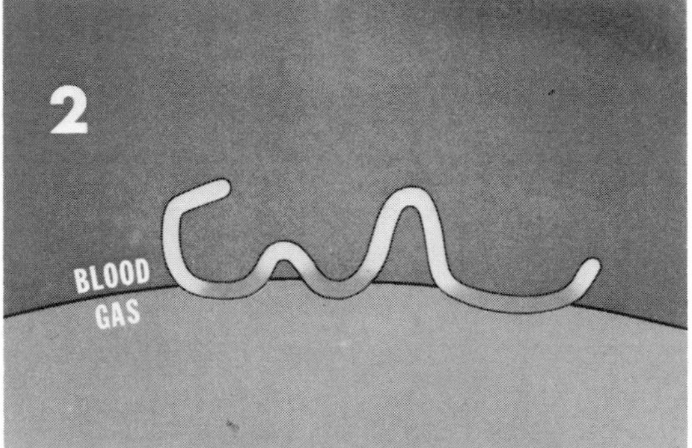

FIGURE 15–1. The first panel (1) depicts schematically a protein in aqueous solution, folded so that the hydrophobic groups are in the center, surrounded by more hydrophilic amino acids. This represents a highly ordered state, but one which minimizes the free energy of the protein in solution. The second panel (2) shows the unfolding that occurs at the blood-bubble interface. The arrangement is less ordered (more entropy) when the hydrophobic groups are surrounded by gas rather than by the folded protein, and thus the total free energy of the protein is less.

which activate the coagulation and complement systems. Bubbling air through cell-free plasma causes decreased coagulation time, presumably through activation of the contact system activator, Hageman factor.[69] In addition to initiating the plasma "intrinsic pathway" of thrombin formation, Hageman factor activates the plasma system for kinin formation, with resultant pain, vasodilatation, edema formation, and leukocyte chemotaxis, and also activates the plasma fibrinolysis system.[70] The activation of the complement system by the presence of bubbles has been demonstrated in rabbit serum and is also seen after cardiopulmonary bypass.[71, 72] The net effect of the activation of these systems is to extend any mechanical blockage of the circulation with progressive clotting and to further damage tissue by a reduction of local blood flow, the formation of edema and, possibly, toxic oxygen species, and by the attraction of leukocytes to the area.[52] The activated proteins will also distribute systemically and contribute to leukocyte trapping in the lungs[71] and probably to damage in sites remote from the original bubble formation.

Human studies have shown an increased hematocrit and decreased platelet count following decompression which are consistent with the development of edema and the activation of thrombin.[73] These changes further impair the flow in the microcirculation because they increase blood viscosity.[74] Leukocytes and platelets have been shown by electron microscopy to adhere to circulating bubbles[75]; this may lead to further impairment of the circulation by the formation of plugs. Both leukocytes and platelets have been shown to accumulate in areas of low blood flow after bubble-induced central nervous system injury.[76, 77] Thus, intravascular bubble formation can lead to a progressive process of clotting, which worsens any ischemia produced by the original mechanical blockage of the circulation. These effects are probably most important in the central nervous system form of decompression sickness, where small areas of reduced blood flow can produce severe disability.

CLINICAL PATTERNS OF DECOMPRESSION SICKNESS

The varied presentation of decompression sickness among the caisson workers who constructed the Dartford Tunnel led Golding and colleagues[51] to divide their cases into Type I, or "pain only," bends and Type II cases, which presented with symptoms other than pain or with abnormal signs. This classification has been refined by Elliott and Kindwall[78] such that Type I decompression sickness may now be defined as including musculoskeletal pain, cutaneous and lymphatic manifestations, and some nonspecific symptoms such as malaise, anorexia, and fatigue. The Type II category includes cases with any central nervous system defect, cardiorespiratory involvement, and peripheral neuropathy. This classification is based loosely on the perceived severity of the problem and on the response to treatment; Type I symptoms require no treatment or a brief repressurization, and Type II generally represents a more severe illness that poses greater problems in treatment. These divisions are not exclusive. It is not unusual for a Type I presentation to progress to a Type II illness, particularly when the onset of decompression sickness occurs soon after exposure. It is also common for both the patient and the physician to overlook minor neurological abnormalities in the presence of a painful limb bend, especially when the pain is severe. It is therefore important that patients with an apparently minor limb bend are not only carefully examined for neurological signs on presentation but are also routinely re-examined during treatment.

Type I Decompression Sickness

Musculoskeletal Pain

The onset of aching pain in a limb is the most classic and common manifestation of decompression sickness. The limb bend most frequently presents during decompression or soon after surfacing (95 per cent within 6 hours of surfacing), but the onset has been reported 36 or more hours after the dive. The first symptom may be a sensation that "something is wrong" or a subconscious desire to move the affected limb. Initially, the deep, aching pain is characteristically dull and vaguely localized. Over time it may progress to a more intense, throbbing pain, the location of which can be accurately indicated by the patient, although the area is not usually tender and, except in severe cases, movement of the affected joint does not exacerbate the pain. Often, divers will report much less intense sensations of fleeting aches and odd feelings, known collectively as the "niggles," prior to the development of a more classic type of pain or as the only symptom after a dive.

There are usually no physical signs associated with a limb bend, although the power of the local muscle groups may be lessened due to pain, and the adjacent skin may occasionally show a "peau d'orange" appearance associated with lymphatic obstruction. Any synovial joint may be affected, with the possible exception of the sternoclavicular joint, which has never been reported to be involved. When the pain is well localized, it is often described as being adjacent to rather than within the joint. In short dives on compressed air (bounce diving), the upper limbs are affected two to three times as frequently as the lower limbs, with the shoulder being the most common site. In contrast, it is the lower limbs that tend to predominate following caisson work, aviation, and deep oxy-helium dives, with symptoms around the knee most common.[79] When more than one site is affected, they are not usually symmetrically distributed.

The most striking feature of this pain is its rapid relief on recompression. To differentiate between the pain of bends and possible alternative causes is sometimes difficult, and recompression may be the only means of confirming the pain as that of decompression sickness. Musculoskeletal strain or injury is a likely alternative cause of pain after a dive because divers frequently perform hard manual labor on the bottom. This type of injury does not respond as promptly, if at all, to pressure. Pain due to ischemia (for example, because of tight tank straps) does not respond to pressure either, and the brief increase in the intensity of ischemic pain that accompanies the re-establishment of the circulation is not seen when bends are recompressed. Furthermore, when it is possible to increase the local hydrostatic pressure around a painful joint, as may be achieved for example by inflating an encircling sphygmomanometer cuff, the pain of bends may be temporarily relieved, unlike that associated with other causes. Finally, it is a frequent observation that if the recompression is inadequate, pain often returns to exactly the same site upon subsequent decompression.

The nature of the pain of a limb bend offers a number of clues as to its etiology. The rapid relief on the application of pressure and, in particular, the return to the same site if the recompression is inadequate, make ischemia secondary to an arterial gas embolism an unlikely cause. The pain is more probably produced by bubbles trapped within a tissue. Direct evidence for the presence of static bubbles in decompression has been forthcoming from the use of ultrasonic imaging in guinea pigs.[80] Preliminary studies employing this technique in human decompressions indicate that the presence of static bubbles may correlate with clinical decompression sickness.[81, 82] The means by which static bubbles cause pain are not entirely clear. One possibility is that bubbles are formed in a slow, but well-innervated, noncompliant tissue, and pain results from the physical deformation of nerve endings within the tissue.[83] The periarticular location of this pain and the widely recognized observation that the presence of gas bubbles within a joint space is not painful per se suggest that the tendinous capsules and muscle insertions are the site of the painful bubble formation. Evidence from animal studies shows that tendon has a low blood flow[84, 85] and even that flow may be intermittent[86]; thus, the rate of gas clearance is limited and would predispose it to bubble formation. Moreover, tendon is well innervated and pain, very similar to that caused by decompression sickness, can result if its interstitial pressure is raised by injecting Ringer's solution.[87] Bubble-induced complement activation, which has been shown to occur in blood,[72] may also be a response to bubble formation within tissues, leading to local inflammation and the generation of pain-producing kinins. However, the absence of physical signs of inflammation and the rapid resolution of symptoms with recompression imply that the major source of local pain is most likely to be due to the mechanical distortion of nerve endings rather than to their irritation by inflammatory substances.

Decompression Complications Affecting the Skin

The skin is often affected during and after decompression, and there are two distinct manifestations. The first type of problem is a transient multifocal pruritus affecting the trunk, ears, wrists, and hands. This problem most commonly occurs after dives in a hyperbaric chamber, where the diver's skin is directly exposed to high inert gas pressures, rather than after "wet" dives. This is also commonly associated with short, deep profiles. This syndrome is due to absorption of gas into the sweat glands and skin pores with resultant local bubble formation upon decompression. There may be an associated scarlatiniform rash, but this condition is not a harbinger of more serious sequelae and resolves without intervention.

An interesting feature of this pruritus is its occurrence in conditions for which there is no change of pressure but rather a sudden change of inert gas making up the chamber atmosphere, or if the diver breathes one inert gas when his skin is exposed to an atmosphere containing another. This isobaric counterdiffusion is an exception to the rule that decompression is needed to produce decompression sickness; it is due to the fact that diffusion of a new inert gas into tissue can occur faster than the previous one leaves, leading to transient tissue overpressure and bubble formation.[88] This syndrome is only seen in unusual circumstances but may involve the vestibular system as well, leading to more serious sequelae.

The second type of skin problem in decompression is what is classically referred to as cutaneous decompression sickness. The syndrome commences with itching, which may be intense. The pruritic areas, usually limited to the trunk, are first reddened by vasodilation in the dermis, then vascular stasis results in a characteristic mottling of the skin. If the skin is examined at this stage, confluent rings of pallor are seen surrounding areas of cyanosis, which blanche to the touch (cutis marmorata). This is quite different from the peau d'orange lesion from skin lymphatic obstruction which may be associated with the musculoskeletal pain of limb bends. Recompression will promptly relieve the itching, although if left alone the condition resolves over a period of days; thus, treatment is more for comfort than to avoid possible complications. In aviators, in whom this condition is rare, two cases have been reported whereby this form of cutaneous decompression sickness preceded neurocirculatory collapse. Careful observation of these cases is prudent.[89] Cutaneous decompression sickness is thought to be due either to obstruction of the skin's venous drainage by bubbles or to vasospasm that is provoked by the presence of bubbles within skin.[90]

There have been rare reports of bubbles forming in the lymph nodes and the parotid gland after decompression, with resultant swelling and pain.[78] These symptoms are usually considered minor, and therapy is undertaken only if the symptoms warrant it.

Constitutional Symptoms

Fatigue is a frequent sequel to hyperbaric exposures, even if the workload has been light. It is usually transient and therefore ignored. Occasionally, however, the exhaustion is sufficiently marked to provoke comment, and then it is often a forerunner or accompaniment of more serious signs of decompression sickness.[91] Rarely, fatigue is the only presenting symptom of decompression sickness. Other constitutional symptoms include malaise and anorexia. A number of mechanisms have been proposed for the cause of these symptoms, including adrenocortical exhaustion,[92] subclinical pulmonary gas embolism,[93] and involvement of cerebral structures concerned with wakefulness by decompression sickness.[94] If brain involvement is responsible for the exhaustion and anorexia seen after certain dives, these signs may warrant early and vigorous treatment as a Type II decompression sickness.

Type II Decompression Sickness

Type II decompression sickness may occur alone or in combination with musculoskeletal pain. One series estimated that about 30 per cent of Type II bends was accompanied by pain.[84] The three principal targets of this condition are the pulmonary, nervous, and vestibular systems.

Pulmonary Decompression Sickness ("Chokes")

As Table 15–1 shows, this is a relatively rare condition in diving, and it generally occurs with very rapid, emergency ascents. Aviators, however, are more likely to suffer a sudden, severe decompression than divers, and this may account for the greater frequency of pulmonary decompression sickness in this group.[96] The onset is usually heralded by a sensation of substernal discomfort that commences within minutes of reaching the surface. Initially, the pain may be present alone or may be accompanied by a cough, but as it progresses, pain occurs on both inspiration and expiration. Deep breaths worsen the discomfort and may provoke paroxysms of unproductive coughing. The breathing pattern becomes rapid and shallow; cyanosis may develop at this point, as well as signs of right heart failure. At this stage the patient is in cardiovascular shock, and immediate treatment with recompression and hyperbaric oxygen is essential. Fluid resuscitation and pressor agents may also be required.

This disorder is almost certainly caused by the direct and indirect effects of massive pulmonary gas embolism. In experimental animals, pulmonary arterial pressure and right ventricular pressure rise, and cardiac output and arterial pO_2 fall after a severe decompression stress.[97, 98] This occurs in concert with the detection of bubbles in the pulmonary artery,[99] and these symptoms are quite similar to the effects of a shower of any pulmonary emboli. The surface activity of bubbles may cause the trapping of leukocytes in the lung, their resultant release of vasoactive substances and proteolytic enzymes, and production of toxic oxygen species.[100] The syndrome resembles the adult respiratory distress syndrome (ARDS), which has been reported as a consequence of accidental venous air embolism.[101]

Neurological Decompression Sickness

Clinical Findings

The incidence of neurological involvement in decompression sickness varies from one population to another. In general, the incidence is highest in sport divers, most notably among the irresponsible minority who dive without adequate training or supervision. In commercial and military diving, Type II decompression sickness is more commonly associated with bounce than saturation diving, and the involvement of the central nervous system is more common following short, deep dives than longer, shallow ones.[102, 103] The risk of decompression sickness varies from table to table and even between dive profiles within a given table.[104] Add to this situation the likelihood that minor bends go unreported and one finds that any assessment of the true incidence is most unreliable. A bends rate of about 1 per cent is expected in most tables, with the proportion of Type I illness being about 86 per cent in military populations[105] and Type II as much as 80 per cent among sport divers.[106]

One problem in assessing many series of neurological decompression sickness is that the findings are presented in such a way that it is not possible, with confidence, to locate the lesions that cause the signs and symptoms. Another problem is that the timing and quality of the physical examination of patients has been quite variable. It is often the case that divers delay reporting their symptoms, and there is inevitably a further delay before any examination or treatment. Hence, transient signs and symptoms may be missed. The situation is worst in the case of civilian sport divers, although significant delays may occur in commercial and occasionally in military diving accidents. It is unusual for any diver to undergo a specialist neurological examination prior to treatment, if only because the urgency of commencing treatment precludes it.

Where careful neurological examination has been undertaken and reported, even though this may be after treatment, the pattern of neurological injury may differ from classical descriptions. Historically, early reports strongly implicated the spinal cord as the primary site of central nervous system injury in decompression sickness, with the lower thoracic and upper lumbar cord being most frequently involved.[107, 108] This observation has been borne out by some more recent series.[91, 95, 106] On the other hand, there is also evidence to indicate that the brain may be hit with at least equal frequency,[109–113] and two series[110, 114] report a considerable incidence of peripheral nerve involvement.

In view of the above, it is not possible to describe a representative case of neurological decompression sickness. Cerebral decompression sickness may present with a wide variety of symptoms such as a change in personality, loss of recent memory, an acute psychosis, headache, dysphasia, visual disturbances, or more peripheral sensory losses, pareses, and plegias. Spinal cord lesions may be preceded or accompanied by loin pain. A characteristic and sinister march of events is the onset of a blunting of sensation in the legs with paresthesia, progressing to motor weakness, paraplegia, and a loss of bowel and bladder sphincter control. One feature of severe spinal cord injury, often overlooked, is the remarkable rapidity with which its onset can become manifest. In a recent series of 26 cases, for example, 19 (71.3 per cent) reported onset times within 4 minutes, and 23 (88.5 per cent) had reported within 20 minutes of surfacing.[115] Less complete spinal lesions may present more slowly and as a Brown-Séquard syndrome.

When describing the symptoms of decompression sickness involving the nervous system, it is useful to remember that the hallmark of the spinal cord lesion is signs distributed up to a level on the trunk or hip, and that loss of power or sensation or both confined to one limb is often better localized to the cortex. Any neurological symptom must be taken seriously, however, even if unaccompanied by signs.

Pathogenesis

Few topics in the study of decompression sickness have generated more research effort and controversy than the mechanism of central nervous system injury. The following is but a brief résumé, and interested readers may wish to refer to more detailed reviews.[52, 68]

Arterial Gas Emboli. From the earliest days of research into the subject, there have been proponents of the view that the primary event in neurological decompression sickness is the arterial embolism of gas bubbles[1, 2, 28, 116] and that consequent CNS ischemia results in the neurological manifestations and pathological findings of the disease. This approach is attractive for its simplicity, but there are a number of features of the condition which this mechanism fails to explain. Among other objections to the hypothesis, Hallenbeck and co-workers point out that in all other embolic conditions of the central nervous system, it is the brain that is the principal target.[93] One reason why the brain apparently escapes injury in decompression sickness may be that gas bubbles are less damaging to the brain than other emboli. The evidence for this is not good. One carotid artery Doppler study of patients undergoing open-heart surgery reported that all patients received significant numbers of gaseous emboli, yet the incidence of psychiatric and neurological symptoms was low.[117] On the other hand, more recent reports suggest a rather higher incidence.[118, 119] Spinal symptoms following such surgery are rarely reported. Considering that the spinal cord appears to be more resistant to ischemia than the brain,[120] one would expect that cerebral symptoms would predominate in decompression sickness if an arterial embolic phenomenon were entirely responsible. It is conceivable that cerebral embolism occurs in decompression sickness but remains clinically silent, whereas all spinal emboli result in symptomatic lesions due to limited redundancy in the cord. For example, it is generally cerebral rather than spinal lesions that escape clinical detection in multiple sclerosis.[121, 122] It may be that this has occurred to some extent in decompression sickness, since there is a growing realization that some more subtle cerebral lesions may go unrecognized in divers.[49, 112, 113, 123–127] It seems unlikely however, that unrecognized disease offers a complete explanation for the considerable disparity between the ratio of lesions in the spinal cord and cerebrum in decompression sickness compared with other embolic diseases of the CNS. For, if the normally tiny ratio[128] was occurring in decompression sickness but was apparently increased to even 50 per cent due to silent cerebral lesions, such massive cerebral injury would be sustained by divers and compressed-air workers that it is hard to believe it has remained silent for so long! Although it is unlikely that simple blockage of arteries by gas accounts for the prominence of spinal cord involvement in decompression sickness, Palmer's conception, which emphasizes a combination of bubble triggered rheological disturbances and local conditions acting in concert with the impact of arterial emboli on the spinal circulation, deserves further consideration.[39]

Venous Infarction. In a paper exploring a number of possible mechanisms of CNS decompression sickness, Haymaker and Johnson[129] proposed that venous engorgement of the spinal cord, due to the presence of bubbles in the spinovertebral venous system and back pressure from bubble-laden lungs through anastomotic venous channels, might contribute to the injury. Using animal models of decompression sickness, Hallenbeck, Bove, and Elliot initiated studies that have provided convincing evidence that the venous drainage of the spinal cord is indeed compromised by bubbles and the products of the blood-bubble interaction following a spinal cord–damaging dive.[130–133] Several other laboratories have obtained evidence supporting this mechanism in animals[134] and humans.[135, 136] However, Hills and James[137] point out that this theory also suffers from shortcomings, namely, that venous stasis could occur as either a cause or an effect of spinal cord injury, and that it is difficult to understand how such an extensive venous lake as the epidural vertebral venous system could be blocked sufficiently to cause spinal cord dysfunction and, if it were, why lesions should be largely limited to the white matter. Finally, they point out that, as with limb bends, if recompression is inadequate, then spinal symptoms return to their original distribution. Such an observation limits the validity of any etiology based on vascular obstruction, since once the blockage has presumably been cleared by recompression and the patient rendered asymptomatic, the probability of an identical vascular obstruction occurring with premature decompression is presumably very small. It should be noted, however, that since the epidural vertebral venous system is more of a lake than a unidirectional conduit, bubble obstruction could be partially relieved by recompression only to reoccur as the bubble re-expands upon surfacing. It could also lead to the same signs and symptoms because the bubble nucleus would not have been swept away, as it might be by the more continuous flow of the peripheral veins.

The Autochthonous Bubble Hypothesis. This mechanism, which is based upon the concept that tissue injury is caused by the consequences of bubble nucleation and growth within the tissue, has a long history. It was discussed by Bert[116] and Boycott, Damant, and Haldane,[28] and in both instances it was rejected as a mechanism for spinal cord dysfunction in decompression sickness in favor of an intravascular pathophysiology. It was again proposed, on purely theoretical grounds, by Keyser,[138] but it was not until the work of Hills and James in the early 1980's that the hypothesis received serious scientific attention.[137] Following a study of the mechanical properties of dura mater and spinal cord tissue, they proposed that bubbles form within myelin or between the nerves of the cord and, in so doing, raise the tissue pressure sufficiently to exceed the arteriolar closing pressure and thus to provoke ischemia.

This mechanism has suffered, however, from a paucity of evidence that extravascular bubbles ever form in the spinal cord. Some early histological studies reported air lacerations[139] and stippling[140] within the white matter of caisson workers and divers which rapidly succumbed from decompression sickness. More recently, there was a report of the neuropathological study of a diver who suffered a similar fate, which described and illustrated round, nonstaining spaces in the brain and spinal cord.[136] In animal studies, abnormalities of spinal cord myelin have been described that may be interpreted as evidence of autochthonous bubble injury,[141] and recently numerous overt, nonstaining, space-occupying lesions in spinal cord myelin have been demonstrated by both light and electron microscopy[142] (Fig. 15–2). In this recent work, it is proposed that autochthonous bubbles may impair spinal cord function by three mechanisms: the mechanical disruption of conducting tissue, the effect of pressure on adjacent axons,[143, 144] and by ischemia. It is considered that the ischemia is likely to be localized to the tissue immediately surrounding these bubbles, since current estimates of their volume indicate that they are unlikely to result in the global ischemia described by Hills and James. It is further postulated that these bubbles are rarely described because they are short-lived.[145] It is considered likely that they impose shearing forces on the delicate microcirculation of the white matter during nucleation and growth and, therefore, may be precursors of the scattered, punctate hemorrhages that are a common histopathological feature of the disease.[146]

Whatever the pathogenesis of spinal cord decompression sickness, there is some evidence that clinical recovery of function is not necessarily dependent upon the restoration of normal spinal cord architecture. The postmortem findings in human and animal cases of spinal cord decompression sickness, which have made a considerable or apparently complete recovery and die from an unrelated cause, demonstrate considerable scarring and residual demyelination.[148–152] It is possible that a significant proportion of the recovery seen in spinal cord decompression sickness treated without recompression[153] and following incompletely successful therapy with recompression and oxygen[154] is due to the recruitment of alternative pathways within the spinal cord. There is good evidence that such a process occurs during the functional recovery from surgical section of the spinal cord.[155]

Vestibular Decompression Sickness: the "Staggers"

A relatively common presentation of decompression sickness is as a syndrome of dizzi-

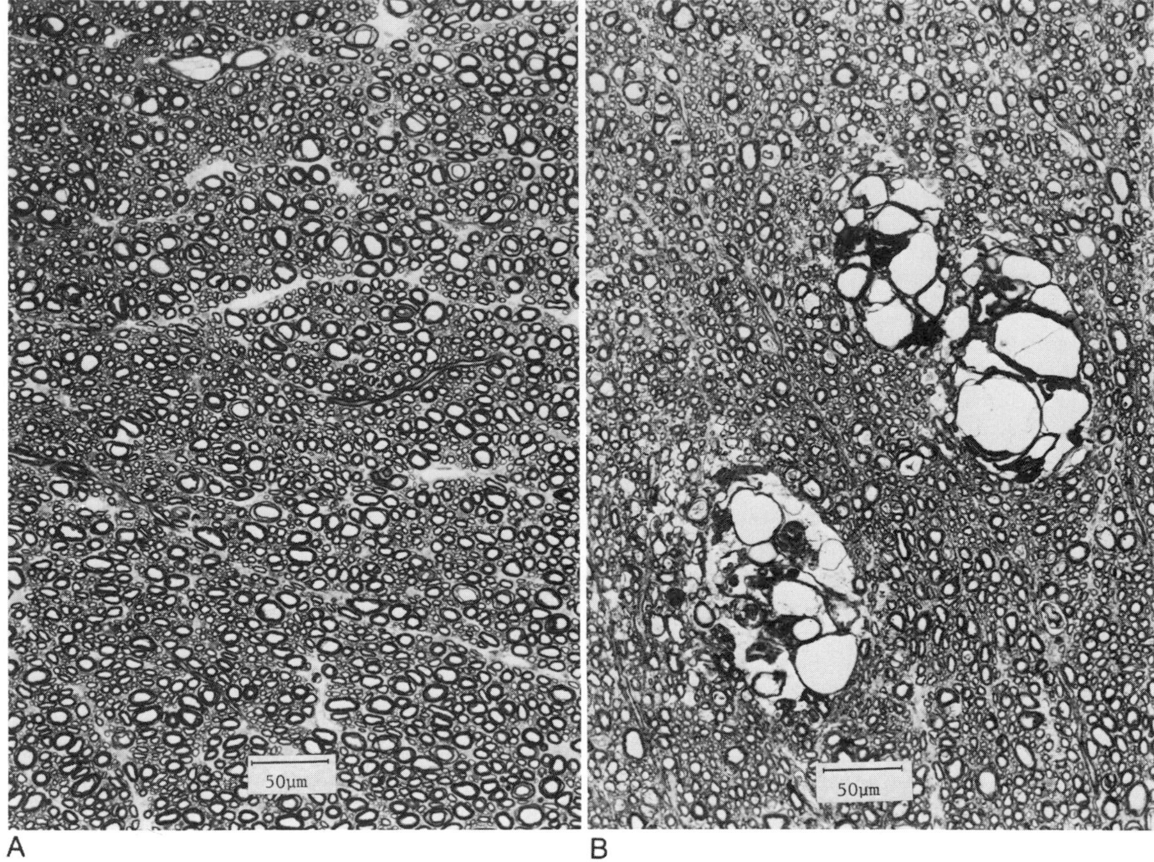

FIGURE 15–2. Two views of canine spinal cord white matter stained with multiple stain solution (bar = 50 µm). Panel *A* control, Panel *B* spinal cord rapidly fixed after the onset of decompression sickness. Note: large nonstaining spaces contain disrupted myelin figures and some compression of normal surrounding tissue. (Methodology described in Francis TJR, Pezeshkpour AH, Dutka AJ, et al: Is there a role for the autochthonous bubble in the pathogenesis of spinal cord decompression sickness? J Neuropathol Exp Neurol 47:475–487, 1988.)

ness, nausea, vomiting, nystagmus, and, occasionally, hearing loss and tinnitus. The incidence of these symptoms varies from as little as 13 per cent to as much as 72 per cent of cases of Type II decompression sickness. This syndrome is more prevalent in saturation than in bounce diving. The typical presentation is of the sudden onset of vertigo, with or without tinnitus and hearing loss, upon decompression. A few of these cases have been reported after gas switching at depth[156] and are probably due to the isobaric counterdiffusion mentioned above. The pathology of the lesion in experimental animals consists of rupture of the delicate membranes in the semicircular canals and cochlea, with bleeding and, as healing occurs, new bone formation.[157] The forces generated by decompression must be considerable because this is occasionally accompanied by petrous bone fractures.[158] New bone formation has also been documented in pathological specimens from active divers.[159]

It is unclear how much of the very common problems of hearing loss in commercial and military divers after many years of service may be due to decompression sickness. These individuals also invariably work in a very noisy environment, and the long-term effects of noise trauma and decompression sickness are indistinguishable. In addition, repeated ear "squeeze" can result in hearing loss as well.

CONCLUSION

Decompression sickness is a complex condition that presents a considerable challenge to health care workers involved with diving. Its manifestations are protean, and its cause, although seemingly simple, has many subtle ramifications. With any symptom occurring soon after diving, think of the possibility of decompression sickness and refer the patient to a recompression facility as soon as possible. A high index of suspicion and a liberal use of recompression in doubtful cases will help to reduce the morbidity and mortality associated with diving.

REFERENCES

1. Gersh I, Catchpole HR: Decompression sickness: Physical factors and pathologic consequences. *In* Fulton JF (ed): Decompression Sickness. Philadelphia, WB Saunders Company, 1951, pp 165–181.
2. Behnke AR: Decompression sickness. Milit Med 117:257–271, 1955.
3. Hills BA: Decompression Sickness. Vol 1: The Biophysical Basis of Prevention and Treatment. Chichester, John Wiley & Sons, 1977, pp 167–168.
4. Kety SS: Theory and application of exchange of inert gases at lungs and tissue. Pharmacol Rev 3:1–41, 1951.
5. Larsen OA, Lassen NA, Quaade F: Blood flow through human adipose tissue determined with radioactive xenon. Acta Physiol Scand 66:337–345, 1966.
6. Mitchell HH, Hamilton TS, Steggera FR, Bean HW: The chemical composition of the adult human body and its bearing on the biochemistry of growth. J Biol Chem 158:625–637, 1945.
7. Sandler AN, Tator CH: Review of the measurement of the spinal cord blood flow. Brain Res 118:181–198, 1976.
8. Brante G: Studies on lipids in the nervous system with special reference to quantitative chemical determination and topical distribution. Acta Physiol Scand 18(suppl 63):1–189, 1949.
9. Scheinberg P, Meyer JS, Reivich M, et al: Cerebral circulation and metabolism in stroke. Stroke 7:213–233, 1976.
10. Norton WT, Poduslo SE, Suzuki K: Subacute sclerosing leucoencephalitis. II. Chemical studies including abnormal myelin and an abnormal ganglioside pattern. J Neuropathol Exp Neurol 25:582–597, 1966.
11. Rothe CF, Friedman JF: Control of the cardiovascular system. *In* Selkurt EE (ed): Physiology. 3rd ed. Boston, Little, Brown & Company, 1971, pp 371–394.
12. Shepherd JT: Circulation to skeletal muscle. *In* Shephert JT, Abboud FM, Geiger SR (eds): Handbook of Physiology. Sec 2, Vol III, Part I. Bethesda, American Physiological Society, 1983, pp 319–370.
13. Hermansson K, Osteg G, Walgast M: The cortical and medullary blood flow at different levels of renal nerve activity. Acta Physiol Scand 120:161–169, 1984.
14. D'aoust BG, Smith KH, Swanson HT: Decompression-induced decrease in nitrogen elimination in awake dogs. J Appl Physiol 41:348–355, 1976.
15. Hills BA: Effect of decompression per se on nitrogen elimination. J Appl Physiol 45:916–921, 1978.
16. Kindwall EP, Baz A, Lightfoot EN, et al: Nitrogen elimination in man during decompression. Undersea Biomed Res 2:285–297, 1975.
17. Haymaker W, Davidson C: Fatalities resulting from exposure to simulated high altitudes in decompression chambers: A clinico-pathologic study of five cases. J Neuropathol Exp Neurophysiol 9:29–59, 1950.
18. Weathersby PK: Personal communication, 1986.
19. Rugman F, Meecham J: Spinal decompression sickness at unusually shallow depth. J Soc Occup Med 35:103–104, 1985.
20. Gray JS: Constitutional factors affecting decompression sickness. *In* Fulton JR (ed): Decompression Sickness. Philadelphia, WB Saunders Company, 1951, pp 187–190.
21. Rattner BA, Gruenau S, Altland PD: Cross-adaptive effects of cold, hypoxia, or physical training on decompression sickness in mice. J Appl Physiol 47:412–417, 1979.
22. Vann RD, Clark HG: Bubble growth and mechanical properties of tissues in decompression. Undersea Biomed Res 2:185–194, 1975.
23. Hemmingsen EA: Supersaturation of gases in water: Absence of cavitation on decompression from high pressures. Science 197:1493, 1970.
24. Weathersby PK, Homer LD, Flynn ET: Homogeneous nucleation of gas bubbles in vivo. J Appl Physiol 53:940–946, 1982.
25. Evans A, Walder DN: Significance of gas micronuclei in the etiology of decompression sickness. Nature 222:251–252, 1969.
26. Vann RD, Grimstad J, Nielsen CH: Evidence for gas nucleii in decompressed rats. Undersea Biomed Res 7:107–112, 1980.
27. Bayne CG, Hunt WS, Johanson DC, et al: Doppler bubble detection and decompression sickness: A prospective clinical trial. Undersea Biomed Res 12:327–332, 1985.
28. Boycott AE, Damant GCC, Haldane JS: The prevention of compressed air illness. J Hyg 8:342–443, 1908.
29. Weathersby PK, Homer LD: Current concepts of inert gas exchange and decompression. *In* Bachrach A (ed): Underwater Physiology VII. Bethesda, Undersea Medical Society, 1981, pp 687–698.
30. Harvey EN: Decompression sickness and bubble formation in blood and tissues. Bull NY Acad Med 21:505–536, 1945.
31. Hemmingsen BB, Steinberg NA, Hemmingsen EA: Intracellular gas supersaturation tolerances of erythrocytes and resealed ghosts. Biophys J 47:491–496, 1985.
32. Paganelli CV, Strauss RH, Yount DE: Bubble formation within decompressed hen's eggs. Aviat Space Environ Med 48:48–49, 1977.
33. Bennett RA: Fine structure of decompression sickness. *In* Schilling CW, Beckett MW (eds): Underwater Physiology VI. Proceedings of the 6th Symposium on Underwater Physiology, San Diego, 1975. Bethesda, FASEB, 1978.
34. Gersh I, Hawkinson GE, Jenney EH: Comparison of vascular and extravascular bubbles following decompression from high pressure atmospheres of oxygen, helium-oxygen, argon-oxygen and air. J Cell Comp Physiol 26:63–74, 1945.
35. Boyle R: New pneumatical experiments about respiration. Philos Trans R Soc Lond 5:2011–2031, 2031–2056, 1670.
36. Cockett ATK, Nakamura RM, Franks JJ: Recent findings in the pathogenesis of decompression sickness (dysbarism). Surgery 58:384–389, 1965.
37. Hamilton PT, Haldane JS, Bacon HS, Lees E: Deep Water Diving. CN1549. London, Her Majesty's Stationary Office, 1907.

38. Palmer AC: The pathology of spinal cord lesions in goats. *In* James PB, McCallum RI, Rawlins JSP (eds): Report of the Proceedings of Symposium on Decompression Sickness—VIII Annual Congress of the EUBS. Cambridge, 1981, pp 46–52.
39. Palmer AC: The neuropathology of decompression sickness. *In* Cavanagh JB (ed): Recent Advances in Neuropathology. 3rd ed. New York, Churchill Livingstone, 1986, pp 141–162.
40. Gersh I, Hawkinson GE, Rathbun EN: Tissue and vascular bubbles after decompression from high pressure atmospheres—correlation of specific gravity with morphological changes. J Cell Comp Physiol 24:35–70, 1944.
41. Buckles RG: The physics of bubble formation and growth. Aerosp Med 39:1062–1069, 1968.
42. Heimbecker RO, Koven I, Richards K: Role of gas embolism in decompression sickness. *In* Defense and Civil Institute of Environmental Medicine, Conference Proceedings, December 1973, pp 218–226.
43. Lynch PR, Brigham M, Tuma R, Wiedeman MP: Origin and time course of gas bubbles following rapid decompression in the hamster. Undersea Biomed Res 12:105–114, 1985.
44. Evans A, Barnard EEP, Walder DN: Detection of gas bubbles in man at decompression. Aerosp Med 43:1095–1096, 1972.
45. Spencer MP, Campbell SD: Development of bubbles in venous and arterial blood during hyperbaric decompression. *In* Lambertsen CJ (ed): Underwater Physiology V. Bethesda, FASEB, 1976.
46. Spencer MP, Campbell SD, Sealey JL, et al: Experiments on decompression bubbles in the circulation using ultrasonic and electromagnetic flowmeters. J Occup Med 11:238–244, 1969.
47. Gardette B: Correlation between decompression sickness and circulating bubbles in 232 divers. Undersea Biomed Res 6:99–107, 1979.
48. Nashimto I, Gotoh Y: Relationship between precordial doppler ultrasound records and decompression sickness. *In* Shilling CW, Beckett MW (eds): Underwater Physiology VI. Bethesda, FASEB, 1978, pp 497–501.
49. Powell MR, Johanson DC: Ultrasound monitoring and decompression sickness. *In* Shilling CW, Beckett MW (eds): Underwater Physiology VI. Bethesda, FASEB, 1978, pp 503–510.
50. Eatock BC, Nishi RY: Analysis of doppler ultrasound data for the evaluation of dive profiles. *In* Bove AA, Bachrach AJ, Greenbaum LJ (eds): Underwater Physiology IX. Bethesda, Undersea and Hyperbaric Medical Society, 1987, pp 183–195.
51. Golding FC, Griffiths P, Hempleman HV, et al: Decompression sickness during construction of the Dartford Tunnel. Br J Indust Med 17:167–180, 1960.
52. Hallenbeck JM, Andersen JC: Pathogenesis of the decompression disorders. *In* Bennett PB, Elliott DH (eds): The Physiology and Medicine of Diving. 3rd Ed. San Pedro, Best Publishing Company, 1982, pp 435–460.
53. Newman TJ, Bove AA: Severe refractory Type II decompression sickness resulting from combined no-decompression dives and pulmonary barotrauma. *In* Bove AA, Bachrach AJ, Greenbaum LJ (eds): Proceedings of the IX International Symposium on Underwater and Hyperbaric Physiology. Bethesda, Undersea and Hyperbaric Medical Society, 1987, pp 985–991.
54. Ring GC, Blum S, Kurbatov T, et al: Size of microspheres passing through the pulmonary circuit in the dog. Am J Physiol 200:1191–1196, 1961.
55. Butler BD, Hills BA: The lung as a filter for microbubbles. J Appl Physiol 47:537–543, 1979.
56. Hills BA, Butler BD: Size distribution of intravascular air emboli produced by decompression. Undersea Biomed Res 8:163–174, 1981.
57. Butler BD, Hills BA: Transpulmonary passage of venous air emboli. J Appl Physiol 59:543–547, 1985.
58. Spencer MP, Oypma Y: Pulmonary capacity for dissipation of venous gas emboli. Aerosp Med 42:822–827, 1971.
59. Niden AH, Aviado DM: Effects of pulmonary embolism on the pulmonary circulation with special reference to arterio-venous shunts in the lung. Circ Res 4:67–73, 1956.
60. Butler BD, Katz J: Vascular pressures and passage of gas emboli through the pulmonary circulation. Undersea Biomed Res 15:203–209, 1988.
61. Butler BD, Hills BA: Effect of excessive oxygen upon the capability of the lungs to filter gas emboli. *In* Bachrach AJ, Matzen MM (eds): Underwater Physiology VII. Bethesda, Undersea Medical Society, 1981.
62. Meister SG, Grossman W, Dexter L, Dalen JE: Paradoxical embolism: Diagnosis during life. Am J Med 53:292, 1972.
63. Thompson T, Evans W: Paradoxical embolism. Q J Med 23:135, 1930.
64. Mellemgaard K, Lassen NA, Georg J: Right to left shunt in normal man determined by the use of tritium and krypton 85. J Appl Physiol 17:770–782, 1962.
65. Lynch JJ, Schuchard GH, Gross CM, Wann LS: Prevalence of right-to-left atrial shunting in a healthy population: Detection by valsalva maneuver constrast echocardiography. Am J Cardiol 53:1478–1480, 1984.
66. Lee WH, Hairston P: Structural effects on blood proteins at the gas-blood interface. Fed Proc 30:1615–1620, 1971.
67. Lee WH, Krumhaar D, Fonkalsrud EF, et al: Denaturation of plasma proteins as a cause of morbidity and death after intracardiac operations. Surgery 50:29–39, 1961.
68. Haymaker W: Decompression sickness. *In* Lubarsh O, Henke F, Rassle R (eds): Handbuch der Speziellen Pathologischen: Anatomie und Histologie. Vol XIII, Pt 1. Berlin, Springer-Verlag, 1957, pp 1600–1672.
69. Hallenbeck JM, Bove AA, Elliott DH: The bubble as a non-mechanical trigger in decompression sickness. *In* Ackles KN (ed): Proceedings of a Symposium on Blood Bubble Interactions. Defense and Civil Institute Environmental Medicine Report No. 73-CP-960, Downsview, Ontario, 1973.
70. Ogston D, Bennett B: Surface mediated reactions in the formation of thrombin, plasmin, and kallikrein. Br Med Bull 34:107–112, 1978.
71. Chenoweth DE, Cooper SW, Hugli TE, et al: Complement activation during cardiopulmonary bypass. N Engl J Med 304:497–503, 1981.
72. Ward CA, Koheil A, McCulloch D, et al: Activation of complement at the plasma-air or serum-air interface of rabbits. J Appl Physiol 60:1651–1658, 1986.
73. Philp RB, Ackles KN, Inwood MJ, et al: Changes in the hemostatic system and in blood and urine chemistry of human subjects following decompression from a hyperbaric enviroment. Aerosp Med 43:498–505, 1972.

74. Hallenbeck JM: Some aspects of the pathophysiology of decompression sickness. *In* Weekly Update: Hyperbaric and Undersea Medicine. Vol 1, No. 10. Princeton, Biomedia, 1978.
75. Philp RB, Inwood MJ, Warren BA: Interactions between gas bubbles and components of the blood: Implications in decompression sickness. Aerosp Med 43:946–953, 1972.
76. Hallenbeck JM, Dutka AJ, Tanishima T, et al: Polymorphonuclear leukocyte accumulation in brain regions with low blood flow during the early postischemic period. Stroke 17:246–253, 1986.
77. Obrenovitch TP, Kumaroo KK, Hallenbeck, JM: Autoradiographic detection of ^{111}In labelled platelets in brain tissue sections. Stroke 15:1049–1056, 1984.
78. Elliott DH, Kindwall EP: Manifestations of the decompression disorders. *In* Bennett PB, Elliott DH (eds): The Physiology and Medicine of Diving. 3rd Ed. San Pedro, Best Publishing Company, 1982.
79. Elliott DH, Hallenbeck JM, Bove AA: Acute decompression sickness. Lancet 2:1193–1199, 1974.
80. Daniels S, Davies JM, Paton WDM, Smith EB: The detection of gas bubbles in guinea-pigs after decompression from air saturation dives. J Physiol 308:369–385, 1980.
81. Daniels S, Davies JM, Paton WDM, Smith EB: Recent experiments using ultrasonic imaging to monitor bubble formation in divers. *In* Bachrach AJ, Matzen MM (eds): Underwater Physiology VIII. Bethesda, Undersea Medical Society, 1984.
82. Rubissow GR, MacKay RS: Decompression study and control using ultrasonics. Aerosp Med 45:476–478, 1974.
83. Nims LF: A physical theory of decompression sickness. *In* Fulton JF (ed): Decompression Sickness. Philadelphia, WB Saunders Company, 1951, pp 192–222.
84. Hopper G, Davies R, Tothil P: Blood flow and clearance in tendons: Studies with dogs. J Bone Joint Surg 66B:441–443, 1984.
85. Weidman KA, Simoner WT, Wood MB, et al: Quantification of regional blood flow to canine flexor tendons. J Orthop Res 2:257–261, 1984.
86. Hills BA: Intermittent flow in tendon capillary bundles. J Appl Physiol 46:696–702, 1979.
87. Inman VT, Saunders JB: Referred pain from skeletal structures. J Nerv Ment Dis 99:660–667, 1944.
88. Lambertsen CJ, Idicula J: A new gas lesion in man, induced by "isobaric gas counterdiffusion." J Appl Physiol 39:434–443, 1975.
89. Davis JC, Sheffield PJ, Schucknecht L, et al: Altitude decompression sickness: Hyperbaric therapy results in 145 cases. Aviat Space Environ Med 48:722–730, 1970.
90. Dennison WL: A review of the pathogenesis of skin bends. U.S. Naval Submarine Medical Center Report No 660. New London, CT, 1971.
91. Kidd DJ, Elliott DH: Clinical manifestations and treatment of decompression sickness in divers. *In* Bennett PB, Elliott DH (eds): The Physiology and Medicine of Diving and Compressed Air Work. London, Baillere Tindall and Cassell, 1969, pp 464–490.
92. Dewey WA: Decompression sickness—an emerging recreational hazard. N Engl J Med 267:759–820, 1962.
93. Hallenbeck JM, Bove AA, Elliott DH: Decompression sickness studies. *In* Lambertsen CJ (ed): Underwater Physiology V. Bethesda, FASEB, 1976, pp 273–286.
94. Rozsahegyi I, Roth B: Participation of the central nervous system in decompression. Ind Med Surg 35:101–110, 1966.
95. Slark AG: Treatment of 137 cases of decompression sickness. J Roy Nav Med Serv 50:219–225, 1964.
96. Malette WG, Fitzgerald JB, Cockett ATK: Dysbarism: A review of 35 cases with suggestions for therapy. Aerosp Med 33:1132–1139, 1962.
97. Bove AA, Hallenbeck JM, Elliott DH: Circulatory responses to venous air embolism and decompression sickness in dogs. Undersea Biomed Res 1:207–220, 1974.
98. Francis TJR, Dutka AJ, Clark JB: An evaluation of dexamethasone in the treatment of acute experimental spinal decompression sickness. *In* Bove AA, Bachrach AJ, Greenbaum LJ (eds): Underwater and Hyperbaric Physiology IX. Bethesda, Undersea and Hyperbaric Medical Society, 1987, pp 999–1013.
99. Neuman TR, Spragg R, Howard R, Moser K: Cardiopulmonary consequences of decompression stress. Am Rev Resp Dis 117:162, 1978.
100. Tate RM, Repine JE: Neutrophils and the adult respiratory distress syndrome. Am Rev Resp Dis 128:552–559, 1983.
101. Ence TJ, Gong H: Adult respiratory distress syndrome after venous air embolism. Am Rev Resp Dis 119:1033–1038, 1979.
102. Lanphier EH, Lehner CE: Spinal cord bends, scuba diving and basic issues. Undersea Biomed Res 12(suppl):30, 1985.
103. Lehner CE, Hei DJ, Palta M, et al: Accelerated onset of decompression sickness in sheep after short, deep dives. *In* Bove AA, Bachrach AJ, Greenbaum LJ (eds): Underwater and Hyperbaric Physiology IX. Bethesda, Undersea and Hyperbaric Medical Society, 1987, pp 197–206.
104. Weathersby PK, Survanshi SS, Hays JR, McCallum ME: Statistically based decompression tables. III. Comparative risk using US Navy, British and Canadian standard air schedules. Medical Research Progress Report of the Naval Medical Research Institute, NMRI 86–50. Bethesda, July 1986.
105. Behnke AR: A review of physiologic and clinical data pertaining to decompression sickness. Project X-443, Report No. 4. Bethesda, Naval Medical Research Institute, 1947.
106. Desola AJ, San Pedro AG: Epidemiological study of 146 dysbaric diving accidents. *In* Desola AJ (ed): Diving and Hyperbaric Medicine. Proceedings of the IX Congress of the European Undersea Biomedical Society. Barcelona, 1984.
107. Heller R, Mager W, von Schrotter H: Luftdruckerkrankungen mit Besonderer Berucksichtigung der Sogenannten Caissonkrankheit. Vienna, Alfred Holder, 1900.
108. Hill L: Caisson Sickness and the Physiology of Work in Compressed Air. London, Arnold, 1912, pp 74–98.
109. Dick PK, Massey EW: Neurologic presentation of decompression sickness and air embolism in sports divers. Neurology 35:667–671, 1985.
110. Erde A, Edmonds C: Decompression sickness: A clinical series. J Occup Med 17:324–328, 1975.
111. Kelly PJ, Peters BH: The neurological manifestations of decompression accidents. *In* Hong SK (ed): International Symposium on Man in the Sea. Bethesda, Undersea Medical Society, 1975, pp 227–232.
112. Peters BH, Levin HS, Kelly PJ: Neurologic and psychologic manifestations of decompression sickness in divers. Neurology 27:125–127, 1977.

113. Vaernes RJ, Eidsvik S: Central nervous dysfunction after near miss accidents in diving. Aviat Space Environ Med 53:803–807, 1982.
114. Rivera JC: Decompression sickness amongst divers: An analysis of 935 cases. Milit Med 129:314–334, 1963.
115. Hyashi K, Kitano M, Kawashima M, Hayashi K: Twenty six cases of complete transverse injury of the spinal cord in decompression sickness. *In* Miller JN, Parmentier JL (eds): Rehabilitation of the Paralysed Diver. Thirtieth Undersea Medical Society Workshop. Bethesda, Undersea Medical Society, 1985, pp 94–99.
116. Bert P: La Pression Barometrique: Recherches de Physiologies Experimentale. Paris, Masson, 1878. (Translated by Hitchcock MA and Hitchcock FA, Columbus, OH, College Book Company, 1943.)
117. Gallagher EG, Pearson DT: Ultrasonic identification of sources of gaseous microemboli during open heart surgery. Thorax 28:295–305, 1973.
118. Shaw PJ, Bates D, Cartlidge NEF, et al: Early neurological complications of coronary artery bypass surgery. Br Med J 291:1384–1387, 1985.
119. Shaw PJ, Bates D, Cartlidge NEF, et al: Neurological complications of coronary bypass surgery: Six month followup study. Br Med J 293:165–167, 1986.
120. Kobrine AI, Evans DE, Rizzoli HV: Relative vulnerability of the brain and spinal cord to ischaemia. J Neurol Sci 45:65–72, 1980.
121. Gebarski SS, Gabrielsen TO, Gilman S, et al: The initial diagnosis of multiple sclerosis: Clinical impact of magnetic resonance imaging. Ann Neurol 17:469–474, 1985.
122. Gilbert JJ, Sadler M: Unsuspected multiple sclerosis. Arch Neurol 40:533–536, 1983.
123. Edmonds C, Boughton J: Intellectual deterioration with excessive diving (punch drunk divers). Undersea Biomed Res 12:321–326, 1985.
124. Edmonds C, Hayward L: Intellectual impairment with diving: A review. *In* Bove AA, Bachrach AJ, Greenbaum LJ (eds): Underwater and Hyperbaric Physiology IX. Bethesda, Undersea and Hyperbaric Medical Society, 1987, pp 877–886.
125. Gorman DF, Edmonds CW, Parsons DW, et al: Neurologic sequelae of decompression sickness: A clinical report. *In* Bove AA, Bachrach AJ, Greenbaum LJ (eds): Underwater and Hyperbaric Physiology IX. Bethesda, Undersea and Hyperbaric Medical Society, 1987, pp 993–998.
126. Melamed Y, Ohry A: The treatment and the neurological aspects of diving accidents in Israel. Paraplegia 18:127–132, 1980.
127. Smyth E: Deep sea diving may cause loss of memory. New Scient 1439:8, 1985.
128. Blackwood W: Discussion on vascular disease of the spinal cord. Proc R Soc Med 51:543–547, 1958.
129. Haymaker W, Johnson AD: Pathology of decompression sickness: A comparison of the lesions in airmen with those in caisson workers. Milit Med 117:285–306, 1955.
130. Hallenbeck JM: Cinephotomicrography of dog spinal vessels during cord-damaging decompression sickness. Neurology 26:190–199, 1976.
131. Hallenbeck JM, Bove AA, Elliott DH: Mechanisms underlying spinal cord damage in decompression sickness. Neurology 25:308–316, 1975.
132. Hallenbeck JM, Bove AA, Moquin RB, Elliott DH: Accelerated coagulation of whole blood and cell-free plasma by bubbling in vitro. Aerosp Med 44:712–714, 1973.
133. Hallenbeck JM, Sokoloff L: Blood flow studies during spinal cord–damaging decompression sickness in dogs. *In* Schilling CW, Beckett MW (eds): Underwater Physiology VI. Bethesda, FASEB, 1978, pp 579–585.
134. Wolkiewiez J, Martin PJ, Lapoussiere JM, Kermarec J: Spinal cord accidents. Med Aeronaut Spat Med Subaquat Hyp 18:313–317, 1979.
135. Martin PJ, Wolkiewiez J, DeBoucha P, Teulieres L: Med Aeronaut Spat Med Subaquat Hyp 20:72–76, 1981.
136. Kitano M, Hayashi K, Kawashima M: Three autopsy cases of acute decompression sickness. Consideration of pathogenesis about spinal cord damage in acute decompression sickness. Jpn Orthop Traum 26:402–408, 1977.
137. Hills BA, James PB: Spinal decompression sickness: Mechanical studies and a model. Undersea Biomed Res 9:185–201, 1982.
138. Keyser TJ: Compressed air disease with notes on a case and discussion of etiology from the standpoint of physical laws. Cleve Med J 15:250–255, 1916.
139. Brooks H: Caisson disease: The pathological anatomy and pathogenesis with an experimental study. Long Is Med J 1:149–158, 1907.
140. Blick G: Notes on diver's paralysis. Br Med J 2:1796–1798, 1909.
141. Sykes JJW, Yaffee LJ: Light and electron microscopic alterations in spinal cord myelin sheaths after decompression sickness. Undersea Biomed Res 12:251–258, 1985.
142. Francis TJR, Pezeshkpour AH, Dutka AJ, et al: Is there a role for the autochthonous bubble in the pathogenesis of spinal cord decompression sickness? J Neuropathol Exp Neurol 47:475–487, 1988.
143. Kobrine AI, Evans DE, Rizzoli HL: Experimental acute balloon compression of the spinal cord. J Neurosurg 51:841–845, 1979.
144. Tarlov IM, Klinger H: Spinal cord compression studies. II. Time limits for recovery after acute compression in dogs. Arch Neurol Psychiatr 71:271–290, 1954.
145. Francis TJR: A current view of the pathogenesis of spinal cord decompression sickness in an historical perspective. *In* Vann RD (ed): Proceedings of a Symposium on the Physiological Basis of Decompression. Bethesda, Undersea and Hyperbaric Medical Society, 1988 (in press).
146. Calder IM: Dysbarism: A review. Foren Sci Int 30:237–266, 1986.
147. Casey HW, Bancroft RW, Cooke JP: Residual pathologic changes in the central nervous system of a dog following rapid decompression to 1 mm Hg. Aerosp Med 37:713–718, 1966.
148. Mastaglia FL, McCallum RI, Walder DN: Myelopathy associated with decompression sickness: A report of six cases. Clin Exp Neurol 19:54–59, 1983.
149. Lichtenstein BW, Zeitlin H: Caisson disease: A histologic study of late lesions. Arch Pathol 22:86–98, 1936.
150. Palmer AC, Blakemore WF, Greenwood AG: Neuropathology of experimental decompression sickness (dysbarism) in the goat. Neuropathol Appl Neurobiol 2:145–156, 1976.
151. Palmer AC, Calder IM, McCallum RI, Mastaglia FL: Spinal cord degeneration in a case of "recovered" spinal decompression sickness. Br Med J 283:888, 1981.
152. Palmer AC, Calder IM, Hughes JT: Spinal cord damage in active divers. Undersea Biomed Res 15(Suppl):70, 1988.

153. Saumarez RC, Bolt JF, Gregory RJ: Neurological decompression sickness treated without recompression. Br Med J 1:151–152, 1973.
154. Workman RD: Treatment of bends with oxygen at high pressure. Aerosp Med 39:1076–1083, 1968.
155. Nathan PW, Smith MC: Effects of unilateral cordotomies on the motility of the lower limbs. Brain 96:471–494, 1973.
156. Farmer JC, Thomas WG, Youngblood DG, Bennet PB: Inner ear decompression sickness. Laryngoscope 86:1315–1327, 1976.
157. Landolt JP, Money K, Topliff EDL, et al: Pathophysiology of inner ear dysfunction in the squirrel monkey in rapid decompression. J Appl Physiol 49:1070–1082, 1980.
158. Fraser WD, Landolt JP, Money K: Semicircular canal fractures in squirrel monkeys resulting from rapid decompression. Acta Otolaryngol 95:95–100, 1983.
159. Money K, Buckingham IP, Calder IM, et al: Damage to the middle ear and inner ear in underwater divers. Undersea Biomed Res 12:77–84, 1985.

Chapter 16

Pulmonary Barotrauma

MARK E. BRADLEY

Pulmonary barotrauma with air embolism ranks second to drowning as a cause of death in the recreational diving community.[1] Novice and relatively inexperienced divers appear to be at greatest risk. Activities such as emergency ascent training and buddy breathing practice especially carry a risk of air embolism.[2,3]

CAUSES OF PULMONARY OVERINFLATION

Pulmonary overinflation may be caused by excessive intrapulmonary pressure during positive pressure breathing or by the failure of expanding lung gases to escape during ascent. Excessive intrapulmonary pressure during positive pressure breathing can occur when the demand regulator of the underwater breathing apparatus is at a level in the water lower than that of the lung. During ascent, expanding lung gases may be prevented from escaping by voluntary or involuntary breath holding, or by local pulmonary obstructions, such as bronchospasm, pulmonary cysts, viscid pulmonary secretions, or broncholiths, which trap gas.[4] Additionally, there may be intrinsic characteristics of lung tissue and physiology which predispose to pulmonary barotrauma. These are discussed in the next section.

MECHANICS OF LUNG RUPTURE

Experimentally, it has been shown that transpulmonic pressures (defined as intratracheal pressure minus intrapleural pressure) of 95 to 110 cm of H_2O are sufficient to rupture alveolar septa and allow gas to escape into interstitial spaces.[5,6] This extra-alveolar gas can travel along perivascular sheaths and cause mediastinal emphysema and pneumothorax.[7] It can also enter the pericardium, the retroperitoneum, and the subcutaneous tissues of the neck. When intrathoracic pressure drops during the first breath after pulmonary barotrauma, extra-alveolar gas can pass into torn blood vessels, migrate to the left side of the heart, and enter the arterial circulation as bubble emboli.[8]

Pulmonary compliance may be a potential factor for pulmonary barotrauma. Colebatch, et al[9] reported that divers with stiff lungs (i.e., with reduced pulmonary compliance) are at an increased risk for pulmonary barotrauma. In relatively stiff lungs, a nonuniform distribution of lung elasticity may increase susceptibility to barotrauma because the more compliant zones of the lungs are subjected to excessive strain. Overly forceful attempts to exhale during rapid ascent may also produce lung rupture. During forced expiration at low lung volumes, airways tend to narrow and act as check valves. Immersion in water tends to increase this phenomenon. Airway closure with air trapping has been observed in human subjects during head-out immersion. Because of this, it has been postulated that vigorous exhalation at low lung volumes could actually predispose divers to air trapping and contribute to alveolar rupture during rapid ascent.[10]

PATHOPHYSIOLOGY OF ARTERIAL GAS EMBOLISM

Our understanding of the pathophysiology of arterial gas embolism is based on extensive experimental studies and clinical observations made during the last 50 years. Additionally, studies of thromboembolic stroke, which shares many features of the pathophysiology of gas embolization, have extended our knowledge of this area.

Gas that enters the disrupted pulmonary vessels reaches the left heart chambers via the pumonary veins and is ejected into the arterial circulation as foamy particulates that distribute according to their relative buoyancy in blood. In the erect position, the brain receives the bulk of the embolic gas, while the coronary vessels are primarily embolized in the inverted position.

Air injected into the cerebral circulation distributes until it blocks arteries 30 to 60 microns in diameter. As the amount injected is increased, the air distributes widely in the brain, even if the gas is confined to one internal carotid.[11] There is an immediate marked rise in cerebrospinal fluid pressure[12] caused by an increase in cerebral blood volume due to an immediate reactive hyperemia.[13, 14] Systemic arterial hypertension is a concomitant of air embolism. This hypertension can be quite profound and is mediated by enormous increases in circulating plasma catecholamines and possibly by release of vasopressin.[15] The widely dilated cerebral arteries in the hyperemic areas lose autoregulation and respond passively to changes in blood flow.[13, 14] The result is that the systemic hypertension increases cerebral blood volume still further. The cerebrospinal fluid pressure declines over the next 30 to 60 minutes.[14] Blood flow studies reveal that the hyperemic areas are juxtaposed to areas of very low blood flow.[16] This phenomenon may result from an interaction between constituents of blood and damaged endothelium, thereby promoting a process of impaired cerebral reperfusion. This may be partly responsible for the phenomenon of delayed deterioration frequently seen in individuals who experience cerebral air embolism. When brain function is monitored using EEG or evoked responses there is immediate cessation of neuronal function.[14] These changes in blood flow and function and the pattern of heterogenous flow distribution within small areas are typical of ischemic brain.

Loss of blood supply to brain tissue causes an immediate decrease in neuronal ATP[17] and an increase in lactate.[18] Thus, the total energy available is reduced, and excessive synaptic activity will increase ischemic damage by reducing energy that would otherwise be available for maintenance of cellular integrity. Seizures use a very large amount of energy and are known to exacerbate the damage in ischemia. Thus, the prevention of seizures, agitation, and hyperthermia in the postembolization period is critically important. The lactate produced by ischemic brain may be an important element in causing neuronal damage.[19] Studies have shown that an increased glucose level, which is the major determinant of the amount of lactate produced by the ischemic brain, is associated with increased infarction.[19] Control of blood glucose is therefore critical after cerebral air embolism, and the use of glucose solutions is best avoided in the first twelve hours postembolization.

With cerebral gas embolism there is an immediate opening of the blood-brain barrier.[20] Permeability to relatively large molecules is maximal in 30 to 60 minutes and then rapidly declines over 4 to 5 hours. Permeability to smaller molecules is promptly increased postembolism and remains abnormal for up to 24 hours. As a consequence of the opening of the blood-brain barrier, vasogenic edema is prominent but relatively short lived and probably not amenable to steroid therapy, since it takes several hours before steroids have any beneficial effect on this type of edema.[21] Because of the ischemia, swelling of neurons and astrocytes (cytoxic edema) also occurs and may continue after 3 hours, resulting in elevated brain water content for up to 24 hours. Steroids have no effect on this form of edema.[22]

As an integral part of recompression therapy for arterial gas embolism, hyperbaric oxygen can reduce cerebral edema by improving oxygenation, causing constriction of cerebral vessels,[23] and by reducing glucose metabolism.[24]

With arterial gas embolism, there may be major effects on cardiac function. Experimental studies[25] in which air was infused into the left ventricle suggest that cardiac arrest can be produced by two mechanisms. The first of these mechanisms is gaseous embolization of the coronary arteries. Experimental animals in this group develop hypotension, depression of left ventricular contractile force, EKG evidence of myocardial ischemia or injury, and subsequent death. The second mechanism involves embolization of the cerebral circulation resulting in severe hypertension and marked arrhythmias, which in humans would probably take the form of ventricular fibrillation.

CLINICAL MANIFESTATIONS OF ARTERIAL AIR EMBOLISM

Virtually all cases of arterial gas embolism develop signs or symptoms within 5 minutes of ascent.[26] After careful analyses of the signs and symptoms, Elliott and colleagues[27] and Greene[28] have suggested that patients with this disorder can be divided into two categories based on the clinical presentation. In the first category, the initial presentation is that of apnea, unconsciousness, and cardiac arrest. This immediate cardiovascular collapse occurs in 4 to 5 per cent of patients with cerebral gas embolism and is thought to result from cardiac arrhythmias or coronary artery embolization; these individuals are frequently unresponsive to cardiopulmonary resuscitation.

In the second category, the initial presentation is that of neurological signs and symptoms but with preservation of spontaneous respiration and pulse. These individuals may manifest a wide spectrum of neurological signs and symptoms, which in descending order of frequency include: coma, stupor and confusion, unilateral motor changes, convulsions, vertigo, visual distrubances, unilateral sensory changes, collapse, headache, unilateral motor and sensory changes, bilateral motor changes, and bilateral sensory changes. Fortunately, the majority of individuals in this category recover fully with prompt recompression therapy. However, 20 to 32 per cent of patients in this category undergo a seondary deterioration during hyperbaric therapy.[26] This relapse most commonly occurs some 20 minutes to 2 hours after the initial embolization. Signs and symptoms of secondary deterioration include headache, progressive stupor, confusion, and visual disturbances, including blindness and convulsions. Any number of processes may be responsible for this secondary deterioration.[24] These include formation of edema, increased intracranial pressure, further embolization, or release of vasoactive substances from damaged lungs. Any of these pathological events could contribute to a slowing of cerebral flow, but recent work suggests that an interaction between blood factors and damaged vascular or neural tissue can result in a progressive shutdown of cerebral blood flow.

There are certain pathognomonic diagnostic features of arterial gas embolism which have been reported. These include marbling of the skin of the upper body, gas emboli in the retinal vessels, x-ray evidence of gas in cerebral blood vessels, and sharply defined areas of pallor on the tongue. Recent reports of computed tomography and magnetic resonance imaging for diagnosis of brain and spinal lesions are also promising.[29]

OTHER CLINICAL MANIFESTATIONS OF EXTRA-ALVEOLAR GAS

Mediastinal Emphysema

Mediastinal emphysema is usually associated with mild substernal pain and is often described as a dull ache or a feeling of tightness that is worse on inspiration, coughing, or swallowing. Pain may radiate to the shoulders, neck, or back. Unless extensive, this condition is not usually associated with shortness of breath, tachypnea, or other signs of respiratory distress. Mediastinal emphysema is often accompanied by subcutaneous emphysema, and a crunching sound that is synchronous with cardiac action may be noted (Hamman's sign). The chest X-ray is diagnostic.

Subcutaneous Emphysema

The signs and symptoms of subcutaneous emphysema include swelling and crepitation in the neck and supraclavicular fossae, sore throat, a change in voice timbre, and dysphagia. Radiographs of the region of the neck may be helpful in detecting cases involving only small amounts of subcutaneous air.

Pneumopericardium

Evidence of this condition may be apparent radiographically, but historically this has not been a clinically significant condition in diving.

Pneumothorax

Pneumothorax is a relatively uncommon phenomenon, occurring only in about 10 per cent of cases of pulmonary barotrauma.[30] The onset of pneumothorax is often heralded by a sharp pain in the side of the chest during ascent. Recompression can convert a simple pneumothorax to a tension pneumothorax. During recompression, the tear in the visceral pleura may remain open, allowing compressed gas to enter the pleural space. During ascent, the gas that has entered the pleural space will expand, and the simple pneumothorax will become a tension pneumothorax. Manifestations of tension pneumothorax include cyanosis, tachypnea, tachycardia, and hypotension during ascent.

The diagnosis of pneumothorax is made on the basis of diminished or absent breath sounds, increased percussion note, and decreased respiratory excursions on the affected side. Tracheal shift may be present. The chest x-ray in full inspiration is confirmatory. However, x-rays are not available in the chamber, and diagnosis of pneumothorax may not be easy because high noise levels and changes in sound quality make use of a stethoscope difficult.

REFERENCES

1. McAniff JJ: U.S. underwater diving fatality statistics, 1970–78. Report No. URI-SSR-80-13, 1980.
2. Denney MK, Read RC: Scuba-diving deaths in Michigan. JAMA 192:220–222, 1965.
3. Lansche JM: Deaths during skin and scuba diving in California during 1970. Calif Med 116:18–22, 1972.
4. Leibow AA, Stark JE, Vogel J, et al: Intrapulmonary air trapping in submarine escape casualties. U.S. Armed Forces Med J 10:265–289, 1959.
5. Malhotra MC, Wright CAM: Arterial air embolism during decompression and its prevention. Proc R Soc Med B154:418–427, 1960.
6. Schaeffer KE, Nulty WP, Carey C, et al: Mechanisms in development of interstitial emphysema and air embolism on decompression from depth. J Appl Physiol 13:15–29, 1958.
7. Macklin MT, Macklin CC: Malignant interstitial emphysema of the lungs and mediastinum as an important occult complication in many respiratory diseases and other conditions: An interpretation of the clinical literature in the light of laboratory experiment. Medicine 23-258–281, 1944.
8. Polack B, Adams H: Traumatic air embolism in submarine escape. U.S. Navy Med Bull 30:165–177, 1932.
9. Colebatch HJH, Smith MM, Ng CKY: Increased elastic recoil as a determinant of pulmonary barotrauma in divers. Respir Physiol 26:55–64, 1976.
10. Dahlback GO, Lundgren CEG: Dynamic factors in pulmonary air-trapping during immersion. Forsvarsmedicin 9:247–250, 1973.
11. Babcock R, Netsky MG: Respiratory and cardiovascular responses to experimental cerebral emboli. Arch Neurol 2:556–565, 1960.
12. Evans DE, Kobrine A, Weathersby PK, et al: Cardiovascular effects of cerebral air embolism. Stroke 12:338–344, 1981.
13. De La Torre R, Meredith J, Netsky MG: Cerebral air embolism in the dog. Arch Neurol 6:307–316, 1962.
14. Fritz H, Hossman KA: Arterial air embolism in the cat brain. Stroke 10:581–589, 1979.
15. Evans DE, Weihl AC, David TD, et al: Effects of cerebral air embolism on circulating catecholamines and angiotensin. Undersea Biomed Res 6(Suppl)30, 1979.
16. Hallenbeck JM, Leitch DR, Dutka AJ, et al: PGI_2, indomethacin and heparin promote post-ischemic neuronal recovery in dogs. Ann Neurol 12:797–809, 1982.
17. Levy D, Duffy T: Cerebral energy metabolism during transient ischemia and recovery in the gerbil. J Neurochem 28:63–70, 1976.
18. Scheinberg P, Meyer J, Reivich M, et al: Cerebral circulation and metabolism in stroke. Stroke 7:213–233, 1976.
19. Plum F: What causes infarction in the ischemic brain? Neurology 33:222–233, 1983.
20. Lee JC, Olszewski J: Effect of air embolism on permeability of cerebral blood vessels. Neurology 9:619–625, 1959.
21. Shapiro H: Intracranial hypertension. Anesthesiology 43:445–471, 1975.
22. Fishman R: Brain edema. N Engl J Med 293:706–711, 1975.
23. Nakajima S, Meyer J, Amano T, et al: Cerebral vasomotor responsiveness during 100% oxygen inhalation in cerebral ischemia. Arch Neurol 40:271–276, 1983.
24. Hallenbeck JM: Prevention of post-ischemic impairment of microvascular perfusion. Neurology 27:3–10, 1977.
25. Evans DE, Hardenburgh E, Hallenbeck JM: Cardiovascular effects of arterial air embolism. *In* Workshop on Arterial Air Embolism and Acute Stroke. Undersea Medical Society Report No. 11-15-77, 1977.
26. Pearson RR, Goad RF: Delayed cerebral edema complicating cerebral air embolism: Case histories. Undersea Biomed Res 9:283–296, 1982.
27. Elliott DH, Harrison JAB, Barnard EEP: Clinical and radiographical features of 88 cases of decompression barotrauma. *In* Shilling CW, Beckett MW (eds) Proceedings of the Sixth Symposium on Underwater Physiology. Bethesda, FASEB, 1978, pp 527–535.
28. Greene KM: Causes of death in submarine escape training casualties: Analysis of cases and review of the literature. Admiralty Marine Technology Establishment Report No. AMTE (E) R 78-402, 1978.
29. Warren LP, Djang WT, Moon RE, et al: Neuroimaging of scuba diving injuries to the CNS. Am J Roentgenol 151:1003–1008, 1988.
30. Moses J: Casualties in individual submarine escape. Navy Sub Med Res Lab Rpt No 438, 1964.

Chapter 17

Aseptic Necrosis of Bone

DENNIS N. WALDER

Aseptic necrosis of bone is one of the many terms used to describe the changes seen in the bones of some humans following exposure to increased ambient pressure. Therefore, it is a condition that occurs in both compressed-air workers and divers. It does not affect every bone in the body or indeed all of any one bone, but rather it seems to be limited to a few specific and circumscribed sites (Fig. 17–1).

The important sites are those adjacent to the joint surfaces of the shoulder and hip joints, where lesions are called *juxta-articular*. The normal load carried at such sites may result in collapse of the dead bone and disruption of the normally smooth bearing surfaces (Fig. 17–2). This in turn can lead to nonspecific compensatory changes in and around the joint surfaces to result in a secondary arthritis. From the patient's point of view, such a sequence of events results in movements of the affected joint becoming painful and limited. In the early stages, prior to collapse of the articular surface, the condition is typically symptom-free and is usually first detected by routine bone scanning or radiography.

In addition to juxta-articular lesions there are those that occur away from the articular surface either deep in the head or neck of a bone or in its shaft. These are called *head, neck, and shaft lesions*. The shaft lesions are most frequently found at the lower end of the femur and at the upper end of the tibia. Histological examination of the human material available indicates that in addition to the necrosis of bone which occurs there is also evidence of fatty marrow necrosis. Dead fat cells release breakdown products, which stimulate new bone formation,[1] and fatty acids, which combine with calcium to give rise to the diffuse calcified markings typically seen on the radiographs of shaft lesions (Fig. 17–3).

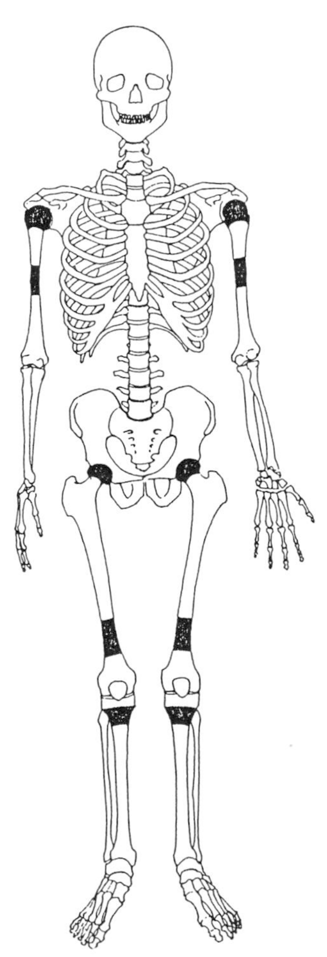

FIGURE 17–1. Common sites of lesions in divers and compressed-air workers.

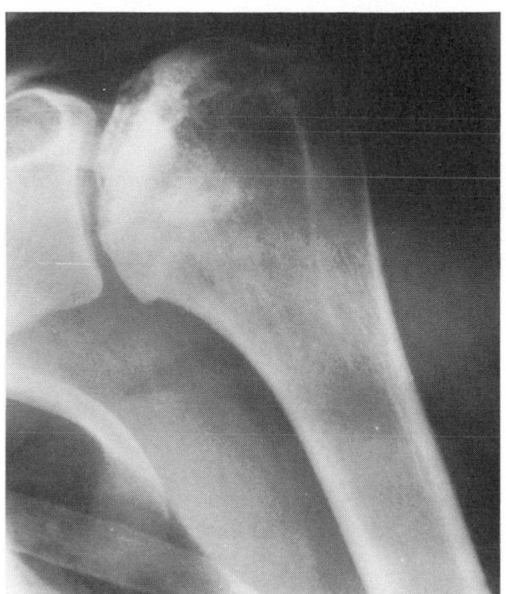

FIGURE 17–2. Radiographic appearance of a juxta-articular lesion affecting head of left humerus. Collapse of the articular surface has occurred.

CLASSIFICATION

To standardize the systems used by different centers to describe the radiographic appearances of bone lesions seen in compressed-air workers and divers, the Medical Research Council (MRC) Decompression Sickness Panel in Great Britain has drawn up a classification (Table 17–1) that has proved to be extremely useful. To assist radiologists in recognizing the various lesions mentioned in the classification, a limited number of radiological atlases[2] were distributed from the MRC Decompression Sickness Team in Newcastle. Many of the x-rays from it have been reproduced by Ilford[3] and can also be found in a book by Davidson.[4] As mentioned above, with the passage of time symptomless juxta-articular lesions may progress to structural failure, with associated pain and limitation of movement, and then may develop osteoarthritic changes. It is therefore necessary to keep a running record of an individual's bone lesion state.

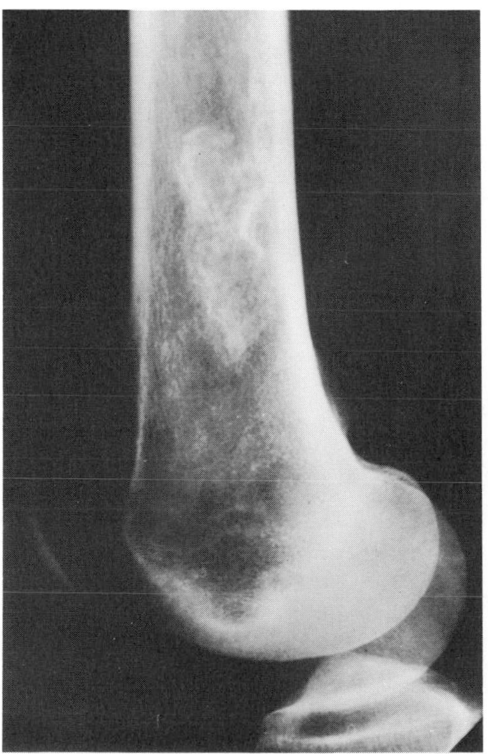

FIGURE 17–3. Radiographic appearance of a shaft lesion in lower end of femur.

RADIOGRAPHY AND OTHER METHODS OF DIAGNOSIS

It must be realized that the only changes that can be seen by x-ray examination are changes in the amount of calcium salts present in the bone. There is no difference in the radiographic appearance of a bone examined today when alive and tomorrow when dead. Neither does the length of time that elapses between death and the examination affect the radiographic appearance. The bones of a man x-rayed many years after death may be practically indistinguishable from those x-rayed on the day of death. As the amount and distribution of calcium salts in the bone of a living man are seen to change after a bone is damaged, it is clear that there must be some form of circulation surrounding that damage and perhaps extending into it at places.

TABLE 17–1. Classification of Bone Necrosis in Compressed-Air Workers and Divers

Juxta-articular lesions

- A1. Dense areas, with intact articular cortex
- A2. Spherical segmental opacities
- A3. Linear opacity
- A4. Structural failure
  - a. Translucent subcortical band
  - b. Collapse of articular cortex
  - c. Sequestration of cortex
- A5. Osteoarthritis

Head, neck, and shaft lesions

- B1. Dense areas
- B2. Irregular calcified areas
- B3. Translucent areas

When, for example, established aseptic necrosis of bone lesions affecting the head of the humerus or femur are examined under the microscope, it is found that the original trabeculae no longer contain living osteocytes in their lacunae, but that these dead trabeculae have been covered by a layer of new bone containing living osteocytes (Fig. 17–4). This represents the body's attempt to repair the damaged bone and can only occur in the presence of a satisfactory blood supply.

These changes come about slowly; from the evidence available at present, it is thought that a lesion cannot be detected radiologically until some 3 to 4 months after the causal incident. This is, of course, a severe disadvantage when trying to attribute the damage to a particular dive.

This is not the only limitation of radiological studies. When it has been possible to compare the histological state of a bone with previous radiographs,[5] it was found, as might be expected from the previous discussion, that the radiograph does not always reveal the full extent of the lesion (Fig. 17–5). Furthermore, it is not yet possible to predict from the radiological appearance whether a specific early juxta-articular lesion will progress to give collapse of the articular surface in a few months, as illustrated in Figure 17–2 or whether it will, like the majority of lesions, remain stable for many years and never cause further involvement of the bone or any signs or symptoms.

Occasionally, the radiographic appearance of a diver's bones gives rise to the suspicion that a lesion may exist but the evidence is not conclusive. In such cases, further radiographic studies in a year's time should be undertaken to confirm whether a lesion is developing. If a suspected lesion is accompanied by pain on movement, there may well be a breakdown of the articular surface continuity, which may only be revealed by tomography. If it is important to make an earlier diagnosis, Zinn[6] has pointed out that trochanteric bone biopsy and bone phlebography are both useful methods.

Further diagnostic techniques are those using bone-seeking radioactive isotopes. These have been employed very successfully in the detection of other bone abnormalities,[7] and there is some evidence of their potential value in the early diagnosis of aseptic necrosis of bone.[8] However, one difficulty is that they appear to be almost too sensitive and may indicate lesions that spontaneously heal and never progress to give radiological change or indeed any disability. More experience is required before such techniques can be adopted universally as alternatives to radiological surveillance of divers.[9] It will also be essential to confirm that the body dose of irradiation to each individual is no greater than that at present allowed for conventional radiography. Fortunately, simple radiological surveys, such as are recommended here, seem to be sufficient to make a diagnosis in the vast majority of cases.

THE SIZE OF THE PROBLEM

It is important to put into perspective the problem of aseptic necrosis of bone as it affects divers. There can be no doubt that those exposed to pressurized environments, such as in

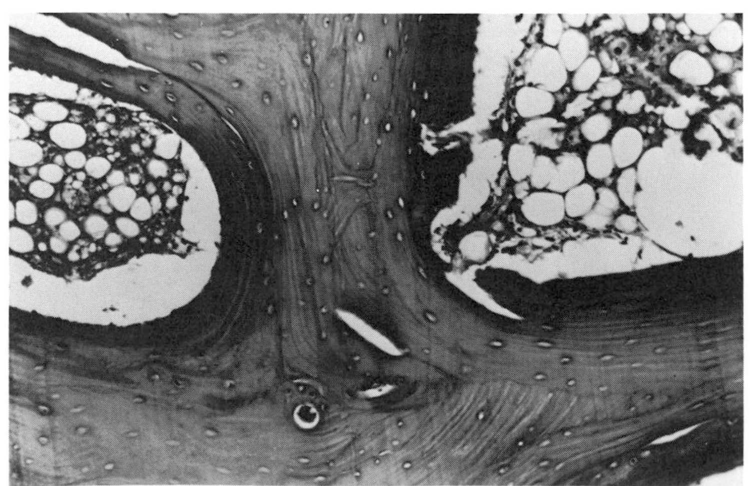

FIGURE 17–4. Photomicrograph (X 125) showing dead trabeculum with empty lacunae onto which a layer of appositional new bone has formed with vital osteocytes in its lacunae.

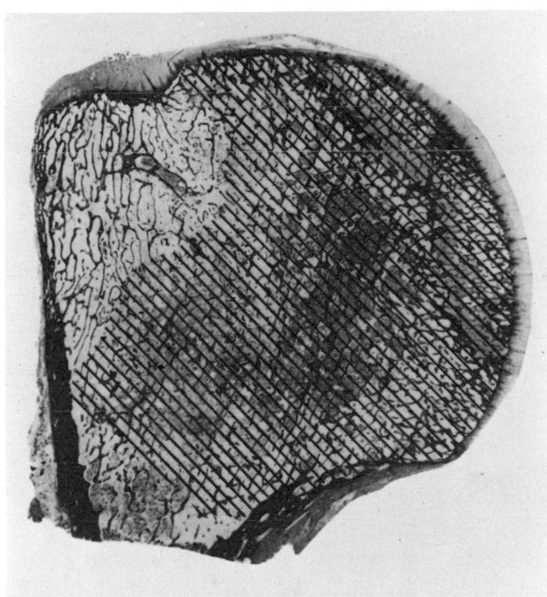

FIGURE 17–5. Photomicrograph (X 2) of head of humerus showing aseptic necrosis. Beneath the articular cartilage is an area of necrotic bone bounded by a line of fibrous tissue. The hatched area beyond this line shows evidence of dead trabeculae, which have been covered by living bone. This represents the full extent of the original damage.

civil engineering compressed-air work and diving, run a risk of bone damage. In one study,[10] a bone radiographic survey was carried out in two groups of manual laborers employed in tunneling work. One group worked in compressed air many times over a period of years, whereas the other group did similar jobs at atmospheric pressure. There was eventually a 26 per cent prevalence of bone lesions in the 171 compressed-air workers, but none of the 120 members of the other group developed a lesion.

For divers there have been widely differing reports of the prevalence of bone necrosis. Ohta and Matsunaga[11] reported a prevalence as high as 50 per cent in Japanese diving fishermen. A survey by Harrison and Elliott[12] of Royal Navy clearance divers showed an overall figure of 5 per cent, although most of the lesions were found in divers who had engaged in experimental diving (dives in which the decompression schedules used were not of proven adequacy[13]). Adams and Parker's report in 1974[14] of U.S. Navy divers suggested that the prevalence might be as high as 30 per cent, although it is possible that these figures included both bone islands and other minor bone changes, so that the true prevalence may have been more in line with that of the British Navy. The figure for the 4980 North Sea commercial divers x-rayed in Great Britain in 1981 was 4.2 per cent[15] and remains at about that level.

THE DISTRIBUTION OF BONE LESIONS IN DIVERS

The lesions of aseptic necrosis of bone are found at the same sites in compressed-air workers and divers (see Fig. 17–1), but the frequency with which the sites are affected seems to differ from one report to another. In the British experience the most common site for lesions is the lower end of the femur, followed by the shoulder joint. The hip joint is rarely affected in divers, although it is quite commonly involved in compressed-air workers. Such observations have led to speculation as to why this should be and whether it can provide some additional clue about the etiology of aseptic necrosis of bone.[16] Unfortunately, the Japanese experience with divers[17] is more like that of the British compressed-air workers, with lesions in the head of the femur seen at just about half the frequency of those in the head of the humerus.

RADIOGRAPHIC MONITORING OF DIVERS' LONG BONES

Not only is it important for an individual diver to know that one's bones are free from necrosis, but it is also important for an employer to be aware of any pre-existing bone abnormalities in a potential employee.

Obviously there is a radiation hazard associated with every radiographic examination, and this must be kept to an acceptable limit. It has been calculated that the long bone survey recommended by the British MRC Decompression Sickness Panel could be carried out safely every 6 months, although it is emphasized that a gonad protector must be used.

Experience so far at the MRC Decompression Sickness Central Registry in Newcastle upon Tyne indicates that the prevalence of bone necrosis in nonsaturation air diving to depths of up to 50 meters is low (0.8 per cent). Furthermore, the Registry has no record of the condition ever having been seen in divers who never dived deeper than 30 meters. It does not seem, therefore, to be justifiable to carry out routine radiographic studies on amateur and sport divers who do not usually exceed 30 meters.

The extent of the radiological examination recommended by the MRC Decompression Sickness Panel to study bone lesions in professional divers is shown in Table 17–2. The full survey should be carried out before starting work, thereafter not more often than annually, unless for some special reason the presence of a suspected lesion requires more frequent monitoring.

Differential Diagnosis

There are many conditions in addition to hyperbaric exposure which can lead to aseptic necrosis of bone in humans (Table 17–3). Most of them can be identified by special tests. For example, alcaptonuria is associated with the presence of homogentisic acid in the urine, sickle cell anemia by the presence of abnormal hemoglobin S in the blood, and so on. The presence of chronic alcoholism is rather more difficult to establish, but in any case the evidence is tenuous that alcoholism is a significant factor that must be excluded in divers with bone lesions.

Bone Islands

The bone island is seen radiographically as an isolated area of increased density. The shape is usually round or oval—the longer diameter varying between 2 and 15 mm—and the margins may be well defined or irregular and indistinct.

In 1973 Conti and Sciarli[18] suggested that bone islands might be more common in divers than in others, and indeed it is possible that some authors have classified them as bone lesions. Later, Davidson and colleagues,[19] reviewing the radiographs of 100 Royal Navy divers and the radiographs of 100 nondiving Navy personnel matched for age and rank, were unable to substantiate this finding and said that bone islands are no more common in divers than in nondivers. The areas compared were those normally radiographed in the MRC Panel's recommendations for diver bone surveys. The presence of bone islands is something that in the past radiologists have rightly dismissed as insignificant, and hence no mention has usually been made of them in routine radiological reports.

ADVICE

What advice should the doctor give to a diver found to have a bone lesion? This is a difficult question to answer because factual evidence on which to base the advice is still limited. Certainly juxta-articular and shaft lesions should be considered separately.

At the moment, it seems reasonable (certainly in Great Britain where the basis of successful litigation is different from that in the United States) to take the view that, although a shaft lesion represents a failure to protect the diver from the consequences of diving, shaft lesions almost never result in disability, so that the individual may continue to dive. Some caution is necessary because Mirra and co-workers[20] have suggested that neoplastic changes have occurred in some shaft lesions, although the risk as far as we know at present is very low. Those with shaft lesions should therefore be informed of the lesions' existence and advised to report to their doctors if any symptoms should ever arise in the affected limb. This possibility will have to be watched for very carefully in the future.

TABLE 17–2. The Radiography of the Bones of Compressed-Air Workers and Divers

1. Good definition of the trabecular structure of the bone is essential.
2. The gonads must be protected from ionizing radiation by the use of a lead shield.
3. Projections required:
   a. Anteroposterior projection of each shoulder joint.
      The patient is placed in a supine position with the trunk rotated at an angle of approximately 45° to bring the shoulder to be radiographed in contact with the table. This arm is partially abducted and the elbow is flexed. Center 1 inch below the coracoid process of the scapular and cone to show as much humerus as possible. Bring the lateral diaphragm to show only the head and shaft of the humerus.
   b. Anteroposterior projection of each hip joint.
      The patient is placed in a supine position with the feet at 90° to the table top. The edge of the gonad protector should be as near the femoral head as possible but not in any way obscuring it. Center the cone over the head of the femur, that is, 1 inch below the midpoint of a line joining the anterior superior iliac spine and the upper border of the pubic symphysis.
   c. Anteroposterior and lateral projections of each knee.
      Center at the level of the upper border of the patella. The field should include the lower third of the femur and the upper third of the tibia and fibula.

TABLE 17–3. Conditions Reported to be Associated with Aseptic Necrosis of Bone

Hyperbaric exposure	Trauma
Steroid therapy	Rheumatoid arthritis
Sickle cell anemia	Gout
Diabetes	Ionizing radiation
Chronic alcoholism*	Syphilis
Cirrhosis of the liver	Alcaptonuria
Hepatitis	Arteriosclerosis
Pancreatitis	Hyperlipidemia
Gaucher's disease	

*Unproven.

If the lesion is juxta-articular, the situation is quite different. Each and every juxta-articular lesion is potentially disabling as there is a 10 to 40 per cent chance that the articular surface will progress to collapse. Even if the potential disability of one major joint was acceptable, the risk that a continuation of diving might result in a second major joint becoming affected cannot be excluded. For these reasons, it seems sensible to recommend that the presence of a juxta-articular lesion should be taken as a contraindication to future diving. Although the possibility of developing further lesions might be reduced by limiting the diving to depths of say 50 meters, the risk would still be present. In any case, in the author's view, such a limitation in Great Britain at present would be impracticable because of the great pressures on individuals to dive to any depth in the North Sea when required.

THE CAUSE OF ASEPTIC BONE NECROSIS IN DIVERS

It is not difficult for those who accept the bubble hypothesis of decompression sickness to believe that aseptic bone necrosis results from the blockage of some critical nutrient blood vessels to bone by gas bubbles liberated at decompression. However, because there is no clear correlation between reported attacks of decompression sickness and the subsequent development of bone lesions,[16] several other mechanisms have been suggested to account for the occurrence of bone necrosis in divers. Jones and Sakovich[21] believe that fat embolism may be an important factor, and Philp, Inwood, and Warren[22] think that the blood vessels to bone may be obstructed by platelet thrombi. Hills[23] put forward the unorthodox idea that gas-induced osmosis may be the etiological agent and that aseptic bone necrosis occurs during compression, as opposed to the generally accepted idea that the decompression is responsible.

There can be little doubt that much more would be known about the cause of bone lesions if it were not so difficult to induce the condition in laboratory animals by simulated diving. This is probably related to the short circulation time in animals smaller than humans, as this would mean that tissue gas tensions would not persist long enough to maintain bubble emboli beyond the time (6 to 12 h) required for osteocytes to be irretrievably damaged.[24] In addition, the regenerative capacity of bone in small animals is probably better than that for humans. In recent years, there have been reports of bone changes in mice,[25] rats,[26] and miniature pigs[27] following hyperbaric exposure, but the lesions described in mice and rats do not appear to be radiologically identical to those seen in humans. Certainly, the extent of the initiating insult (rapid decompression) has in all these reports been so severe that the mechanism involved in producing the experimental lesion in the animal may not be the same as that in humans.

An interesting approach to this problem has been the intra-arterial injection into rabbits of spherical glass particles to simulate bubble emboli. By using this technique, lesions of the femoral heads similar to those seen in humans have been produced in rabbits.[28] This appears to confirm that the difficulty in producing bone lesions in small animals does lie in the short persistence time of bubble emboli in these species.

One possible factor in the etiology of bone necrosis, which until recently has been largely overlooked, is the raised partial pressure of oxygen to which divers and compressed-air workers are exposed. In 1972 Puleo and Sobel[29] did point out that a modification of the collagen of bone could occur as a result of exposure to high partial pressures of oxygen. This however would not explain why only some parts of the skeleton are affected. A new hypothesis involving oxygen has recently been proposed.[30]

It is known that the sites in the skeleton at which lesions occur are those at which fatty marrow is found in the mature adult human. If the fat cells of the marrow should enlarge—as a result of exposure to raised partial pressures of oxygen—they would embarrass the circulation to the overlying bone because the nutrient vessels lie, with the fatty marrow, within the rigid marrow cavity. Any increase in the volume of fat cells would result in compression of blood vessels and impairment of the circulation to the marrow and bone. Not only would this delay the clearance of dissolved gas from the tissues, but any bubble in the circulation would be preferentially trapped in the nutrient vessels of the bone, where it would enlarge because of the existing high gas partial pressures and would persist to result in the death of osteocytes and the necrosis of the bone.

Pooley and Walder[31] have shown that fat cells do increase in volume when exposed to raised partial pressures of oxygen. Furthermore, an analysis of the data held in the Newcastle upon Tyne Decompression Sickness Central Registry[32] showed that most bone necrosis occurs in humans who have breathed oxygen at partial pressures of greater than 0.6 bar for more than 4 hours. Thus both these findings support the hypothesis that, although the final ischemic episode that results in bone death may be a bubble, its critical location and its persistence may be determined by the duration and partial pressure of oxygen breathed during the exposure to hyperbaric conditions.

TREATMENT

As shaft lesions are not expected to produce symptoms or to result in disability, no treatment is indicated. The treatment of aseptic necrosis of bone at juxta-articular sites is not yet entirely satisfactory.

A general principle of treatment applied by orthopedic surgeons to damaged joints before the articular surface has collapsed is to relieve the affected joint of weight bearing in order to give the underlying bone a chance to heal. In the case of aseptic necrosis of bone in divers, this would mean a period of rest lasting for several months. Unfortunately, at present there is no way of determining which lesions are going to break down and which will never give rise to pain or limitation of movement. In general, therefore, conservative treatment is neither practicable nor very satisfactory.[33]

Attempts to treat advanced lesions in which the articular surface has already become disrupted have included (1) inserting a bone graft via a drill hole through the underlying living bone into the area of dead bone in order to provide a pathway for revascularization,[34] (2) gouging out the necrotic bone from beneath the cartilage and packing the cavity with fresh cancellous bone chips,[35] or (3) realigning the shaft of the bone to change the line of weight bearing as in a McMurray's osteotomy. None of these methods has met with great success.

The most satisfactory method of treating the seriously affected joint may be to arthrodese the joint or to replace the damaged head of the bone by a prosthesis. Although the use of prostheses is well established for middle-aged and older patients, questions about the durability of the prosthesis become of great importance when it is to be used in the treatment of active young individuals, such as divers.

REFERENCES

1. Walder DN, Stothard J: Bone necrosis: Reimplantation of anoxic autologous marrow. Undersea Biomed Res 5:39–40, 1978.
2. MRC Decompression Sickness Central Registry: Radiographic appearances of bone lesions in compressed air workers. Newcastle upon Tyne, 1968.
3. Davidson JK, Griffiths PD: Caisson disease of bone. X-ray Focus 10:2–11, 1970.
4. Davidson JK: Dysbaric osteonecrosis. *In* Davidson JK (ed): Aseptic Necrosis of Bone. New York, American Elsevier Publishing Company, 1976.
5. McCallum RI, Walder DN: Bone lesions in compressed air workers. J Bone Joint Surg 48B:207–235, 1966.
6. Zinn WM: Conclusions. *In* Zinn WM (ed): Idiopathic Ischaemic Necrosis of the Femoral Head in Adults. Stuttgart, Theieme, 1971, pp 213–214.
7. Citrin DL, Greig WR, Calder JF, et al: Preliminary experience of bone scanning with 99m Tc-labelled polyphosphate in malignant disease. Br J Surg 61:73–75, 1974.
8. Cox PT, Walder DN: Strontium scanning in caisson disease of bone. *In* Lambertsen CJ (ed): Proceedings of the 5th Symposium on Underwater Physiology. Bethesda, Undersea Medical Society, 1972, pp 177–184.
9. Walder DN (ed): Early Diagnosis of Dysbaric Osteonecrosis. Bethesda, Undersea Medical Society, 1981.
10. MRC Decompression Sickness Panel: Decompression sickness and aseptic necrosis of bone. Br J Ind Med 28:1–21, 1971.
11. Ohta Y, Matsunaga H: Bone lesions in divers. J Bone Joint Surg 56B:3–16, 1974.
12. Harrison JAB: Aseptic bone necrosis in naval clearance divers. Proc R Soc Med 64:1276–1278, 1971.
13. Elliott DH: The role of decompression inadequacy in aseptic bone necrosis of naval divers. Proc R Soc Med 64:1278–1280, 1971.
14. Adams GM, Parker GW: Dysbaric osteonecrosis in U.S. Navy divers. Undersea Biomed Res 1:A20, 1974.
15. Report by the MRC Decompression Sickness Central Registry and Radiological Panel: Aseptic bone necrosis in commercial divers. Lancet 2:384–388, 1981.
16. Walder DN: Caisson disease of bone in Great Britain. *In* Wada J, Iwa T (eds): Proceedings of the Fourth International Congress on Hyperbaric Medicine. London, Bailliere Tindall, 1970, pp 83–87.
17. Kawashima M, Torisu T, Hayashi K, et al; Avascular necrosis in Japanese diving fishermen. *In* Trapp WG, Banister EW, Davison AJ, Trapp PA (eds): Proceedings of the 5th International Hyperbaric Congress. Burnaby, Simon Fraser University, 1974, pp 855–862.
18. Conti V, Sciarli R: Bone lesions in the autonomous diver. Forsvarsmedicin 9:525–527, 1973.
19. Davidson JK, Harrison JAB, Jacobs P, et al: The significance of bone islands, cystic areas and sclerotic

areas in dysbaric osteonecrosis. Clin Radiol 28:381–393, 1977.

20. Mirra JM, Bullough PG, Marcove RC, et al: Malignant fibrous hystiocytoma and osteosarcoma in association with bone infarcts. J Bone Joint Surg 56A:932–940, 1974.
21. Jones JP, Sakovich L: Fat embolism of bone. J Bone Joint Surg 48A:149–164, 1966.
22. Philp RB, Inwood MJ, Warren BA: Interactions between gas bubbles and components of the blood: Implications in decompression sickness. Aerosp Med 43:946–953, 1972.
23. Hills BA: Gas induced osmosis as an aetiological agent for inert gas narcosis, gouty arthritis and aseptic bone necrosis induced by exposure to compressed air. Revue Physiol Subaquat Medecin Hyperbar 2:3–7, 1970.
24. Woodhouse CF: Dynamic influences of vascular occlusion affecting the development of avascular necrosis of the femoral head. Clin Orthop 33:119–128, 1964.
25. Chryssanthou C, Kalberer J, Kooperstein S, et al: Studies on dysbarism. II. Influence of bradykinin and "bradykinin-antagonists" on decompression sickness in mice. Aerosp Med 35:741–746, 1964.
26. Wunche O, Scheele G: Bone cysts in albino rats following decompression from high pressure. Arch Orthop Unfallchir 77:7–16, 1973.
27. Stegall PJ, Smith KH, Hildebrandt J: Aseptic bone necrosis and hematologic changes in miniature pigs as a result of compression/decompression exposures. Fed Proc 31:653, 1972.
28. Cox PT: Simulated caisson disease of bone. Forsvarsmedicin 9:520–524, 1973.
29. Puleo LE, Sobel HH: Oxygen modified collagen and its possible pathological significance. Aerosp Med 43:429–431, 1972.
30. Walder DN: Dysbaric osteonecrosis: A new hypothesis. *In* Sheraki and Matsuoka (eds): Proceedings 3rd International Symposium of U.O.E.H. Japan, 1983, pp 283–286.
31. Pooley J, Walder DN: Changes in cell volume following hyperbaric exposure: A manifestation of oxygen toxicity. *In* Bachrach AJ, Matzen MM (eds): Underwater Physiology VII. Bethesda, Undersea Medical Society, 1980, pp 45–53.
32. Trowbridge WP: An appraisal of the computer data storage project at the Newcastle upon Tyne Decompression Sickness Central Registry. Thesis, University of Newcastle upon Tyne, England, 1982.
33. Romer U, Wettstein P: Results of treatment of 81 Swiss patients with II NFH. *In* Zinn WM (ed): Idiopathic Ischaemic Necrosis of the Femoral Head in Adults. Stuttgart, Theieme, 1971, pp 205–212.
34. Phemister DB: Treatment of the necrotic head of the femur in adults. J Bone Joint Surg 31A:55–66, 1949.
35. Wagner H: Treatment of idiopathic necrosis of the femoral head. *In* Zinn WM (ed): Idiopathic Ischaemic Necrosis of the Femoral Head in Adults. Stuttgart, Theieme, 1971, pp 202–204.

Chapter 18

Ear and Sinus Problems in Diving

JOSEPH C. FARMER, JR.

HISTORICAL CONSIDERATIONS OF DIVING OTOLOGY

Numerous articles concerning ear and sinus problems in diving have appeared since the latter part of the nineteenth century. In 1873, A. H. Smith[1] listed severe deafness and vestibular problems among other injuries in compressed-air workers in his description of "caisson disease." Alt[2, 3] in 1897 described injuries to the middle and inner ears during compression and decompression in caisson workers at Nussdorf. Alt further described inner ear pathology in animals after rapid decompression and was the first to suggest that inner ear injuries in diving could occur during compression, in association with inadequate middle ear pressure equilibration, and during decompression, during which injuries were thought to be secondary to interference with the inner ear blood supply by nitrogen bubbles developing in the labyrinthine vasculature. Vail[4] in 1929 also noted middle and inner ear injuries in compressed-air workers and performed animal studies indicating that the inner ear damage during compression was related to inadequate middle ear pressure equilibration, with resulting stasis and hemorrhage in the inner ear. He also hypothesized that such injuries during decompression were related to nitrogen bubbles, causing emboli and necrosis in the inner ear.

By 1940, discussion of ear problems in the diving literature[5–7] was largely devoted to the prevention and treatment of barotitis media, generally believed to be reversible and not to result in serious disability. Diving-related inner ear injuries were thought to be rare; when symptoms suggestive of inner ear injuries were described, they were usually believed to be caused by central nervous system decompression sickness. However, since the 1940's, as activity in commercial, military, and sport diving to deeper depths has increased, reports of diving-related ear problems have become more frequent. Indeed, middle ear barotrauma during descent has been recognized to be the most common diving medical problem. Also, reports of inner ear disturbances with some permanent sequelae during all types and phases of diving have appeared. An entire book, *Otological Aspects of Diving* by Edmonds, et al[8] in 1973 was devoted to diving otology and contained a detailed review of the various causes of otological problems in diving. In 1974, Kennedy[9] published a review of the literature which summarized the vertigo and dysequilibrium that occurred during diving. Lundgren[10] in 1965 and Ingelstedt and colleagues[11] in 1974 described and demonstrated inadequate middle ear pressure equilibration and subsequent vertigo during ascent.

In the 1970's, the first writings since the early works by Alt and Vail began to emphasize inner ear injuries in diving. Freeman and Edmonds in 1972[12] and Edmonds, et al in 1974[13] described labyrinthine window ruptures and subsequent inner ear injury associated with inadequate middle ear pressure equilibration during the compression phase of shallow diving. Stucker and Echols[14] in 1971 suggested that inner ear injuries during diving could occur from nitrogen bubble emboli forming in the internal auditory artery system during decompression. Rubenstein and Summitt[15] in the same year described

10 cases of isolated vestibular and/or cochlear injuries occurring during or shortly after decompression. Buhlmann and Gehring[16] in 1976 described additional instances of otological injury in humans related to decompression from deep helium oxygen diving. Farmer and co-workers[17] in 1976, enlarging on the 10 cases of Rubenstein and Summitt, presented an additional 13 cases of isolated vestibular and/or cochlear injuries occurring during or shortly after decompression. Specific recommendations for the management of inner ear decompression sickness were reviewed. Animal studies by McCormick and colleagues[18] in 1973 demonstrated intralabyrinthine bubble formations and hemorrhages along with decreases in cochlear function in guinea pigs subjected to rapid decompression. Landolt, et al[19] in 1977 described vestibular dysfunction and inner ear pathology in monkeys after rapid decompression. Further studies by Venter and co-workers in 1983,[20] enlarging on the work of Landolt, demonstrated actual fractures of the bony endosteal layers of the semicircular canals in the inner ears of monkeys with inner ear decompression sickness. Lambertson and Idicula[21] in 1975 described inner ear vestibular dysfunction and injury occurring in divers while at stable deep depths soon after beginning the breathing of different inert gases. This was recognized as a manifestation of the counterdiffusion phenomenon.

In 1977, Farmer[22] reviewed diving inner ear injuries and pointed out that the pathophysiology and treatment of these problems differed depending upon the phase of diving in which the injuries occurred. Persistent inner ear injuries were classified into: (1) injuries occurring during compression (inner ear barotrauma), (2) injuries occurring at stable deep depths, (3) inner ear injuries related to decompression sickness, and (4) sensorineural hearing loss secondary to excessive noise exposure in diving.

RELATED ANATOMY AND PHYSIOLOGY

A complete review of the anatomy and physiology of the ear, nose, and sinus is beyond the scope of this chapter; however, certain points should be made to better understand otological and paranasal sinus problems in diving.

The external auditory canal (Fig. 18–1) is a self-cleaning blind tube lined by squamous epithelium that is continuous with the squamous epithelium on the outer layer of the tympanic

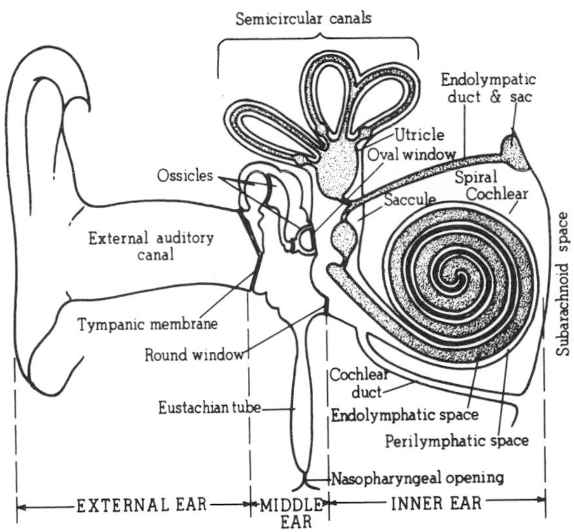

FIGURE 18–1. Simplified diagram of the external, middle, and inner ear showing air within the external auditory canal, middle ear, and eustachian tube. The fluid-filled inner ear is subdivided into the perilymphatic and endolymphatic spaces, which connect indirectly with the subarachnoid space via the cochlear duct and endolymphatic duct and sac, respectively.

membrane. The keratinized epithelial cells are constantly migrating from the eardrum and inner two-thirds, or bony ear canal, outward to the cartilaginous canal, or outer one-third, where they are mixed with cerumen, a colorless, odorless material containing long and short chain fatty acids. The fatty acids in cerumen have a protective function, that of primarily maintaining a slightly acid pH. When cerumen is exposed to air, oxidation and the typical brown color occurs.

The middle ear cleft is an irregularly shaped space that communicates with air cells in the mastoid, petrous, and zygomatic portions of the temporal bone. The total gas volume of this complex varies among individuals depending upon the pneumatization of these areas. The evolution of an air-containing external and middle ear has presented humans with a device that efficiently transforms airborne sound into the fluid-filled inner ear, where it is transduced into electrical signals. Proper function of this mechanism requires that the external ear canal be patent, that both the external ear canal and middle ear be air containing, and that pressure differentials between these structures and the ambient atmosphere as well as the inner ear be avoided. With the pressure changes encountered in diving, a pressure-sensitive middle ear becomes a liability, for with an intact tympanic membrane the only communication for pressure equilibration between the middle ear cleft and the ambient atmosphere is through the eustachian tube. This tube is approximately 35 to 38 mm in length in the adult and is directed downward, forward, and medially from the middle ear to the nasopharynx. The nasopharyngeal ostium is normally closed except when opened by a positive middle ear pressure or when opened by the muscular action of the pharyngeal and palatine muscles upon the surrounding tubal cartilage during swallowing. During descent, active attempts must be made to open this ostium by contracting these muscles; the ostium and tube usually open passively during ascent.

The inner ear (Fig. 18–1) consists of a system of perilymph-filled bony channels within the temporal bone. Membranous structures containing endolymph are located in these channels. Perilymph is biochemically similar to extracellular fluid, whereas endolymph is biochemically similar to intracellular fluid. A resting electrical charge exists between perilymph and endolymph. When acoustical energy enters the cochlea, displacement of the basilar membrane occurs, and the electrical charge depolarizes with activation of the neural auditory pathways.

The membranous inner ear structures are divided into two parts: the vestibular system containing the semicircular canal, utricle, and saccule; and the auditory system containing the spiral cochlea. These two systems are interconnected and are separated by the thinnest multicellular membranes in the body. The blood supply to both systems is through the internal auditory artery, which originates from the basilar or the inferior cerebellar artery. This is an end artery that supplies only the membranous inner ear and has no collaterals with other vessels. Alterations in cerebrospinal fluid (CSF) pressure are transmitted to both the endolymph and perilymph fluid compartments, and significant pressure differences between these spaces are usually avoided.

Thus, any maneuver that increases CSF pressure, such as a Valsalva maneuver, can cause an increased pressure in the inner ear fluid compartments with bulging of the round window membrane into the middle ear. With marked pressure changes, possible round window rupture and/or rupture of inner ear membranes can occur and, as will be described later, does occur in diving, even during shallow exposures.

Respiratory epithelium with a rich vascular supply lines the eustachian tube, the nasopharynx, the nose, and the paranasal sinuses. This epithelium is constantly secreting a mucous blanket, which is moved through the sinus ostia into the nasal cavity by the beating of the microscopic cilia on the mucosal cell surface. Once in the nasal cavity, this mucus is combined with the mucus secreted in the nose and is swept by ciliary action to the nasopharynx. About one liter per day of mucus is secreted by a healthy adult; about one-half of this is evaporated by the inspired and expired air stream. Also, the mucous blanket has cleansing, filtrating, bacteriostatic, and protective functions. Alterations in these functions and obstruction of the airways and sinus ostia can result from chronic inflammatory disease, which is commonly due to one or more of the following underlying factors: allergy, chronic irritation from smoking, prolonged use of nose drops, and chronic obstruction from internal and/or external nasal deformities or from mass lesions. Frequently, acute and/or chronic nasal and sinus infections are due to the congestion and airway obstruction from one or more of these underlying factors and/or the physiological nasal congestion and increased mucous discharge with cold weather exposure. Also, inflammatory nasal and sinus diseases occasionally result in inadequate eustachian tubal function and otitis media in the absence of atmospheric pressure changes, and exposure to the pressure changes frequently produces middle ear or even inner ear barotrauma as well as barotrauma to the paranasal sinuses.

SYMPTOMS OF OTOLOGICAL DYSFUNCTION

The common symptoms of otological dysfunction are ear fullness or pain, tinnitus, hearing loss, and vertigo. It is not within the scope of this chapter to present a complete discussion of each of these symptoms; however, a brief review is in order.

Ear Fullness and Pain

Ear fullness, or the sensation of a blocked ear, commonly occurs from occlusion of the external auditory canal or from high or low middle ear pressure relative to ambient pressure. The resultant tensing of the eardrum and increased ossicular chain impedance cause a decrease in sound transmission to the inner ear. The patient feels that the ear has become occluded. With marked pressure differentials, pain occurs from sensory pain receptors in the eardrum and middle ear mucosa. Increased pain will be felt with eardrum rupture.

Hearing Loss

Hearing loss is classified into three types:

1. Conductive hearing loss results from dysfunction of any component of the sound conduction system, i.e., the external auditory canal and/or the middle ear transformer (the eardrum or ossicular chain). Complete airtight occlusion of the external auditory canal, such as from a cerumen plug, will cause a conductive hearing loss. Partial occlusion or nonairtight seals of the canal usually do not result in hearing loss unless the occluding material lies against the eardrum and impedes vibration. Conductive hearing loss can also occur from any process that interferes with the transmission of sound energy into the inner ear or impedes the movement of the eardrum and ossicles. Such processes can include inflammation and swelling of the eardrum or middle ear mucosa; middle ear effusion or exudates; changes in middle ear gas density, such as is seen in nontraumatic hyperbaric exposures; pressure differentials across the eardrum; fixation of the ossicles, such as from otosclerosis; loss of elasticity of the eardrum and ossicular fixation from scarring or repeated infections; large eardrum perforations; and interruption of the ossicular chain.

2. Sensorineural or nerve hearing loss results from dysfunction in the inner ear, auditory nerve, or brainstem cochlear nuclei. Such dysfunction can result from occlusion of the cochlear blood supply with ischemia; mechanical disruption of inner ear or brainstem structures from trauma or bubbles; leakage of perilymph from round window rupture with inner ear membrane breaks; idiopathic hydrops, or excess fluid pressure in the endolymphatic space (Meniere's disease); inflammatory disease in the inner ear (labyrinthitis); idiopathic degenerative processes such as presbycusis; or trauma-induced degeneration of cochlear structures from excessive noise exposure.

3. Mixed or combined conductive sensorineural hearing losses result from simultaneous dysfunction in the middle and inner ear. This can be seen in co-existing middle and inner ear barotrauma, middle and inner ear otosclerosis, or the development of acute middle or inner ear dysfunction with pre-existing disease in the other area.

Tinnitus

Tinnitus, or spontaneous noise in the ear, is difficult to quantitate. It can occur with middle ear disease that results in a conductive hearing loss but is usually seen with inner ear or central auditory pathway disease. With the former, tinnitus is thought to represent the sounds of cochlear and cranial blood flow which are perceived because the conductive hearing loss results in a loss or a decrease of the masking effect of the usual background noise. With inner ear disease, tinnitus is thought to be due to the spontaneous firing of injured but viable auditory neurons or cochlear hair cells. However, this is not well understood, for destructive labyrinthectomies or eighth cranial nerve sections in patients with recurrent vertigo, tinnitus, and nonfunctional hearing—while usually relieving the vertigo—have frequently not resulted in relief of the tinnitus.

Evaluation of Hearing Loss

The determination of the type of hearing loss is essential in the evaluation and management of any patient with suspected otological dysfunction. This is best done with soundproof booth audiometry by a certified audiologist. However, in some instances, such testing is not available or is impractical, and some preliminary information can be gained by testing with a 512 Hz or 1024 Hz tuning fork in quiet surroundings. A 256 Hz fork can be used, but the examiner has to be careful that the patient does not respond to vibratory sensations, which are more prominently perceived at the lower frequencies.

Weber Test

The struck tuning fork is placed on the forehead or on the upper incisor teeth, and the patient is asked if the sound is louder in either ear or if it is of the same intensity in both ears. With a conductive hearing loss, a sound source placed on either of these midline skull locations will be heard louder in the affected ear; with a sensorineural hearing loss, such sounds will be heard louder in the unaffected ear. With equal hearing in both ears, i.e., normal hearing or bilaterally equal hearing losses, the sound will not lateralize.

Rinne Test

A vibrating tuning fork is alternately placed against the patient's mastoid tip and then held about two inches from the ear canal. The patient is asked to ascertain in which position the sound is louder or heard longer. In a normal hearing ear, or in an ear with a pure sensorineural hearing loss, bone-conducted sound will be heard less loudly and for a shorter time than air-conducted sound. This phenomenon is due to the enhancement of airborne sound by the middle ear transformer, i.e., the eardrum and ossicular chain. With a moderate or severe conductive hearing loss, bone-conducted sound will become equal to or louder than air-conducted sound depending upon the degree of loss. With mild conductive hearing losses, normal results can be obtained.

SCHWABACH TEST

An examiner who knows his own hearing thresholds first places a vibrating tuning fork on the patient's mastoid tip. At the precise moment the patient no longer hears the sound, the fork is placed on the examiner's mastoid tip. If the sound is then heard by the examiner, decreased bone conduction or a nerve hearing loss in the patient's tested ear is suggested.

In general, tuning fork tests are difficult to adequately perform, particularly by untrained or inexperienced examiners. Patient suggestibility, decreased alertness, discomfort, and excessive background noise can adversely affect the results. Also, presence of mixed hearing losses, either unilateral or bilateral, can make interpretation of the results difficult. Adequate audiometry by certified audiologists should be obtained as soon as possible to supplement and confirm the results of tuning fork testing. Individuals who dive regularly should have routine periodic audiometry to detect unnoticed hearing losses and to provide baseline data for future reference.

Vertigo

The central vestibular system is programmed during the first year of life to associate unequal firing rates from the vestibular end-organs, primary vestibular neurons, or brain stem vestibular nuclei with linear and angular acceleration. When sudden unilateral disease affects these structures, the cerebral cortex interprets this as vertigo with rotation, pitching, yawing, or rolling. This type of dizziness must be differentiated from other less specific symptoms of balance disturbances, such as dizziness, lightheadedness, unsteadiness, and presyncopal sensations. If a dizzy patient does not have vertigo, the dizziness is unlikely to be related to primary or secondary vestibular dysfunction. Exceptions to this include individuals with slowly expanding intracranial lesions, who usually describe continuous, progressive unsteadiness with no or brief and mild vertiginous sensations. Another exception is the patient with bilateral vestibular end-organ disease such as that caused by ototoxic drug exposures, who will usually have nonvertiginous unsteadiness that can become quite severe with the loss of a second balance system input, such as decreased vision in dark surroundings or decreased proprioception with peripheral neuropathy.[23]

When vertigo is present, adequate evaluations must be performed to differentiate end-organ from central vestibular dysfunction and to properly determine whether such affected individuals are suited for further diving after apparent recovery. This involves a systematic approach to the evaluation and management of dizzy patients. To develop this type of approach, several general points should be emphasized.[24]

1. The first distinction that should be made is whether a dizzy individual is experiencing nonvestibular dizziness or true vestibular vertigo, defined as a specific alteration of spatial orientation involving the sensation of motion, usually rotary, of either the subject or his environment. Most human maladies and many medications are associated with dizziness. However, if the dizzy individual does not have vertigo, his dizziness is unlikely to be related to primary or secondary vestibular system dysfunction, either in the peripheral end-organ or in the central vestibular pathways.
2. Vestibular dysfunction will usually be accompanied by classical labyrinthine nystagmus with a defined quick and slow component. If by visual observation and by electronystagmography a dizzy patient does not have such accompanying nystagmus, the dizziness is unlikely to be due to vestibular system dysfunction.
3. Nystagmus resulting from nonacute end-organ vestibular dysfunction is frequently suppressed by visual fixation and, therefore, is not observable. Thus, electrical recordings of ocular motion in the dark or with eyes closed, i.e., electronystagmography, is important in the evaluation of a dizzy patient.
4. Vestibular system dysfunction is frequently accompanied by nausea, vomiting, visual disturbances, presyncope, or other symptoms. Thus the presence of these symptoms does not necessarily mean a more extensive central nervous system injury.
5. Once it has been determined that dizziness is likely due to vestibular system dysfunction, the next distinction is whether the pathology is located in the end-organ or in the central vestibular system. In some cases, this determination is not difficult for there are other

accompanying neurological symptoms or signs that point to a centrally located lesion. However, in many cases, such accompanying symptoms or signs are lacking, and this determination becomes more difficult. The presence of accompanying auditory symptoms or the finding of injury to the tympanic membrane or middle ear on otoscopic examination is more frequently, but not always, associated with end-organ injury. The presence of vertical nystagmus almost always means central pathology.

6. Further evaluations such as electronystagmography, pure tone and speech audiometry, temporal bone and skull radiography, and complete otological and neurological examinations should be done as soon as feasible.

7. After an acute unilateral vestibular end-organ injury, vertigo characteristically subsides over a varying time period of several days to four to six weeks. This improvement in symptoms usually results from central nervous system compensation and less frequently from functional recovery of the injured inner ear. Thus, a disappearance of symptoms does not usually mean that the injured part of the vestibular system has been restored to its previous healthy state. Individuals who have compensated from permanent end-organ vestibular injury or destruction frequently have no dizziness. Some may experience transient, brief vertigo and/or loss of spatial orientation with certain positions or motions. These symptoms can be intensified with loss of some proprioception and vision during underwater conditions. Therefore, all divers who experience vestibular injuries should be evaluated by specialists after their symptoms have disappeared. Only in this way can rational judgments be made regarding an individual's suitability for exposure to future situations in which vertigo or spatial orientation might endanger his life or the lives of others.

Vertigo in Diving

Vertigo is one of the most hazardous symptoms to occur during diving. It is frequently accompanied by hearing loss and tinnitus. It is described in multiple phases of diving.[8] However, many of the reports are not well documented, do not differentiate vertigo from nonvertiginous dysequilibrium, or discuss vertigo only as an incidental observation. Possible causes suggested for vertigo in divers include decompression sickness, hypoxia, hypercarbia, nitrogen narcosis, seasickness, alcoholic hangovers, sensory deprivation, hyperventilation, impure breathing gas, unequal caloric stimulation, and difficulties with middle ear pressure equilibration. One can readily appreciate that these causes can encompass a wide variety of pathological mechanisms, the management of which will be vastly different depending upon which mechanism is involved. Also, as noted above, the dizziness experienced in some of these entities is usually not true vertigo.

Edmonds and co-workers[8, 25] have undertaken a complete review of the various causes of dizziness in diving. Their classification is basically broken down into those causes of vertigo due to unequal vestibular stimulation, including caloric stimulations, barotrauma, and decompression sickness; and those due to unequal vestibular responses to equal stimuli, such as the result of one vestibular apparatus being more sensitive than the other. Affected individuals might have vertigo with caloric stimulation resulting from equal amounts of cold water entering the external ear canals. Also included in this group are divers who experience vertigo resulting from a unilateral hypofunctioning vestibular end-organ in situations in which equal and symmetrical pressure changes occur in the middle ear cavities during ascent and descent. In addition, Edmonds' classification includes dizziness noted with nitrogen narcosis; the dizziness, nausea, and tremor described in the high pressure nervous syndrome; and the dizziness noted during oxygen toxicity and sensory deprivation. A modification of this classification is offered which separates diving otological injuries into those with usually transient otological dysfunction and those with permanent otological inner ear injury.

TRANSIENT OTOLOGICAL DYSFUNCTION IN DIVING

Middle Ear Barotrauma (Barotitis Media)

The most common diving medical problem is middle ear barotrauma resulting from inadequate pressure equilibration between the middle ear and the external environment. During compression, the nasopharyngeal ostium of the eustachian tube, which is normally closed, can fail to open if the diver does not make active attempts to clear the ears by swallowing or if local inflammation and swelling prevent opening. Thus, middle ear pressure becomes negative relative to the increasing ambient pressure (Fig. 18–2). If a diver descends 2.6 feet and fails to equilibrate middle ear pressure, there

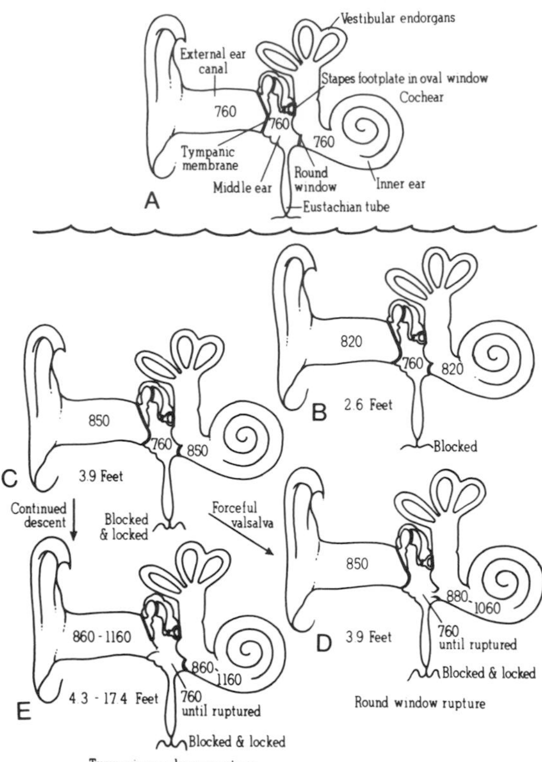

FIGURE 18–2. Otological barotrauma of descent. Theoretical sequence of changes in the right ear of a diver who does not equilibrate middle ear pressure during descent. Pressures are shown in mm Hg. (*A*) Surface condition with equal pressures (760 mm Hg) throughout and a patent eustachian tube with a normally closed nasopharyngeal ostium. (*B*) Depth of approximately 2.6 feet after diver failed to open the eustachian tube upon entering the water. Pressure differential of 60 mm Hg exists. Tympanic membrane and round window are bulging into the middle ear. Diver notices pain and pressure in the ear with a conductive hearing loss and possible vertigo. (*C*) Depth of approximately 3.9 feet with 90 mm Hg pressure differential and blocked and locked eustachian tube. (*D*) Forceful Valsalva maneuver can lead to rupture of the round window with resulting leak of perilymph into the middle ear. The exact pressure differentials at which rupture occurs in humans are unknown. Studies in cats[27] have indicated that round window ruptures occur when a pressure of 120 to 300 mm Hg is added to the cerebrospinal fluid space at 1 ata. (*E*) Continued descent can lead to tympanic membrane rupture at pressure differentials of 4.3 to 17.4 feet.[26] The actual rupture point is quite variable.

is a pressure differential of 60 mm of mercury (Fig. 18–2B). Significant mucosal congestion and edema occurs. This further narrows the eustachian tubal lumen, and subsequent ear clearing or pressure equilibration becomes more difficult. Also, with increasingly negative middle ear pressure, opening of the eustachian tube becomes more difficult because of the nasopharyngeal valve effect. At a pressure differential of approximately 90 mm of mercury, equivalent to a descent of 3.9 feet, it is usually impossible to open the tube voluntarily (Fig. 18–2C). Fullness and pain usually occur at the pressure differential of 60 mm of mercury, and the tympanic membrane has been found to rupture at pressure differentials ranging from 100 to 500 mm of mercury[26] (Fig. 18–2E). With a forceful Valsalva maneuver under these conditions, the existing pressure differential between the inner ear and middle ear becomes greater, and round window rupture with leakage of perilymph and inner ear injury or inner ear membrane breaks (inner ear barotrauma—see the following section) can occur (Fig. 18–2D). Animal studies have demonstrated round window ruptures when CSF pressure has been increased 120 to 300 mm of mercury.[27]

Clinical Presentation

Symptoms of middle ear barotrauma consist initially of a sensation of ear blockage. With further descent and greater pressure differential, frank ear pain occurs. A conductive hearing loss is always present but may not be a primary complaint because of ear pain. Mild tinnitus and vertigo occur. With eardrum rupture pain usually is severe, and vertigo can be seen from a caloric effect if water enters the middle ear. If hearing loss, tinnitus, and vertigo are severe in association with a no decompression dive, possible inner ear barotrauma with round window rupture or other inner ear injury should be suspected.

The presence of pre-dive nasal dysfunction, such as congestion and discharge, makes the occurrence of inadequate eustachian tubal function and subsequent middle ear barotrauma more likely. Likewise, a history of otitis media, mastoiditis, or previous mastoid or middle ear surgery is suggestive of inadequate eustachian tubal function in the absence of the atmospheric pressure changes associated with diving. Such individuals are certainly more likely to have inadequate eustachian tubal function with exposure to the greater atmospheric pressure changes encountered in diving. Also, divers who undertake rapid descent or who do not attempt to equilibrate middle ear pressures every one to two feet of descent are likely to have eustachian tube mucosal congestion and middle ear barotrauma during subsequent dives within the next several days.

Physical Signs

The physical signs of middle ear barotrauma are noted on otoscopic examination. One should remain aware that the pathological changes occur in the entire middle ear and are not confined to the eardrum. These changes include edema and hemorrhage in the middle ear mucosa as well as inflammation and collections of serous fluid and/or blood in the middle ear cleft.

Six grades of middle ear barotrauma have been described previously.[8]

Grade 0—Symptoms without otoscopic signs.

Grade 1—Diffuse redness and retraction of the tympanic membrane.

Grade 2—Grade 1 changes plus slight hemorrhage within the tympanic membrane.

Grade 3—Grade 1 changes plus gross hemorrhage within the tympanic membrane.

Grade 4—Dark and slightly bulging tympanic membrane due to free blood in the middle ear; a fluid level might be present.

Grade 5—Free hemorrhage into the middle ear with tympanic membrane perforation. Blood can be seen outside or within the ear canal.

This classification well describes the pathological changes present; however, the otoscopic findings in middle ear barotrauma frequently include combinations of changes in different grades. Eardrum scarring from previous perforations or surgery plus nondiving-related middle ear disease can obscure the middle ear findings. Occasionally minimal signs or no signs may be seen, only to have obvious signs of negative middle ear pressure with eardrum injection and retraction and middle ear inflammation or effusion develop over the next 24 hours. Also, treatment is not completely dependent upon which of these grades is present.

Treatment

Recommended treatment varies depending upon the type of middle ear barotrauma. Three types of barotrauma are described.

Type 1 Middle Ear Barotrauma. Cases with post-dive symptoms but without otoscopic signs either immediately or 24 hours post-dive. The recommended treatment for Type 1 cases is as follows:

1. Avoid any further diving until (a) any pre-existing nasal symptoms have cleared, (b) individual can easily autoinflate both ears at the surface, and (c) all ear symptoms have cleared.
2. Systemic decongestants such as Sudafed, 30 to 60 mg orally, 3 times daily, and longacting topical nasal decongestants such as Afrin nose drops, 2 to 3 drops into each nostril twice daily with the head extended while supine, can be used. The nose drops should not be used longer than 7 days. Nasal adrenergic sprays are not as effective as drops. Systemic antihistamines and steroid nasal sprays usually do not result in benefit unless pre-existing nasal allergy is present.

Type 2 Middle Ear Barotrauma. Cases with symptoms plus otoscopic findings and no eardrum perforation. The recommended treatment is as follows:

1. Rest and avoid further diving until complete resolution is seen by otoscopic examination and the diver can easily autoinflate both ears at the surface. This usually requires 3 to 14 days depending upon the severity of the injury.
2. Use systemic and topical nasal decongestants as described above. Short courses of systemic steroids have been used with reported benefit; however, the well-described contraindications and complications of systemic steroids should be noted.
3. Systemic antibiotics can be used prophylactically. This is controversial; however, eustachian tubal function is usually poor because of middle ear and tubal mucosal inflammation and swelling. Under these conditions, secondary middle ear bacterial infection is more likely. If purulent nasal discharge and/or cough with purulent sputum production is present, systemic antibiotics should be given.
4. With an intact eardrum, topical ear drops containing antibiotics, steroids, or anesthetic agents are of no benefit since these substances do not readily cross the outer, squamous epithelial layer of the tympanic membrane. An inert, oily preparation such as Auralgan, warmed to body temperature and instilled into the ear, may provide partial pain relief.
5. Pain relief is best achieved with systemic analgesics; however, the use of narcotics is generally not needed.

Type 3 Middle Ear Barotrauma. Cases with symptoms and otoscopic findings that include eardrum perforations. The suggested treatment is as follows:

1. Avoid further diving until a complete otological evaluation has been performed and the middle ear process has resolved with healing or surgical repair of the eardrum. Most of these perforations heal spontaneously and surgical repair is not necessary. Persistence of poor eustachian tubal function and/or middle ear inflammation from secondary infection will delay healing.

2. If significant amounts of blood or other debris are in the ear canal, ear cleansing with 1.5 per cent hydrogen peroxide at body temperature should be done. This solution can be prepared by mixing commercially available 3 per cent hydrogen peroxide with approximately equal amounts of warm water to approach body temperature. This solution is instilled 3 to 4 times daily with a small rubber bulb ear syringe or a 20 to 50 ml hypodermic syringe connected to soft plastic tubing. Once blood, purulent material, and other debris have been cleared from the ear canal, the peroxide irrigations can be discontinued. Solutions containing alcohol or acids should not be used when an eardrum perforation exists because of significant irritating effect on the middle ear mucosa.

3. Most commercial antibiotic ear drop preparations contain drugs that are ototoxic to the inner ear. These should not be used in the presence of an eardrum perforation. Also, otic solutions containing topical anesthetics are usually inadequate for analgesia.

4. Systemic and topical nasal decongestants should be employed as described above.

5. If purulent discharge is found in the nose, tracheal bronchial tree, or draining from the ear, these drainages should be cultured and systemic antibiotics should be administered. Prophylactic antibiotics may be given in the absence of purulent discharge because of the increased possibility of secondary middle ear or mastoid infection from contaminated water.

6. If the eardrum does not heal after one to two weeks of appropriate therapy, the patient should be referred to an otolaryngologist. In addition, further diving should be avoided until healing of the eardrum has occurred and adequate middle ear ventilation is present. The diver should be cautioned that an eardrum perforation occurring under water is potentially a very serious problem. Fortunately, most eardrum perforations resulting from middle ear barotrauma heal spontaneously, and surgical repair is not required. Poor eustachian tubal function resulting from nasal or sinus disease can impair healing.

7. The best treatment of middle ear barotrauma is caution and prevention. An adequate pre-diving otolaryngological examination emphasizing nasal and eustachian tubal function should be done. Particular attention should be paid to those individuals who have pre-existing symptoms or signs of middle ear and/or nasal disease. Frequent bouts of ear infection or drainage, or both, a history of middle ear surgery, the presence of a healed or persistent eardrum perforation, and the existence of a cholesteatoma all suggest poor eustachian tubal function during nondiving conditions. Such individuals are unlikely to be able to tolerate the pressure changes encountered in diving.

Other important factors in the prevention of middle ear and possible inner ear barotrauma include avoiding diving in the presence of significant nasal congestion or discharge, not continuing descent without adequate ear clearing every two feet, slowing descent rates, and avoiding a forceful modified Valsalva maneuver at depth.

Divers should be aware of techniques of equilibrating middle ear pressure which are safer than a modified Valsalva maneuver. The simplest maneuver is a modified yawn and swallow. This maneuver is accomplished by thrusting the lower jaw anteriorly and slightly opening the jaw while maintaining the lips pursed around the regulator. This may be followed by a swallow if ear clearing has not occurred. Another relatively nontraumatic way of ventilating the middle ear is called the Frenzel maneuver. With the nose, mouth, and glottis voluntarily closed, the tongue is used as a piston to compress air in the nasopharynx and thus into the eustachian tube. The mass of the tongue is strongly driven backward and acts to compress the nasopharyngeal air space through the soft palate. Another method of middle ear pressure equilibration consists of the activation of the palatal muscles by raising the soft palate. With experience, this technique can be mastered without the need to swallow or move the jaw. The Toynbee maneuver consists of swallowing with the mouth and nose closed; this produces an initial slight increase followed by a decrease in nasopharyngeal pressure.

These techniques for eustachian tubal opening and middle ear pressure equilibration during diving are safe in that they are unlikely to induce significant changes in pulmonary, alveolar, arterial, central venous, cerebrospinal fluid, or labyrinthine fluid pressures which occur with the modified Valsalva maneuver. Thus, dangerous overpressures in these spaces and subsequent pulmonary or inner ear barotrauma are less likely. Also, these maneuvers, in contrast to the modified Valsalva maneuver, are more effective for they involve contraction of the tensor palatini muscle, which acts to open the nasopharyngeal orifice of the eustachian tube. Thus, less nasopharyngeal pressure is required for tubal opening.

External Ear Canal Barotrauma (External Ear Squeeze, Reverse Ear Squeeze)

External ear canal obstruction can result in barotrauma to the canal and eardrum with ascent or descent during diving. With such blockage, ear canal pressure becomes negative during descent or positive during ascent relative to ambient and middle ear pressures. The resulting tissue damage includes congestion, hemorrhage, outward or inward bulging, and possible rupture of the tympanic membrane. The common causes of external ear canal obstruction are cerumen, foreign bodies, the use of ear plugs, and the use of tight-fitting diving hoods.

The treatment of external ear canal barotrauma is similar to that for middle ear barotrauma. If significant swelling of the external ear canal has occurred, the treatment described for otitis externa in the following section is useful. Again, if tympanic membrane rupture has occurred, ototoxic ear drops should be avoided.

The best treatment of external ear squeeze is prevention. External ear canal patency during pressure changes must be assured. Accumulated masses of cerumen, which can essentially obstruct the ear canal, should be removed by washing the ear in a lukewarm water solution using a rubber bulb syringe. Care should be taken before such washing to ensure that a tympanic membrane perforation does not exist. The use of tight-fitting hoods, solid ear plugs, or head phones, which can completely seal the ear canal, should be avoided.

Otitis Externa

After middle ear barotrauma, otitis externa is the second most common diving medical problem. It is a painful, sometimes debilitating malady encountered in all types of diving. The pathophysiology is related to the effects of moisture and/or humid atmospheres upon cerumen and the canal skin. The external ear canal is lined with squamous epithelium and has a slightly acid pH. Cerumen is produced in the outer cartilaginous ear canal and contains water-soluble bacteriostatic fatty acids in addition to oil-soluble fatty acids. These factors, along with the constant outward migration of the squamous epithelium, provide a natural cleansing mechanism and usually protection from infection in this skin-lined cul de sac. Excessive exposure to water and/or humid atmospheres produces maceration of the squamous epithelium and can dissolve or dilute the water-soluble fatty acids of cerumen, resulting in a shift of pH toward alkalinity and providing a good medium for bacterial growth. Other contributing factors include collections of cerumenous debris, local trauma, the presence of seborrheic dermatitis, poorly fitting or improperly cleaned ear plugs, and swimming in polluted water. Bony external auditory canal exostoses can also contribute to otitis externa. These hard lumps in the bony ear canal are not uncommon in swimmers and divers and are believed to be due to repeated cold water exposures. The mechanism is unknown; supposedly, the very thin tissue of the external canal overlying the periosteum may render the underlying bone vulnerable to ischemic cold injury, with subsequent reactive hyperemia and repair by exostosis formation.

In divers, the prolonged exposure to water and/or humid conditions frequently results in an alteration of the normal skin flora to a greater number of gram-negative bacteria. Thus, *Pseudomonas* and *Proteus* species, in addition to staphylococcus organisms, are frequently found in otitis externa. Other organisms include diphtheroids, *E. coli*, *Aerobacter*, and *Streptococcus faecalis.*[25] Fungi such as *Aspergillus* and *Candida* can also be seen but are usually only noted after prolonged treatment with topical antibacterial agents. Otitis externa is particularly seen in divers exposed for prolonged periods to saturation hyperbaria in chambers with high ambient temperature and humidity.

The symptoms of otitis externa in divers are similar to those seen in the nondiving population and include initial irritation with itching or burning. Later, there is thin white discharge and pain that is frequently quite severe. Examination reveals an inflamed, swollen, and extremely tender external auditory canal. With progression, erythema of the surrounding pinna and skin, cervical lymphadenitis, and complete obstruction of the ear canal with subsequent abscess formation and possible involvement of bone and cartilage can occur. Fortunately, this later complication is rare and is practically never seen in the absence of other debilitating illnesses such as poorly controlled diabetes, an unlikely problem in the usual diving population.

The best treatment of otitis externa is prevention. Ear canals should be cleaned of cerumenous debris and local trauma should be avoided. Adequate control of any seborrheic condition should be achieved before diving. If ventilated ear plugs are to be used, they should be properly fitted and cleaned. A useful prophylactic topical ear solution during exposures to humid and aqueous environments will contain a buffered weak acid such as 2 per cent acetic acid and aluminum acetate. This is commercially available as otic Domeboro solution and should be used after showers, swimming, or diving. Alcohol and alcohol-boric acid preparations have been used as prophylactic measures with variable success. However, alcohol will dissolve the cerumen fat-soluble fatty acids considered to be protective; also, solutions that contain alcohol can be irritating to the ear canal skin, particularly that which is inflamed. Therefore, these solutions are less desirable than a weak, buffered acetic acid preparation. The prophylactic use of antibiotic ear drops is not recommended since they are not usually effective and may enhance the chances of infection with a resistant organism. Once otitis externa is present, treatment principles include cleansing of the external auditory canal, specific therapy to provide topical antibiotics and a more normal canal pH, and relief of pain. Cleansing is best accomplished by ear irrigation using lukewarm tapwater or 1.5 per cent hydrogen peroxide as described above, with care being taken to dry the ear canal afterwards. A stream of warm air from a hair dryer, blown into the canal, is useful for this purpose. If an eardrum perforation exists, irrigation of the ear with water should be avoided and suction with gentle cotton wipes used instead. Narcotics usually are required for adequate pain relief.

More specific therapy includes the use of an ear drop preparation that has a slightly neutral or acid pH and contains topical antibiotics. Several ear drop preparations also contain steroids, which are not contraindicated and are thought by some to aid pain relief because of the anti-inflammatory action. Adequate amounts of these agents should be used three to four times daily. Frequently, swelling of the ear canal prevents these medications from being easily instilled into all of the involved areas of the ear canal skin. In these cases, a cotton wick or commercially available methylcellulose sponge wick should be inserted and the medications instilled onto the wick several times daily. These wicks can usually be removed in two to four days once the canal swelling has subsided. Systemic antibiotics can be used in the management of severe cases. However, the causative bacterial organisms are frequently *Proteus* or *Pseudomonas*, which are resistant to many antibiotics. Therefore, for the management of severe cases, appropriate cultures are important in the choice of systemic antibiotics.

All swimming and diving should cease until the otitis externa has cleared. This usually requires at least five to seven days and can significantly disrupt a one-week diving trip, which only adds to the distress caused by the disease.

Transient Vertigo Resulting from Unequal Middle Ear Pressure Equilibration (Alternobaric Vertigo)

Transient vestibular dysfunction secondary to asymmetrical middle ear pressure equilibration has been described by Lundgren,[10] Vorosmarti and Bradley,[28] and Terry and Dennison.[29] Lundgren attributed such vertigo to a unilateral increase in middle ear pressure during ascent with resulting unequal vestibular end-organ stimulation. Indeed, some individuals who have experienced alternobaric vertigo at depth can produce vertigo and vestibular nystagmus by performing a modified Valsalva maneuver and unequally inflating the middle ears at one ata. Many of these individuals have encountered difficulty during diving with middle ear pressure equilibration, usually unilaterally. Disappearance of the vertigo has been noted with stopping the ascent or descending again or shortly after a sudden hissing of air into one ear. Further work by Tjernstrom[30] and Inglestedt, et al,[11] using a technique for indirectly measuring middle ear pressure changes with simultaneous electronystagmographic recordings, has shown true vestibular nystagmus with an overpressure in one middle ear during decompression in a pressure chamber.

The exact frequency of alternobaric vertigo is not known. A more recent work by Lundgren, et al,[31] involving a questionnaire answered by 2053 Swedish divers, indicates that of 453 divers who had experienced vertigo during diving, 343 were likely to have had alternobaric vertigo. The vertigo was noted to last from a few seconds up to 10 minutes. Divers who had experienced vertigo had logged more dives than those without vertigo and had reported middle ear pressure equilibration difficulties more frequently. These divers also noted that the pressure equilibration difficulties were more dominant in one ear. The occurrence of vertigo during underwater exposures, even those to shallow depths, can be quite hazardous. The resulting spatial disorientation with possible nausea and vomiting may explain some of the previously unexplained deaths of experienced scuba divers. The best treatment is that of prevention. First, the individual should not dive if difficulties with ear clearing exist or if a Valsalva maneuver at one ata produces vertigo. Second, divers should take precautions to adequately equilibrate middle ear pressure every two feet of descent. If a diver notices any ear fullness, blockage, or vertigo during compression, further descent should be stopped and the diver should ascend until the ears can be cleared. If vertigo is noted during ascent, and if gas supplies and other conditions permit, the ascent should be stopped and the diver should descend until the symptoms disappear. Diving with a trained companion and avoiding the beginning of an ascent when gas supplies are almost depleted are excellent rules that should not be violated.

Transient Vertigo Due to Caloric Stimulation

During most diving conditions, the vestibular end-organs are stimulated equally and vertigo does not occur. Edmonds, et al[8, 25] described caloric vertigo in divers resulting from unequal vestibular stimulation and unequal vestibular responses to equal stimuli. Vestibular nystagmus was demonstrated when cold water entered one ear, particularly when the divers were in a position in which the horizontal semicircular canal was in a vertical orientation, that is, supine with the head elevated 30° or prone with the head depressed 30°. Usually, water immersion results in an equal flow of cold water into both external auditory canals, with subsequent symmetrical vestibular end-organ stimulation and an absence of vertigo. Obstruction of one ear canal with cerumen, foreign bodies, exostoses, otitis externa, ear plugs, or diving hoods can increase the chances of unequal entry of cold water into the external auditory canals and caloric stimulation. A tympanic membrane perforation may also result in unequal entry of cold water into the middle ear and caloric stimulation vertigo.

Transient Dizziness Associated with High Pressure Nervous Syndrome (HPNS)

Transient symptoms suggestive of vestibular system dysfunction (vertigo, dizziness, and nausea) have been reported in association with high pressure nervous syndrome (HPNS).[32–34] Later studies[35–38] have indicated that these symptoms are not accompanied by demonstrable electronystagmographic nystagmus but are associated with decrements in postural equilibrium and bilaterally equal increases in the vestibulo-ocular reflex. Thus, such symptoms during HPNS are believed to be related to dysfunction in more centrally located structures and not to unilateral end-organ and/or primary vestibular neuron dysfunction.

Alternobaric Facial Paralysis

Transient unilateral facial paralysis in association with ipsilateral middle ear overpressure during ascent has been described in divers by Molvaer[39] and Becker[40] and in flyers by Bennett and Liske.[41] The divers also experienced alternobaric vertigo with an overpressure in the ear on the same side as the facial paralysis. In each instance, the paralysis subsided within one hour after onset. Becker[40] postulated that the middle ear overpressure during ascent compressed the horizontal portion of the facial nerve through a dehiscent bony fallopian canal. Also, excessive middle ear pressure during ascent may result in gas bubbles entering a nondehiscent fallopian canal through the fenestrum of the chorda tympani nerve.

Because alternobaric facial paralysis is an infrequent problem and appears to be transient, the possibility of unreported cases exists. The best treatment is prevention and should focus upon equilibration of middle ear pressure and measures to prevent inadequate ear clearing during exposures to altered atmospheric pressures as described above.

PERMANENT OTOLOGICAL INJURY IN DIVING

As discussed in the section on historical considerations, inner ear injury in diving was recognized in the latter part of the nineteenth century and in the early part of the twentieth century. In the 1930's and 1940's, safety procedures for air diving improved, and the frequency of inner ear injuries in diving decreased. Indeed, most of the diving literature concerning decompression sickness noted symptoms suggestive of inner ear injury in association with what was thought to be central nervous system decompression sickness, whereby the inner ear symptoms are relegated to secondary importance and are usually considered to be related to lesions located in the central nervous system. Hearing loss, tinnitus, or vertigo occurring during or shortly after decompression in the absence of other symptoms suggesting decompression sickness were often not treated, since isolated inner ear decompression sickness was not recognized. These conclusions reached during that time are understandable, for isolated inner ear injuries are not usually life-threatening unless a diver notes severe vertigo, nausea, and vomiting while under water. Also, it was not generally recognized by the diving community that the vestibular symptoms resulting from permanent destruction of one vestibular end-organ in otherwise healthy individuals would usually subside in four to six weeks from central nervous system compensation, even though no recovery of inner ear function had occurred. In addition, the frequency of isolated inner ear decompression sickness appears to be much greater with deeper mixed gas diving than with air diving, the major diving medium used in the 1930's and 1940's.

Beginning in the 1960's and 1970's with more frequent diving and with mixed gas diving to deeper depths, reports of permanent inner ear injury in multiple phases of diving appeared. The pathogenesis and management of diving inner ear injuries differed depending upon the phase and type of diving in which the injury occurred. These injuries have been classified as:[17, 22, 42–44] (1) injuries during descent or compression (inner ear barotrauma); (2) inner ear injuries at stable deep depths (isobaric otological barotrauma); (3) injuries occurring during ascent, during or shortly after decompression (inner ear decompression sickness); (4) sensorineural deafness related to high background noise during diving.

Injuries Occurring During Descent or Compression (Inner Ear Barotrauma)

Inner ear injuries occurring in association with relatively shallow diving and those in which the otological symptoms begin during the compression phase of deeper diving have been termed inner ear barotrauma. These injuries were first documented and named by Freeman and Edmonds in 1972[12] and were related to labyrinthine window ruptures by Edmonds, et al[13] in 1974. In these cases there was difficulty with ear clearing during descent and/or evidence on otoscopic examination of middle ear barotrauma. The depth and duration of the dives made decompression sickness unlikely. The sensorineural deafness was noted to be total or partial and occurred with or without varying degrees of vestibular dysfunction. Goodhill, et al[45] proposed that these injuries were secondary to oval and/or round window ruptures and postulated implosive and explosive mechanisms for these ruptures occurring in relationship to diving and nondiving stresses. The explosive mechanism depicted in Figure 18–2D suggests that, with inadequate middle ear pressure equilibration during descent, middle ear pressure becomes negative relative to intralabyrinthine fluid pressure as well as ambient pressure. Straining or a modified Valsalva maneuver in an attempt to clear the ear results in a further increase in the pressure differential between the labyrinth and the middle ear as a result of transmission of increases in CSF pressure to the inner ear. There is rupture of the round or oval window membrane into the middle ear and a subsequent perilymph fistula. Studies by Harker and co-workers[27] have shown that increased CSF pressure results in bulging of the round window membrane in cats, with ruptures occurring when CSF pressure is increased at levels ranging from 120 to 300 mm Hg. The implosive mechanisms suggest that, with sudden Valsalva maneuver resulting in middle ear ventilation, the rapid increase in middle ear pressure can produce rupture of the round or oval window into the intralabyrinthine space. Another possible implosive mechanism suggests that, in the presence of a negative middle ear pressure, there is inward displacement of the eardrum, ossicular chain, and stapes footplate. With a significant negative middle ear pressure, the footplate can sublux into the vestibule and an oval window fistula can occur.

Inner ear barotrauma in association with middle ear barotrauma with subsequent inner ear auditory and/or vestibular dysfunction may occur in diving without labyrinthine window rupture. Hemorrhage into the basal turn of the cochlea was noted in the animal studies by Vail in 1929.[4] Kelemen[46] noted hemorrhage in the middle and inner ears of the temporal bones of two drowning victims. No evidence of inner ear membrane tears or round or oval window fistulae were seen. Simmons[47, 48] postulated that the pressure changes encountered with inadequate middle ear pressure equilibration during the descent phase of diving may result in intralabyrinthine membrane breaks with or without labyrinthine window rupture. Indeed, Gussen[49] in 1981 noted a Reissner's membrane break without labyrinthine window rupture in the temporal bone of a woman who suffered severe ear pain with subsequent hearing loss, tinnitus, and vertigo after an airplane trip.

On the basis of these studies, Parell and Becker[50] divided the causes of 14 cases of inner ear injury related to scuba diving into hemorrhage within the inner ear, labyrinthine membrane tear, and perilymph fistula. Inner ear hemorrhage cases presented with absent or transient vestibular symptoms and moderate sensorineural hearing loss and have excellent hearing recovery without surgery. Cases with labyrinthine membrane tear presented with similar symptoms and findings, except that a localized persistent hearing loss in one or two frequencies was noted on recovery audiograms. The four cases of labyrinthine window fistula were noted to have vestibular symptoms in addition to sensorineural hearing loss. In one case, the fistula occurred in a round window that was more vertical in position so that most of the membrane could be directly seen on exploratory tympanotomy, a finding previously noted by Pullen, et al[51] and by Singleton.[52] Most labyrinthine window ruptures associated with diving involved the round window. A few cases have been noted to involve the oval window.[53]

Any diver who presents with signs of inner ear injury—vertigo, sensorineural hearing loss, loud tinnitus—after dives in which decompression sickness is unlikely should be suspected of having inner ear barotrauma and possible labyrinthine window fistula. Unless other signs indicating pulmonary overpressure accidents and air embolization are present, divers suspected of suffering inner ear barotrauma should not be subjected to recompression therapy, since such therapy exposes the patient to the same pressure changes that contributed to the otological injury. Instead these divers should be placed on bed rest with head elevation, and care should be taken that CSF and inner ear pressures are not increased. Valsalva maneuvers, coughing, nose blowing, and straining at defecation should be avoided.[13, 45] Medications that supposedly increase intracranial and inner ear blood flow are generally not effective in this regard and may result in a decrease of intracranial blood flow due to shunting of the axial circulation to the periphery and skin. Anticoagulants are potentially harmful because of possible hemorrhage from traumatized otological tissues. Ear drops containing ototoxic antibiotics should be avoided. A complete evaluation by an otolaryngologist to include otoscopic examination, proper audiometric testing, a complete neurological examination, and tests of vestibular function and the possible presence of an otological fistula should be accomplished as soon as feasible.

The need for exploratory tympanotomy in the management of diving-related inner ear barotrauma is controversial. Certainly if a fistula is present and there are no signs of improvement with conservative therapy, surgical repair of the fistula is indicated. However, as noted above, inner ear barotrauma related to diving may not be associated with an active fistula. Even the diagnosis of a perilymphatic fistula in nondiving-related cases is controversial. Seltzer and McCabe[54] noted a wide variety of signs and symptoms ranging from unilateral tinnitus and aural fullness to sudden and profound hearing loss, roaring tinnitus, and whirling vertigo in 91 patients with documented perilymphatic fistula. Twenty-three per cent of the fistulae were associated with head trauma, barotrauma, direct ear trauma, or acoustic trauma. Kohut, et al[55] point out that any one of a combination of the following criteria in a patient with an otherwise healthy ear would be highly suggestive of a perilymphatic fistula: a sensorineural hearing loss of sudden onset, fluctuating nature, or rapid progression; a positive Hennebert's sign or symptom (deviation of the eyes or dysequilibrium with changes in external ear canal pressure); dysequilibrium with loud noise exposure; positional nystagmus; and/or constant dysequilibrium of varying severity between attacks of spontaneous vertigo.

Some authors have advocated immediate exploratory surgery in all suspected cases of labyrinthine window fistula.[51] Others have suggested reserving surgery for those who do not improve after 48 to 72 hours of bed rest with head elevation.[45] Caruso and colleagues[53] reasoned that, although the majority of labyrinthine window ruptures may heal spontaneously with conservative treatment, such treatment may be associated with progressive hearing loss. They recommend that when the diagnosis is fairly certain, surgery should be performed without delay to prevent further inner ear deterioration. Most authors[56–58] advise that an initial trial of medical management as described above should be undertaken and exploratory surgery reserved for those who demonstrate no improvement after 5 to 10 days or if inner ear function worsens in the interim.

Otological Problems Occurring at Stable Deep Depths

Inner ear problems occurring at stable deep depths have been described on one occasion by Sundmaker.[59] These episodes were noted at the University of Pennsylvania in late summer of 1971. Three divers who had been breathing an oxyhelium atmosphere at a simulated depth of 600 feet in a pressure chamber noted the sudden onset of vertigo, nausea, and nystagmus shortly after starting to breathe by mask a gas mixture containing a second inert gas (neon or nitrogen). Follow-up evaluations after the dive revealed permanent end-organ vestibular dysfunction in two of the three affected subjects. No changes in auditory function were noted. The likely mechanism of these injuries appears to be related to the counterdiffusion of different inert gases with different solubilities between inner ear fluid compartments, with gas bubbles forming at tissue interfaces, such as the partitions in the inner ear between the perilymphatic and endolymphatic spaces.[21] This bubble formation produces displacement and/or disruption of the inner ear structures and occurs without changes in total ambient pressure. Blenkarn, et al[60] and Graves, et al[61] have noted gas-filled blister formations in skin following the sequential exposure to various inert gases at constant ambient pressures. These eruptions are believed to represent gas bubble formations in the deeper layers of the skin resulting from the counterdiffusion of different inert gases across tissue interfaces. Farmer[22] suggested that these inner ear injuries occurring shortly after inert gas changes at stable deep depths could be related to increased pressure in the endolymphatic space resulting from an osmotic flux of water due to more rapid accumulation of the dissolved new inert gas in endolymph.

Until the exact mechanism of these injuries at stable deep depths has been established, changes between inert gases at deep depths should be avoided if possible.

PERMANENT OTOLOGICAL INJURIES OCCURRING DURING ASCENT OR DECOMPRESSION (INNER EAR DECOMPRESSION SICKNESS)

As noted in the introduction, Smith[1] in 1873, Alt[2, 3] in 1897, and Vail[4] in 1929, indicated that inner ear injuries could occur during decompression and were possibly related to nitrogen bubble formations in the labyrinthine vasculature. The possibility of inner ear injury during diving was largely discounted until the 1960's and 1970's when there were more frequent exposures to deeper depths using mixed helium atmospheres and when isolated inner ear decompression sickness was recognized. Buhlmann and Waldvogel[62] in 1967 described 82 decompression accidents from a series of chamber dives ranging in bottom depths from 11 ata to 23 ata and noted that the only neurological symptoms of the entire series consisted of vertigo, nausea, vomiting, and tinnitus in 11 divers, with hearing loss present in 2 of these divers. Rubenstein and Summitt[15] in 1971 described 10 cases of isolated inner ear decompression sickness after diving. Farmer, et al[17] included these 10 cases and added 13 more cases of isolated inner ear decompression sickness occurring during or shortly after decompressions from 4 air and 19 helium-oxygen dives. None of these cases was associated with symptoms of middle ear barotrauma during compression, otological symptoms at the maximum depth, uncontrolled or rapid ascents, nor with other symptoms or signs suggestive of central nervous system decompression sickness. Ten of the divers had vertigo only, seven had hearing loss and tinnitus, and six exhibited hearing loss, tinnitus, and vertigo. A significant correlation between prompt recompression treatment and recovery was noted. The 11 divers who were recompressed within 42 minutes after the onset of the otological symptoms experienced relief during recompression, and subsequent studies revealed no residual inner ear dysfunction. Three divers were recompressed within 60 to 68 minutes after symptom onset; one of these individuals experienced relief of symptoms, with the remaining two having only partial or no relief and demonstrating significant residual inner ear dysfunction. In the remaining cases, recompression treatment was either delayed longer than 68 minutes after symptom onset or was not given, and the divers experienced residual inner ear dysfunction.

Thirteen of the 19 helium dives in this series involved a switch to an air atmosphere at depths ranging from 60 to 150 feet during the latter stages of decompression. Farmer and coworkers[17] postulated that the sudden decrease in helium partial pressure during such an air switch possibly contributed to the formation of helium gas bubbles in inner ear tissues during decompression. Another speculated pathophysiological mechanism involved the formation of bubbles at inner ear tissue boundaries resulting from the counterdiffusion of two different inert gases between inner ear fluid compartments, similar to the counterdiffusion mechanism suggested by Graves, et al[61] and by Lambertson and Idicula[21] to explain inner ear injuries noted at stable deep depths after inert gas changes.

Animal studies have shown interesting findings regarding the pathophysiology of inner ear decompression sickness. McCormick and colleagues[18, 63] in 1975 showed that guinea pigs subjected to rapid decompression developed bubble formation and hemorrhages in labyrinthine fluid spaces and decreases in cochlear potentials. They also observed that these deficits in inner ear electrical function could be lessened by treating the animals with heparin prior to the dives, indicating that a key mechanism of inner ear decompression sickness may be hypercoagulation in the inner ear microvasculature as described by Philp.[64] The most extensive animal studies of inner ear decompression sickness have been performed in Toronto and are reviewed by Landolt, et al.[65] These investigations have revealed that the inner ear in squirrel monkeys, apparently similar to the inner ear in humans, is susceptible to decompression sickness. Clinical observations plus electronystagmographic recordings and post-dive histological studies revealed that the injuries occurred during the latter stages of decompression and were related to specific inner ear histological findings. Shortly after the injuries, varying degrees of hemorrhage and blood-protein exudate in the inner ear fluid spaces and tissues were noted. The inner ears of monkeys killed 38 to 383 days following decompression showed the appearance of connective tissue and new bone growth that tended to obliterate the damaged regions of the semicircular canals. An interesting biophysical mechanism to explain these changes involves the production of significant pressures by bubble enucleation and growth within osteoplastic cell cavities of the endosteal bone immediately surrounding the semicircular canals. During the latter stages of decompression, significant pressure differentials will occur between these bony cellular spaces and the adjacent perilymphatic spaces with a sudden implosive fracture of the endosteal bone into the canal space. The implosive nature of such fractures was postulated to cause a pressure wave bolus to move rapidly along the canal with tearing of the endosteum and loosening of the attachments of the membranous semicircular ducts to the canal wall with initial bleeding and a later stimulus for subsequent new bone growth. Indeed, Money, et al[66] in 1986 reported similar changes in the inner ear of a professional diver who died of unrelated causes 56 days after suffering left inner ear decompression sickness that did not respond to prompt recompression. He was noted to have a persistent total loss of left vestibular function and partial left sensorineural deafness. His temporal bone histology revealed ectopic bone growth and fibrosis in the left ear semicircular canal similar to that seen in the squirrel monkeys sacrificed 38 days or longer after inner ear decompression sickness.

Management of Inner Ear Decompression Sickness

As a result of the human investigations, the following measures were proposed by Farmer and colleagues[17] in 1976 and, thus far, appear to be appropriate:

1. Inner ear symptoms that begin during or shortly after the decompression phase of dives in which decompression sickness is possible should be considered forms of decompression sickness and should be recompressed promptly.
2. Divers who experience such symptoms during or shortly after a switch to an air environment during decompression from a deep helium-oxygen exposure should be switched back to the presymptom helium-oxygen atmosphere and recompressed promptly.
3. The optimum treatment depth has not been established. Obviously the lesser of the depth of relief or the bottom depth would be an appropriate end point. However, in some cases, bubble formation in the inner ear will have caused structural deformities, such as those described in animal studies[65] and in one human study[66] by Landolt and co-workers; thus, relief of inner ear symptoms will not be seen even though an adequate depth of recompression to drive the bubbles back into solution has been achieved. Also, returning to the bottom depth in some diving situations may be hazardous or impractical. Therefore, it was arbitrarily suggested in 1976[17] that the optimum treatment depth in these situations should be 3 atm deeper than the depth at which symptoms occurred. When symptom onset occurs after surfacing, prompt recompression using tables suitable for the treatment of central nervous system decompression sickness should be instituted. These recommendations thus far seem to be adequate; however, future studies are needed to more precisely define the optimum recompression profile.
4. The use of other measures in the treatment of otological decompression sickness, such as anticoagulants and low molecular weight dextran, have not been adequately evaluated. Anticoagulation could cause additional harm, particularly if inner ear hemorrhage has occurred as indicated in the animal studies. Therefore, anticoagulation is not recommended. Drugs that supposedly increase intracranial and inner ear blood flow are generally not effective in this regard and result in shunting of blood to the periphery; therefore, these agents are not recommended. Conversely, fluid replacement and

other measures such as the administration of oxygen-enriched treatment gases, as advocated in the treatment of decompression sickness, are indicated. Whether or not steroids and salicylates are beneficial in the management of inner ear decompression sickness is not known. If significant hemorrhage has occurred, the use of salicylates could possibly be undesirable because of an additional anticoagulation effect. Also, salicylates are potentially ototoxic.

5. Diazepam (Valium), 5 to 15 mg intramuscularly, has been noted to result in significant relief of vertigo, nausea, and vomiting, which can be quite severe during otological decompression sickness. This drug can suppress the accompanying nystagmus and may thus mask a sign of optimum treatment. In many cases, however, the symptoms are so severe that relief is preferred. Monitoring of the respiratory rate and blood pressure after parenteral admission of Valium is recommended.

6. A complete otoneurological examination with audiometry and electronystagmography as soon as possible after adequate recompression therapy is essential. A disappearance of vestibular symptoms within 4 to 6 weeks after the injury does not usually mean that recovery of inner ear function has occurred, for central nervous system compensation will occur. Thus, individuals who have completely lost inner ear vestibular function on one side usually become asymptomatic, provided a normal inner ear is present on the opposite side and normal central nervous system vestibular function is present.

7. Divers who suffer permanent inner ear dysfunction as a result of inner ear decompression sickness should not be returned to diving. Some believe further inner ear injury to the same ear is more likely and could result in extreme danger at depth from the associated vertigo and possible nausea and vomiting. Also, injury to the opposite inner ear during future diving could result in significant disability for nondiving activities, particularly occupational and life skills involving communication and balance.

The persistence in either ear of a pure tone audiometric threshold greater than 25 db in the frequency ranges of 500 to 2000 Hz, a speech discrimination score of less than 90 per cent, or electronystagmographic abnormalities indicating persistent inner ear vestibular dysfunction should disqualify the individual for future diving.

Differential Diagnosis of Inner Ear Barotrauma and Inner Ear Decompression Sickness[43, 44]

In some instances, the differential diagnosis of inner ear barotrauma and inner ear decompression sickness is difficult. An accurate, prompt diagnosis is important because the proper treatment of these two entities is significantly different. Prompt recompression therapy is essential in the appropriate management of inner ear decompression sickness; recompression therapy should be avoided in cases with inner ear barotrauma. Decompression sickness can occur even when the decompression tables are accurately followed; thus, the differential diagnosis may be difficult if the related dive involves an exposure close to the no decompression limits. Also, divers occasionally do not know when during the dive the symptoms began, and signs of middle ear barotrauma suggesting inner ear barotrauma or other signs of decompression sickness may not be present. Usually, an accurate history and physical examination will allow the physician to differentiate these two entities; however, in cases when the differential diagnosis is difficult, the major factors to be considered include the following:

1. The time of symptom onset. Otological symptoms occurring during compression most likely represent inner ear barotrauma; otological symptoms starting during or shortly after decompression are most likely related to inner ear decompression sickness.

2. Knowledge of the dive type and profile. Inner ear dysfunction associated with shallow dives where decompression sickness is unlikely, with rapid descent, or the lack of conscious efforts to adequately equilibrate middle ear pressure during descent are more likely to be related to inner ear barotrauma. Also, inner ear barotrauma seems to be more common with air diving, whereas inner ear decompression sickness appears to be more common with deeper mixed gas diving.

3. The presence or absence of associated symptoms. Ear pain, blockage, or fullness during compression are more likely to be related to inner ear barotrauma. Other symptoms of decompression sickness are more likely to be associated with inner ear decompression sickness.

4. The presence or absence of associated physical findings. Findings indicating middle ear barotrauma are more likely to be associated

with inner ear barotrauma. Divers who exhibit inner ear symptoms and who have other signs of decompression sickness, such as other neurological deficits, should be suspected of having inner ear decompression sickness.

OTOLOGICAL INJURIES RELATED TO HIGH BACKGROUND NOISES DURING DIVING CONDITIONS

Coles and Knight[67] in a survey of Royal Navy divers concluded that high frequency sensorineural deafness seen in the usual diving population could be explained on the basis of previous nondiving noise exposures. Divers with no history of previous excessive noise exposure had high frequency hearing losses similar to the overall nondiving population when allowances were made for age. However, investigations by Summitt and Reimers[68] and Murray[69] have demonstrated excessive noise levels ranging from 98 to 120 dbA in pressure chambers from the inflow of gases during compression from the ventilators and in diving helmets from the inflow of breathing gases. Acceptable damage risk criteria for noise exposure limits at the surface suggest that these levels during diving in pressure chambers and in diving helmets may cause noise-induced hearing losses with exposures as brief as 15 minutes. It is not known whether the previously noted reversible and depth-related conductive hearing losses, secondary to decreased sound transmission by the eardrum and ossicles in compressed gases,[70–72] are sufficient to provide attenuation from excessive noise during diving. Smith[73] at the Naval Submarine Medical Research Laboratory in New London indicated that auditory threshold shifts are smaller during noise exposures at depth than during comparable noise exposures on the surface. Thus, some protective attenuation by the temporary conductive hearing losses caused by the compressed gas environment may be present. However, temporary threshold shifts were noted by Summitt and Reimers[68] in the air helmet dives. This would indicate that these conductive hearing losses do not provide sufficient attenuation to protect divers from these noise levels.

In any case, the existing noise exposure limits for exposures at 1 ata would seem inappropriate for application to hyperbaric exposures. Until more data are available regarding the actual damage risk from excessive noise in diving, chambers and helmets should be designed to operate as quietly as possible.

INTRACRANIAL CONSEQUENCES OF OTOLOGICAL BAROTRAUMA

Goldmann[74] described in 1986 an interesting case of pneumocephalus secondary to otological barotrauma. A 26-year-old healthy male scuba diving instructor noted left ear pain while ascending to the surface after a 60-foot freshwater dive. Upon reaching the surface, his left ear pain suddenly disappeared and he developed a severe left vertex headache. After several hours of surface interval, he subsequently dove again to 60 feet and noted the headache improved at depth; however, upon ascent the headache returned with increasing severity. Upon presentation, the physical examination was unremarkable with the exception of left middle ear barotrauma. Skull x-rays revealed a subdural pneumocephalus localized to the left side of the cranium; a CT scan of the brain revealed air in the subdural space, and a nuclear magnetic resonance scan of the brain 16 days after the incident revealed a small amount of blood in the left epidural space near the base of the skull with blood in both mastoids, greater on the left side. He was treated conservatively with prophylactic antibiotics with gradual resolution of his headache and a normal follow-up CT scan one month later. Usually during ascent expanding gas in the middle ear passively is cleared by the eustachian tube. However, if a greater than 2 to 3 foot pressure differential occurs between the middle ear space and the ambient pressure during descent, swelling and congestion of the eustachian tube and middle ear mucosa will impede passive clearing of the middle ear during ascent, with subsequent increased middle ear pressure similar to that noted with alternobaric vertigo as described above. This increased pressure is distributed throughout the middle ear cleft and mastoid air cell system. Frequently the bony roof of the middle ear attic area, which also forms the floor of the middle cranial fossa, is thin with dehiscences in approximately 22 per cent of normal human temporal bones as described by Ferguson, et al.[75] Thus, this area may have provided a route for the escape of expanding gas into the intracranial space.

PARANASAL SINUS BAROTRAUMA

Paranasal sinus barotrauma has been described in flyers[76, 77] and in divers.[78, 79] The mechanisms and pathophysiology are related to inadequate pressure equilibration between the air-containing paranasal sinus cavities during ascent, descent, or both. Usually adequate ventilation and pressure equilibration between the middle ear and paranasal sinuses are dependent, to a large degree, upon nasal function. Inflammation and congestion of the nasal mucosa, nasal structural deformities, or mass lesions, can result in blockage of the paranasal sinus ostia. Such blockage occurring in the absence of ambient atmospheric pressure changes leads to a series of changes within the sinuses consisting of absorption of pre-existing air and decreased intrasinus pressure; swelling, engorgement, and inflammation of the sinus mucosa; and collection of transudate in the sinus cavity. When such blockage occurs during descent in diving or flying, the decrease in intrasinus pressure becomes greater, and the resulting pathological changes are more severe with hemorrhage into the mucosa and often into the sinus cavity. Paranasal sinus barotrauma also occurs during ascent whereby the pathological mechanism is frequently related to a one-way valve blockage of the sinus ostium by inflamed mucosa, cyst, or polyps located within the sinus. Thus, pressure equilibration may occur during descent but may be impaired during ascent.

Fagan and colleagues[79] reported in 1976 a series of 50 consecutive cases of documented paranasal sinus barotrauma in divers. In 68 per cent of the divers, symptoms developed during or immediately after descent; symptoms occurred after ascent in 32 per cent. Pain was the predominant symptom. The frontal sinus was most often involved. This is likely due to the fact that the nasofrontal duct is longer and more tortuous, whereas the communications between the maxillary, ethmoid, and sphenoid sinuses and the nasal cavity are short ostia. The second most common symptom was epistaxis occurring in 58 per cent of the cases. Thirty-two per cent of the patients noted a history of previous paranasal sinus barotrauma, and 50 per cent had a history of recent upper respiratory tract infections. A history of chronic nasal and sinus problems was also reported by 50 per cent of the patients, and associated signs of middle ear barotrauma were noted in 48 per cent. Symptoms in addition to pain and epistaxis include pain in the upper teeth, occasional paresthesias, and decreased sensation over the infraorbital nerve distribution, as reported by Neuman and co-workers in 1975.[80] The presence of purulent nasal discharge indicates secondary infection.

Chronic paranasal sinus disease can predispose to paranasal sinus and middle ear barotrauma during atmospheric pressure changes. The common underlying etiologies of such chronic diseases are: (1) allergy, either intrinsic or extrinsic; (2) chronic irritation from smoking, excessive or prolonged use of nose drops or nasal sprays, or exposure to toxic or irritating chemical vapors; (3) mechanical obstruction from internal and external nasal deformities, polyps, or neoplasia; and (4) vasomotor causes from chronic tension, stress, or anxiety.

In many patients with chronic paranasal sinus disease, more than one of these causative factors is involved. Exposure to cold dry air normally results in increased nasal blood flow with congestion and increased mucous secretion. Thus, worsening of the underlying conditions is frequently seen during the winter months. Secondary bacterial infection not uncommonly occurs and is indicated by the appearance of purulent discharge. Frequently there is also associated chronic inflammation of the lower respiratory tract, such as seen in patients with allergies (asthma) or chronic irritation from smoking.

Treatment of paranasal sinus barotrauma includes the use of topical and systemic vasoconstrictor agents to promote nasal mucosal shrinkage and opening of the sinus ostia, with purulent nasal discharge. Cultures and appropriate antibiotics are also indicated. Future atmospheric pressure changes should be avoided until recovery, which usually requires 7 to 14 days. Most of the patients in the series reported by Fagan, et al[79] required no treatment; those who did responded to nasal decongestants alone, and only occasional patients required antibiotics. No patient required sinus lavage or surgery. Individuals who have symptoms persisting for long periods, who have decreased transillumination of a maxillary or frontal sinus, or who have indications of systemic disease or a chronic underlying paranasal sinus disease should be referred for sinus x-rays and otolaryngological evaluation.

Systemic and topical adrenergic drugs can improve paranasal sinus and middle ear ventilation. However, caution should be observed for rebound phenomenon, especially with topical nose drops, which can lead to greater nasal congestion and increased difficulty with middle ear and paranasal sinus cavity pressure equilibration. The topical nasal decongestants also cause varying degrees of paralysis in the mucosal microscopic cilia and dissolution of the protective mucous blanket. Thus, prolonged use of these agents can result in chronic nasal irritation and mucosal inflammation, with increased problems of middle ear and paranasal sinus pressure equilibration. Antihistamines, either in combination or singly, can unpredictably cause drowsiness. Also, adrenergic drugs, either singly or in combination, can cause systemic, undesired adrenergic effects as well as excessive drying of the nasal and paranasal sinus mucosa and, thus, may be detrimental in some conditions. Individuals who must use decongestants and/or antihistamines, either systemic or topical, in order to equilibrate middle ear pressure during diving should be warned that they are not ideal diving candidates, and consideration should be given to trying to identify a chronic and possibly correctible underlying cause as described above before returning to diving. At the time of a pre-diving physical, individuals with a history of possible chronic paranasal sinus or nasal disease, such as chronic nasal congestion or discharge, chronic purulent discharge, frequent upper respiratory infections, a previous history of middle ear disease, or a past history of nasal or paranasal sinus surgery, all occurring in the absence of altered atmospheric pressure changes, are certainly less likely to be able to adequately equilibrate paranasal sinus or middle ear pressure when exposed to pressure changes encountered in diving and should be thoroughly evaluated before being cleared to dive.

SUMMARY OF OTOLARYNGOLOGY GUIDELINES FOR THE MEDICAL EXAMINATION OF SPORTS SCUBA DIVERS

Neblett[81] has well summarized the guidelines for the medical examination of sports scuba divers. Some of those related to otolaryngology are reviewed in the previous sections of this chapter.

Ear

History

A history of ear drainage, middle ear effusions, or middle ear infections in the past three years indicates poor eustachian tubal function and an increased likelihood of middle ear barotrauma. The presence of frequent or chronic respiratory tract membrane disease as noted above also increases this likelihood.

A history of previous ear surgery should alert the physician to possible continuing borderline or poor eustachian tubal function. Individuals who have undergone a previous simple repair of a tympanic membrane perforation can be considered for diving if the eardrum has remained healed and if the ear can easily be autoinflated or cleared at the surface. Those who have undergone a previous simple mastoidectomy that has healed well with adequate eustachian tubal function can also be considered for diving. However, those who have undergone a mastoidectomy, which involves removal of the posterior external auditory canal wall (a radical or modified radical mastoidectomy), should not undertake diving. A caloric response with vertigo, nausea, and vomiting is more likely if water enters such a cavity. Also, such patients are more likely to have poor eustachian tubal function. Patients who have undergone stapedectomy or stapedotomy surgery should not dive because of the increased risk of an oval window fistula and inner ear injury with middle ear pressure changes. Individuals who have a history suggestive of Meniere's disease, characterized by recurrent bouts of vertigo and/or hearing loss with tinnitus, or other inner ear disease with recurrent bouts of vertigo should not dive, since the occurrence of vertigo with possible nausea and vomiting while under water can result in drowning. Also, the presence of such pathological changes in the inner ear may increase the likelihood of inner ear injury with diving. These are appropriate contraindications even if the audiometric and vestibular results at the time of the examination are not disqualifying.

Physical Examination

The prerequisites for diving include an intact tympanic membrane and the ability to easily autoinflate each ear by a gentle modified Valsalva or Toynbee maneuver. Movement of the tympanic membrane should be visible. Contraindications to diving, in addition to a tympanic membrane perforation, would include the presence of or need for ventilation tubes which indicates inadequate eustachian tubal function in the absence of significant atmospheric pressure changes. Eardrums frequently exhibit whitish plaques of varying size. If the drum is intact, moves well, and the patient can autoinflate, diving may be considered. A thin flaccid tympanic membrane (monomeric or dimeric eardrum) indicates poor eustachian tubal function and an increased likelihood of tympanic membrane perforation as well as middle ear barotrauma with diving. The presence of a cholesteatoma, or a skin-lined sac within the middle ear, indicates chronic middle ear disease and poor eustachian tubal function and should be a contraindication to diving. Also, water may enter and contaminate a cholesteatoma sac with infection and further bone erosion.

Stenosis or atresia of the ear canal as well as chronic or acute external otitis until healed should be contraindications to diving. Patients who have cerumen impactions should not dive until the cerumen is removed. Individuals with marked narrowing of the canal from ear canal osteomas should be cautioned about diving.

Laboratory Investigations

The presence in either ear of a pure tone audiometric threshold worse or greater than 25 db in the frequency range of 500 to 2000 Hz, a speech discrimination score of less than 90 per cent, or electronystagmographic abnormalities indicating inner ear vestibular dysfunction should disqualify an individual for future diving. Such inner ears may be more susceptible to future inner ear barotrauma, inner ear decompression sickness, or both. Injury to the opposite inner ear during future diving could result in significant disabilities.

Returning to diving after diving-related otological injury is discussed under each specific entity.

Nose and Paranasal Sinuses

Candidates being considered for suitability for scuba diving should have patent nasal airways and should not have either acute or significant chronic nasal or sinus symptoms. Conditions that cause nasal obstruction such as polyps, septal deviations, or chronically edematous nasal mucosa as seen with allergies or chronic irritations increase the chance of middle ear and paranasal sinus barotrauma. Patients who require frequent or chronic usage of oral and topical decongestants, antihistamines, or steroids should be carefully evaluated. Such individuals are at an increased risk for barotrauma. Many have underlying respiratory tract allergies that involve the lower as well as the upper respiratory tract; bronchial asthma would be a contraindication for diving. Individuals who require the use of decongestants in order to dive should be cautioned about rebound phenomena and adrenergic side effects; they should be advised to abort dives if adequate middle ear pressure equilibration does not easily occur every two feet of descent. The use of these drugs does not usually allow safe pressurization in the presence of an acute upper respiratory tract infection; diving should be delayed until the acute episode has subsided.

Larynx

Any patient who has intermittent and chronic aspiration suggesting an incompetent larynx should not be cleared for diving. The presence of a laryngocele should also disqualify a patient for diving until the problem is corrected. The existence of a tracheotomy or tracheostomy is an absolute contraindication to swimming as well as diving.

REFERENCES

1. Smith AH: The Effects of High Atmospheric Pressure, Including the Caisson Disease. Brooklyn, Eagle Print, 1873, pp 1–53.
2. Alt F: Pathologie der Luftdruckerkrankungen des Gehororgans. Verh Dtsch Otol Ges 6:49–64, 1897. (English translation by Mrs. A Woke, NMRI, 1972.)
3. Alt F, Heller R, Mager W, vonSchrotter H: Pathologie der Luftdruckerkrankkungen des Gehororgans. Mschr Ohrenheilk 21:229–242, 1897. (English translation by Mrs. A Woke, NMRI, 1972.)
4. Vail HH: Traumatic conditions of the ear in workers in an atmosphere of compressed air. Arch Otolaryngol 10:113–126, 1929.
5. Behnke AR: Physiologic effect of pressure changes with reference to otolaryngology. Trans Am Acad Ophthalmol Otol 49:63–71, 1944.
6. Shilling CW, Everley IA: Auditory acuity in submarine personnel, Part III. US Navy Med Bull 40:664–686, 1942.
7. Taylor GD: The otolaryngologic aspects of skin and scuba diving. Laryngoscope 69:809–858, 1959.
8. Edmonds C, Freeman P, Thomas R, et al: Otological Aspects of Diving. Sydney, Australian Medical Publishing Company, 1973.
9. Kennedy RD: General history of vestibular disorders in diving. Undersea Biomed Res 1:73–81, 1974.
10. Lundren CEG: Alternobaric vertigo—a diver's hazard. Br Med J 2:511–513, 1965.
11. Ingelstedt S, Ivarsson A, Tjernstrom O: Vertigo due to relative overpressure in the middle ear: An experimental study in man. Acta Otolaryngol 78:1–14, 1974.
12. Freeman P, Edmonds C: Inner ear barotrauma. Arch Otolaryngol 95:556–563, 1972.
13. Edmonds C, Freeman P, Tonkin J: Fistula of the round window in diving. Trans Am Acad Ophthalmol Otol 78:444–447, 1974.
14. Stucker FJ, Echols WB: Otolaryngologic problems of underwater exploration. Milit Med 136:896–899, 1971.
15. Rubenstein CJ, Summitt JK: Vestibular derangement in decompression. *In* Lambertsen CJ (ed): Underwater Physiology, Proceedings of the Fourth Symposium on Underwater Physiology. New York, Academic Press, 1971, pp 287–292.

16. Buhlman AA, Gehring H: Inner ear disorders resulting from inadequate decompression—"vertigo bends." *In* Lambertsen CJ (ed): Underwater Physiology, Proceedings of the Fifth Symposium on Underwater Physiology. Bethesda Federation of American Societies for Experimental Biology, 1976, pp 341–347.
17. Farmer JC, Thomas WG, Youngblood DG, Bennett PB: Inner ear decompression sickness. Laryngoscope 86:1315–1326, 1976.
18. McCormick JG, Philbrick T, Holland W, Harrill JA: Diving induced sensorineural deafness: Prophylactic use of heparin and preliminary histopathology results. Laryngoscope 83:1483–1501, 1973.
19. Landolt JP, Money KE, Topliff EDL, et al: Vestibulocochlear dysfunction in squirrel monkeys in simulated diving experiments. Med Aeronaut Spat Med Subaquat Hyperbar 16:377–381, 1977.
20. Venter RD, Ho BN, Johnson WR, et al: Fracture studies on semicircular canals of the inner ear. Undersea Biomed Res 10:225–240, 1983.
21. Lambertsen CJ, Idicula J: A new gas lesion syndrome in man, induced by "isobaric gas counterdiffusion." J Appl Physiol 39:434–443, 1975.
22. Farmer JC, Jr: Diving injuries to the inner ear. Ann Otol Rhinol Laryngol 86(Suppl 36, no 1, pt 3):1–20, 1977.
23. Farmer JC, Jr: Otolaryngology. *In* Sabiston DC (ed): Essentials of Surgery. Philadelphia, WB Saunders Company, 1987, pp 686–705.
24. McCabe BF: Vestibular physiology: Its clinical application in understanding the dizzy patient. *In* Paparella MM, Schumrick DA (eds): Basic Sciences and Related Disciplines. Vol 1. Otolaryngology. Philadelphia, WB Saunders Company, 1973, pp 318–328.
25. Edmonds C, Lowry C, Pennefather J: Diving and Subaquatic Medicine. 2nd Ed. Mosman, Australia, Diving Medical Center, 1981, pp 393–406.
26. Keller AP: A study of the relationship of air pressures to myringopuncture. Laryngoscope 68:2015–2029, 1958.
27. Harker L, Norante J, Rzu J: Experimental rupture of the round window membrane. Trans Am Acad Ophthalmol Otol 78:448–452, 1974.
28. Vorosmarti J, Bradley JJ: Alternobaric vertigo in military divers. Milit Med 135:182–185, 1970.
29. Terry L, Dennison WL: Vertigo amongst divers. Special Report 66–2. Groton CT, USN Submarine Medical Center, 1966.
30. Tjernstrom O: On alternobaric vertigo—experimental studies. Forvarsmedicin 9:410–415, 1973.
31. Lundgren C, Tjernstrom O, Ornhagen H: Alternobaric vertigo and hearing disturbances in connection with diving: An epidemiologic study. Undersea Biomed Res 1:251–258, 1974.
32. Buhlmann A, Matthys H, Overrath H, et al: Saturation exposures at 31 ata. Aerosp Med 41:394–402, 1970.
33. Bennett PB, Towse EJ: The high pressure nervous syndrome during a simulated oxygen-helium dive to 1500 feet. Electroencephalogr Clin Neurophysiol 31:383–393, 1971.
34. Brauer RW: Seeking man's depth level. Ocean Ind 3:28–33, 1968.
35. Adolfson JA, Goldberg L, Berghage TE: Effects of increased ambient air pressures on standing steadiness in man. Aerosp Med 43:520–524, 1972.
36. Braithwaite WR, Berghage TE, Crothers JC: Postural equilibrium and vestibular response at 49.5 ata. Undersea Biomed Res 1:309–323, 1974.
37. Farmer JC, Thomas WG, Smith RW, Bennett PB: Vestibular function during HPNS (abstract). Undersea Biomed Res 1:A–11, 1974.
38. Gauthier GM: Alterations of the human vestibulo-ocular reflex in a simulated dive at 62 ata. Undersea Biomed Res 3:103–112, 1976.
39. Molvaer OL: Alternobaric facial palsy. Med Aeronaut Spat Med Subaquat Hyperbar 18:249–250, 1979.
40. Becker GD: Recurrent alternobaric facial paralysis resulting from scuba diving. Laryngoscope 93:596–598, 1983.
41. Bennett D, Liske E: Transient facial paralysis during ascent to altitude. Neurology 17:194–198, 1967.
42. Farmer JC: Otological and paranasal sinus problems in diving. *In* Bennett PB, Elliott DH (eds): The Physiology and Medicine of Diving. 3rd Ed. London, Bailliere Tindall, 1982, p 507.
43. Farmer JC: Inner ear barotrauma, pp 414–416, and Inner ear decompression sickness, pp 312–316. *In* Shilling CW, Carlston CB, Mathias RA (eds): The Physician's Guide to Diving Medicine. New York, Plenum Press, 1984.
44. Farmer JC, Gillespie CA: Otologic medicine and surgery of exposures to aerospace, diving, and compressed gases. *In* Alberti PW, Ruben RJ (eds): Otologic Medicine and Surgery. New York, Churchill Livingstone, 1988, pp 1753–1802.
45. Goodhill V, Harris I, Brockman S: Sudden deafness in labyrinthine window ruptures. Ann Otol Rhinol Laryngol 82:2–12, 1973.
46. Kelemen G: Temporal bone findings in cases of salt water drowning. Ann Otol Rhinol Laryngol 92:134–136, 1983.
47. Simmons FB: Theory of membrane breaks in sudden hearing loss. Arch Otolaryngol 88:41–48, 1968.
48. Simmons FB: Fluid dynamics in sudden sensorineural hearing loss. Otolaryngol Clin North Am 11:55–61, 1978.
49. Gussen R: Sudden hearing loss associated with cochlear membrane rupture. Arch Otolaryngol 107:598–600, 1981.
50. Parell GJ, Becker GD: Conservative management of inner ear barotrauma resulting from scuba diving. Otolaryngol Head Neck Surg 93:393–397, 1985.
51. Pullen FW, Rosenberg GJ, Cabeza CH: Sudden hearing loss in divers. Laryngoscope 89:1373–1377, 1979.
52. Singleton GT: Diagnosis and treatment of perilymph fistulas without hearing loss. Otolaryngol Head Neck Surg 94:426–429, 1986.
53. Caruso BG, Winkelmann PE, Correia MJ, et al: Otologic and otoneurologic injuries in divers: Clinical studies on nine commercial and two sport divers. Laryngoscope 87:508–521, 1977.
54. Seltzer S, McCabe F: Perilymph fistula: The Iowa experience. Laryngoscope 94:37–49, 1986.
55. Kohut RI, Hinojosa R, Budetti JA: Perilymph fistula: A histopathologic study. Ann Otol Rhinol Laryngol 95:466–471, 1986.
56. Singleton GT, Karlan MC, Post KN, Bock DG: Perilymph fistulas: Diagnostic criteria and therapy. Ann Otol Rhinol Laryngol 87:797–803, 1978.
57. Althaus SR: Perilymph fistulas. Laryngoscope 91:538–562, 1981.
58. Love JT, Waguespack RW: Perilymph fistulas. Laryngoscope 91:1118–1128, 1981.
59. Sundmaker W: Vestibular function. *In* Lambertsen C (ed): Special Summary Program, Predictive Studies III. Philadelphia, University of Pennsylvania, 1973.
60. Blenkarn G, Aquadro C, Hills B, Saltzman H: Urticaria following the sequential breathing of various inert gases at a constant pressure of 7 ata: A possible manifestation of gas induced osmosis. Aerosp Med 42:141–146, 1971.

61. Graves D, Idicula J, Lambertsen C, Quinn J: Bubble formation in physical and biological systems: A manifestation of counterdiffusion in composite media. Science 179:582–584, 1973.
62. Buhlmann A, Waldvogel W: The treatment of decompression sickness. Helv Med Acta 33:487–491, 1967.
63. McCormick JG, Holland WB, Brauer RW, Holleman IL: Sudden hearing loss due to diving and its prevention with heparin. Otolaryngol Clin North Am 8:2:417–430, 1975.
64. Philp RB: A review of blood changes associated with compression-decompression: Relationship to decompression sickness. Undersea Biomed Res 1:117–150, 1974.
65. Landolt JP, Money KE, Radomski MW, et al: Inner ear decompression sickness in the squirrel monkey: Observations, interpretations, and mechanisms. *In* Bachrach AJ, Matzen MM (eds): Underwater Physiology VII, Proceedings of the 8th Symposium on Underwater Physiology. Bethesda, Undersea Medical Society, 1984, pp 211–224.
66. Money KE, Buckingham IP, Calder IM, et al: Damage to the middle and the inner ear in underwater divers. Undersea Biomed Res 12:77–84, 1985.
67. Coles R, Knight J: Aural and audiometric survey of qualified divers and submarine escape training instructors. Med Res Counc Ser (Lond) Report RNPL 61/1011, 1961.
68. Summitt J, Reimers J: Noise: A hazard to divers and hyperbaric chamber personnel. Aerosp Med 42:1173–1177, 1971.
69. Murray T: Noise levels inside Navy diving chambers during compression and decompression. Nav Sub Med Cntr, Report No 643, 1970.
70. Fluur E, Adolfson J: Hearing in hyperbaric air. Aerosp Med 57:783–785, 1966.
71. Farmer J, Thomas W, Preslar M: Human auditory response during hyperbaric helium-oxygen exposures. Surg Forum 22:456–458, 1971.
72. Thomas W, Summitt J, Farmer J: Human auditory thresholds during deep saturation helium-oxygen dives. J Acoust Soc Am 55:810–813, 1974.
73. Smith PF: Development of hearing conservation standards for hazardous noise associated with diving operations. Nav Sub Med Cntr Report No 1029, 1983.
74. Goldmann RW: Pneumocephalus as a consequence of barotrauma. JAMA 255:3154–3156, 1986.
75. Ferguson BJ, Wilkins RH, Hudson WR, Farmer JC: Spontaneous CSF otorrhea from tegmen and posterior fossa defects. Laryngoscope 96:635–644, 1986.
76. Wright B, Boyd H: Aerosinusitis. Arch Otolaryngol 41:193–203, 1945.
77. Campbell P: Aerosinusitis, a resume. Ann Otol Rhinol Laryngol 54:69–83, 1945.
78. Idicula J: Perplexing case of maxillary sinus barotrauma. Aerosp Med 43:891–892, 1972.
79. Fagan P, McKenzie B, Edmonds E: Sinus barotrauma in divers. Ann Otol Rhinol Laryngol 85:61–64, 1976.
80. Neuman T, Settle H, Beaver G, Linaweaver PG: Maxillary sinus barotrauma with cranial nerve involvement: Case report. Aviat Space Environ Med 46:314–315, 1975.
81. Neblett LM: Otolaryngology and sport scuba diving: Update and guidelines. Ann Otol Rhinol Laryngol 94(suppl 115):2–12, 1985.

Chapter 19

Neurological Consequences of Diving

HUGH D. GREER

THE TARGET ORGAN

The nervous system is the principal target of diving injury. Bert recognized this when he wrote about decompression sickness in 1877.[1] Virtually all the "bends" literature before 1975 described 'pain only' versus 'CNS' decompression sickness. Hallenbeck sorted out the pathophysiology of spinal cord decompression sickness in that year and called attention to the rarity of brain decompression sickness in divers.[2, 3] At about the same time, Peters and colleagues[4] presented evidence that brain involvement does occur, often unrecognized or overshadowed by the more dramatic paraplegia of spinal cord injury. Others have written of divers being "punchy" after multiple exposures.[5, 6]

In dramatic contrast, air embolism attacks the brain directly and immediately, presenting as acute stroke with focal hemispheric or brain stem injury. Seizure, aphasia, and hemiparesis are common, and cortical blindness occurs disproportionately often. The frequent occurrence of cardiorespiratory arrest suggests that the posterior circulation is often embolized.[7–9]

Encephalopathy from hypoxemia is a grim feature of drowning or of air supply failure from any cause and is not peculiar to divers.

The peripheral nerves are infrequently injured by decompression sickness. The facial, trigeminal, and median nerves each have anatomical peculiarities that provide opportunity for discrete single bubble hits.

The common denominator is the exquisite vulnerability of nerve cells to ischemia. It is generally recognized that nerve cells lose function after a few minutes of hypoxia and that cell death occurs shortly thereafter. Nerve cells have no anaerobic metabolism. They require a constant supply of oxygen and glucose from the blood in order to function and survive. The homeostatic limits are narrow. Loss of consciousness occurs when P_aO_2 falls to 20 to 30 torr and when glucose falls to 20 to 30 mg per cent. The former limit is frequently approached in long breath-hold dives. The mechanisms of ischemia are different in decompression sickness, air embolism, and asphyxia, but the basic unit is the neuron. The onset, course, and outcome of each illness are largely determined by the duration of neural ischemia.

BRAIN

In decompression sickness, brain dysfunction is often manifested by confusion, drowsiness, fatigue, and indifference. The pain and paraplegia of spinal cord decompression sickness occurs earlier and more often and attracts the most attention. However, examiners and companions often call attention to decreased mentation; retrospective analyses indicate that cognitive and psychological defects do result from decompression sickness.

Peters reported the study of 20 divers in 1977. Ten of the divers had definite events of neurological decompression sickness. Neuropsychological testing demonstrated evidence of cerebral, cerebellar, or brain stem injury in seven of the 10 divers with history of decompression sickness. None of the control divers showed such abnormalities.[4] Vaernes and Eidsvik[5] reported similar findings in 1982. Both studies relate to known events of decompression sickness, in which brain injury was part of the picture.

Edmonds tested the "punchy diver" hypothesis in a retrospective study of Australian abalone divers who commonly made long, shallow water, compressed-air dives and were casual about decompression obligations. They did not, however, describe a high incidence of definite decompression sickness, were rarely treated for it, and did not recognize nor admit to cognitive dysfunction. Testing with a battery of psychometric instruments, Edmonds found evidence of intellectual impairment in 11 of 24. Although half of the overall group had reported incidents of decompression sickness, the recognized events did not correlate with the finding of dementia.[6] A prospective study, not yet reported, is in process in Norway.[10]

Most of our knowledge in this area is based on clinical information. Calder and Palmer[11] have recently reported autopsy evidence of diffuse cerebral white matter pathology in divers.

The association of spinal cord and brain decompression sickness is seen in the following case history:

A 28-year-old commercial diver made a series of dives in 50°F water. On the fourth day of the job, during ascent from a 272/39 foot dive, he developed pain in both elbows, hips, ankles, shoulders, and knees. Standard surface decompression was altered to USN table 6, and symptoms resolved completely by the end of the treatment. He did not dive on the following day but on the next day he made a similar dive to 272 feet. He completed in-water and surface decompression but an hour later developed abdominal pain, lumbosacral pain, and weakness of his legs, such that he had to drag himself back to the chamber.

He was treated on USN table 6 with two extensions at 60 feet. He walked from the chamber pain-free but exhausted. The next morning, he drove to visit friends and became lost in familiar surroundings. He ran his automobile off the road several times, fortunately without injury. On the following day, two days after completion of treatment, he flew home by commercial air. When he arrived, he was again sleepy, confused, and had recurrence of back pain. A long course of retreatment was carried out with improvement in pain but with persistent ataxia, extensor toe signs, absent abdominal reflexes, absent reflexes in the left upper extremity, decreased pain, temperature, and vibratory sense below the T6 level, and with continuing complaint of decreased concentration, memory, and word finding. The neurologist who examined him at that time saw evidence of cord lesions at two levels. Psychometric testing indicated difficulties with concentration, word finding, arithmetic, and short-term memory. His family found him changed in personality.

This case illustrates widespread decompression sickness, involving multiple joints, the spinal cord, and the brain itself. The problem was probably aggravated by flying after his treatment for decompression sickness.

Brain injury from arterial gas embolism, principally a hazard to scuba divers, is anatomically discrete and stroke-like. The onset is commonly heralded by seizure or cardiorespiratory arrest as the expanding bubbles occlude major arterial supply.[7] Hemispheric lesions cause seizures from cortical ischemia or direct mechanical pressure. Hemiparesis, aphasia, and cortical blindness are seen with great frequency, all indicating emboli to the hemispheres. Cardiorespiratory arrest implies brain stem hypoxia.[8, 9] Bilateral cortical blindness also suggests that the posterior circulation is frequently embolized. Arterial gas embolism is a major cause of death in scuba diving.[12] Many such cases come to necropsy. The arterial lesions may frequently escape the coroner's attention.

Unless the coroner is forewarned and does the necropsy with tissues submerged, bubbles may not be seen. In addition, most such patients have had prolonged arrest, resuscitation, and have suffered whole brain hypoxia. Acute ischemic changes in the distribution of a specific artery are thus obscured. Many patients who succumb to typical events of arterial gas embolism are given a coroner's diagnosis of drowning.

Of the survivors, many do exceedingly well. There are a surprising number of accidents in which arterial gas embolism is manifested by seizure, hemiparesis, coma, even respiratory arrest, whereby the subject recovers spontaneously without recompression treatment. With recompression, however, response is often dramatic and immediate.[9] A patient in full arrest may regain consciousness and alertness as the chamber is being pressurized, indicating that a simple reduction in bubble diameter is sufficient to restore circulation in the deficient area and to allow bubbles to pass through the microcirculation, or at least to be redistributed downstream in the vascular tree.[13]

Immediate response to treatment is not always complete, and some patients are left with stroke-like neurological deficit, such as hemiparesis, dysphasia, or visual field defect. Even in these cases, long-term disability is relatively less than that seen following ischemic stroke.

Two factors may contribute to the relatively good outlook for recovery in survivors of arterial gas embolism: (1) Most diving accident victims are young in contrast to stroke victims. Cardiopulmonary function is healthier, collateral vessels are larger and more abundant, and, perhaps most important, more brain cells are available for retraining. The brain cell attrition that occurs with aging reduces plasticity of cortical function because it reduces the number of new synapses that can be established. (2) The embolus is gas, not clot, and when it is eventually absorbed, with or without treatment, downstream flow may be restored. This is in contrast to thrombosis, in which the vessel is permanently lost.

When arterial gas embolism and decompression sickness occur together, injury can be severe. Scuba divers are particularly vulnerable to this combination because of the structure of the life support system. When the scuba diver close to the no decompression limit in a deep dive runs out of air, the stage is set for a damaging chain of events. An out-of-air ascent from depth carries a high risk of pulmonary overpressure. If arterial gas embolism occurs, bubbles are introduced into an already supersaturated system and decompression sickness is induced. Alternatively, the victim of arterial gas embolism who convulses may induce decompression sickness from mechanical shear forces in a saturated system. The diver may convulse, be hemiparetic on surfacing, and then develop the abdominal pain and leg weakness of spinal cord decompression sickness. This grievous combination may occur even without violation of safe diving practices. The following is an example.

A scientific diver made an 85-foot, 25-minute dive in the mid-Atlantic. He made a normal controlled ascent and stopped briefly at 10 feet to exhale before surfacing. Observers confirmed that his ascent rate was not rapid. As he climbed into the inflatable boat, he suddenly lost motor control and became unconscious. He awakened in a few minutes, quadriplegic and insensate in all four extremities. He then had a prolonged generalized seizure. When he next regained consciousness, he had excruciating pain across his chest. He was returned to the ship and treated with oxygen. The vessel got underway immediately and steamed for port, but it was nine hours after the accident before helicopter evacuation could be accomplished. The diver was treated with USN table 6A, extended, but with little response. He was transferred to a saturation chamber and treated for seven days. At the end of treatment, he had sensory loss to T4, weakness in both hands, flaccid paraplegia from the mid-thoracic region, and no sphincter control. There was gradual improvement during several months of rehabilitation. A year later, he was able to walk with forearm crutches, had moderate weakness of foot extensors, and had regained sphincter control.

Several years before this event, this diver had surfaced from a dive and had a brief episode of unilateral weakness. He was thought to have had an "undeserved" embolism from which he made a complete recovery. He had been treated for asthma in childhood but had not had symptomatic asthma as an adult.

Several points are illustrated here:

1. Cerebral air embolism occurred in spite of good diving practice. The diver made a normal ascent, yet symptoms occurred immediately after surfacing; he lost consciousness and convulsed.

2. Spinal cord decompression sickness was precipitated by air embolism. The thoracic sensory level establishes the diagnosis as spinal cord disease. The introduction of air bubbles into the blood stream via the arterial circulation precipitated bubbling in a partially saturated solution. The dive did not exceed the no decompression limits but was sufficient to incur a considerable nitrogen load. Bubbling was further favored by the mechanical effect of the prolonged generalized seizure.

3. Childhood asthma never goes away and continues to be a hazard to divers, even if apparently arrested and asymptomatic in adulthood. There are a number of documented cases of undeserved arterial gas embolism in this setting.

SPINAL CORD

The anatomy of the spinal cord, which protects it so well from minor trauma, renders it uniquely susceptible to decompression sickness. The mechanical structure of the vertebral column shields the cord from most injury. The redundant collateral arterial supply assures that the cord will be nourished directly from the aorta even when less favored tissues are allowed to become ischemic.

The venous drainage of the cord, slowed and made pendular by respiratory pressure changes, makes it uniquely vulnerable to venous infarction. Hallenbeck demonstrated this in dog experiments.[3] Arterial insufficiency may play a part as well, particularly in the relative watershed area of the dorsal root entry zone.[14]

This vulnerability causes a unique spinal cord disease, clinically different from any other neurological syndrome. Spinal decompression sickness presents a clinical picture of diffuse multilevel cord disease. Extrinsic pressure on the cord, such as is seen in compression fracture or metastatic tumor, results in paraparesis with sensation loss to the level of the lesion. A meningioma, compressing the cord from one side, may produce a Brown-Séquard lesion with loss of motor function, vibratory and joint sense on the compressed side, and loss of pain and temperature sense on the contralateral side. Anterior spinal artery thrombosis, most often following trauma to the thoracic aorta, causes injury to the anterior cord with resultant paraparesis, pain, and temperature loss, sparing the posterior columns that carry position and vibratory sense. Spinal decompression sickness, by contrast, attacks the cord at multiple levels and at random sites. Fiber tracts may be interrupted at different levels, and a nip may be taken out of the root entry zone here and there. The clinical result may be a painful transverse mid-lumbar myelopathy, but may as well be a combination of pain, sensory loss, and motor weakness at multiple sites all along the neuraxis.

While the recovery from spinal decompression sickness is often gratifying, there may be residual symptoms and findings unique among neurological diseases.[15, 16] The sensory loss found in mid-lumbar decompression sickness may be patchy. A physician accustomed to dealing with spinal cord trauma or compression expects to find a level of sensory loss at or slightly below the level of the lesion. In decompression sickness, by contrast, there may be patches of preserved sensory function interspersed between areas of dense anesthesia.

During recompression treatment, an anesthetic patch may be observed to shrink in area, perhaps to disappear, only to reappear on decompression. This sequence is so unlike any other neurological disease that the author did not believe it until it was demonstrated to him by Van Meter, Pilmanis, and others.

Spinal decompression sickness may also produce a chronic pain syndrome with paroxysmal features. The author has seen several patients who have been treated for spinal decompression sickness with nearly complete recovery but who have had recurrent paroxysmal bouts of pain in the distribution of the original insult. The following case is pertinent:

An experienced commercial diver made an heliox dive in the Gulf and decompressed on a proprietary 225/60 table. He shifted to air at 100 feet, then to 50/50 nitrox. After finishing surface decompression, he had pain in the left side of his chest, which increased and then subsided. Two days later, he made a second and similar dive and again experienced pain in the chest, worse than on the first occasion. He made a third and similar dive to the same profile on the next day. On descent, he became quite chilled when he shifted to heliox at 100 feet and remained so for the rest of the dive. On ascent, he felt warmer when he shifted back to air at 100 feet but became chilled again with the shift to 50/50 nitrox.

When he emerged from the surface decompression chamber, he had a wide band of pain across his chest and abdomen, extending from neck to groin. He felt weak and exhausted. He was evacuated by helicopter to a recompression facility where he arrived about 12 hours after surfacing. Table 6A did not give relief and he continued to complain of pain radiating from his mid-thorax into the right knee. Repeated treatments were carried out for eight days and the pain gradually subsided. During this hospitalization, neurological examination showed minimal decrease in vibratory and position sense in the feet, with intact pain perception in the arms, but decreased pain perception from T4 to T12 bilaterally. Motor function was intact and reflexes unremarkable. Auditory- and somatosensory-evoked potential responses were normal.

Pain had subsided by the time of discharge, 10 days post-dive. There was still altered sensation over the trunk. Several days later, he began to experience numbness of the 3rd and 4th fingers on the left hand and electric shock–like sensations shooting down his arm from the level of the mid-humerus into the fingers. These lasted for a few minutes, subsided, then returned. There was sharp pain in the elbow. He had similar sensation in the right arm with episodes occurring once or twice a day, or every other day, for two months. The pains lasted for minutes to hours.

On one occasion, while driving, he had the onset of shooting pains so severe that he became nauseated and vomited. His arm pain extended from the shoulder to the elbow, and below the elbow his arm felt as though it were being massaged. He returned to the hyperbaric facility, where his right hand was noted to be sweating profusely. This was confirmed with cornstarch testing, and the area of increased sweating extended to the elbow. He was treated with carbamazepine, which suppressed the pain but caused nausea and diarrhea. When he discontinued medication, the pain recurred. Codeine and meperidine were necessary for pain relief. For several days, his left arm and hand felt clumsy and he dropped things.

He was unsteady on his feet, particularly in diminished light, and had fallen on one occasion. He did not have vertigo or disturbance of bowel, bladder or sexual function, and he did not complain of weakness. There was no previous history of decompression sickness.

Neurological examination eight months after the

injury demonstrated normal gait, reflexes, and strength. Abdominal reflexes were present and symmetrical. The anal reflex was decreased on the left. There was an unusual sensory loss extending from T4 on the right and T5 on the left down to T12, right, and T10, left. There was slight decrease of pain perception on the left side of perineum. Vibratory and joint sense were normal (Fig. 19–1).

This case illustrates spinal decompression sickness with bilateral thoracic and lumbar myelopathy. The findings are remarkable in that motor function was entirely spared and minimal disturbance was seen in the posterior columns. The paroxysmal tic-like character of the pain, its relationship to the original site of injury, and its response to carbamazepine speak for a lesion in the dorsal root entry zone. This is clinically consistent with the experimental lesions produced by Palmer.[14] It most resembles the syndrome of "tonic painful seizures" described in multiple sclerosis, it is thought to represent an MS plaque in the dorsal horn of the cervical cord.[17]

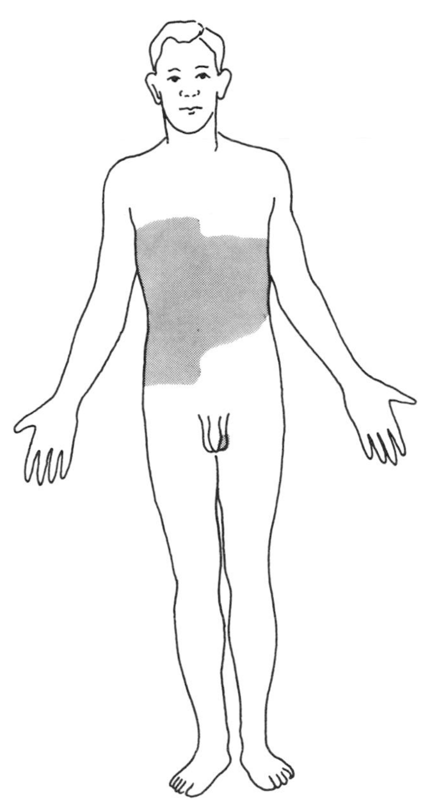

FIGURE 19–1. Pattern of pain and temperature loss in a diver with persistent paroxysmal limb pain following decompression sickness. The girdle-like anesthesia is consistent with multiple level lesions in the dorsal root entry zone.

PERIPHERAL NERVES

Peripheral nerve injuries are rare in diving. Those that occur in decompression sickness involve nerves that traverse a tightly confined area in which a bubble may cause mechanical compression. These include the facial nerve in the facial canal,[18] the trigeminal nerve as it traverses the foramen ovale and rotundum, and the median nerve as it enters the hand beneath the carpal tunnel.[20] Scarcely any others are so affected.

Facial baroparesis may result from a single bubble hit but has also been seen in reverse squeeze on ascent. Both instances are benign and resolve in hours to weeks.[21, 22] Peripheral mononeuropathy from decompression sickness has been described in the oculomotor (3rd) nerve and in branches of the trigeminal nerve.[19] Traumatic peripheral neuropathy from a weightbelt has been reported to cause "scuba diver's thigh" in the distribution of the lateral cutaneous nerve.[23]

The definition of peripheral nerve injury is important. It means nerve injury outside the spinal cord, peripheral to the dorsal root ganglion. Peripheral nerves are purely nerve fibers; no nerve cells are present. Injury to the peripheral nerve causes pain, dysesthesia, sensory loss, and weakness only in the distribution of that nerve. Such injuries in decompression sickness are usually "neuropraxic." The axon fibers are preserved, the insulating myelin is lost, and the outlook for recovery is good.

Some attention should be devoted to the precise diagnosis of peripheral nerve injury and its differentiation from Type I or "pain only" decompression sickness and Type II or spinal decompression sickness. The point here is that spinal decompression sickness with pain, dysesthesia, anesthesia, and weakness is common in the upper extremities as well as the lower ones. If the venerable concept of pain only bends is to be honored, it must be strictly applied to pain only in a single joint. Multiple joint pain and bilateral pain must be regarded as serious decompression sickness. *If there are physical findings*, such as weakness or loss of sensation, nerve tissue must be involved. This nearly always means the spinal cord. However, if physical findings prove injury to a single peripheral nerve, such as the median nerve in the carpal tunnel, the diagnosis reverts to Type I decompression sickness. Symptoms resulting from a single lesion in the limb, whether in the elbow, joint, or carpal tunnel, are of equal significance. Therefore, if one is satisfied that the weakness or sensory loss is anatomically located in a single nerve outside the cord, a lesser diagnosis is justified.

Finally, the anatomical diagnosis influences intensity of treatment. It requires some fortitude for the physician to change treatment and commit a patient and a chamber crew to additional hours of treatment. The more precise the anatomical diagnosis, the easier becomes the decision.

Is lesser treatment justified? Probably not. The diagnosis of decompression sickness demands treatment. It has been common practice for diving supervisors, both naval and commercial, to treat Type I with USN table 5 and Type II with USN table 6. Table 5 takes 2 hours and 15 minutes and table 6 takes 4 hours and 45 minutes, a difference of 2 hours and 30 minutes. A lesser diagnosis, therefore, shortens the task and allows everyone to go home sooner. Because inadequate treatment may allow recurrence of symptoms, many authorities, believing that the use of table 5 results in an unacceptable recurrence rate, have recommended that it be abandoned. It has not been. It is included in the latest edition of the USN Diving Manual with the statement that it is to be used for pain only decompression sickness if symptoms resolve in 10 minutes at 60 feet. If symptoms persist beyond that time, treatment is extended to table 6.[24, 25]

Therefore, why bother to determine the type of decompression sickness? If the level of treatment is determined by response to treatment, is it really necessary to make fine anatomical distinction between spinal cord and peripheral nerve or even between Type I and Type II? The author's view is that the diagnosis of decompression sickness requires treatment on table 6 as a minimum. The cost of retreatment and the results of inadequate treatment far exceed the cost of 2.5 hours early on. The distinction between Type I and Type II should not determine the choice of initial treatment.

There are other considerations. Both the course of treatment and long-term management may be influenced by anatomical diagnosis. The patient who presents with spinal decompression sickness demands maximal treatment directed at the prevention of permanent cord damage. If the patient fails to make a complete recovery with standard treatment, i.e., single table 6, he is permanently disqualified from diving.[26] If, however, the patient has a median neuropathy or peripheral facial palsy, a complete recovery is likely in a matter of weeks and the individual will be able to return to diving. The following case illustrates the difficulty in classifying symptoms into Type I or Type II.

Contact was made from an oil rig off the Kenai Peninsula in Alaska. The diver (also the company owner) had made two decompression dives on the previous day. On day two, he dove to 127 for 78 on air. He decompressed using a 130/80 table and surface decompression with oxygen. He surfaced from the chamber without incident, but awakened 2 hours and 20 minutes later with severe pain inside the left wrist, extending 6 inches above the wrist joint and into the fingers. He was treated on table 5 with relief before 60 feet. On conclusion of treatment, he went back to work on deck. After the shift he retired only to awaken in 3 hours with recurrent pain and numbness in the first three fingers of the left hand. He was treated again, this time using table 6A, and again had immediate relief under pressure. Numbness waxed and waned. When he surfaced, the pain recurred to some extent.

Instructions for examination of the hand were given by radiotelephone. There was no weakness of intrinsic muscles of the hand, but there was decreased sensation in the 2nd, 3rd, and 4th fingers. He was treated yet again on table 6 and surfaced without recurrent pain. The numbness persisted. Final treatment was table 5 on the third day. The patient was evacuated to Anchorage where he was examined by a neurologist. I talked to the neurologist by telephone. She found weakness in the short abductor of the hand. Nerve conduction study of the median nerve was normal. The diver's symptoms subsided without residual effects. He was ready to return to work in one week.

It was concluded that the diver had a discrete lesion in the median nerve, probably in the carpal tunnel at the wrist, and that this was resolved entirely with treatment. Type I decompression sickness, the cause of a single lesion in one limb, was the diagnosis. Note that this did not meet the more limited definition of pain only; the diver had both sensory loss and weakness, and a distinction had to be made to exclude spinal cord disease.

END ORGANS

Vestibular decompression sickness is principally a heliox phenomenon, occurring almost exclusively when decompressing divers make the 170-foot switch from heliox to air. This probably represents a counterdiffusion phenomenon. At the moment the valve is turned, the diver is enormously supersaturated with helium, which off-gases rapidly across a 6 ata gradient. Even though helium has excellent diffusion characteristics, some bubbling may occur and decompression sickness may result.

The selectivity of this phenomenon for the vestibular system is explained by the anatomy of the semicircular canals. The tiny counterdiffusion bubbles confined in the semicircular canals bend the hair cells and cause vertigo. A similar phenomenon surely occurs in the spinal fluid but causes no symptoms, because the bubbles there have no such fragile receptors to stimulate.

PRE-EXISTING NEUROLOGICAL DISEASE

Although the most important limiting conditions that pose problems for the physician interested in diving medicine relate to conditioning and cardiovascular and pulmonary functions, questions are occasionally raised about several neurological problems.

Epilepsy

About one half of one per cent of the population has epilepsy. It most often begins in childhood, but the risk continues indefinitely. A majority of patients with epilepsy are under treatment with medication. With good management, such patients are able to finish school, compete in the job market, participate in sports, and drive. Some will want to dive.

Patients with uncontrolled seizures are obviously unsuited for diving, driving, or any other activity that exposes them to risk should they lose consciousness. A seizure under water carries great hazard for drowning, uncontrolled ascent, and embolism. It exposes other members of the dive party and the rescue party to additional hazard. Should a serious accident not result, the diver's companions will still be faced with a diagnostic dilemma. Conventional doctrine holds that a seizure in water or after surfacing is presumptive evidence of air embolism. Treatment is obligatory. Parenthetically, this is analogous to the dilemma that occurs when an insulin-dependent diabetic has altered consciousness after diving.

The fitness-to-dive decision is less clear-cut in patients with well-controlled epilepsy. Several considerations are important here: (1) Does diving increase the likelihood of seizures in an epileptic patient? (2) Should a patient under treatment with anticonvulsant medication be allowed to dive? (3) Should an individual who has outgrown epilepsy be allowed to dive?

Epileptics are said to have a lowered seizure threshold. This means that they are more susceptible to seizures than the general population, and stimuli that induce seizures in some percentage of the general population will be more likely to do so in those who have epilepsy. Examples of such stimuli are prolonged sleep deprivation, alcohol and sedative withdrawal, visual stimulation with rapidly flashing lights, and hyperventilation. The latter is of particular interest to divers. Hyperventilation at atmospheric pressure is routinely used to test for seizure susceptibility. Breath-hold divers regularly hyperventilate before a drop.

The effect of hyperbaric oxygen on epileptic populations has not been studied. However, it is well established that high partial pressures of oxygen may induce seizures in normal individuals. Navy diving standards require that candidates undergo an oxygen tolerance test in which they breathe pure oxygen in a chamber for 30 minutes at a depth equivalent to 60 feet of seawater. This test is designed to screen out those candidates who are susceptible to oxygen toxicity. About one per cent of healthy candidates have grand mal seizures under these conditions. The oxygen tolerance test is based on the assumption that all divers will be subject to increased pO_2 in their work or perhaps in treatment, and that the test will help to eliminate susceptible candidates.[27] Both these assumptions are defensible. It is likely, although not proven, that epileptics have an increased risk of oxygen convulsions.

The well-controlled epileptic leads a fairly normal life, with no apparent physical handicap. In most jurisdictions, an epileptic can obtain a conditional driver's license if seizure-free for one year, and in almost all jurisdictions for two years.[28, 29] However, an epileptic individual cannot get a pilot's license or a commercial driver's license and would not meet physical requirements for military or commercial diving.[24]

As a sport diver, an epileptic may voluntarily put his own life at risk. Should a seizure occur under water, the individual may drown or suffer an embolism. Both of these accidents have occurred in nonepileptic patients with oxygen convulsions. These are personal risks. There is yet another. The diver who has trouble under water exposes to risk other members of the diving and search parties. As a student, an epileptic individual imposes an unusual obligation and liability on the instructor. Value judgments must be made. The law takes notice of the epileptic driver, not because of the risk to the individual, but because of the risk to the public; the public safety is greatly endangered by an automobile driver who has a seizure.

With the diver, the public risk is much less but not negligible.

The law generally accepts that a seizure-free interval of two years under treatment constitutes control sufficient to operate a motor vehicle. The risk of recurrent seizures in the controlled subject is nevertheless several times that of the general population.[30] Because the risk of seizures after two years of control are small, public policy recognizes that driving has great social and economic importance and accepts the risk.

The controlled epileptic also pays a price in side effects of medication. Virtually all anticonvulsive medications have some sedative effect. There is great variation among individuals, with respect to both dosage and susceptibility to sedation. The average dose of medication for epilepsy usually produces only mild sedation. It is nevertheless measurable on performance testing. This has a bearing on divers. All sedative medications can be expected to increase the hazard of nitrogen narcosis, in the same manner as does alcohol.

About 20 per cent of children with epilepsy outgrow the disorder by age 21. Those who have been seizure-free for five years without medication are generally regarded as cured for legal purposes except for the requirements of flying and of special military service. The risk of recurrent seizures in this population is nevertheless considerably greater than random.[31] Based on these considerations, the author has recommended the following:

1. The diagnosis of epilepsy, properly established, is disqualifying for military and commercial diving without exception.
2. Individuals who have been seizure-free for five years and take no medication have a small statistical risk of recurrent seizures. There is no definite evidence that diving will increase the risk of recurrence, but these individuals should be advised to avoid hyperventilation and cautioned that elevated partial pressures of oxygen may precipitate seizures.
3. Individuals with controlled epilepsy (taking medication, seizure-free for two years, therefore meeting the requirements of most driving jurisdictions) are nevertheless advised not to dive. While driving is important to livelihood, diving is not. The risk, to both the individual and his companions, is inconsistent with the pursuit of sport.[32]

Spinal Surgery

Although indications for spinal surgery continue to be a matter of dispute, many operations are done. Since the advent of lumbar laminectomy and anterior interbody fusion, many thousands of Americans have had one or more of these operations. Many want to dive. There are two considerations, one theoretical and the other practical.

1. An operation that compromises the paravertebral venous plexus might be expected to increase the likelihood of decompression sickness. Such compromise certainly occurs in lumbar laminectomy in which coagulation of bleeders in the venous plexus is routine. Anterior interbody fusion, which approaches the spinal canal without laminectomy, has relatively less bearing on the paravertebral plexus. I think this theoretical consideration may be important but I know of no proven instances in which decompression sickness has been attributed to previous laminectomy.
2. Spinal surgery causes spinal disability. Under the best circumstances, a patient recovers from spinal surgery with altered structure. If the operation is entirely successful and the patient is symptom-free, the individual nevertheless emerges with a skeleton that has been physiologically and structurally altered. In Workers' Compensation Appeals Board parlance in the State of California, a patient who has had such surgery is usually regarded as "disabled for heavy work." This means in the same parlance that he has lost 30 per cent of his previous capacity for lifting, pulling, pushing, and so forth.

Diving is hard work. A spinal structural disability certainly is disqualifying for military and commercial divers. Whether a sport diver should be disqualified on this basis depends on how much pulling and hauling must be done on the surface. Someone else can lift bottles or dress the diver out, but the individual will not necessarily have help to climb the ladder into the boat or to heave over the gunwale after surfacing.

Migraine

Queries about the history of migraine frequently appear on divers' medical evaluations. I am not sure why this is so. Migraine is an exceedingly common phenomenon. Probably more than half of the world's population will have some experience with migraine during their lives. Perhaps 5 per cent will see a doctor about it.[33] Many of these people certainly dive. Even those with frequent migraine do not usually experience an increased incidence of headache related to diving nor are they unusually vulnerable to decompression sickness.

Vasodilating headache can be induced by elevated levels of carbon dioxide, just as it can be ameliorated by high pO_2. Decompression with falling pO_2 can provoke migraine, at least theoretically. Subjects with severe or complex migraine, in which the prodromal event is hemianopsia or hemiplegia, may present a diagnostic dilemma. Consideration of decompression sickness or air embolism might even result in an unnecessary recompression treatment. There is, however, little evidence to suggest that migraine poses a significant hazard to divers. Subjects with migraine of such severity as to interfere with diving will usually sort themselves out of a program.

Cerebral Palsy, Paraplegia, Multiple Sclerosis, and Muscular Dystrophy

These disparate illnesses are considered here because in the past patients with these diagnoses have learned diving and certainly more will do so. The issue here is principally physical stamina. Beyond that, each case must be considered individually. Cerebral palsy patients, for instance, have an increased incidence of epilepsy. The previous discussion applies here. If they have not had seizures, are adequately conditioned, and can pass the swimming tests, there should be no blanket contraindication.

Paraplegic patients require special thought. In traumatic paraplegia from spinal cord injury, there is at least a theoretically increased risk of spinal cord decompression sickness, because of injury to the circulation of the spinal cord. Spinal cord disease, whether from trauma or demyelinization (multiple sclerosis), is evidence of structural abnormality. The individual who undertakes diving with an altered spinal cord would seem to be at greater risk for decompression sickness because some of the population of nerve fibers would already be lost.

Multiple sclerosis is a distressingly common disease. Diving and the exposure to a hyperbaric environment probably would not make it worse. Several years ago, there was a brief flurry of interest in the use of hyperbaric oxygen to treat multiple sclerosis. Studies have shown it to have little effect, positive or negative.[34, 35] Multiple sclerosis patients, however, have limited stamina, and vigorous physical exercise usually serves them poorly. Most neurologists advise multiple sclerosis patients to avoid exhaustion, and this also means the avoidance of chilling.

Muscular dystrophy occurs in different forms. Those with generalized progressive dystrophy of the Erb-Duchenne type are severely handicapped and surely will not be divers. Some patients with limited disease (limb girdle, facioscapulohumeral dystrophy) may have sufficient strength to dive effectively. Diving will not make them worse. Patients with myotonic dystrophy are likely to do poorly when chilled.[36]

Risking repetition, the main criteria must be physical stamina and agility. Patients with preexisting neurological disease or other handicaps need not be disqualified from diving if they are well conditioned and sufficiently capable in the water of functioning independently. If their handicaps are so severe as to require regular assistance from other divers or instructors, common sense must prevail.

REFERENCES

1. Bert P: Barometric Pressure: Researches in Experimental Physiology (1877). Translated by Hitchcock MA, Hitchcock FA, Columbus Book Co., 1943. Reprinted, Undersea Medical Society, Bethesda, 1978.
2. Hallenbeck JM, Bove AA, Elliott JH: Mechanisms underlying spinal cord damage in decompression sickness. Neurology 25:308, 1975.
3. Hallenbeck JM: Cinephotomicrography of dog spinal vessels in decompression sickness. Neurology 26:190–199, 1976.
4. Peters VH, Leven HD, Kelley PJ: Neurologic and psychologic manifestations of decompression sickness in divers. Neurology 27:136, 1977.
5. Vaernes RJ, Eidsvik S: Central nervous functions after near-miss accidents in diving. Aviat Space Env Med 53:803, 1982.
6. Edmonds C, Boughton J: Intellectual deterioration with excessive diving. Undersea Biomed Res 12:1321, 1985.
7. Elliott DH, Harrison AB, Barnard EP: Clinical and radiological features of 88 cases of decompression barotrauma. *In* Shilling CW, Beckman MW (eds): Proceedings of the Sixth Symposium of Underwater Physiology. Bethesda, FASEB, 1978, p 527–535.
8. Gillen HW: Symptomatology of cerebral gas embolism. Neurology 18:507–512, 1968.
9. Neuman TS, Hallenbeck JM: Barotraumatic cerebral air embolism and the mental status examination: A report of four cases. Ann Emerg Med 16:220–223, 1987.
10. Dick A: Personal communication, 1987.
11. Palmer AC: Neuropathology of brain in decompression sickness. European Underwater Biology Society Proceedings, Palermo, September, 1987 (in press).
12. McAniff JJ: US underwater diving fatality statistics 1970–1978. University of Rhode Island Report URI SSR 80–13, September 1980.
13. Gorman DF, Browning DMN: Cerebral vasoreactivity and arterial gas embolism. Undersea Biomed Res 13:317, 1986.
14. Palmer AC, Blakemore WF, Greenwood AG: Neuro-

pathology of experimental decompression sickness in the goat. Neuropathol Appl Neurobiol 2:145, 1976.
15. Linaweaver PG, Greer HD: The natural history of decompression sickness. *In* Miller JN, Parmentier JL (eds): Rehabilitation of the Paralyzed Diver. Bethesda, Undersea Medical Society, 1985, p 7–19.
16. Hayaski K, Kitano M, Kawashima M, et al: Twenty six cases of complete transverse injury to the spinal cord. *In* Miller JN, Parmentier JL (eds): Rehabilitation of the Paralyzed Diver. Bethesda, Undersea Medical Society, 1985, p 94–99.
17. Shibasaki H, Kuroiwa Y: Painful tonic seizures in multiple sclerosis. Arch Neurol 30:47–51, 1974.
18. Eidsvik S, Molvaer O: Facial baroparesis: A report of 5 cases. Undersea Biomed Res 12:456–465, 1985.
19. Hart BL, Dutka AJ, Flynn ET: Pain only decompression sickness affecting the orbicularis oculi. Undersea Biomed Res 13:461–464, 1985.
20. Greer HD: Peripheral mononeuropathy in decompression sickness. Undersea Medical Society, North Pacific Meeting, Santa Barbara, November, 1983.
21. Molvaer OI: Alternobaric facial palsy. Med Aeronaut Spat Med Subaquat Hyperbare 18:249–250, 1979.
22. Becker GD: Recurrent alternobaric facial paralysis resulting from scuba diving. Pressure 13:6, 1982.
23. Greenhouse AH: Scuba diver's thigh. West J Med 145:668, 1986.
24. USN Diving Manual, Rev 1. San Pedro, Best Publishing Company, 1985, p 8–27.
25. Leitch DR, Hallenbeck JM: Oxygen in the treatment of decompression sickness. Undersea Biomed Res 12:269, 1985.
26. Davis JC (ed): The Return to Active Diving After Decompression Sickness or Arterial Gas Embolism. Bethesda, Undersea Medical Society, 1980, p 8.
27. Butler FK, Knafele ME: Screening for oxygen tolerance in US Navy divers. Undersea Biomed Res 13:91–110, 1986.
28. Hoeber C (ed): Epilepsy and the Law. New York, Harper and Row, 1966, p 63.
29. Livingston B: Participation of epileptic patients in sports. JAMA 224:236, 1973.
30. Emerson DS: Stopping medication in children with epilepsy. N Engl J Med 306:831–836, 1981.
31. Thurston JH: Prognosis in childhood epilepsy. N Engl J Med 306:1125–1129, 1981.
32. Greer HD: Epilepsy and diving. Skin Diver 33:44, 1984.
33. Ziegler DK, Hasaanein RS, Couch JR: Characteristics of life headache histories in a non clinic population. Neurology 27:265–269, 1977.
34. Fischer BH, Marks M, Reich T: Hyperbaric oxygen treatment of multiple sclerosis. N Engl J Med 308:81–86, 1983.
35. Bass BH: Hyperbaric oxygen therapy in chronic stable multiple sclerosis: Double blind study. Neurology 36:988, 1986.
36. Greer HD: *In* Vorosmarti J (ed): Fitness to Dive. Bethesda, Undersea Medical Society, 1987, p 80.

Chapter 20

Pulmonary Disorders in Diving

TOM S. NEUMAN

The problem of advising individuals with pulmonary disorders on the risk of diving is a particularly vexing one. Whereas most physicians can understand the risk of not being fit enough if caught in a stong current or of not being able to equalize if one has trouble clearing one's ears, it is difficult to understand the increased risk of air embolism because of abnormal distribution of ventilation or altered airway function.

ASTHMA

Asthma is probably the most common pulmonary disorder we are asked to evaluate in a diver or diving candidate. Fortunately, most physicians have a basic understanding of asthma, even though the participants of the CIBA Foundation study group on the "Identification of Asthma" concluded, "asthma could not be defined on the information at present available."[1] For practical purposes, it might be more useful to define asthma as a disorder(s) "characterized by increased responsiveness of the airways (i.e., hyperreactivity) to various stimuli and by resultant smooth muscle contraction and obstruction."[2] Yet asthma can still be subclassified, and most current classifications attempt to define syndromes based upon specific precipitating factors and specific patterns of response. These classifications are important because the natural history of these syndromes appear to be different, and therefore the recommendations of diving physicians might as well be different.

One of the more common asthma syndromes is atopic asthma. This is characterized by onset in childhood and by association with allergic rhinitis or allergic dermatitis. Attacks may be precipitated by various sensitizing agents. Children who develop this asthma syndrome in the first few years of life do not necessarily have persistent asthma into adult life. In one study, only 15 per cent of 10-year-old children whose asthma began before the age of two had persistent wheezing.[3] If the precipitating cause of attack was infection, it was found that 50 per cent of children were considered to be cured when re-examined 20 years later.[4] Adults do not seem to fare as well with asthma. There is a much lower percentage of individuals who become free of disease with time,[5–7] and the proportion of severe to mild cases seems to rise steeply with age.[8]

In many patients, however, attacks cannot be ascribed to a specific precipitating agent or event. This syndrome is called intrinsic asthma; however, there is a great deal of overlap between groups, and many individuals present a mixed picture.[9, 10]

Another important syndrome is exercise-induced asthma. The cause of this syndrome, most frequently seen in the young, was for many years unclear. Evidence now suggests that the underlying cause is not hyperventilation, hypocapnea, and so forth, but rather cold stimulus to the tracheobronchial tree in susceptible individuals.[11, 12]

Other less common syndromes are the aspirin sensitivity triad (nasal polyps, urticaria, and asthma following aspirin ingestion) and occupational asthma.

Thus, asthma is not a single disease, and there is a tremendous degree of heterogeneity among asthmatic patients. As already mentioned, the factors that precipitate attacks vary tremendously. But equally important, the actual location of obstruction seems to vary with different patients depending upon what one believes various pulmonary function tests measure.

Most importantly, there is considerable difference in the degree of airway obstruction reversibility demonstrated by asthmatics. Some asthmatics demonstrate completely normal pulmonary function tests (PFTs) "including measurements of pulmonary mechanics and of regional ventilation distribution"[13] between attacks. Others, although asymptomatic, continue to show evidence of airway obstruction even after vigorous therapy. Under such circumstances, the distinction between chronic obstructive pulmonary disease (COPD) and reactive airway disease (RAD), i.e., asthma, becomes blurred.

As a result of these marked differences in prognosis, intermorbid pulmonary function, and baseline pulmonary function, recommendations concerning diving should take into consideration the individual patient's specific asthma syndrome and history.

The major concern in permitting an asthmatic to dive is that such an individual might be dangerously susceptible to pulmonary barotrauma and cerebral air embolism even during a normal ascent. This concern is based upon an understanding of pulmonary physiology and extrapolations based upon that understanding. Liebow, et al[14] have demonstrated that under certain conditions partial pulmonary obstruction in large airways can lead to arterial gas embolism (AGE). Similarly, Schaefer and colleagues[15] have demonstrated that overpressurization of the lung can lead to AGE; Colebatch and coworkers[16] have shown that decreased compliance is associated with AGE. All of these factors are operative in asthmatics. Coupled with this, some asthmatics have significant noncommunicating air spaces as demonstrated by differences in measured lung volume compared by helium dilution techniques and whole body plethysmography.[17] Additionally, the acute asthmatic is usually hyperinflated; and as has been demonstrated, not only is overpressurization required to produce AGE, but overinflation is required as well.[15] More sophisticated studies on asthmatics reveal that even in asymptomatic individuals, marked abnormalities of ventilation/perfusion ratios can exist. This study demonstrated that as many as half of the lung units were perfused by completely closed airways that were ventilated only by collaterals.[18]

Thus, there is a wealth of physiological data that suggest it would be unsafe for the active asthmatic to dive. Examining accident statistics, one finds that perhaps as many as 50 per cent of air embolisms are not associated with panic, out-of-air, or breath-holding ascents.[19] In other words, apparently half of arterial gas embolisms occur in divers ascending normally and not holding their breath. This suggests that undetected underlying lung disease may play a role in these accidents. In contrast to these findings, analysis of pulmonary function in approximately 40 cases of air embolism at the Marine Science Center on Catalina Island over a five-year period revealed only one asthmatic.[20]

Thus, there are sound theoretical reasons to suggest that diving with asthma predisposes divers to AGE; and accident statistics suggest that underlying lung disease might play a role in as many as 50 per cent of AGE cases.

What then are reasonable recommendations in light of these data? First, asthma is a contraindication to diving. Second, all individuals who have current active asthma are advised not to dive. Third, any individual who seems to have outgrown his asthma and has not had any bronchospasm, wheezing, or chest tightness and has not used any bronchodilator recently may be a candidate for diving if a complete battery of PFTs are normal. If any question still exists, more complete testing may be performed.[21] (See section on special tests.)

These are superficially extremely conservative recommendations, especially in light of observations that asthmatics do not seem to be overrepresented in accident statistics.[22–35] Yet at present there are no data available to accurately assess the numbers of asthmatics who do dive, and, as a result, their true risk is unknown. Considering the potentially catastrophic consequences of an air embolism, it seems appropriate to recommend that asthmatics not dive. In the future, should data become available that define the risk of asthma and diving more clearly, more liberal recommendations might be possible.

CHRONIC OBSTRUCTIVE PULMONARY DISEASE (COPD), CHRONIC BRONCHITIS, AND EMPHYSEMA

The question of diving with COPD is in many ways similar to advising the individual who has asthma. The same theoretical arguments apply to the individual with COPD concerning increased risk for AGE, except that the person with COPD never has airway function return to normal. Thus, the diver or diver candidate with COPD is not just at increased theoretical risk when an attack takes place; rather that individual is at increased theoretical risk at all times.

From a practical point of view, by the time individuals with chronic lung disease become symptomatic they are usually incapable of sustaining the exercise necessary to dive, and as a result, it is extremely rare to see a diver with significant COPD. Additionally, COPD is generally a disease that takes decades of tobacco smoke exposure to develop, so it is a disease of older individuals, once again making divers with COPD rare in a diving medicine practice. Finally, by the time COPD can be detected clinically, such major physiological alterations have occurred that there is little argument that such individuals be advised not to dive. Thus, the question of advising someone with COPD is really the question of advising someone who is asymptomatic but who has abnormal PFTs, much like the asthmatic who might develop pulmonary function abnormalities during a dive. Those with COPD of any severity may also have a component of reactive airway disease; their pulmonary obstruction varies with external stimuli, and the obstruction is treated with similar bronchodilating drugs. Thus, individuals with clear-cut laboratory evidence of COPD should be advised not to dive. In practice, this is defined as PFTs more than two standard deviations from normal (Table 20–1). Unfortunately, the exact definition of normal is still unclear, and as a result, individuals with mild disease may overlap predicted normal values between two standard deviations and the mean.[36] As a result, individuals whose isolated values may be low normal should undergo more extensive testing if their clinical history is suggestive of chronic lung disease.

TABLE 20–1. Approximate Lower Limits of Normal at Fifth Percentile Level

PARAMETER	PERCENT OF PREDICTED
VC	Below 75
FRC	Below 70 or above 130
RV	Below 65 or above 135
TLC	Below 80 or above 120
FEV_1	Below 80
FEV_1/FVC %	Below 85
FEF_{25-75}	Below 65

From Clausen J: Pulmonary function testing. *In* Bordow RA, Moser KM (eds): Manual of Clinical Problems in Pulmonary Medicine. 2nd Ed. Boston, Little, Brown & Company, 1985.

PNEUMOTHORAX

By definition, a pneumothorax is a collection of air within the pleural space. Pneumothorax can be classified in several ways, but for the purposes of advising a diving candidate who has had a pneumothorax, it is best to look at pneumothoraces as either spontaneous, iatrogenic, or traumatic.

Spontaneous pneumothorax occurs in a patient without any antecedent trauma and without previous physician intervention. In a young, otherwise healthy individual without any apparent underlying lung disease, the pneumothorax is usually caused by the rupture of congenital subapical blebs. This individual is usually a male between 20 and 30 years of age who is tall, thin, and a cigarette smoker.[40] Another mechanism for the occurrence of pneumothorax is overdistention of distal air spaces by partial bronchial obstruction acting as a one-way valve. Eventually this results in disruption of the air spaces, and air dissects back along bronchovascular planes to the mediastinum. As the process continues, air can either dissect into the soft tissues of the neck (causing subcutaneous emphysema) or rupture into the pleural space resulting in a pneumothorax.[41] It is this latter mechanism that is thought to be the etiology of subcutaneous emphysema in patients suffering from asthma.

Spontaneous pneumothorax can also occur due to more severe underlying lung disease. Any of the diffuse interstitial lung diseases seem to predispose to a pneumothorax—eosinophilic granuloma, sarcoidosis, pneumoconiosis, interstitial pneumonitis—and spontaneous pneumothorax is also common in patients with COPD (especially bullous emphysema[42]).

Once an individual suffers a spontaneous pneumothorax, recurrent pneumothoraces are likely. In one study,[43] approximately 40 per cent of individuals without apparent underlying lung disease who had one pneumothorax had a second. The average time span between the first and second episode was approximately one and a half years (range 4 to 35 months). Approximately one third of those who had a second pneumothorax went on to have a third. In another study[44] of individuals (again without apparent underlying lung disease) treated with tube thoracostomy for spontaneous pneumothorax, approximately 50 per cent had an ipsilateral recurrence. The average time span to recurrence was 2.3 years. Approximately two thirds of those who had a second pneumothorax went on to have a third.

A traumatic pneumothorax can be due to either blunt or penetrating trauma. In the case of blunt trauma, rib fractures cause lacerations of the lung surface, although there are other mechanisms that can produce pneumothorax. In penetrating trauma, the pneumothorax can be due to lung injury or to direct leak from the chest wall.

Iatrogenic pneumothoraces are generally seen after invasive thoracic procedures such as subclavian line placement, thoracentesis, transthoracic needle aspiration of the lung, and of course thoracotomy. Iatrogenic pneumothorax is also commonly due to high positive-pressure ventilation.

Any form of pneumothorax can be complicated by conversion to a tension pneumothorax. This entity occurs when the rent in the pleura acts as a one-way valve and air is continually introduced into the pleural space. This progressively leads to complete collapse of the involved lung and to shifting of the mediastinum to the uninvolved side with compression of the contralateral lung and compromise of venous return to the heart. Tension pneumothorax can rapidly result in death even in otherwise normal individuals.[45]

The above information provides a firm theoretical basis for advising divers who have had previous spontaneous pneumothoraces not to dive. Should a pneumothorax occur under water, changes in atmospheric pressure while surfacing could cause a simple pneumothorax to become a tension pneumothorax. This in turn could result in death. The previous information also suggests that reoccurrences can occur after several years, and the mere fact that a pneumothorax has not occurred for 2 to 3 years does not ensure that it will not reoccur in the future. Finally and equally important, the presence of subpleural blebs (the cause of most spontaneous pneumorthoraces) strongly suggests that there will be areas of the lung which are poorly ventilated, trap air, and are at risk for causing AGE. For these reasons, a history of spontaneous pneumothorax with or without underlying lung disease is considered a contraindication to diving.[46–50]

Traumatic pneumothoraces due to isolated injury to the chest wall should not pose any risk to a diver; however, most traumatic pneumothoraces are asssociated with underlying lung injury as well. If the injury was severe enough to lead to radiographic changes, it may well have led to areas of air trapping. As a result, most authorities agree such individuals should be advised not to dive, although extensive diagnostic and hyperbaric chamber testing might define those at greatest risk.[51]

Iatrogenic pneumothoraces can be due to pulmonary surgery or nonpulmonary procedures. Those pneumothoraces that are due to nonpulmonary procedures (i.e., subclavian line placement, cardiac or mediastinal surgery, and so forth, during which the pleura was opened) should not be a contraindication to diving. If pulmonary surgery was the cause of the pneumothorax, it is not the pneumothorax per se that may increase the diver's risk but rather the underlying lung disease. Additionally, with the almost universal use of the stapling device for suture lines in pulmonary parenchyma, surgeons generally do not need to follow anatomical planes with precision. This in turn may lead to distortion of architecture and to areas of air trapping.[51] As a result, individuals who have had previous pulmonary surgery should be advised not to dive. In general, any lung disease, procedure, or event that can result in air trapping is considered a contraindication to diving.

However, the above arguments are theoretical, as is the case with asthmatics and individuals with COPD. There has not been in the available United States diving fatality statistics a single reported death attributed to a tension pneumothorax or an arterial gas embolism that was ascribed to a previous spontaneous pneumothorax or previous thoracic surgery.[46–50] As mentioned previously, in survivors of AGE, underlying pulmonary problems have not been frequently noted.[20] As a result, these contraindications to diving must be considered in light of the diver's maturity, level of understanding, responsibility, and willingness to accept presumably increased risk.

SPECIAL TESTS

Methacholine or Histamine Challenge

This test has considerable utility evaluating a patient with a questionable history of asthma. Notwithstanding, a limited number of unusual asthmatics unresponsive to methacholine[17]—essentially all asthmatics—"consistently show hyperreactivity to nonspecific agents."[2] Thus, in a patient with a clear-cut history of asthma, there is no point in bronchial provocation since that individual will have a positive response. Indeed, in such a setting, bronchial provocation testing might even be dangerous. On the other hand, if the history is questionable and if episodes are not clearly bronchospastic, then methacholine challenge can be useful in identifying patients with asthma. Methacholine challenge is probably not, however, indicated to make the diagnosis of exercise-induced asthma. In that setting, pre- and postexercise PFTs are more specific and certainly less dangerous. Unfortunately, although methacholine testing is extremely sensitive, it is not specific for bronchospastic asthma. Some patients with a so-called cough asthma have normal PFTs and no history of episodic wheezing but have positive methacholine challenge testing. Their sole manifestation of asthma is a relatively prolonged period of coughing following an upper respiratory infection.[37] Many other individuals with so-called "twitchy" airways have PFT abnormalities following upper respiratory infection and can have a positive response to methacholine for as long as two months after the acute infection.[38] Thus, although useful, a positive bronchial provocation challenge is not equivalent to the diagnosis of asthma.

Specialized Pulmonary Function Testing

Since there is considerable overlap between mild disease and low normal functioning in routine pulmonary function testing, on occasion more sophisticated tests may be indicated. In circumstances in which divers or candidates have PFTs below the 5 per cent probability of normalcy, such testing is probably not warranted since the diagnosis of COPD is secure; however, if an individual has low normal PFTs and has a heavy smoking history or another reason to clinically suspect early COPD, a more complete evaluation of static lung volumes can reveal a pattern of obstructive lung disease. Such evaluation may require helium dilution and body plethysmography and can at times determine whether significant noncommunicating air space is present.

Ventilation Scanning

Finally, on rare occasion ventilation scanning with radioactive xenon may be useful to determine whether areas of the lung are poorly ventilated and therefore at risk to develop pulmonary overinflation. Generally, a single breath scan in this setting is inadequate. A full study utilizing wash-in, equilibrium, and, most importantly, wash-out scanning is required to detect poorly ventilated areas. Typically, patients with very poorly ventilated lung zones may fill apparently normally with radioactive gas during a single slow inhalation. This abnormality can be best detected by observing delayed clearance of radioactivity during the wash-out phase of the study.[39]

REFERENCES

1. Report of the Working Group on Definition of Asthma. *In* Porter R, Birch J (eds): Identification of Asthma. CIBA Foundation Study Group No. 38, January 13–14, 1971. Edinburgh, Churchill-Livingstone, 1971.
2. Ramsdell J: Asthma: Clinical presentation and diagnosis. *In* Bordow RA, Moser KM (eds): Manual of Clinical Problems in Pulmonary Medicine. 2nd Ed. Boston, Little, Brown & Company, 1985.
3. William H, McNickol KN: Prevalence, natural history and relationship of wheezy bronchitis and asthma in children: An epidemiologic study. Br Med J 4:321, 1969.
4. Rackeman FN, Edwards MC: Asthma in children: A follow-up study of 688 patients after an interval of 20 years. N Engl J Med 246:815, 1952.
5. Derrick EH: The significance of the age of onset of asthma. Med J Aust 1:1317, 1971.
6. Ogilvie AG: Asthma: A study in prognosis of 1000 patients. Thorax 17:183, 1962.
7. Smith J: Survey of rural children with asthma and hay fever. J Allergy Clin Immunol 47:28, 1971.
8. Pearson RSB: Natural history of asthma. Acta Allergol 12:277, 1958.
9. Bernstein IL, Siegal SC, Brandon ML, et al: A controlled study of cromolyn sodium, sponsored by the Drug Committee of the American Academy of Allergy. J Allergy Clin Immunol 50:235, 1972.
10. Lindblad JR, Farr RS: The incidence of positive intradermal reactions and the demonstration of skin sensitizing antibody to extracts of ragweed and dust in humans without history of rhinitis or asthma. J Allergy Clin Immunol 32:392, 1961.
11. Deal EC, McFadden ER, Ingram RH, Strauss RH: Heat loss vaporization of water and exercise-induced asthma. Am Rev Respir Dis 117(4):328, 1978.
12. Zebellos RJ, Shturman-Ellstien R, McNally JF, et al: The role of hyperventilation in exercise-induced bronchoconstriction. Am Rev Respir Dis 118:277, 1978.
13. Bates D, Macklem P, Christie R (eds): Spasmodic asthma. *In* Respiratory Function in Disease. 2nd Ed. Philadelphia, WB Saunders Company, 1971.
14. Liebow AA, Stark JE, Vogel J, Schaeffer KE: Intrapulmonary air-trapping in submarine escape training casualties. U.S. Armed Forces Med J 10:265, 1959.
15. Schaefer KE, McNulty WP, Carey C, Liebow AA: Mechanisms in development of interstitial emphysema and air embolism on decompression from depth. J Appl Physiol 13:15, 1958.
16. Colebatch HJH, Smith MM, Ng CKY: Increased elastic recoil as a determinant of pulmonary barotrauma in divers. Respir Physiol 26:55, 1976.
17. Farr RS, Spector SL: Management of the difficult asthmatic. *In* Stein M (ed): New Directions in Asthma. Park Ridge, IL, American College of Chest Physicians, 1975.
18. Wagner PD, Dantzker DR, Iacovoni VE, et al: Ventilation-perfusion inequality in asymptomatic asthma. Am Rev Respir Dis 118:511, 1978.

19. Dick AP, Massey EW: Neurologic presentation of decompression sickness and air embolism in sport divers. Neurology 35:667, 1985.
20. Sipsey J: Correlation of dive injury/accident/illness due to medical/physical problems, or is there a lack of problems due to present absolute/relative contraindications for diving. UMS Workshop on Physical Standards for Diving, Bethesda, Maryland, May 15–16, 1986.
21. Neuman TS: Pulmonary considerations. I. Asthma, COPD: Need for special testing? UMS Workshop on Physical Standards for Diving, Bethesda, Maryland, May 15–16, 1986.
22. Schench HV, McAniff JJ: United States underwater fatality statistics, 1972. U.S. Department of Commerce, NOAA. U.S. Government Printing Office Report No. URI-73-8, December 1973.
23. Schench HV, McAniff JJ: United States underwater fatality statistics, 1973. U.S. Department of Commerce, NOAA. U.S. Government Printing Office Report No. URI-SSR-75-9, May 1975.
24. Schench HV, McAniff JJ: United States underwater fatality statistics, 1974. U.S. Department of Commerce, NOAA. U.S. Government Printing Office Report No. URI-SSR-75-10, April 1976.
25. Schench HV, McAniff JJ: United States underwater fatality statistics, 1975. U.S. Department of Commerce, NOAA. U.S. Government Printing Office Report No. URI-SSR-77-11, March 1977.
26. Schench HV, McAniff JJ: United States underwater fatality statistics, 1976. U.S. Department of Commerce, NOAA. U.S. Government Printing Office Report No. URI-SSR-78-12, December 1978.
27. McAniff JJ: United States underwater fatality statistics, 1970–78. National Underwater Accident Data Center, University of Rhode Island. Report No. URI-SSR-80-13, September 1980.
28. McAniff JJ: United States underwater fatality statistics, 1970–79. National Underwater Accident Data Center, University of Rhode Island. Report No. URI-SSR-80-14, August 1981.
29. McAniff JJ: United States underwater fatality statistics, 1970–80, including a preliminary assessment of 1981 fatalities. National Underwater Accident Data Center, University of Rhode Island. Report No. URI-SSR-82-15, December 1982.
30. McAniff JJ: United States underwater fatality statistics, 1970–81, including a preliminary assessment of 1982 fatalities. National Underwater Accident Data Center, University of Rhode Island. Report No. URI-SSR-83-16.
31. McAniff JJ: United States underwater fatality statistics, 1970–82, including a preliminary assessment of 1983 fatalities. National Underwater Accident Data Center, University of Rhode Island. Report No. URI-SSR-84-17.
32. Kizer KW: Dysbaric air embolism in Hawaii. Seventh Annual Conference on the Clinical Application of Hyperbaric Oxygen; Memorial Hospital Medical Center, Long Beach, California, June 9–11, 1982.
33. Walker D: New Zealand diving-related fatalities, 1981–82. SPUMS Journal 14(2):12, 1984.
34. Fraundorfer RM: Diving fatalities in New Zealand, 1982–1985 (abstract). SPUMS Journal 15(4):21, 1985.
35. Walker D: Provisional report on diving-related fatalities in Australian waters, 1984. SPUMS Journal 15(3):17, 1985.
36. Clausen J : Pulmonary function testing. *In* Bordow RA, Moser KM (eds): Manual of Clinical Problems in Pulmonary Medicine. 2nd Ed. Boston, Little, Brown & Company, 1985.
37. Corrao WM, Braman SS, Irwin RS: Chronic cough as the sole presenting manifestation of bronchial asthma. N Engl J Med 300:633, 1979.
38. Fedullo P: Chronic cough. *In* Bordow RA, Moser KM (eds): Manual of Clincal Problems in Pulmonary Medicine. 2nd Ed. Boston, Little, Brown & Company, 1985.
39. Fedullo PF: Radioisotopic techniques. *In* Bordow RA, Moser KM (eds): Manual of Clinical Problems in Pulmonary Medicine. 2nd Ed. Boston, Little, Brown & Company, 1985.
40. Editorial. Br Med J 2:1407–1408, 1976.
41. Clausen JL: Pneumothorax. *In* Bordow RA, Moser KM (eds): Manual of Clinical Problems in Pulmonary Medicine. 2nd Ed. Boston, Little, Brown & Company, 1985.
42. Stradling P, Poole G: Conservative management of spontaneous pneumothorax. Thorax 21:145–149, 1966.
43. Seremetis MG: The management of spontaneous pneumothorax. Chest 57:65–68, 1970.
44. Gobbel WG, Rhea WG, Nelson IA, Daniel RA: Spontaneous pneumothorax. J Thorac Cardiovasc Surg 46:331–345, 1963.
45. Noble D: Some particulars of treatment in a case of pneumothorax. Br Med J 2:425–426, 1873.
46. Becker GD, Parell GJ: Medical examination of the sport scuba diver. Otolaryngol Head Neck Surg 91:246, 1983.
47. Neblett LM: Otolaryngology and sport scuba diving: Update and guidelines. Ann Otol Rhinol Laryngol 94(1):2, Supplement 115, 1985.
48. Edmonds C, Lowry C, Pennefeather J (eds): Medical standards. *In* Diving and Subaquatic Medicine. 2nd Ed. Mosman, Australia, Diving Medicine Center, 1981.
49. Kindwall EP: Medical examination of the diver. *In* Strauss R (ed): Diving Medicine. New York, Grune and Stratton, 1976, pp 341–347.
50. Physician's Guide to Diving Medicine. Undersea Medical Society, Bethesda, Maryland, 1984.
51. O'Hara V: Pulmonary considerations. II. Pneumothorax, chest surgery, etc. UMS Workshop on Physical Standards for Diving, Bethesda, Maryland, May 15–16, 1986.

Chapter 21

Cardiovascular Disorders and Diving

ALFRED A. BOVE

The principal effects of diving on the cardiovascular system are a result of the work and exercise involved. Since exercise requires increased skeletal muscle activity, and since skeletal muscle requires increased oxygen and fuel to produce increased activity, the heart and circulation are affected by all levels of exercise. The cardiovascular system normally demonstrates an immediate response to exercise.[1, 2] This response includes local alterations in blood flow and vascular resistance, which evoke reflexes that stimulate the heart to provide an increased cardiac output.

From the cardiovascular standpoint, exercise is any activity that raises the resting oxygen consumption above basal levels (Fig. 21–1). Thus, the heart and cardiovascular system respond to swimming, walking with heavy gear, climbing ladders, and performing heavy labor relating to diving as forms of exercise that require an increased output.[3] The principle that most tissues and organs contain a functional reserve is well accepted and applies also to the heart.[3, 4] Thus, the heart at rest is working at a small percentage of its maximal capacity, and measurement of maximal cardiac performance may be necessary to accurately assess limitations imposed by heart disease. Reduction of the maximal capacity of the heart and circulation occurs early in heart disease and may be undetected for long periods of time unless the patient or physician tests the reserve and finds it diminished, or unless cardiac impairment progresses to the point where the loss of reserve is significant enough to affect resting cardiac performance.

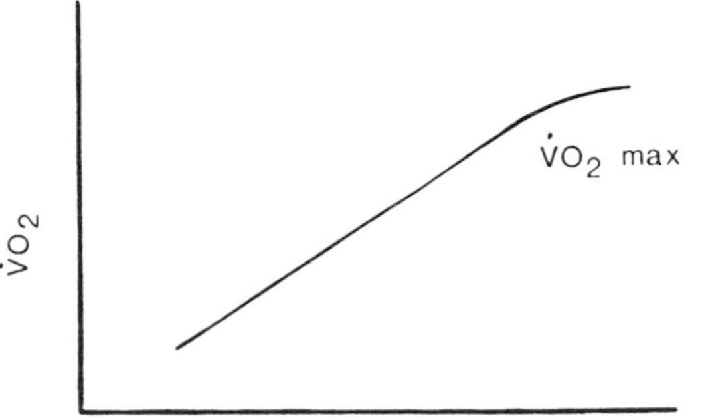

FIGURE 21–1. ***Schematic plot of oxygen consumption versus work load.*** **The linear portion of the curve indicates that oxygen consumption is directly related to work load to a point where O_2 consumption is maximum. At this point, further increases in work load are not accompanied by increased VO_2, and the subject becomes anaerobic.**

Numerous authors[5–11] have pointed out the need to measure cardiovascular reserve when assessing the cardiovascular system, and exercise stress testing has become a useful clinical means of assessing cardiovascular reserve. Although exercise testing is often used to detect coronary disease, its application in testing for cardiac reserve is also important and useful.[6–8] With the addition of measurements of left ventricular performance during exercise using radionuclide techniques,[12, 13] it is now possible to assess overall exercise capacity, to measure specific responses of the heart to exercise, and to identify abnormal cardiovascular responses.[14, 15] The physical stress imposed by diving can be simulated by these standard clinical tests, and assessment of capability to dive can be made from the results.

In dealing with patients with heart disease, it is important to understand the relationships among external physical work, myocardial oxygen consumption, and blood flow to the myocardium. Understanding these relationships will provide the basis for assessing the performance of individuals with heart disease and for determining their ability to dive.

CARDIAC WORK, OXYGEN CONSUMPTION, AND BLOOD FLOW

It is generally accepted that the heart does not greatly increase its extraction of oxygen as its work demands increase. Usually only a small increase in oxygen extraction occurs (e.g., an increase of 2 ml of oxygen per 100 ml of blood from a baseline of 10), whereas large increases in myocardial blood flow provide the increased oxygen needs when myocardial work load, increase[16] (Fig. 21–2).

Studies on the physiology of the coronary arteries by Johnson and Wiggers in 1935–1940[17] and later by Sarnoff and co-workers[18] demonstrated the relationship of blood flow to cardiac work. It was found that increased cardiac work could arise from increases in arterial pressure with little change in the amount of blood flow passing through the heart (pressure work), or from increases in blood flow with almost constant pressure (volume work). It is possible to experience diving environments that produce either primarily pressure work or primarily volume work on the heart. For example, isometric work associated with heavy lifting raises the arterial blood pressure and causes an increased pressure load on the heart, whereas the work associated with swimming causes an increased flow demand on the heart and results in a volume load. The studies of Sarnoff, et al[18] demonstrated that a pressure work load is more demanding in terms of myocardial oxygen consumption than an equivalent volume load. It is important to remember this difference when considering the diver with hypertension.

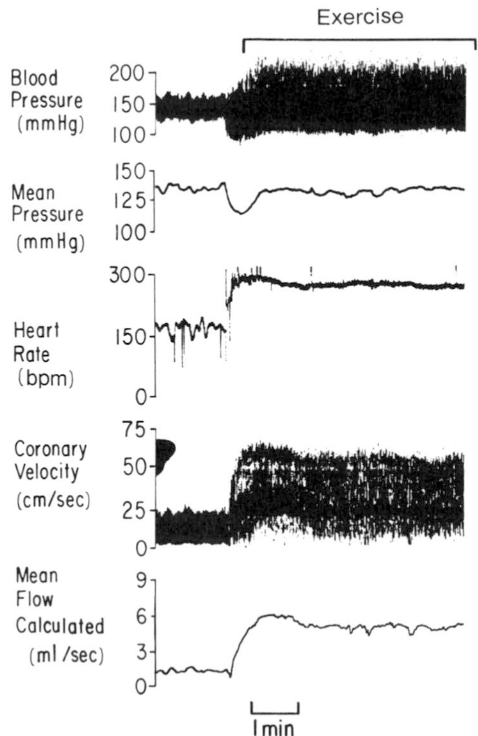

FIGURE 21–2. Hemodynamic changes during exercise in a chronically instrumented dog. As heart rate and blood pressure rise, coronary flow *(lower panel)* increases due to increased cardiac work. (From Van Citters RL, Franklin DL: Cardiovascular performance of Alaska sled dogs during exercise. Circ Res 24:33, 1969.)

Work by Gregg and co-workers[19, 20] detailed the relationships among cardiac contraction, oxygen consumption, and myocardial blood flow. From these studies it has become evident that the myocardium depends on increasing blood flow to supply oxygen demands; when flow restrictions occur due to coronary stenosis, the myocardium cannot obtain adequate oxygen by increasing oxygen extraction, and oxygen deficits occur during exercise.[21]

Chronic pressure or volume overload–induced hypertrophy of the myocardium, coronary artery disease, and congenital heart disease all may affect myocardial oxygen consumption, myocardial blood flow, and blood flow distribution to the myocardium.[22, 23] Better understanding of these blood flow principles will significantly aid in assessing the diver with heart disease.

CORONARY ARTERY DISEASE

Coronary artery disease is the most prevalent, life-threatening disease in the United States. Two million Americans per year are afflicted with new onset of the disease, and over 500,000 per year die from coronary artery disease.[24] From the physiological standpoint, the basic abnormality of coronary disease is partial or complete obstruction of one or more epicardial coronary arteries (Fig. 21–3). Complete or partial occlusion of one or more coronary arteries limits the blood flow that can be delivered to the myocardium, and in the presence of increased myocardial demand or of additional coronary vasoconstriction, myocardium becomes ischemic. If ischemia is prolonged or severe enough, there will be death of myocar-

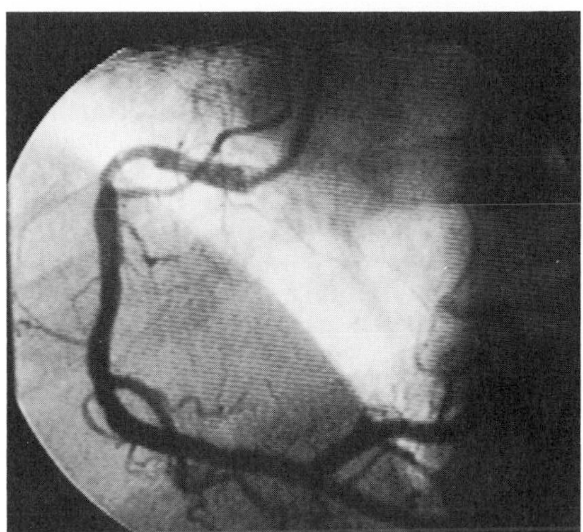

FIGURE 21–3. Coronary angiogram of the right coronary artery demonstrating a proximal 70 per cent stenosis. Lesions of this type limit blood flow during exercise and can develop further constriction from coronary spasm stimulated by such environmental factors as cold.

dial cells, i.e., myocardial infarction. The basic principle that should guide the physician in caring for patients with coronary disease who wish to dive is that each individual must be evaluated to assure that myocardial ischemia is prevented during diving. This principle can be applied to all patients with coronary disease. Patients with moderate to severe left ventricular failure from ischemic heart disease should not dive.

Coronary stenosis limits the blood flow that can pass through the stenosed artery.[25] The total resistance to flow in the coronary artery includes the resistance of the peripheral vascular bed plus the resistance of the stenosis.[26] As long as the stenosis is mild, flow can be controlled by the resistance of the peripheral coronary vascular bed, and the normal coronary blood flow response to increased work load will occur. When a stenosis becomes significant (greater than 50 per cent reduction in cross-sectional area), resistance of the stenosis at high flow rates becomes significant and will limit the ability of the peripheral coronary circulation to control flow.[27] As the stenosis becomes more severe, its resistance becomes a significant component of the total resistance to flow, and ultimately a stenosis that causes 85 to 90 per cent narrowing is the dominant factor controlling flow through the coronary artery.[28] When stenosis produces 90 per cent narrowing, peripheral coronary regulation has little or no effect on blood flow under states of increased demand. In this situation, the maximal possible flow through the coronary artery may be adequate only to supply the myocardial demands at rest. Any amount of physical stress will induce myocardial ischemia. It is evident from the stenosis versus flow characteristics of the coronary artery shown in Figure 21–4 that resting studies used to detect the presence of myocardial ischemia may not reveal a severe underlying stenosis. In the presence of coronary stenosis it may be necessary to stress the myocardium to demonstrate the imbalance between myocardial flow capability and myocardial oxygen demand. Before approval for diving, the physician must be certain that diving-induced exercise stress will not produce ischemia (Fig. 21–5).

There are several consequences of an imbalance between myocardial oxygen supply and demand during diving. Angina pectoris or serious ventricular arrhythmias may occur; the ischemic myocardium may develop an acute local or global reduction in contractile capability. The signs and symptoms that accompany this latter response include onset of a third heart sound, development of marked dyspnea, development of basilar rales, fall in blood pressure with exercise, and early fatigue. Reduced contractile performance and possible increases in diastolic stiffness induced by ischemia may combine to produce congestive heart failure. Coronary disease of this severity precludes diving.

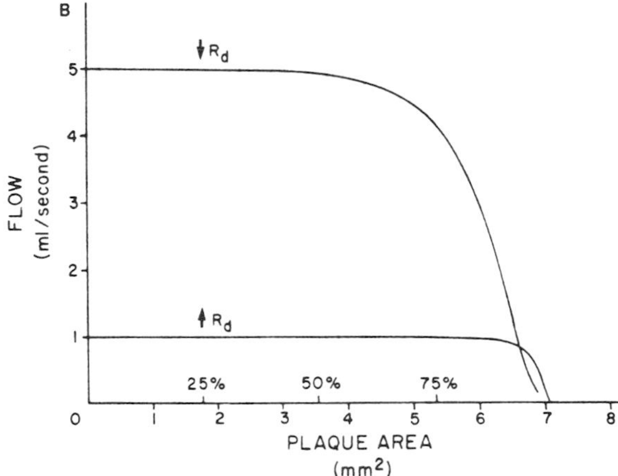

FIGURE 21–4. ***Coronary blood flow versus cross-sectional area of typical coronary plaque (theoretical analysis).*** **As the plaque narrows, the artery resistance stays nearly stable until the reduction in the plaque area reaches 75 per cent, when flow is limited during increased flow demand. At rest, narrowing must reach 80 to 85 per cent cross-section reduction before coming symptomatic** ***(lower curve).*** **(From Santamore WP, Bove AA: A theoretical model of a compliant arterial stenosis. Am J Physiol 248:H274, 1985.**

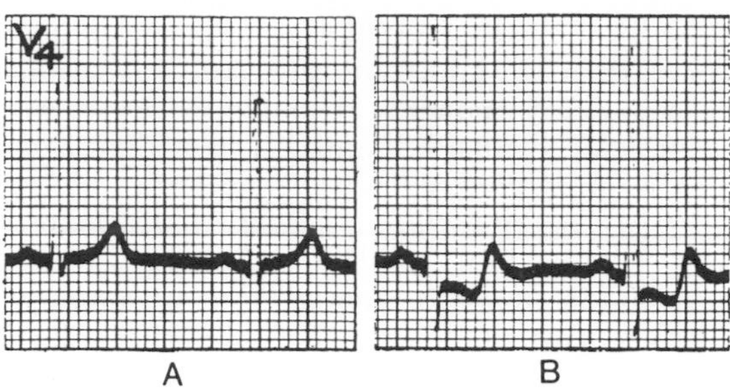

FIGURE 21–5. ***Typical electrocardiographic changes of ischemia due to exercise.*** **The ST segment is depressed from baseline with a down sloping configuration typical of myocardial ischemia *(right panel).***

An important component of coronary disease is the presence in some patients of coronary vasomotion (spasm) that produces instability of coronary stenoses under external stimuli, such as emotional and other stresses that cause catecholamine release.[28] Coronary vasomotion of this type can produce signs and symptoms of unstable angina. Several studies[37, 38] have suggested that coronary vasomotion or coronary spasm may be induced by cold exposure or exercise. Both stresses are common in diving, and patients demonstrating vasomotor-induced ischemia should not be approved for diving. Occasionally 24-hour or long-term electrocardiographic monitoring with an appropriate search for alterations in S-T segment may be needed to find periodic episodes of asymptomatic ischemia. Maseri and co-workers[31] have demonstrated that patients who have a vasotonic component to their myocardial ischemia may show ischemic changes on the electrocardiogram in the absence of symptoms. When this type of response is present, clear documentation of the response must be obtained prior to approval for diving, since the periodic ischemic episodes may coincide with exposures to physical stress or cold stress related to diving.

The most troublesome patient with coronary disease is the one who has no symptoms or arrhythmias but who develops marked ischemia detected only by electrocardiogram or by 24-hour ECG monitoring (silent ischemia). These patients require careful evaluation of exercise capacity prior to diving. Patients with asymptomatic ischemia may be at greater risk for sudden death since they develop no premonitory symptoms when severe myocardial ischemia is occurring.

CARDIOVASCULAR DRUGS AND DIVING

Many sport diving candidates take a variety of cardiac and blood pressure medications. It is therefore necessary to understand the response of patients taking such medications to exercise and diving.

Patients on large doses of antihypertensive medication may have significant inhibition of normal control mechanisms of the vascular system and may have poor exercise tolerance. Medications that inhibit blood pressure rise during exercise may result in exertional syncope. Because of these effects, diving candidates using these drugs require careful attention for evidence of inadequate blood pressure response during exercise. Limitations to moderate exercise due to dyspnea, weakness, dizziness, or palpitations should alert the physician to do careful exercise screening prior to approval for diving.

Patients taking beta adrenergic blocking drugs may also have unique problems with exercise. These patients may have significant inhibition of the heart rate response to exercise; therefore, measurement of heart rate does not provide the index of exercise work load which is generally found in the patients who have normal autonomic responsiveness[32, 33] (Fig. 21–6). Because of this difference, one must carefully observe these patients for subjective responses to exercise using perceived exercise scores[34] (Table 21–1). When stress testing a patient on beta-blocking drugs, a relative maximum heart rate can be achieved by comparing the perceived exercise score with that measured when the patient has significant fatigue. If the subject can achieve 13 mets of exercise under

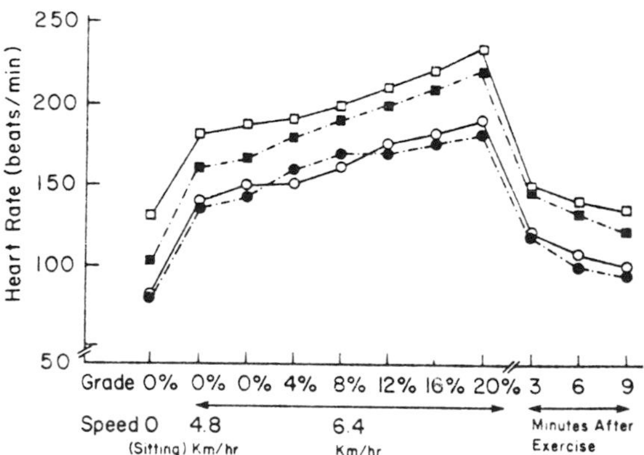

FIGURE 21–6. Heart rate response to exercise in a group of trained dogs receiving propranolol (circles), and not receiving propranolol (squares). Two curves represent trained animals (filled symbols) and nontrained animals (open symbols). Note that heart rate at all levels of exercise is reduced in both trained and untrained animals when treated with the beta blocker (Adapted from Lawlor MR, Bove AA: Effects of chronic β-adrenergic blockade on hemodynamic and metabolic responses to endurance training. Med Sci Sports Exer 17:393–400, 1985; by the American College of Sports Medicine.)

TABLE 21–1. Perceived Exertion Scale Used for Subjective Analysis of Exercise Capacity

6	
7	very, very light
8	
9	very light
10	
11	fairly light
12	
13	somewhat hard
14	
15	hard
16	
17	very hard
18	
19	very, very hard
20	

beta blockade without severe fatigue, then diving can be approved. Heart rate response to exercise, however, does not indicate a poor physiological response in this case.

There is some suggestion that beta adrenergic blockade will inhibit maximum exercise performance. Diving should not provoke maximum work demand. However, it is important to advise divers taking beta blockers to avoid extreme exercise since their maximum capacity may be inhibited by beta blockade.

Stress testing should be done in the presence of beta blockade when determining exercise capacity for a diver taking this medication. Here it is important to test exercise capacity in the presence of the usual therapeutic regimen. If the diver taking beta blockers can sustain exercise to 13 mets, then diving should be safe.

Patients on nitrate medications generally have severe enough coronary disease that diving is contraindicated. Table 21–2 summarizes the effect of common cardiac drugs in diving.

TABLE 21–2. Important Cardiovascular Drugs and Diving

DRUG	DIVING PROBLEMS
Antiarrhythmics	None (evaluate cause of drug use)
Antibiotics	None (caution on photosensitivity with tetracyclines)
Antihypertensives	Reduced exercise capacity; orthostatic hypotension
Aspirin	None
Beta blockers	Reduced exercise capacity; Raynaud's phenomenon
Coumadin	Risk of bleeding with trauma
Digitalis	None (evaluate cause of drug use)
Diuretics	None (caution about hydration in hot climates)

CONGESTIVE HEART FAILURE

Although patients with heart failure should not dive, an occasional diver with compromised cardiac function may develop acute heart failure during a dive as an initial manifestation of disease.

Patients with reduced cardiac function may develop syncope while diving because of an inability to generate an appropriate cardiac output, vasodilation in skeletal muscle, and lowering of blood pressure. The response may be obscured by the absence of venous pooling during water immersion, and syncope will occur when exiting the water. Any diver candidate with suspected compromise of cardiac function should have a thorough analysis of cardiac performance prior to approval for diving. If the subject has reduced left ventricular function (ejection fraction < 0.5) or requires drug therapy for heart failure, significant cardiac reserve is lost and the subject should not dive.

VALVULAR AND CONGENITAL HEART DISEASE

With patients who have valvular heart disease or some form of congenital heart disease, the physician must understand the effects of increased physical activity and central blood shifts due to water immersion on the heart's overload state as a result of the valvular or congenital lesion. The presence of an abnormality per se is not a contraindication to diving. In the case of intracardiac shunts and significant stenotic valvular or vascular lesions, diving is contraindicated.

Pathophysiological Principles

In considering the pathophysiology of congenital and valvular heart disease, one should be cognizant of the myocardial consequences of the lesions. Overload lesions of the heart can be classed as either pressure or volume types.[35] Pressure overload lesions include the concentric left ventricular hypertrophy that results from aortic stenosis,[36] whereas volume overload of the left ventricle can occur from aortic or mitral regurgitation[37, 38] or in the right ventricle from atrial septal defect.[39] The response of the myocardium to these overload states depends on whether the overload is a pressure or volume type. The myocardium appears to adapt specifically to handle the type of load imposed.

In either type of hypertrophy the increased muscle mass that occurs in response to chronic overload demands an increased myocardial blood flow.[40] Thus, the blood flow to either the pressure or volume overloaded hypertrophied heart is increased above normal resting levels. Maximum blood flow appears to be limited by a relative undergrowth of the vascular bed in relationship to the amount of contracting muscle tissue. Experimental evidence suggests that in pressure overload hypertrophy there is a reduction in the capillary to myocardial cell volume ratio, thus leaving the myocardium with the inability to adequately perfuse all areas of heart muscle under high load states.[41] Because of this relative underperfusion, it is likely that zones of ischemia may occur in severe pressure overload hypertrophy. The subendocardial ischemia found on the exercise ECG in aortic stenosis and in chronic hypertension with hypertrophy in the absence of coronary atherosclerotic narrowing is one example of abnormal flow distribution in hypertrophied myocardium. Such response should also be expected under the stress of diving. The flow and capillary to cell ratio in chronic volume overload hypertrophy is less well documented. There is some evidence that, like the changes found in pressure overload hypertrophy, there is a reduction in the capillary to cell volume ratio, suggesting that regions of the volume overloaded heart may also be underperfused when flow demand is high.

In all instances the first areas to be rendered ischemic during diving in hypertrophied hearts will be the subendocardial zones of the myocardium. This occurs for several reasons: first, the forces in the subendocardial layers of the myocardium are higher, thus requiring somewhat greater oxygen demand from the cells of the endocardial regions; second, the resistance vessels of the subendocardium are most distant from the supplying arteries that reside in the epicardium. Early hypertrophy, which may even be undetected by electrocardiogram, can be associated with evidence of subendocardial ischemia detected by exercise stress testing.[42] Fortunately, the changes induced in the endocardium by maldistribution of blood flow during exercise are often detected by the exercise stress test, which can be used to evaluate the presence or absence of ischemia in patients who have volume or pressure overloads due to acquired or congenital heart disease. Although there are specific contraindications, it is possible to allow selected patients with congenital or valvular heart disease to dive (Table 21–3). The basic principle of simulating the diving exposure in the controlled environment of the exercise stress test with electrocardiographic and blood pressure monitoring should be followed. This information is then used to determine individual exercise capacity. By approaching the patient with valvular or congenital heart disease in this manner, it is possible to allow some candidates to dive if the lesion is small and no right to left shunts exist. The candidate should be able to tolerate 13 mets of exercise (oxygen consumption of about 42 ml/min·kg) to dive safely.

Circulatory Considerations in Valvular and Congenital Disease

Certain specific circulatory abnormalities that are present in acquired valvular and congenital heart disease need special consideration when evaluating diving candidates. Patients with circulatory obstruction, such as is found with aortic stenosis, mitral stenosis, aortic coarctation, or pulmonic stenosis, have limitations to exercise because of the narrowed segment of the circulation. When an imbalance occurs between peripheral circulatory demand and cardiac output, blood pressure will fall and the patient will develop syncope. Indeed, this mechanism may be one of the causes for sudden death in patients with aortic stenosis. Patients with these abnormalities should not be approved for diving. This

TABLE 21–3. Congenital and Valvular Heart Disease and Diving

CONDITION	DIVING PROBLEM
Aortic stenosis	Exercise syncope; sudden death
Aortic insufficiency	None (heart failure if severe)
Mitral stenosis	Exercise-induced pulmonary edema
Mitral insufficiency	None (heart failure if severe)
Pulmonic stenosis	None (reduced exercise tolerance if severe)
Pulmonic insufficiency	None
Tricuspid stenosis	None (reduced exercise tolerance if severe)
Atrial septal defect	Paradoxical arterial gas embolism
Ventricular septal defect	Paradoxical arterial gas embolism
Patent ductus arteriosus	None (heart failure if severe)
Mitral valve prolapse	None (arrhythmias may accompany)

approach to the diving candidate is similar to that taken for competitive sports.[43]

Patients with regurgitant or shunt lesions are generally less likely to develop syncope or hypotension with diving but are more likely to develop pulmonary congestion and evidence of severe dyspnea from combined exercise and water immersion.

Considerations mentioned above apply to both valvular regurgitation and shunt lesions such as atrial and ventricular septal defects. In patients with minimal or no symptoms who have either atrial or ventricular septal defects, if pressures in the central circulation are normal, the shunt will be directed from left to right and no arterial desaturation occurs. Any patient with a right to left shunt and arterial hypoxemia will normally have severely limited exercise capacity.[44]

In diving candidates with atrial or ventricular septal defects, there is a risk of paradoxical embolism of gas bubbles that occur in the venous circulation during decompression.[45] Since intraatrial and intraventricular shunts can be bidirectional at different phases of the cardiac cycle,[46] presence of an atrial or ventricular septal defect is a contraindication to diving.

Mitral valve prolapse, found in 8 to 15 per cent of the healthy, normal population, is not a contraindication to diving. Mitral regurgitation or accompanying arrhythmias should be considered independently.

Patent Foramen Ovale

A study by Moon and colleagues published in 1989[46a] suggests that the incidence of decompression sickness in sport divers may be increased in those with a patent foramen ovale. Echocardiographic studies with bubble contrast were performed in 30 divers with decompression sickness. In 18 with serious decompression sickness, 61 per cent had evidence of shunting across a patent foramen ovale during a Valsalva maneuver. In studies of normal volunteers, the incidence of Valsalva-induced right-to-left shunting across a patent foramen ovale, demonstrated by similar echocardiographic techniques in nondiving normal subjects[46b] and in patients with a stroke history,[46c] was reported to be 8.5 per cent. Moon and associates suggested that right-to-left shunting across a patent foramen ovale may increase the incidence of decompression sickness by allowing asymptomatic bubbles to enter the arterial circulation. At present, these results are suggestive but not conclusive. No recommendations can be made regarding screening for patent foramen ovale; however, when decompression sickness occurs following an apparently safe dive schedule, echocardiographic studies with bubble contrast and a Valsalva maneuver may be helpful diagnostically.

CARDIAC ARRHYTHMIAS

Patients with or without heart disease may develop a variety of arrhythmias during diving. The importance of the arrhythmia varies depending on the type and on the patient's history. Most arrhythmias are benign and will cause no effects on the diver. Serious arrhythmias are a contraindication to diving.

Supraventricular Arrhythmias

Premature atrial beats, supraventricular tachycardia, and atrial fibrillation may be associated with diving. Episodic supraventricular tachycardia and atrial fibrillation in the young adult population is usually associated with a normal heart[47]; however, in the presence of these arrhythmias, one should carefully evaluate the individual to rule out mitral stenosis, hyperthyroidism, and hypertension. Rarely, pulmonary emboli may produce atrial arrhythmias in this asymptomatic population, and this diagnosis should also be considered. Generally, premature atrial contractions are of no consequence and are found frequently in normal persons. Often stress, alcohol, and caffeine alone or in combination are the cause of supraventricular arrhythmias. In the absence of organic heart disease, and when removal of these stimuli abolishes the arrhythmia, diving can be permitted. In normal individuals, therapy for the arrhythmia may produce more troublesome symptoms than the arrhythmia itself. Thus, care in selection of both therapy and the patient requiring therapy is necessary. After ruling out significant cardiac disease or systemic illness, such as hyperthyroidism or hypertension, and after evaluating for ingestion of cardiac excitatory agents, such as caffeine (coffee, cola drinks, and various combination over-the-counter analgesics), catecholamine-like drugs (such as those found in anti-allergy medications), alcohol, and nicotine, prevention of episodic tachycardia can be accomplished with digitalis. If adequately controlled, sport diving may be considered.

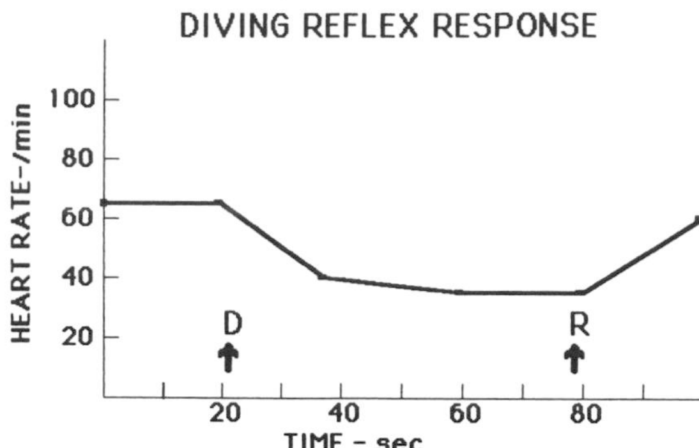

FIGURE 21–7. Heart rate response to breath-held facial immersion in one diver. Note the rapid fall in rate immediately following facial immersion (D). Heart rate remains reduced until removing the face from water (R).

Ventricular Arrhythmias

Ventricular arrhythmias, manifest as isolated premature ventricular contractions, are found in normal individuals in the absence of heart disease; for diving candidates, these should be assessed for their behavior during exercise. Normally, premature contractions that demonstrate a multifocal pattern, R on T phenomenon, or frequent coupling of sequential premature beats should be considered as serious and should disqualify the diving candidate.

Vagotonic Arrhythmias

Well-conditioned candidates may have augmented vagal tone and a resting bradycardia.[48] Often vagal tone may be so high that resting heart rates in the 30's and 40's are present. These are normally well tolerated because of the appropriately increased stroke volume, and, normally, athletes do not show significant symptoms because of the bradycardia. Variants of vagotonic rhythms include first degree heart block and Wenckebach-type second degree heart block. Although these rhythms are often benign in a well-trained candidate, a test with exercise to abolish the rhythm should be done prior to approval for diving. Failure of these changes to reverse with exercise should raise suspicion of organic heart disease, and diving should not be approved. Diving bradycardia (Fig. 21–7) is a unique vagotonic response to water immersion which can result in heart rates of 40 to 50/min in some divers. Rarely, a diving candidate will demonstrate profound bradycardia and syncope with every exposure to water immersion. These appear to be hypervagotonic syndromes and can be treated with anticholinergic medication. This author believes that this rare but profound response is a contraindication to diving.

CONDUCTION ABNORMALITIES AND PACEMAKERS

Patients with conduction system abnormalities normally demonstrate evidence of cardiac disease as the cause of these abnormalities. Congenital heart disease, certain valvular heart diseases (aortic stenosis with valvular and A-V ring calcification), cardiomyopathy, and coronary heart disease all may be associated with chronic conduction system abnormalities. Most patients with acquired complete heart block are limited in their capacity to exercise because of inability to increase cardiac output. Patients with acquired complete heart block should be treated along standard clinical lines; most commonly a permanent pacemaker is implanted to provide adequate cardiac output and heart rate. Diving candidates with pacemakers should not be permitted into commercial, military, and scientific diving. Sport diving must be individualized. If no other heart disease is present, and if the pacemaker is tested against pressure up to 130 fsw and exercise tolerance is good, the candidate might be allowed to dive.

PRE-EXCITATION SYNDROMES

Patients with short P-R intervals, with and without QRS abnormalities, may develop rapid tachycardia at rest or during exercise.[49, 50] However, many patients with short P-R intervals are asymptomatic. The finding of a short P-R on the electrocardiogram is not in itself a contraindication to diving. Patients with a history of paroxysmal tachycardia should be evaluated for the presence of the pre-excitation syndrome; if recurrent paroxysmal or exercise-induced tachycardia is a significant symptom, then appropriate diagnostic and therapeutic procedures should be followed. Exercise syncope may be induced by tachyarrhythmias, and evaluation of the electrocardiogram during exercise will aid in this diagnosis. Symptomatic Wolff-Parkinson-White syndrome is a contraindication to diving.

CARDIAC SURGERY

Coronary Bypass Surgery and Angioplasty

Patients with successful coronary bypass surgery or angioplasty who wish to undertake sport diving need not be denied this activity, although commercial or military diving should not be approved. Coronary anatomy, degree of vascularization, and exercise tolerance (exercise test) should be reviewed. If the diver can exercise to 13 mets with no ischemia or angina, with normal blood pressure response, and with no serious arrhythmia, limited sport diving may be considered.

Valvular Surgery

Prosthetic cardiac valves create two important problems in divers and potential divers. In high output states related to exercise, there may be a significant gradient across the valve, and with high heart rates, the valve poppet may not open and close completely, thus aggravating the gradient or producing significant valve regurgitation. Because of these limitations, patients who have prosthetic cardiac valves should not dive. However, individual exceptions for carefully constrained sport diving can be made. The use of center opening valves, including heterograft valves with tissue leaflets that open with larger orifices and have less mass, provides the possibility for greater cardiac output and, therefore, greater exercise capacity.

The second consideration in divers with prosthetic cardiac valves is anticoagulation. Because diving often results in minor trauma, anticoagulation is likely to produce excess bleeding in situations that produce blunt trauma, injury, or bruising. Heterograft valves provide a significant advantage in this regard since patients with heterograft aortic valves can be followed without anticoagulation after an initial period for recovery from surgery.[51] Patients with heterograft mitral valves often are maintained on anticoagulation. Divers and diving candidates with prosthetic heart valves must also be evaluated for cardiac function. Often chronic valvular disease results in decreased ventricular function and a state of chronic heart failure, which will compromise exercise performance when diving. To resolve questions about exercise capacity with prosthetic valve patients, an exercise test to 13 mets is a good screening tool.

REFERENCES

1. Nadel ER: Circulatory and thermal regulations during exercise. Fed Proc Fed Am Soc Exp Biol 39:1491–1497, 1980.
2. Astrand PO, Cuddy TE, Saltin B, Stenberg J: Cardiac output during submaximal and maximal work. J Appl Physiol 19:268–274, 1964.
3. Mitchell JH: Regulation in physiological systems during exercise. Fed Proc Fed Am Soc Exp Biol 39:1479–1480, 1980.
4. Folkow B: Role of sympathetic nervous system. *In* Larson OA, Malmborg RO (eds): Coronary Heart Disease and Physical Fitness. Baltimore, University Park Press, 1975, pp 68–73.
5. Master AM: The two-step electrocardiogram: A test for coronary insufficiency. Ann Intern Med 32:842–863, 1950.
6. Bruce RA, McDonough JR: Stress testing in screening for cardiovascular disease. Bull NY Acad Med 45:1288–1305, 1969.
7. Bruce RA, Hornstein TR: Exercise stress testing in evaluation of patients with ischemic heart disease. Prog Cardiovasc Dis 11:371–391, 1969.
8. Ellestad MH, Wan MKC: Predictive implications of stress testing. Circulation 51:363–369, 1975.
9. Naughton JP, Haider R: Methods of exercise testing. *In* Naughton JP, Hellerstein HK (eds): Exercise Testing and Exercise Training in Coronary Heart Disease. New York, Academic Press, 1973, pp 79–91.
10. Redwood DR, Epstein SE: Uses and limitations of stress testing in the evaluation of ischemic heart disease. Circulation 46:1115–1131, 1972.
11. Matingly TW: The postexercise electrocardiogram. Am J Cardiol 9:395–409, 1962.
12. Mann DL, Mackler PT, Bove AA: Reduced left ventricular contractile reserve in aged subjects. Clin Res 29:220A, 1981.
13. Rerych SK, Scholz PM, Sabiston DC, Jones RH: Effects of exercise training on left ventricular function in normal subjects: A longitudinal study by radionuclide angiography. Am J Cardiol 45:244–252, 1980.
14. Zaret BL, Strauss HS, Hurley PJ, et al: A noninvasive scintiphotographic method for detecting regional ventricular dysfunction in man. N Engl J Med 284:1165–1170, 1971.
15. Strauss HW, Zarret BL, Hurley PJ, et al: A scientiphotographic method of measuring left ventricular ejection fraction in man without cardiac catheterization. Am J Cardiol 28:575–580, 1971.
16. Jorgensen CR, Kitamura K, Gobel FL, et al: Hemodynamic correlates of coronary blood flow and myocardial oxygen consumption during vigorous upright exercise in normal humans. *In* Maseri A (ed): Myocardial Blood Flow in Man. Torino, Minerva Medica, 1972, pp 251–259.
17. Johnson JR, Wiggers CJ: The alleged validity of coronary sinus outflow as a criterion of coronary reactions. Am J Physiol 118:38–51, 1937.
18. Sarnoff SJ, Braunwald E, Welch GH: Hemodynamic determinants of oxygen as a criterion of coronary reactions. Am J Physiol 118:38–51, 1968.
19. Gregg DE: Physiology of the coronary circulation. Circulation 27:1128–1177, 1963.
20. Sabiston DC, Gregg DE: Effect of cardiac contraction on coronary blood flow. Circulation 15:14–20, 1957.
21. Ball RM, Bache RJ: Distribution of myocardial blood flow in the exercising dog with restricted coronary artery inflow. Circ Res 38:60–66, 1976.
22. Bove AA, McGinnis AA, Spann JF: Ventriculographic correlates of left ventricular oxygen consumption during acute afterload changes in the intact dog. Fed Proc Fed Am Soc Exp Biol 38:1267, 1979.
23. Buckberg GD, Fixler DE, Archie JP, Hoffman JIF: Experimental subendocardial ischemia in dogs with normal coronary arteries. Circ Res 30:67–81, 1972.

24. American Heart Association: Heart Facts. Dallas, American Heart Association, 1981, pp 10–11.
25. Santamore WP, Bove AA: Alterations in the severity of coronary stenosis: Effects of intraluminal pressure and proximal coronary vasoconstriction. *In* Santamore WP, Bove AA (eds): Coronary Artery Disease. Baltimore, Urban & Schwarzenberg, 1982, pp 157–172.
26. Gould KL, Kelly KO: Hemodynamics of coronary stenosis. *In* Santamore WP, Bove AA (eds): Coronary Artery Disease. Baltimore, Urban & Schwarzenberg, 1982, pp 173–198.
27. Logan SE: On the fluid mechanics of human coronary stenosis IEEE. Trans Biomed Eng BME-22, 237–334, 1975.
28. Prizmetal M, Kenamer R, Nerrliss R, et al: Angina pectoris. I. A variant form of angina pectoris. Am J Med 27:375–388, 1959.
29. Yasue AR, Omote S, Takazawa A, et al: Circadion variation of exercise capacity in patients with Prinzmetal's variant angina: Role of exercise induced coronary spasm. Circulation 59:938–948, 1979.
30. Specchia G, DeServi S, Falcone C, et al: Coronary arterial spasm as a cause of exercise induced ST segment elevation in patients with variant angina. Circulation 59:949–954, 1979.
31. Maseri A, Mimmo R, Cherchia S, et al: Coronary artery spasm as a cause of acute myocardial ischemia in man. Chest 68:625–633, 1975.
32. Lawlor MR, Thomas DP, Michele J, et al: Effect of propranolol on cardiovascular adaptation to endurance training in dogs. Med Sci Sports Exer 14:123, 1982.
33. Thomas DP, Lawlor MR, Michele J, et al: Metabolic adaptations to endurance training in dogs: Effects of chronic propranolol therapy. Med Sci Sports Exer 14:124, 1982.
34. Borg GAV: Perceived exertion: A note on history and methods Med Sci Sports Exer 5:90–93, 1973.
35. Rushmer RF: Cardiovascular Dynamics. 4th ed. Philadelphia, WB Saunders Company, 1976, pp 497–531.
36. Spann JF, Bove AA, Natarajan G, Kreulen TH: Ventricular pump performance, pump function, and compensatory mechanisms in patients with aortic stenosis. Circulation 62:576–582, 1980.
37. Osbakken MD, Bove AA, Spann JF: Left ventricular regional wall motion and velocity of shortening in chronic mitral and aortic regurgitation in man. Am J Cardiol 47:1005–1009, 1981.
38. Osbakken MD, Bove AA, Spann JF: Left ventricular function in chronic aortic regurgitation with reference to end-systolic pressure, volume and stress relations. Am J Cardiol 47:193–198, 1981.
39. Osbakken MD, Bove AA, Coulson RL, et al: Increased passive stiffness of short term pressure overload hypertrophied myocardium in cat. Am J Physiol 237:4676–4680, 1979.
40. Hultgren PB, Bove AA: Myocardial blood flow and mechanics in volume overload-induced left ventricular hypertrophy in dogs. Cardiovasc Res 15:522–528, 1981.
41. Breisch EA, Houser SR, Carey RA, et al: Myocardial blood flow and capillary density in experimental volume overload. Fed Proc Fed Am Soc Exp Biol 40:445, 1981.
42. Wroblewski EM, Pearl FJ, Hammer WJ, Bove AA: False positive stress tests due to undetected left ventricular hypertrophy. Am J Epidemiol 115–412–417, 1982.
43. Starek PJK: Athletic performance in children with cardiovascular problems. Phys Sports Med 10:78–79, 1982.
44. Epstein SE, Beiser GD, Goldstein RE, et al: Hemodynamic abnormalities in response to mild and intense upright exercise following operative correction of atrial septal defect on tetralogy of fallot. Circulation 47:1065–1075, 1973.
45. Bove AA: The basis for drug therapy in decompression sickness. Undersea Biomed Res 9:91–112, 1982.
46. Myizawa K, Smith HC, Wood EH, Bove AA: Roentgen video densitometric determination of left to right shunts in experimental ventricular septal defect. Am J Cardiol 31:627–634, 1973.
46a. Moon RE, Camporesi EM, Kisslo JA: Patent foramen ovale and decompression sickness in divers. Lancet 1:513–514, 1989.
46b. Lynch JJ, Schuchard GH, Gross CM, Wann LS: Prevalence of right-to-left atrial shunting in a healthy population: Detection by Valsalva maneuver contrast echocardiography. Circulation 59:379–384, 1984.
46c. Lechat PH, Mas JL, Lascault G, et al: Prevalence of patent foramen ovale in patients with stroke. N Engl J Med 318:1148–1152, 1988.
47. Zipes DP: Management of cardiac arrhythmias. *In* Braunwald E (ed): Heart disease (3rd ed). Philadelphia, WB Saunders Company, 1988.
48. Scheuer J, Tipton CM: Cardiovascular adaptations to physical training. Annu Rev Physiol 39:221–251, 1977.
49. Wolff L, Parkinson J, White PD: Bundle branch block with short P-R interval in healthy young people prove to paroxysmal tachycardia. Am Heart J 5:685, 1930.
50. Lown B, Ganong WF, Levine SA: The syndrome of short P-R interval, normal QRS complex and paroxysmal heart action. Circulation 5:685, 1952.
51. Levinson GE: Aortic stenosis. *In* Dalen JE, Alpert JS (eds): Valvular Heart Disease. Boston, Little, Brown, 1981, pp 171–230.

Chapter 22

Treatment of Decompression Sickness and Arterial Gas Embolism

JEFFERSON C. DAVIS

Extensive historical reviews of treatment of decompression sickness (DCS) and arterial gas embolism (AGE) have been written.[1–4] Recent studies on pathogenesis,[5–9] treatment protocols,[5, 10–17] and clinical reports[18–27] have created opportunities and challenges that may improve results in difficult cases. Few subjects in medicine engender such controversy as treatment of these disorders. This chapter concentrates on the treatment of decompression disorders occurring in compressed air bounce diving. Commercial, naval, and most scientific diving is fully supported by diving medicine physicians with extensive training and experience, fully equipped on-scene hyperbaric treatment facilities, and a large body of research and clinical experience. This chapter is directed to the physician and chamber team called upon to treat divers who lack that intensive support.

That recompression treatment is mandatory is undisputed, but beyond that, decisions on individual cases center around the following:

- Maximum pressure required
- Treatment gas to be breathed
- Time-pressure profile of treatment
- Treatment procedures for early versus late cases
- Adjunctive drug and fluid treatment
- Repeat hyperbaric treatments for residual manifestations

No one treatment protocol is effective for all cases, and, in some, permanent residual deficits will persist despite any known treatment protocol. There have been no controlled human studies to compare treatment methods. Animal experimentation appears to offer data to answer some controversies, but extrapolation to human cases is done with caution.

What follows is intended to represent practical approaches based on experimental data and actual experience.[28] Treatment of the most difficult cases will be emphasized, but the reader may be encouraged to know that 80 to 90 per cent of all cases of decompression sickness and arterial gas embolism respond promptly to recompression and remain clear of symptoms or signs even after long delays.[20, 26] The clinical course of a large number of cases of decompression sickness or arterial gas embolism has been used to synthesize the following strategies for management from the moment of an accident to hyperbaric chamber treatment.

IMMEDIATE CARE

Arterial Gas Embolism

If a recompression chamber is on scene, the first priority is rapid recompression, and all other measures to be discussed are conducted during chamber treatment. Except in submarine escape training, commercial, naval, or select scientific diving settings, this is rarely possible. More commonly arterial gas embolism occurs during or after surfacing from a scuba dive, from a boat or shore, at a site that is minutes to hours distant from a recompression chamber. The immediate priority is life-saving procedures while efforts are underway to secure the most expeditious transportation to the nearest recompression chamber. Frequently, alteration of consciousness due to arterial gas embolism occurs as the diver is ascending or upon reaching the surface, and near drowning is the immediate and life-threatening first priority. Rescue and cardiopulmonary resuscitation are then the immediate concerns. While there is some disagreement, most diving medicine physicians recommend that the diver suspected of arterial gas embolism be placed in the Trendelenburg position, turned to one side to prevent aspiration of vomitus, and maintained in that position until the victim is under pressure in a recompression chamber. The airway must be protected, and endotracheal intubation may be required. While arrangements are made for transportation to the nearest recompression chamber, treatment for near drowning must be instituted if indicated.

Decompression Sickness

The most common initial problem with suspected decompression sickness is to make the diagnosis. The onset may be insidious and confusing with a frequent problem of denial on the part of the diver, divemasters, or companion divers. Attempts are often made to ascribe limb-bends pain or the back pain of spinal cord DCS to trauma to avoid implication of improper decompression procedures. Aggravating this problem is the fact that DCS does occur following safe dives within the limits of no-decompression tables or within supposedly safe limits of decompression computers. The immediate tendency on scene is to seek another cause for the symptoms since decompression sickness is "impossible" following such a dive. Well-documented cases of decompression sickness have occurred with the no-decompression limits of tables and computers. One of several factors may account for such events:

1. There may be combined pulmonary overpressure accident with seeding of supersaturated venous blood as microscopic gas emboli from the arterial circulation pass through capillary beds or by flow through a physiologically patent foramen ovale from arterial to the venous circulation, there to serve as bubble nuclei.
2. There is individual variability in susceptibility to decompression sickness. No-decompression limits of tables or computers may not be adequate for all divers.
3. Precise depth and time limits may not have been followed during the dive, or pressure gauge inaccuracies may have occurred.

Another common problem confounding initial management of decompression sickness is the lack of specificity and often minor nature of some early symptoms. The diver often attempts to overlook such minor symptoms, believing that minor joint pain, profound fatigue, or mottled skin lesions will clear with time and may not require treatment. A review of Chapter 15 demonstrates the current opinion that such minor symptoms must be viewed as potential forerunners of more serious manifestations. It is relatively easy to make a decision to move a patient to a chamber and treat such minor manifestations when the chamber is within reasonable proximity and transportation is immediately available, but in reality such symptoms may occur in a diver at a site quite remote from a recompression chamber. A diver on a remote island suffering limb-bends pain and no other manifestations will be advised to obtain sea level pressurized air evacuation to the nearest recompression chamber, but such transportation is extraordinarily expensive. For this reason, the diver may decide to "wait out the symptoms." It is true that many cases of limb bends or other so-called minor manifestations of decompression sickness will clear with time and sea level oxygen inhalation; however, an estimated 20 to 30 per cent of such cases left untreated may progress to more serious neurological manifestations. In such a predicament, the diver who is requesting consultation from a diving medicine physician will ask for the probability that the minor manifestations will progress to more serious neurological complications. Unfortunately, the diver must be told that hard statistics do not exist to provide actual risk factors, and whether spontaneous resolution or progression to more serious problems will occur is totally unpredictable. The decision to move a diver suffering more obvious serious manifestations of decompression sickness such as spinal cord decompression sickness, cerebral manifestation of decompression sickness, chokes, or vestibular decompression sickness is easier because the need for movement to the chamber is obvious to all concerned.

TREATMENT EN ROUTE TO THE HYPERBARIC CHAMBER

The treatment procedures selected will depend on the level of medical expertise and the supplies available. While awaiting and during transportation to the nearest recompression chamber, the following procedures may be considered.

Life Support

Cardiopulmonary resuscitation should be instituted if needed. The patient should be positioned on the side with head low for cerebral arterial gas embolism until at treatment pressure in a recompression chamber. It is important to ensure an open airway and to prevent aspiration of vomitus.

Oxygen

One hundred per cent oxygen should be administered by mask or endotracheal tube. When a mask is used, it is important to deliver 100 per cent oxygen with a tight double seal mask. One hundred per cent oxygen administration and maintenance of intravascular volume are considered the most important features of immediate treatment and should be continued until reaching the chamber. The oxygen can be breathed continuously or intermittently for periods up to 16 hours during transportation to a recompression chamber without concern for serious pulmonary oxygen toxicity. The reason 100 per cent oxygen is stressed in regard to decompression sickness is that one is not only trying to deliver oxygen to relatively ischemic, hypoxic tissue, but also to eliminate as much inert gas as possible.

Fluids

In conscious patients oral nonalcoholic liquids such as fruit juices or balanced electrolyte beverages may be given (1 liter in the first hour). In unconscious patients and in patients with vomiting or any manifestations more serious than limb bends, intravenous fluid replacement is preferred. Isotonic solutions should be given to maintain urine output at one to two milliliters per kilogram per hour. With spinal cord involvement, an indwelling urinary catheter should be considered.

Drugs

For any neurological involvement give *hydrocortisone hemisuccinate*, 1 gram intravenously, or *dexamethasone*, 10 to 30 milligrams intravenously. The efficacy of corticosteroids in treatment of cerebral edema has been seriously questioned. However, the indications in decompression sickness may be different, and treatment is directed at the possible inflammatory nature of DCS.[10] Proof of effectiveness is lacking, but corticosteroids have been used for DCS extensively and some reports suggest efficacy.[25]

For intractable vomiting due to labyrinthine decompression sickness or unmanageable agitation, *intravenous diazepam* can be infused through a flowing intravenous catheter. Direct intravenous injection may produce phlebitis. Also, the arterial gas embolism patient may experience seizures, and diazepam may be needed for control.

For its activity to reduce platelet aggregation[29] 0.5 to 1.0 gram of *oral aspirin* has been suggested, but opinion is still divided regarding its efficacy. Except for the risk of gastric irritation, the safety of this drug makes this recommendation reasonable. Other pain-relief medication should not be used to avoid masking of symptoms.

Recent research suggests that *lidocaine* may offer several useful effects.[12] In an animal model of air embolism, it was shown to improve neuronal recovery and dampen the rise of intracranial pressure and catecholamines. It can prevent arrhythmias, which may occur in air embolism, and provide anticonvulsant effects, which can be devastating in air embolism because of the large energy requirements at the time of an ischemic insult. Further studies may add lidocaine to the immediate care armamentarium. Because lidocaine at moderately high doses is seizurogenic in some patients, caution is advised.

Communication

Early contact with the recompression chamber to which the patient is to be transported is mandatory. It is important to be sure the chamber is available and a crew is assembled and awaiting the patient's arrival.

Transportation

A major determinant of successful outcome is shortening the time from onset of decompression sickness or arterial gas embolism to compression chamber treatment. If the distance is too great for surface transportation, air evacuation must be used. It is important that the patient not be exposed to decreased barometric pressure at altitude. The usual cabin altitude of commercial airliners or other pressurized aircraft may be as low as 2000 to 5000 feet, but even this is unsafe for moving a decompression sickness or arterial gas embolism patient who already has incurred gas separation in blood or other tissues. Many aircraft are capable of maintaining sea level cabin pressure up to flight altitudes as great as 18,000 feet. Such aircraft include the military C-9 aeromedical evacuation jet aircraft, the C-130 Hercules, the Cessna Citation, and Lear jet. If the patient is moved by helicopter, the pilots must be instructed to keep the flight altitude as low as safely possible, but not greater than 800 to 1000 feet above ground level. Caution must be exercised when transportation by unpressurized aircraft would require climbing over mountains. It would be better to await a pressurized aircraft than to expose the decompression sickness or arterial gas embolism patient to such decreased pressure. One hundred per cent oxygen and fluid therapy must be maintained in flight. Decompression sickness or arterial gas embolism cases have become much worse or have resulted in a fatal outcome due to exposure to cabin altitudes of even 4000 to 5000 feet.

Recompression treatment in the water using compressed air is to be strictly forbidden. Attempts to administer compressed air in water recompression therapy have resulted in some of the most difficult cases ever treated. Further, inert gas loading of tissues while the patient breathes compressed air in the water results in massive gas separation during final decompression and must be strictly forbidden. Underwater oxygen treatment of decompression sickness is used in certain regions of the Indopacific. In remote conditions with expert and experienced personnel and when procedures have been fully planned and the proper equipment is at hand, this technique can have value.[30]

HYPERBARIC CHAMBER TREATMENT

Arterial Gas Embolism

Significant controversy regarding optimum treatment depth, time, and inspired gas mixtures exists in the undersea and hyperbaric medical community. This difference of opinion is best understood by tabulating the current status:

1. Military and commercial diving operations have a long and successful history of treatment of arterial gas embolism using immediate recompression to 6 ata when a chamber is on-scene. Since the mid 1960's, this treatment has generally been according to a schedule of a rapid recompression to 6 ata followed by hyperbaric oxygen from 2.8 ata to the surface according to U.S.N. Treatment Table 6A[31] (see Appendix 4). The June 1, 1985 U.S. Navy Diving Manual prescribes initial depth of 6 ata in treatment of arterial gas embolism.[32] Either 50 per cent oxygen–50 per cent nitrogen or 40 per cent oxygen–60 per cent nitrogen is recommended during exposure to 6 ata to improve tissue oxygenation and to reduce the addition of nitrogen in tissues.
2. Experimental studies in animals have demonstrated clearing of pial gas bubbles upon reaching 4 ata.[33]
3. Clinical series have been reported with successful treatment with hyperbaric oxygen at 2.8 to 3.0 ata with no initial deep treatment.[19, 22, 23]
4. In their exhaustive studies on an animal model of air embolism, Leitch et al could find no objective benefit in starting treatment deeper than 2.8 ata.[14–17]
5. Extrapolation from animal models with controlled injection of given gas volumes to actual human cases resulting from pulmonary overpressure accidents must be done with caution.
6. Human arterial gas embolism is known to produce at least three clinical presentations.[5] These may depend upon the volume of intravascular gas, the distribution of intravascular gas (coronary vessels, cerebral arteries), and possibly the position of the diver during barotrauma.
   a. Immediate cardiopulmonary arrest. The diver may or may not be responsive to resuscitation even if a chamber is on-scene and recompression is immediate.
   b. Neurological deficits that improve promptly with recompression treatment but recur later may occur in 20 per cent of cases.
   c. The majority of cases treated immediately according to the standard Table 6A starting at 6 ata followed by hyperbaric oxygen from 2.8 ata to the surface respond promptly and remain free of recurrences.

These classic descriptions are for those cases treated within minutes of the pulmonary barotrauma–arterial gas embolism event. The growing problem is that sport scuba divers stricken with AGE rarely have that kind of support. The usual presentation to a chamber is measured in hours from the time of the accident. By then, they present not only with the variable cerebral ischemic neurological deficits but may have also suffered permanent neural tissue damage. Significant improvement with hyperbaric oxygen even after long delays supports the concept that some neurons survive in the "ischemic penumbra"; hence, even late attempts at treatment must be made. There has also been time for the intravascular gas emboli–blood interface to activate the coagulation cascade to add essentially incompressible solid thrombi that will respond to no amount of pressure. An early case of AGE with the chamber on-scene or nearby should undergo treatment at 6 ata on Table 6A, breathing 40 or 50 per cent oxygen at 6 ata, or in the case of monoplace or duoplace chambers, the maximum safe pressure for the chamber with 100 per cent oxygen. Logic would dictate maximum recompression possible at this early stage to resolve intravascular gas before time allows blood-bubble interaction and bubble-induced arteriolar vasoactivity.

After significant delay in reaching chamber treatment, it may be rational to treat with hyperbaric oxygen staring at 2.8 ata and following Table 6 with extensions if needed or even extension to Table 7 (see Appendix 4). What is a significant delay? It is impossible to put precise numbers on such a biological decision, but one could suggest that after a delay of about six hours, treatment with hyperbaric oxygen at 2.8 ata with extensions, repeat examinations, and adjunctive treatment may be more valuable than an initial excursion to 6 ata.

Upon arrival at the chamber, the diver may be receiving cardiopulmonary resuscitation, and it may be apparent that recompression therapy as soon as possible may be the only chance of saving the patient's life. In this case, the initial evaluation is limited to a quick assessment of vital signs, clinical stabilization of the patient, and a rapid assessment of the neurological status for comparison once the patient is at depth. The patient is taken quickly into the recompression chamber and is recompressed to the treatment depth according to time of arrival and equipment available at the center. An arterial gas embolism patient who is stable upon arrival with stable neurological manifestations and one who has had a considerable delay (e.g., 6 hours or more) in reaching the chamber may be afforded the benefit of a complete neurological examination by a neurologist and evaluation of pulmonary status by chest x-ray and careful examination. It is important to determine whether or not the patient is suffering pneumothorax as part of the pulmonary barotrauma incident so that preparations can be made to insert a chest tube in order to allow safe decompression during the treatment procedure in the chamber.

Decompression Sickness

Most commonly the decompression sickness patient will arrive at the chamber sometime after the onset of symptoms in stable condition and can be afforded a more detailed examination and preparation for hyperbaric chamber treatment.

Type I

A patient with mild or severe joint pain of limb bends may not have noticed or may not have been found to have associated neurological manifestations that could in fact exist. It is important to do a detailed neurological examination before putting the patient into the chamber in order to assess progress and determine chamber treatment duration. Attention should be directed particularly to evaluation of sensory losses and especially sensory loss in the perineal region, which may be easily overlooked. Anal sphincter tone must be evaluated. An assessment of motor function and a search for abnormal reflexes must be pursued. Any neurological finding, however subtle, calls for treatment with U.S.N. Table 6 (see Appendix 4), and, in fact, this author and many other experienced diving medicine physicians now suggest that U.S.N. Table 5 should be abandoned and all decompression sickness be treated initially with at least Table 6. By following this approach, subtle neurological manifestations that could have been missed in examination of the limb-bends patient will be treated more adequately, and there will be a lower incidence of recurrence of limb bends during or after decompression. Cutaneous manifestations may include simple pruritus with no visible skin lesions, the mottled skin lesion that may be associated with burning and itching, or localized edema. The former symptom (itches, diver's lice, the creeps) usually occurs following chamber dives and is thought to represent gas separation in the skin itself as a result of direct absorption of inert gas due to high partial pressures exposed directly to the skin. It is usually innocuous and disappears spontaneously within a few minutes without chamber treatment.

The second symptom (mottled skin lesions) is viewed more seriously and should be treated by recompression with Table 6. The exact relationship is not known, but this lesion has been seen in association with severe decompression sickness with progression to life-threatening shock. Because the exact implications are not known and experience is limited, the author prefers to recommend Table 6 for this event.

Localized cutaneous edema in decompression sickness is considered the result of bubble occlusion of the lymphatic drainage. This lymphedema may be associated with pain, and both edema and pain can be resolved with recompression. Treatment according to Table 6 would be appropriate.

Type II

Neurological decompression sickness may include involvement of the spinal cord and/or the brain. An assessment of cranial nerves is important as is an evaluation of the patient's mental status. It is important to ask friends or fellow divers accompanying the patient whether or not the patient's behavior appears to be normal. Subtle changes in behavior can be a reflection of cerebral decompression sickness. In the case of spinal cord decompression sickness, it is important not only to examine for sensory or motor deficits and pathological reflexes, but also to assess anal sphincter tone and urinary bladder function. If time allows it is advisable to obtain full examination by a neurologist who will then be able to provide follow-up examination after treatment. Severe, life-threatening pulmonary decompression sickness (chokes) may require immediate treatment beginning at 6 ata as above for arterial gas embolism because of profound dyspnea and chest pain. Milder cases should respond to standard decompression sickness treatment according to Table 6, with extensions if needed.

Most treatment of decompression sickness and arterial gas embolism is conducted according to treatment tables prescribed in the naval manuals of the world. In order to have key tables immediately available for study with this chapter, the most commonly used tables are included (Appendix 4). However, every treatment chamber should have a full copy of the military diving manual they use on hand at the chamber. U.S. Navy Treatment Table 5 (RN 61) has been used for limb bends treated immediately and which responds to treatment promptly upon arrival at 2.8 ata and remains clear during the treatment schedule. Most experienced diving medicine physicians now recommend the use of U.S. Navy Treatment Table 6 (RN 62) for all decompression sickness in order to reduce the incidence of recurrence of symptoms.

Differential Diagnosis

Any symptoms that occur during or following decompression from a compressed gas dive dictate that one of the decompression illnesses be considered first. However, the act of compressed gas diving does not confer immunity from any other coincidental medical or surgical disorder. A careful history of the dive profile and relative timing of onset of symptoms will be helpful. For example, a diver who suffers an acute myocardial infarction at depth may become incapacitated by pain, shock, or arrhythmia and could suffer a superimposed pulmonary overpressure accident during rescue ascent. Such a confusing case could be expected to fail to respond to cardiopulmonary resuscitation or even recompression treatment, and the final diagnosis may not be evident until autopsy demonstrates coronary artery occlusion.

The diving medicine physician must consider the entire array of possible coincidental medical events. Ill-advised diving by a diabetic patient could lead to similar incapacitation by an unexpected hypoglycemic episode. A diver could suffer a cerebrovascular accident during diving and present as a case indistinguishable from arterial gas embolism.

The history of the dive, ascent pattern, and timing of the onset of symptoms will be helpful to differentiate air embolism from decompression sickness. The immediate onset of arterial gas embolism and more gradual onset of decompression sickness along with the nature of the symptoms and signs may help in the diagnosis. The growing awareness of combined cases of arterial gas embolism and decompression sickness discussed earlier in this chapter must be considered. "When in doubt, recompress" remains a safe course of action.

With decompression sickness, a phenomenon of early but transient symptoms and signs followed by a lucid interval and then recurrence of manifestations must be recognized. The safest action is to provide chamber treatments for decompression sickness manifestations even if initial manifestations seem to have cleared spontaneously. At least, such a patient should be under observation for several hours.

Treatment of Refractory Cases

Even in cases delayed by several hours in reaching the chamber, the standard schedules have an 80 to 90 per cent success rate; thus, attention is directed toward possible options for those situations in which the patient fails to respond to established procedures. There are effective treatment flow charts in use for treatment of decompression sickness and arterial gas embolism.[32, 34] Here we identify problems that commonly arise following any flow chart and following standard tables detailed in diving manuals. The following will be a strategy based on options that the diving medicine physician may choose to follow when confronted with these specific problems.

1. An arterial gas embolism patient at 165 fsw either has not responded to treatment after 30 minutes on Table 6A or deteriorates on attempts to decompress to 2.8 ata. Possible treatment options for this situation include:
   a. Remain at 6 ata for up to 2 hours, and if the patient responds well to fluid resuscitation and steroids, decompress to 2.8 ata according to U.S.N. Table 4 (RN 54) and enter Table 6 using all extensions. An air breathing tender must be locked in at 60 fsw because the original tender must be treated with oxygen during all of the oxygen breathing periods of extended Table 6 with the patient.
   b. The use of a 40 per cent oxygen, 60 per cent nitrogen, or 50-50 oxygen-nitrogen breathing mixture at 6 ata during Table 6A intermittently up to two hours is recommended on all Table 6A treatments if possible. This mixture is almost equivalent to breathing 100 per cent oxygen at 2.8 ata.
   c. If the patient has not responded satisfactorily to 2 hours at 6 ata, the nitrogen-oxygen saturation method of Miller et al[34] may be considered. The equipment and gas supplies needed to adapt any compressed air chamber and the treatment schedules used are set forth in this reference.
2. A patient at 2.8 ata using Table 6 or 6A may fail to respond satisfactorily or deteriorate on attempted decompression despite maximum possible oxygen extensions at 2.8 ata. Possible treatment options include remaining at 2.8 ata for an indefinite period breathing chamber air with oxygen breathing periods according to Table 7 (see Appendix 4) until maximum benefit has apparently been achieved. This option is selected only for those cases with major motor deficits and is not to be undertaken lightly. It is becoming increasingly apparent that 100 per cent oxygen breathing during the treatment tables at 2 to 2.8 ata may be extended significantly beyond that previously thought safe. It is also clear that oxygen breathing during the treatment schedule is indeed the treatment of choice, and one should be prepared to extend treatment schedules using as much oxygen breathing as possible.
3. A patient may respond satisfactorily or partially to an initial treatment on Table 6 or 6A and then suffer recurrence within a few minutes to hours after surfacing or may have a residual deficit that was not fully cleared by the first treatment. Table 6 can be repeated for recurrence after surfacing from the first treatment dive. The time between treatments will depend upon the magnitude of the recurrent symptoms and signs, but generally one may provide treatments as often as every 8 to 12 hours, repeating Table 6 or Table 5 depending upon the severity of symptoms. A modification of Table 5 to provide three oxygen periods at 2.8 ata has proved useful in the author's experience. Steroid therapy and physiotherapy for spinal cord decompression sickness can be used during the period of repeat daily hyperbaric oxygen therapy. This daily hyperbaric oxygen therapy can be continued as long as definite improvement can be seen at depth breathing oxygen with each treatment. There may be regression between treatments, but as long as improvement is seen at depth, it is considered useful to continue repeat hyperbaric oxygen treatments. Proof is lacking that these repeated hyperbaric oxygen treatments improve the long-term outcome, but experience seems to be accumulating that this regimen hastens recovery and leads, in at least some cases, to a better outcome.
4. The patient with persistent serious manifestations at depth, but with pulmonary oxygen poisoning due to the preceding circumstances, may be treated using nitrogen-oxygen saturation therapy or prolonged exposure at 2.8 ata breathing air and oxygen only as tolerated according to U.S.N. Table 7.

The availability of telephone or radio communication from any chamber in the world makes it possible to obtain assistance in difficult cases. Even experienced diving medicine physicians frequently call for other opinions. The diving alert network at Duke University (919-684-8111) is available for consultation on diagnosis, transportation, and treatment of these complex disorders.

Tending the Patient

The level of medical expertise of the individual assigned to accompany the patient inside the chamber must be chosen according to the severity of the case. A critical care physician or anesthesiologist would be the ideal tender for the arterial gas embolism patient requiring full life support. At the other extreme is the limb-bends or fixed neurological deficit patient who can safely be accompanied by a medical technician or nurse. The diving medicine physician may choose to accompany the diver for the initial compression to confirm relief or improvement in objective findings, then lock out, leaving the patient with a technician or nurse. The physician can lock in during progress of the treatment table for repeat examinations or in case of an emergency during treatment.

Intravenous fluid replacement can be continued or instituted during treatment, medications administered on schedule, vital signs monitored, urinary catheterization performed if the need arises, and any other medical or comfort needs attended to. The patient should be encouraged to move about if possible to avoid lying in one position and to avoid pressure points or lack of local tissue perfusion due to pressure during decompression.

Oxygen-induced seizures are uncommon on the 20-minute oxygen–5-minute air break schedules at 2.8 ata, but the tender should be alert for warning signs or symptoms. Oxygen breathing should be interrupted at once for such symptoms as unexplained onset of restlessness, nausea, sweating, air hunger, diaphragmatic flutter, auditory hallucinations, visual changes, muscle twitching, or seizure activity. In the event of a seizure, oxygen is discontinued, the chamber pressure is held stable to avoid pulmonary overpressure accident, and the patient is protected from trauma. The seizure will last from a few seconds to minutes after resuming air breathing, and the patient will exhibit postictal confusion. Treatment procedures following seizures are presented in the diving manuals, but basically the table can be resumed after 15 minutes of air breathing.

Within the limits of standard treatment tables, pulmonary oxygen toxicity symptoms are virtually unknown. However, with extensions of the tables, substernal burning discomfort may occur and call for alterations in the oxygen-air breathing periods or treatment depth to allow continuation of hyperbaric oxygen treatment while avoiding significant pulmonary symptoms.

U.S. Air Force modifications of the standard U.S. Navy Treatment Tables call for continuation of the 20-minute oxygen–5-minute air schedule used at 2.8 ata after reaching 1.9 ata. U.S.N. Tables 6 and 6A use 60 minutes of oxygen with 15-minute air breaks at 1.9 ata. This Air Force modification provides the same number of oxygen breathing minutes at 1.9 ata but on a more intermittent schedule. It was conceived by the author during treatment of a case of chokes in 1968. After full resolution of pulmonary discomfort at 2.8 ata and during the first 90 minutes at 1.9 ata according to the 60-minute oxygen period, recurrence of substernal distress and coughing raised the question of whether it was due to recurrent chokes or to pulmonary oxygen toxicity. Oxygen breathing was interrupted and symptoms resolved within a few minutes. While this is a very uncommon event using the 60-15 protocol, U.S. Air Force Tables were modified as above. Treatment results have remained good and no further pulmonary symptoms have occurred.

Instructions on the tables to prevent decompression sickness among tenders must be followed carefully. Especially when the tender has performed work at depth, as in handling a seizure, the oxygen breathing time at 1.9 ata can be extended liberally.

Adjunctive Treatment

Adjunctive treatment of decompression sickness and arterial gas embolism is generally directed to the events that occur at the blood-bubble interface when free gas is released into the circulation. The activation of the clotting mechanism described in Chapter 15 and a reaction akin to the inflammatory reaction as described by Bove[10] represent the basis for at least some of the recommended adjunctive treatments. Clearly, the primary treatment of decompression sickness and arterial gas embolism is pressure, oxygen, and time, and all other measures are purely adjunctive. Those adjunctive measures discussed above in the immediate care section (fluid replacement, aspirin, steroids) are all directed toward these blood-bubble interaction and inflammatory reactions. Other adjuvants must include the use of the urinary catheter to allow for bladder dysfunction and to help monitor adequacy of fluid replacement and physiotherapy.

Treatment of Residual or Recurrent Manifestations

Frequently with delayed cases and occasionally with those treated promptly, there may be significant improvement during the initial chamber treatment, but residual symptoms or signs persist or recur within the ensuing hours. The initial treatment table should be extended to achieve the best possible response, and the admonition that worsening symptoms or signs during decompression call for immediate return to greater pressure and extension of the treatment table must be followed. However, there may be fixed neurological deficits at the end of the treatment table despite all possible extensions, or manifestations may recur after treatment.

A particularly troublesome and common occurrence, especially during treatment of neurological decompression sickness, is recurrence of symptoms and signs within the hours following apparently successful chamber treatment. Edmonds[30] has suggested the possible explanation that small residual gas bubbles grow when air breathing at sea level allows tissue nitrogen tension to increase. His recommendation is that a regimen of intermittent 30-minute periods breathing 100 per cent oxygen and 30-minute periods of air breathing at ground level be followed for 6 to 8 hours after chamber treatment. Pulmonary function tests should be used to ensure that oxygen toxicity does not develop. This appears to be a sound recommendation and may reduce the incidence of recurrences.

Even without further chamber treatment, experience has shown that with hospitalization, medical treatment for cerebral or spinal cord edema, physiotherapy, and time, improvement can be expected over several months in most cases. Some cases improve only partially or not at all and are presumed to represent those with irreversible neurological damage before reaching hyperbaric chamber treatment.

Repeat hyperbaric oxygen treatments have gained widespread acceptance as part of management of residual or recurrent manifestations. The mechanism of action and solid proof of efficacy remain elusive, but clinical observation of significant improvement during oxygen breathing on repeat treatments strongly suggests benefit. Repeat treatments may be according to Table 6 or Table 5. One modification in use is Table 5 with three oxygen periods at 2.8 ata. Another is the use of repeat treatments at 1.9, 2.0, or 2.4 ata according to standard hyperbaric oxygen schedules of 90 to 120 minutes of oxygen breathing once or twice daily. These repeat treatments are usually continued as long as definite improvement in symptoms or signs is found during the periods of oxygen breathing at depth.

Other measures include repeated neurological evaluation, MRI or CT scanning of spinal cord and brain to seek evidence of damage. It is important to maintain fluid balance to improve tissue perfusion. Physiotherapy should be started for significant motor deficits, and the physical medicine team can be advised to expect generally better results with divers than with traumatic or vascular neurological cases.

Altitude Decompression Sickness

Even without preceding diving, rapid exposure to ambient altitudes above approximately 18,000 feet can result in decompression sickness manifestations indistinguishable from those found among divers. It may result from exposure in an altitude chamber, unpressurized aircraft, or accidental loss of cabin pressure in a pressurized airplane.

Treatment according to Table 6, following the same procedures described for divers, is appropriate. The same treatment is used for cases of decompression sickness resulting from flying after diving. Such cases have occurred at cabin altitudes or on mountains as low as 4000 feet. Prevention is to strictly prohibit flying for at least 12 hours after no-decompression diving. Flight to cabin altitudes above 8000 feet or flying after dives requiring decompression stops require at least a 24-hour interval before flying. Following treatment for decompression sickness or arterial gas embolism, flying should not be undertaken for 72 hours (see below).

Treatment of Decompression Sickness and Arterial Gas Embolism in a Monoplace Chamber

There are literally hundreds of monoplace hyperbaric oxygen treatment facilities around the world today used to treat various indications for hyperbaric oxygen therapy. These chambers have also been used to successfully treat arterial gas embolism and decompression sickness.[22, 23] Controversy regarding monoplace hyperbaric oxygen chambers can be summarized as follows:

Advantages:

1. In favor of these chambers is their widespread availability and the fact that they are most often the nearest chamber to a diving accident.

2. The chambers are often located in a hospital so that full hospital services are available to the patient.

Disadvantages:

1. Treatment time and depth are limited in such chambers by oxygen toxicity, patient isolation, and structural constraints. The decision to keep the difficult case under pressure for hours or days therefore cannot be made.
2. Diagnostic procedures and institution of intensive care as needed while the patient is under pressure to prepare for eventual decompression are not possible (e.g., the occurrence or discovery of a pneumothorax while the patient is under pressure requires insertion of a chest tube before decompression).
3. The large number of these chambers used for other medical indications means that they are often operated by physicians without full military or commercial training and experience in diving medicine. This particular objection can be overcome by training.

Treatment schedules for monoplace chambers have been published[4] and are supplied with manufacturer's instructions and training.

FOLLOW-UP CARE

Post-Treatment Observation

If all symptoms and signs are resolved by the end of a standard treatment table, the diving medicine physician can decide to admit the patient to a hospital for observation or to allow the patient to remain near the chamber as an out-patient. If the latter is chosen, the patient must be accompanied by a responsible person with telephone numbers to reach the chamber team if any changes should occur.

Patients with residual manifestations should usually be hospitalized for evaluation and follow-up treatment as noted above.

Flying After Treatment

Although inert gas elimination by oxygen breathing during treatment should preclude new gas separation at altitude, the possibility of residual gas bubbles in tissues dictates a conservative approach. In general, patients treated for Type II decompression sickness or arterial gas embolism should avoid altitude exposure for 72 hours after treatment. After successful treatment for Type I decompression sickness, flight at cabin altitudes not to exceed 8000 feet may be undertaken after 24 hours.

Return to Diving

Several recommendations have been suggested by naval and commercial diving medical departments.[3, 32] The following will be a more conservative application of those recommendations to sport scuba divers.

1. Following Type I decompression sickness with no neurological manifestations and full resolution upon chamber treatment, return to diving could be allowed after one week free of symptoms.
2. Following spinal cord decompression sickness with full resolution after one treatment table, some diving medicine authorities recommend no return to diving. This is because of the possibility of undetectable focal neural damage with loss of reserve in case of future episodes. For casual scuba divers this approach is recommended. For semi-professional scuba divers such as underwater photographers or others whose livelihood depends on diving, the diver is provided with information on risks, and the following could be recommended: If a complete neurological evaluation reveals no residua, diving could be resumed after 6 weeks. However, the diver should review decompression practices and resume diving with more conservative procedures than before. If neurological decompression sickness recurs, diving should be discontinued.
3. If any residual neurological deficit persists, compressed gas diving should be discontinued.
4. With pulmonary overpressure accident (POA), with arterial gas embolism, or with other manifestations, the inciting circumstances should be reviewed. If the POA was physiologically "deserved," full recovery resulted from treatment, and if a full pulmonary evaluation is normal, return to diving could be recommended. For example, if a diving instructor suffered a POA during rescue of a student and apparently suffered pulmonary overpressure during straining and breath-holding during ascent, the episode was "deserved" or could be expected to happen to any diver under those circumstances. On the other hand a diver who suffered POA during normal ascent from a dive should be suspected of a local air trapping lesion regardless of the findings on pulmonary evaluation and should be permanently disqualified from compressed gas diving.

SUMMARY

While we have dealt with the treatment of decompression sickness and arterial gas embolism representing the most difficult end of the spectrum, it must be noted that most cases do respond well to initial treatment on established treatment schedules. Those with delayed arrival at compression chambers or those with unusually severe barotrauma or violations of decompression procedures represent the most difficult cases to treat. The treatment aspects most likely to be amenable to improvement occur in the interval required to transport victims to recompression chambers and intensive medical care administered initially and en route. Oxygen inhalation, steroids to reduce CNS inflammation, and fluid therapy to maintain intravascular volume and perfusion are stressed. Although pressure, time, and oxygen administered according to established treatment schedules are usually effective when used early in the treatment of decompression sickness and arterial gas embolism, delayed cases must be viewed as serious multi-organ disorders. Vigorous intensive care by a physician, including diagnostic studies, fluid resuscitation, maintenance of acid–base balance, the administration of steroids, and other intensive care required during compression therapy, is of the utmost importance. Serious decompression sickness must be managed by physicians trained in diving medicine and with support of a neurologist and critical care physicians. Standard treatment tables are effective for most cases, but each must be handled individually. The diving medicine physician must be prepared to alter treatment profiles according to response of an individual case.

Finally, divers must be informed that prevention of decompression sickness and arterial gas embolism is still the most important means of avoiding permanent neurological injury. Decompression sickness and arterial gas embolism are serious disorders that sometimes cannot be corrected no matter what the treatment. There is a tendency among divers to believe that any case arriving alive at a recompression chamber can be cured. This erroneous impression fails to recognize that irreversible changes in nervous or cardiovascular systems cannot be undone. Despite any known treatment, in some cases there will be treatment failures or incomplete recovery.

REFERENCES

1. Berghage TE, Vorosmarti J Jr, Barnard EEP: Background. *In* Davis JC (ed): Treatment of Serious Decompression Sickness and Arterial Gas Embolism. Rep 34 WS (SDS). Bethesda, Undersea Medical Society, 1979, pp xi–xvii.
2. Bond GF: Arterial gas embolism. *In* Davis JC, Hunt TK (eds): Hyperbaric Oxygen Therapy. Bethesda, Undersea Medical Society, 1977, pp 141–152.
3. Davis JC, Elliott DH: Treatment of the decompression disorders. *In* Bennett PB, Elliott DH (eds): The Physiology and Medicine of Diving. 3rd Ed. London, Bailliere Tindall, 1982, pp 473–487.
4. Kindwall EP: Decompression sickness. *In* Davis JC, Hunt TK (eds): Hyperbaric Oxygen Therapy. Bethesda, Undersea Medical Society, 1977, pp 125–140.
5. Dutka AJ: A review of the pathophysiology and potential application of experimental therapies for cerebral ischemia to the treatment of cerebral arterial gas embolism. Undersea Biomed Res 12:403–421, 1985.
6. Evans DE, Kobrine A, Weathersby PK, Bradley ME: Cardiovascular effects of cerebral air embolism. Stroke 12:338–344, 1981.
7. Gorman DF, Browning DM: Cerebral vasoreactivity and arterial gas embolism. Undersea Biomed Res 13:317–335, 1986.
8. Hallenbeck JM, Bove AA, Elliott DE: The bubble as a non-mechanical trigger in decompression sickness. *In* Ackles K (ed): Proceedings of a Symposium on Blood Bubble Interactions in Decompression Sickness. Rep 73-CP-960. Downsview, Ontario, Defence and Civil Institute of Environmental Medicine, 1973, pp 129–139.
9. Meldrum BS, Papy JJ, Vigouroux RA: Intracarotid air embolism in the baboon. Effects on cerebral blood flow and the EEG. Brain Res 25:301–315, 1971.
10. Bove AA: The basis for drug therapy in decompression sickness. Undersea Biomed Res 9:91–111, 1982.
11. Catron PW, Hallenbeck JM, Flynn ET, et al: Pathogenesis and treatment of cerebral air embolism and associated disorders. Naval Medical Research Institute Rep 84–20. Bethesda, 1984.
12. Evans DE, Kobrine A, LeGrys DC, Bradley ME: Protective effect of lidocaine in acute cerebral ischemia induced by air embolism. J Neurosurg 60:257–263, 1984.
13. Hallenbeck JM, Leitch DR, Dutka AJ, et al: PGI_2, indomethacin and heparin promote postischemic neuronal recovery in dogs. Ann Neurol 12:797–804, 1982.
14. Leitch DR, Greenbaum LJ Jr, Hallenbeck JM: Cerebral air embolism. I. Is there benefit in beginning HBO treatment at 6 bar? Undersea Biomed Res 11:221–235, 1984.
15. Leitch DR, Greenbaum LJ Jr, Hallenbeck JM: Cerebral arterial air embolism. II. Effect of pressure and time on cortical evoked potential recovery. Undersea Biomed Res 11:237–248, 1984.
16. Leitch DR, Greenbaum LJ Jr, Hallenbeck JM: Cerebral arterial air embolism. III. Cerebral blood flow after decompression from various pressure treatments. Undersea Biomed Res 11:249–264, 1984.
17. Leitch DR, Greenbaum LJ Jr, Hallenbeck JM: Cerebral arterial air embolism. IV. Failure to recover with treatment, and secondary deterioration. Undersea Biomed Res 11:265–274, 1984.
18. Bayne GG: Acute decompression sickness: 50 cases. JACEP 7:351–354, 1979.
19. Bove AA, Clark JM, Simon AJ, Lambertsen CJ: Successful therapy of cerebral air embolism with hyperbaric oxygen at 2.8 ata. Undersea Biomed Res 9:75–80, 1982.
20. Davis JC: Treatment of decompression accidents among sport scuba divers with delay between onset and compression. *In* Davis JC (ed): Treatment of Serious

Decompression Sickness and Arterial Gas Embolism. Rep 34 WS(SDS). Bethesda, Undersea Medical Society, 1979, pp 3–9.
21. Elliott DH, Harrison JAB, Barnard EEP: Clinical and radiological features of 88 cases of decompression barotrauma. *In* Shilling CW, Beckett MW (eds): Proceedings of the Sixth Symposium on Underwater Physiology. Bethesda, Federation of American Societies for Experimental Biology, 1978, pp 527–536.
22. Hart GB: Treatment of decompression sickness and air embolism with hyperbaric oxygen. Aerosp Med 45:1190–1193, 1974.
23. Hart GB, Strauss MB, Lennon PA: The treatment of decompression sickness and air embolism in a monoplace chamber. J Hyperbar Med 1:1–7, 1986.
24. Kizer KW: The role of computed tomography in the management of dysbaric diving accidents. Radiology 140:705–707, 1981.
25. Kizer KW: Corticosteroids in treatment of serious decompression sickness. Ann Emerg Med 10:485–488, 1981.
26. Kizer KW: Delayed treatment of dysbarism: A retrospective review of 50 cases. JAMA 247:2555–2558, 1982.
27. Melamed Y, Ohry A: The treatment and the neurological aspects of diving accidents in Israel. Paraplegia 18:127–132, 1980.
28. Waite CL (ed): Case Histories of Diving and Hyperbaric Accidents. Bethesda, Undersea and Hyperbaric Medical Society, 1988.
29. Jobin F: Acetylsalicylic acid, hemostasis and human thromboembolism. Semin Thromb Hemost 4:199–227, 1978.
30. Edmonds C, Lowry C, Pennefather J: Diving and Subaquatic Medicine. Mosman, NSW, Australia, Diving Medical Centre, 1981, pp 171–180.
31. Van Genderen L, Waite C: Evaluation of rapid recompression-high pressure oxygenation approach to the treatment of traumatic cerebral air embolism. Aerosp Med 39:709–713, 1968.
32. U.S. Navy Diving Manual. NAVSEA 0994-LP-001-9010. Revision 1, Volume 1, Washington, DC, Navy Department, 1985, pp 8–28.
33. Waite CL, Mazzone W, Greenwood M, Larsen R: Dysbaric cerebral air embolism. *In* Lambertsen CJ (ed): Proceedings of the Third Symposium on Underwater Physiology. Baltimore, Williams and Wilkins, 1967, pp 205–215.
34. Miller JN, Fagraeus L, Bennett PB, et al: Nitrogen-oxygen saturation therapy in serious cases of compressed-air decompression sickness. Lancet 2:169–171, 1978.

Chapter 23

Medical Supervision of Diving Operations

EDWARD T. FLYNN, JR.

The vast majority of military, commercial, and sport dives proceed smoothly. Medical problems occur infrequently and are generally minor in nature. This excellent safety record may be attributed to rigorous standards for diver selection, diver training, and equipment design, as well as to careful pre-dive planning and adherence to safe diving procedures. This chapter will focus first on the role of the physician or diving medical technician in the prevention of diving accidents. It will then discuss the common medical problems that are encountered in diving operations and how they are diagnosed. The treatment of the various disorders will not be covered, since this topic has been amply addressed in the preceding chapters.

PREVENTION OF DIVING ACCIDENTS

The most important role of the physician or diving medical technician involved in a diving operation is prevention of diving accidents. This process includes: (1) careful selection and pre-dive physical examination of the divers, (2) careful selection of the appropriate equipment and gas mixtures for the dive, and (3) careful pre-dive planning to anticipate problems and to formulate contingency plans.

The opinions in this chapter are those of the author and do not necessarily reflect the views of the Navy Department or the naval service at large.

Diver Selection

The standards for physical selection of divers are discussed extensively in other chapters of this book. The general requirement is for a vigorous, emotionally stable individual free of cardiovascular, pulmonary, neurological, or otolaryngological disease. The on-scene physician or diving medical technician should perform a pre-dive physical examination to ensure that there are no temporary conditions that disqualify the diver. Such conditions include acute upper or lower respiratory tract infections, sinusitis, otitis media, alcohol or drug intoxication, hangover, excessive fatigue, gastrointestinal upset, recent orthopedic trauma, and sea sickness.

Underwater Breathing Apparatus Selection

Most dives will employ some type of underwater breathing apparatus. The type of apparatus selected and gas mixture used will depend on many factors including the depth of the dive, its anticipated duration, and the need for decompression stops, communication, protection, mobility, and independence. Underwater breathing apparatus (UBA) may be classified along several lines: (1) whether it is self-contained (SCUBA) or has an umbilical gas supply; (2) whether it employs air, oxygen, or mixed gas (i.e., nitrogen-oxygen or helium-oxygen); (3) whether it has an open, a semi-closed, or a closed circuit breathing loop; and (4) whether communications are present or not. Chapter 3 and other standard references[1–3] provide a complete description of these systems. Only a few salient features important to dive planning, accident prevention, and medical diagnosis will be reiterated here.

Air Diving

Air is the most economical gas to use for diving, since it can be compressed on-site and made available in unlimited quantities. Consequently, the overwhelming majority of the world's dives are air dives. Most air is compressed with oil-lubricated compressors; this introduces the possibility of contamination of the diver's air with carbon dioxide (CO_2), carbon monoxide (CO), and various gaseous and particulate hydrocarbons. Even with a perfectly functioning compressor, improper placement of the compressor inlet near exhaust fumes (including those of the compressor itself) can introduce contaminants into the diver's air supply. Nitrogen narcosis is also a problem during air diving. Nitrogen narcosis will begin to limit an air diver's performance at 132 fsw (40 msw). From a practical standpoint, an air depth of 200 fsw (60 msw) should not be exceeded. Absorption of nitrogen by body tissues with the subsequent requirement for decompression stops becomes an increasing problem as dive depth and duration increase. Oxygen toxicity, on the other hand, is almost never a problem during air diving. Nitrogen narcosis and lengthy decompression times generally prevent the diver from diving deep enough and long enough to exceed oxygen exposure limits.

Three UBA systems are commonly used for air diving: demand SCUBA, surface-supplied free-flow helmet systems, and surface-supplied demand helmet systems. Demand SCUBA is the most widely used system and the one almost exclusively used for sport diving. Compressed air from a high pressure cylinder is inhaled through a demand regulator (i.e., one that supplies air on demand) and is subsequently exhaled into the water. The breathing circuit is referred to as "open" because no gas is rebreathed. Duration is limited by the volume of air carried by the diver and is inversely proportional to the diver's depth in the water and his respiratory minute volume. Because of the limited air supply, careful planning is necessary for dives requiring decompression, and no-decompression dives are strongly encouraged. Depth is generally limited to 130 fsw (40 msw) because of the limited air supply. Excessive breathing resistance, with associated alveolar hypoventilation and CO_2 retention, is usually not a problem at this depth with modern regulators.

The classic air diving system is the surface-supplied free-flow helmet. It is also an open-circuit system. Compressed air flows through the helmet continuously at rates up to 180 l/min. The flow rate is adjusted manually by the diver to minimize the accumulation of CO_2 in the helmet. The harder the diver works, the higher the fresh air flow must be to keep the helmet free of CO_2. Unlike SCUBA, the air helmet provides head protection, communications, and an umbilical air supply that allows long duration dives. The principal problem with this system is accumulation of CO_2 in the helmet during heavy exercise. The maximum depth is limited to approximately 200 fsw (60 msw) by nitrogen narcosis.

Recently, demand regulators have been incorporated into surface-supplied helmet systems to create a new type of air diving system. The continuous free flow of air through the helmet is replaced by an oral-nasal mask supplied by a demand regulator. The head protection, communications, and unlimited duration umbilical supply advantages of the former free flow system are preserved. The newer demand regulators generally have a sufficiently low flow resistance that alveolar hypoventilation and CO_2 retention are not a problem for the working diver. Depth is still limited to approximately 200 fsw (60 msw) because of nitrogen narcosis.

Oxygen Diving

Pure oxygen may be used as a diving gas instead of air, but only for very shallow dives. Pure oxygen diving is primarily a military specialty. One hundred per cent oxygen (O_2) is rebreathed in a completely closed-circuit breathing system. No gas escapes from the apparatus, hence there are no bubbles to attract unwanted attention. Fresh oxygen to meet metabolic requirements is supplied from a high pressure cylinder to the rebreathing circuit. Exhaled carbon dioxide is absorbed in a chemical bed. The duration of the apparatus is limited only by the size of the cylinder oxygen supply and the size of the absorbent bed. Central nervous system (CNS) oxygen toxicity is the greatest problem and can be expected if the depth-time limits exceed those shown in Table 23–1. Hypoxia from improper purging of nitrogen from the rebreathing circuit and CO_2 accumulation in the rebreathing circuit from a

TABLE 23–1. Representative Depth-Time Limits for 100% Oxygen Diving

DEPTH (fsw)	MAXIMUM OXYGEN TIME (min)
25	240
30	80
35	25
40	15
50	10

Adapted from U.S. Navy Diving Manual.[2]

failed absorbent bed are additional problems. Decompression sickness (DCS) is not a problem with this apparatus since inert gas absorption does not occur. Depth is limited to 50 fsw (15 msw) because of the risk of oxygen seizures.

Nitrogen-Oxygen Mixed Gas Diving

Semi-closed–circuit nitrogen-oxygen SCUBA was developed to achieve a greater depth capability during clandestine military operations than was possible with 100 per cent oxygen closed-circuit SCUBA. An oxygen-enriched nitrogen-oxygen mixture, ranging from 32 to 60 per cent oxygen, enters the apparatus at a flow rate sufficient to meet the metabolic demand for oxygen. This may be through a constant mass flow of the mixture or through a constant ratio of mixture flow to respiratory minute volume. Exhaled CO_2 is absorbed in a chemical bed. The system is called semi-closed because, while most of the gas is rebreathed, a small amount continually escapes to the water. The duration of the apparatus is essentially independent of depth. Problems with semi-closed systems include CNS oxygen toxicity if oxygen partial pressure–time limits are exceeded, hypoxia if the mixed gas injector system fails, and CO_2 accumulation in the apparatus if the absorbent bed fails. Arterial hypercapnia may also occur in the absence of elevated inspired CO_2 levels if the breathing resistance of the apparatus is high. The hyperoxic gas mixture in the rebreathing circuit contributes to this phenomenon by decreasing the sensitivity of the respiratory control centers to carbon dioxide. On a 32.5 per cent oxygen mixture, depth is limited to 130 fsw (40 msw) by oxygen toxicity considerations.

Recently, completely closed-circuit nitrogen-oxygen SCUBA has been developed for military operations. This highly sophisticated unit maintains a constant partial pressure of oxygen in the breathing mixture, regardless of depth. One hundred per cent oxygen is added to the rebreathing circuit as it is used metabolically. Oxygen addition is controlled by an oxygen sensor and its associated electronics. Exhaled CO_2 is absorbed in a chemical bed. Diluent nitrogen gas is added to the rebreathing circuit during descent. The duration of the unit is limited by the size of the oxygen cylinder and/or absorbent bed and is essentially independent of depth. Problems with this apparatus include failure of the oxygen addition system, resulting in either hypoxia (system fails shut) or CNS oxygen toxicity (system fails open), and exhaustion, channeling, or flooding of the absorbent bed, resulting in CO_2 accumulation. Arterial hypercapnia may also result from excessive breathing resistance. Depth is limited to approximately 150 fsw (45 msw) by nitrogen narcosis considerations.

Nitrogen-oxygen diving is also done for commercial and scientific reasons. Surface-supplied demand helmets are most commonly used. The gas is pre-mixed in high pressure cylinders or blended on-site by mixing oxygen with air (so-called enriched air). The hyperoxic gas mixtures (principally 40 per cent and 32.5 per cent oxygen) are used primarily to gain a decompression advantage. The principal problem is CNS oxygen toxicity if oxygen partial pressure–time limits are exceeded.

Helium-Oxygen Mixed Gas Diving

To dive deeper than 200 fsw (60 msw), it is necessary to switch from nitrogen to helium, a gas that does not have narcotic properties. The reduced density of helium compared with nitrogen also helps alleviate problems with breathing resistance and forestalls the development of alveolar hypoventilation and arterial hypercapnia until very deep depths are attained. Gas contamination problems are unusual in helium-oxygen diving as the component gases are meticulously monitored for purity. CNS oxygen toxicity is of major concern. Oxygen exposure limits, such as those in Table 23–2, should not be exceeded.

Helium-oxygen dives can be divided into those shallower than 300 fsw (90 msw) and those deeper. For dives shallow to 300 fsw, two UBAs are commonly employed: the surface-supplied recirculating helium helmet and the surface-supplied demand helmet. Closed-circuit, constant oxygen partial pressure SCUBA may also be used in specialized applications.

The recirculating helmet is a semi-closed–circuit system. A helium-oxygen mixture enters the helmet through a venturi jet at approxi-

TABLE 23–2. Representative Normal Oxygen Partial Pressure Limits for Surface-Supplied Helium-Oxygen Diving

EXPOSURE TIME (*min*)	MAXIMUM OXYGEN PARTIAL PRESSURE (*ata*)
30	1.6
40	1.5
50	1.4
60	1.3
80	1.2
120	1.1
240	1.0

Adapted from U.S. Navy Diving Manual.[2]

mately 15 l/min, a rate sufficient to meet the metabolic demand for oxygen. The action of the jet recirculates the ambient helmet gas into a CO_2 absorbent bed at a rate approximately 10 times the incoming fresh gas flow, i.e., at 150 l/min. The diver's requirements for oxygen replenishment are met by the incoming fresh gas flow, while requirements for carbon dioxide removal are met by recirculation of helmet gas through the CO_2 absorbent bed. When a single supply gas mixture is used for the entire dive, it must have an oxygen concentration that will not cause hypoxia on the surface or lead to CNS oxygen toxicity on the bottom. The usual standard mixture selected is 84 per cent helium–16 per cent oxygen. Since the recirculating helmet is a semi-closed system, the oxygen concentration in the helmet will be lower than that in the supply gas; the difference between the helmet and supply oxygen concentrations is a direct function of the diver's metabolic rate. Supply mixtures with less than 16 per cent oxygen will lead to hypoxia on the surface if the diver exercises. This constraint on lowering the oxygen concentration prohibits diving beyond 297 fsw (10 ata) for 30 minutes if the 1.6 ata/30 min oxygen toxicity limit of Table 23–2 is to be met. To avoid the limitations of a single gas mixture, gas switching during descent is common. The descent is begun on a higher percentage oxygen mixture to avoid hypoxia on the surface. During descent or once on the bottom, "down-shifting" to a lower oxygen percentage mixture is accomplished to remain within the limits of Table 23–2. Decompression from these helium-oxygen dives may involve a switch to air during ascent and usually also involves a period of oxygen breathing in the water before surfacing. Problems with the recirculating helmet include CNS oxygen toxicity on the bottom and during the oxygen-breathing decompression stops, hypoxia from failure of the injector, and accumulation of CO_2 from failure of the recirculator or the absorbent bed.

Open-circuit demand helmets identical to those used for air diving are also commonly employed for helium-oxygen dives down to 300 fsw (90 msw). An open diving bell is frequently used in conjunction with the helmet for added diver safety. With the demand system, supply and inspired oxygen concentrations are equal. This allows a slightly lower oxygen percentage mixture to be breathed safely at the surface, thereby reducing the risk of oxygen toxicity on the bottom. Nevertheless, down-shifting of gases is often done with this system as well. With multiple gas mixtures on-site, there is the ever present danger of inadvertently shifting the diver to a mixture with too high or too low an oxygen content for the depth.

Saturation Diving

Although the helium recirculating helmet and the open-circuit demand helmet are capable of dives deeper than 300 fsw, the requirements for in-water decompression become prohibitive and the chance for catastrophic decompression sickness in the water becomes significant. Dives deeper than 300 fsw are generally done with saturated divers in a deep diving system (DDS). The DDS consists of a deck decompression chamber (DDC), where the divers live under pressure for up to a month at a time, and a personnel transfer capsule (PTC) or diving bell, in which the divers are transported under pressure to and from the worksite. The divers exit the PTC on umbilically supplied UBAs. These UBAs are usually open-circuit demand helmets fitted with gas reclaiming devices to return expired gas to the PTC or surface for CO_2 removal, oxygen addition, and ultimate return to the diver. The reclaiming devices are fitted with safeguards that prevent sudden depressurization of the helmet and consequent squeeze. While saturated in the DDC, the divers breathe a helium-nitrogen-oxygen mixture with an oxygen partial pressure of 0.4 ata. Gas mixtures for excursion dives outside the PTC are generally helium-oxygen and are chosen to avoid hypoxia during excursions above the depth of the PTC and oxygen toxicity during excursions below the depth of the PTC. Saturation diving techniques using nitrogen-oxygen mixtures may also be used for prolonged shallow jobs. Chapter 5 provides further discussion of saturation diving.

Table 23–3 summarizes the major types of UBAs available, their principal uses, their

TABLE 23–3. Commonly Available Underwater Breathing Apparatus and Associated Medical Problems

TYPE	DEPTH LIMIT (*fsw*)	HYPOXIA	HYPERCAPNIA	OXYGEN TOXICITY	N_2 NARCOSIS	CONTAMINATED GAS	DECOMPRESSION SICKNESS	PRINCIPAL USES
Demand SCUBA	130 N_2O_2*	0	+	+ +	+	+	+	Recreation, search and recovery, scientific diving
	130 air	0	+	0	+	+	+	
Surface-supplied demand helmet	130 N_2O_2*	0	+	+ +	+	+	+	Salvage, ship husbandry, underwater construction
	200 air	0	+	0	+ +	+ +	+ +	
	300 HeO_2†	0	+	+ +	0	0	+ +	
Free-flow air helmet	200	0	+ +	0	+ +	+ +	+ +	Salvage, underwater construction
100% oxygen SCUBA	50	+	+ +	+ + +	0	0	0	Combat swimming
Helium-oxygen recirculating helmet	300†	+	+ +	+ +	0	0	+ +	Submarine rescue, search and recovery, salvage
Semi-closed mixed gas SCUBA	130 N_2O_2*	+ +	+ +	+ +	+	0	+	Combat swimming, mine clearance
	180 HeO_2†	+ +	+ +	+ +	0	0	+ +	
Constant pO_2 mixed gas SCUBA	150 N_2O_2‡	+ + +	+ +	+	+ +	0	+ +	Combat swimming, mine clearance
	300 HeO_2‡	+ + +	+ +	+	0	0	+ +	
Deep dive system with demand helmet	1500 HeO_2§	0	+ +	+	0	0	+	Deep water salvage, deep water search and recovery, deep water construction

*32.5% oxygen.
†16% oxygen.
‡pO_2 = 0.7 ata.
§pO_2 = 0.4–1.6 ata.
0 indicates improbable; + possible; + + probable; + + + very probable

depth limits, and their associated medical problems.

Protective Garment Selection

Beyond the UBA itself, protective garments are the second most important element of the diver's equipment. These garments should be selected to protect against thermal insult, dangerous marine life, cuts and abrasions, and chemical or microbiological pollution.

The requirements for thermal protection in cold water are fairly well defined and are available in several reference sources.[1, 4, 5] Generally, thermal protection consists of wet suits, dry suits, or hot water suits. Wet suits are sufficient for short, shallow operations, even in ice water. They are fast to don, comfortable to wear, allow excellent mobility, and require minimal weighting. Because of compression of the closed-cell foam, the insulative value is reduced at depth. Consequently, they offer the greatest protection near the surface. Dry suits are required for deeper, longer missions. They are more cumbersome, reduce mobility, require more weighting, require a source of inflation gas to avoid suit squeeze on descent and to preserve insulation values, and are subject to leaks. They do, however, offer superior insulation when compared with wet suits. Hot water suits offer the best thermal protection but require support equipment not available at many dive sites. While hot water suits avoid the intense shivering and painfully cold hands and feet occasionally seen with wet and dry suits, the use of these suits can be associated with an insidious, asymptomatic hypothermia that leads to undetected mental incapacitation of the diver. Burns from improperly regulated hot water sources may also occur. On helium-oxygen dives deeper than 400 fsw, respiratory gas heating is required in addition to thermal protection of the body.

The requirement to dive in hot water is rapidly increasing in the commercial diving sector. Typical locations are cooling water outfalls and nuclear reactors. Water temperatures may exceed 50°C. For exposures of less than 1.5 hours at water temperatures below 40°C, open-circuit free-flow air helmet systems may be used effectively.[6] The large flow of incoming cool air provides sufficient convective cooling. Above a water temperature of 40°C, water-cooled suits are required.

For diving in bacterially or chemically polluted waters, a dry suit and helmet breathing system are preferred. The suit should have attached hard sole boots and attachable dry gloves, and the helmet should mate to the suit at the neck in a leakproof manner. The helmet must cover the entire head. Ordinary demand SCUBA regulators are considered unacceptable for this type of diving. They allow seepage of water around the mouth and through the exhaust valve. Full face masks are also considered unacceptable. They leave part of the head exposed and may become dislodged. The helmet should be equipped with a gas reclaimer on the exhaust side or a double exhaust valve to prevent backflow of water. For demand helmets, isolation of the inhalation diaphragm from the water is desirable to prevent contaminated water from seeping through pinhole leaks. Vulcanized rubber suits have proved to be easy to disinfect after exposure to bacterially polluted water. Wet suits and nylon-coated dry suits, on the other hand, have proved to be very difficult to decontaminate. Because of the extreme danger, divers should never be allowed to dive in water contaminated with acetic anhydride, bromine, methyl parathion, acrylonitrile, epichlorohydrin, or chlordane.[6] Techniques for diving in contaminated water have been summarized in recent publications.[6, 7]

Regardless of the need for thermal or pollution protection, divers should always wear leather or rubber gloves to protect the hands from trauma.

Pre-Dive Planning

Proper pre-dive planning constitutes the third important element of accident prevention. Proper scheduling of dives is essential to avoid fatigue, to remain within oxygen limits, and to avoid excessive decompression obligations. Factors to be considered are water temperature, current, work load, and visibility. The most difficult decision will be how to divide the total bottom time required for completion of the mission into discreet individual dive packets to maximize efficiency and safety. A thorough knowledge of the type of equipment to be employed, its operating characteristics, and the required decompression schedule is essential.

Pre-dive planning also includes preparation to diagnose and treat diving accidents if they arise. Proper diagnostic and therapeutic equipment must be on-scene and checked for operability. It is also important to establish communications with back-up medical and recompression facilities and to plan for the transport of a patient to these facilities if such becomes necessary. A frequently overlooked piece of emergency equipment is a source of

100 per cent oxygen which the diver can breathe while undergoing transport to such facilities.

COMMON MEDICAL PROBLEMS IN DIVING OPERATIONS

The medical problems unique to diving have been discussed in great detail in the preceding chapters. Some of these conditions are common; others are rare. A number are related to specific types of diving equipment. One of the most useful ways to organize this information is to review what can go wrong during each phase of the dive. The value of this approach is two-fold. First, knowledge of the phase of the dive in which a problem occurred is one of the most important clues to diagnosis. Second, knowledge of what may happen during each phase of the dive is crucial for anticipating problems and for developing contingency plans.

Medical Problems During Descent

The following medical problems should be considered during descent.

Barotrauma

During descent, barotrauma is by far the most likely injury. Middle ear squeeze is extremely common and occurs more frequently than other forms of barotrauma. Up to 10 per cent of divers may be affected at any given time. The presenting symptom of middle ear squeeze is pain. The diagnosis rests on the characteristic symptoms and the presence of a hemorrhagic tympanic membrane upon surfacing. Barotrauma to the paranasal sinuses is the second most common form of barotrauma during descent but is considerably less frequent than middle ear squeeze. Less than 1 per cent of divers will be affected at any given time. Pain in the involved sinus on descent and a bloody nasal discharge on ascent allow the diagnosis to be made. In the case of maxillary sinus barotrauma, pain may have been referred to the upper molars. Face mask, dry suit, tooth and external ear canal squeezes (reversed ear) are all relatively uncommon. They are easily diagnosed. Lung squeeze is exceedingly rare, due to better buoyancy and descent control in modern equipment and the all-important presence of nonreturn valves in umbilically supplied equipment. Few physicians will ever see this injury.

Frequent and forceful attempts to equalize middle ear pressure during descent may produce transient vertigo, generally just as the diver hits bottom and performs his last equalization maneuver. This condition is referred to as alternobaric vertigo (ABV) of descent. Difficulty "clearing the ears" may also produce actual inner ear injury, a condition known as inner ear barotrauma (IEBT)[8] A perilymph fistula through the oval or round window may or may not be a part of this injury. The symptoms of inner ear barotrauma are sustained neurosensory hearing loss and/or vertigo.

Caloric Vertigo

Transient caloric vertigo may occur on entering the water or during the early phases of descent if cold water enters one external ear canal faster than the other. Obstruction of one ear canal by cerumen, by otitis externa, or by a tight-fitting wet suit hood are common precipitating causes. Sudden transient caloric vertigo may also occur if the tympanic membrane ruptures from barotraumatic injury and cold water enters the middle ear.

Hypercapnia

Transient arterial hypercapnia with attendant cerebral symptoms may occur during very fast descents due to rapid compression of alveolar gas. It may also occur in the older style helmet systems without neck dams. In the latter instance, CO_2 accumulates in the diver's dress while he is on deck before the dive and is then forced into the helmet when he enters the water and is compressed by the descent. This problem is quickly remedied by ventilating the helmet. Hypercapnia is a much more common problem on the bottom. The factors that can lead to hypercapnia in diving will be discussed at length in that section.

Hypoxia

In air diving, hypoxia cannot occur during descent because the oxygen concentration is fixed at 21 per cent, and air diving systems are all open-circuit. In open-circuit mixed gas diving, however, hypoxia may occur at the surface or in the early phases of descent if gas mixtures with too low an oxygen content are supplied to the diver by mistake. There are many instances in which divers have become unconscious in the first few moments of a dive when the gas supply was inadvertently switched to pure helium or nitrogen. Hypoxia near the surface is a particular problem for most semi-closed systems. Heavy exertion near the surface will rapidly lower the inspired oxygen partial pressure below the supply gas oxygen partial pressure, often into the hypoxic range. The risk of hypoxia from this mechanism will lessen as the diver's depth increases.

Oxygen Toxicity

Oxygen toxicity will not be a problem during descent in routine air diving. In mixed gas diving, oxygen poisoning is also quite unlikely to occur during descent because the exposure time is short and the oxygen partial pressure is low until depth is reached. However, oxygen poisoning can occur during descent on a deep dive if the diver is inadvertently breathing 100 per cent oxygen instead of the intended gas mixture.

Contaminated Gas

Gas supplies contaminated with various aliphatic, aromatic, and halogenated hydrocarbons or with CO may lead to problems on descent if the concentrations are sufficiently high. Such contamination can easily result from improper cleaning of cylinders, valving, and pipes if cleaning solvents are not completely removed, or from the faulty operation of compressors. Gas supplies should be routinely checked for the presence of such contaminants. The U.S. Navy has established a limit of 25 parts per million (ppm) for total hydrocarbon vapor (methane equivalents) and 20 ppm for CO.[1] Mixed gas diving mixtures are made from pure gases, so that CO poisoning is very rare on mixed gas dives. The one exception is when air is used to form the mixture. Any gas with a pronounced or abnormal odor should not be used until a definitive analysis can be made.

Medical Problems on the Bottom

Once a stable depth has been reached, barotrauma ceases to be a problem. Delayed onset of vertigo from a labyrinthine window rupture sustained during descent is the one exception to this rule. The following possible problems should be considered.

Hypercapnia

Hypercapnia, with an impaired level of consciousness, is most likely to occur during the bottom phase of the dive. Arterial hypercapnia may come about in two ways. First, CO_2 may be present in the inspired gas due to contamination of the supply gas, inadequate gas flow in helmets, or weak or exhausted CO_2 absorbent beds. For each 1 mm Hg rise in inspired CO_2 partial pressure, arterial CO_2 partial pressure will rise 1 mm Hg if pulmonary ventilation does not increase to compensate. Such compensation may be difficult in a hard-working diver breathing a dense gas. Second, while the inspired gas may be free of CO_2, the diver's pulmonary ventilation may be too low relative to his CO_2 production. This condition is called pulmonary hypoventilation and is common in diving. Hypoventilation at depth results from increased resistance to breathing caused by dense gas flowing through regulators, valves, hoses, and the diver's airway, from dead space in the breathing apparatus, and from an elevated inspired oxygen partial pressure that suppresses respiratory drive. Both pulmonary hypoventilation and CO_2 in the inspired gas may be present simultaneously. Hypercapnia is most likely to occur on the bottom because the breathing resistance is greatest, the inspired oxygen pressure is highest, and the diver's CO_2 production is greatest while working.

Hypercapnia is most likely with closed and semi-closed systems but may happen with open-circuit systems as well. In closed- and semi-closed diving systems, CO_2 can accumulate in the breathing loop due to wet, depleted, or defective CO_2 absorbent or due to improper packing of absorbent canisters. The greatest accumulation will be during exercise when the load on the canister is greatest. With these systems, the diagnosis of hypercapnia is usually made retrospectively, by coupling characteristic symptoms of CO_2 excess with a visual inspection of the faulty absorber.

The helium-oxygen recirculating helmet constitutes a special type of semi-closed unit. Carbon dioxide scrubbing is not breath-powered as it is in other units. Carbon dioxide scrubbing, therefore, depends not only on the adequacy of the absorbent bed, but also on the adequacy of the recirculation flow through the canister. The recirculation flow is a function of the incoming gas supply flow. Since this supply flow is constant and not coupled to the diver's exercise rate, helmet CO_2 levels will rise with exercise and fall with rest. In most systems, the CO_2 levels will also increase as a function of depth. Thus, the helium helmet diver must always contend with an inspired CO_2 level of some degree. If the injector jet becomes partially clogged, CO_2 accumulation in the helmet can become very pronounced. The diagnosis of hypercapnia in a recirculating helmet diver is usually made when symptoms of CO_2 excess disappear upon switching the helmet to an open-circuit free-flow mode of operation, bypassing the need for the canister.

In open-circuit free-flow helmets, the diver must adjust the flow of fresh air through the helmet to match the amount of CO_2 exhaled into the helmet. If the diver fails to do so, significant CO_2 accumulation will occur. For a given work load, greater helmet ventilation is required as the diver descends in order to compensate for the small amount of CO_2 always present in normal air. Most air helmet divers have significant inspired CO_2 levels that contribute to hypercapnia during exercise. The diagnosis of hypercapnia in a free-flow helmet diver can usually be made when symptoms of CO_2 excess disappear when the diver stops work and ventilates the helmet with a large volume of fresh air.

Carbon dioxide in the inspired gas will rarely be a problem in open-circuit demand UBAs using either air or mixed gas. Arterial hypercapnia may occur, however, if the breathing resistance is excessive or if the diver voluntarily skip-breathes to conserve gas.

Hypoxia

The partial pressure of oxygen in air increases in linear proportion to the diver's depth. As a result, hypoxia during air SCUBA diving will not occur on the bottom unless the demand regulator fails completely and the diver becomes asphyxiated. Even in the air free-flow helmet, the air flow rates would have to be reduced to extremely low levels for hypoxia to occur. Barring complete failure of the air supply, severe CO_2 intoxication would occur before hypoxia. Hypoxia is also unlikely in open-circuit mixed gas demand systems. A diver at 132 fsw (5 ata) would have to be switched to a gas mixture containing less than 3 per cent oxygen (15 per cent oxygen surface equivalent) before hypoxia would occur.

Hypoxia is more likely in semi-closed or closed-circuit rigs. In closed-circuit diving gear equipped with oxygen sensors, hypoxia may occur at the bottom if the oxygen sensor fails and new oxygen is not added to the rig. The onset of symptoms will be gradual as the diver breathes down the available oxygen within the breathing circuit. In semi-closed mixed gas systems, complete failure of the injector system will also lead to hypoxia. The onset will be gradual as above. Partial failure of the injector system may or may not lead to hypoxia depending on the degree to which the supply gas flow is reduced, the oxygen content of the supply gas, and the diver's depth and oxygen consumption. When the diver is deep and at rest, the oxygen partial pressure may not fall low enough to produce hypoxia but will be considerably lower than it should be for the depth. In this situation hypoxia can be expected during ascent.

As mentioned, the helium-oxygen recirculating helmet constitutes a special type of semi-closed circuit system. The injector jet responsible for providing oxygen replenishment also powers the venturi recirculator that removes CO_2 from the helmet. Near the surface, partial obstruction of the injector jet will lead predominantly to symptoms of hypoxia, manifested by euphoria. The number of new molecules of oxygen entering the helmet per minute, i.e., the product of the oxygen partial pressure and the flow rate, is too low relative to the oxygen consumption rate. At depth, on the other hand, partial obstruction of the injector jet will lead predominantly to symptoms of hypercapnia, characterized by breathlessness and feelings of suffocation. At depth, the oxygen partial pressure in the supply gas is high and can more than offset the lower flow rate. At 10 ata, the supply gas flow would have to be reduced to less than 10 per cent of the normal value for hypoxia to occur.

Hypoxia may occur on the bottom using certain 100 per cent oxygen rebreathers if proper purging procedures have not been followed. In this instance, the breathing bag contains a significant amount of residual nitrogen derived from air incompletely washed out of the bag and lungs at the beginning of the dive, and from nitrogen washout of body tissues during the dive. Oxygen in the bag can be completely consumed before the bag volume becomes sufficiently small to interfere with tidal respiration or to prompt new oxygen addition. Onset of hypoxia is gradual as the last volumes of oxygen are consumed from the bag.

In breath-hold diving, excessive hyperventilation may drive body stores of carbon dioxide so low that hypoxia will occur during the breath-hold before there is an adequate stimulus for terminating the breath-hold and breathing.[9] This accident occurs most frequently during competitive breath-holding in swimming pools.

Oxygen Toxicity

CNS oxygen toxicity on the bottom would not be expected during routine air diving because the depth and time restrictions imposed by nitrogen narcosis and decompression do not allow a sufficient dose of oxygen to be breathed. The probability of CNS oxygen toxicity in mixed gas diving depends on the oxygen partial pressure level and the length of time spent at depth. The tendency to develop hypercapnia at depth and the fact that the diver is working favor the development of oxygen poisoning. CNS oxygen toxicity is more likely when oxygen partial pressure–time limit curves are approached or exceeded. The sudden onset of involuntary muscle twitching, visual disturbances, nausea, vertigo, or a feeling that something very bad is about to happen should prompt this diagnosis. Development of hiccoughs may be indicative of oxygen toxicity.

Contaminated Gas

Gas supplies contaminated with CO or hydrocarbons (e.g., methyl chloroform, trichloroethylene) may lead to serious problems at depth. In the case of CO contamination of a gas mixture with a fixed oxygen percentage, such as air, the partial pressure of both CO and oxygen will rise linearly with depth. This leads to complex effects. The rise in oxygen partial pressure will offset the rise in CO partial pressure (pCO) such that the equilibrium carboxyhemoglobin level that can be obtained with the mixture at depth will be approximately the same as if the mixture had been breathed on the surface. This reduces the potential toxicity of the elevated pCO. However, the rate at which equilibrium is approached will be accelerated in proportion to the elevated pCO.[10] This is because more molecules of CO are available for uptake from each breath. Thus, the diver would be expected to get sicker faster on the bottom than on the surface but to have comparable illness at equilibrium were it not for still another effect, the ability of the elevated oxygen partial pressure on the bottom to maintain oxygen transport in the face of inactivated hemoglobin. With heavy CO contamination of the air supply, it is almost certain that symptoms of CO intoxication will appear on the bottom. With lesser levels of contamination, however, intoxication may be delayed until ascent when the protective effect of oxygen is lost. In contrast, symptoms due to other gas contaminants are most likely to appear on the bottom. The partial pressure of these contaminants is at the highest value that will be seen during the dive, time is available for absorption, and their toxicity is not offset by the elevated oxygen pressure. Special care must be taken not to introduce contaminants into the sealed environment of a saturation diving system. This can be a problem with underwater welding. It can also happen when prohibited items are locked into the DDC or when a diver working in chemically polluted water (e.g., an oil spill) reenters the PTC at the end of a dive.

Nitrogen Narcosis

In both air and nitrogen-oxygen diving, nitrogen narcosis will begin to produce significant cerebral symptoms when the nitrogen partial pressure exceeds 4.0 ata. Progressive intoxication and performance impairment will occur with increasing nitrogen partial pressures beyond that point. At a nitrogen partial pressure of 8.0 ata, the diver will be severely affected. If a helium-oxygen diver is suddenly switched to air because of a failure of the helium-oxygen supply, a much greater degree of narcosis will be experienced than if a dive to the same depth was made on air. This is a transient phenomenon, but it can be momentarily incapacitating. Narcosis is not a problem on helium-oxygen dives. Helium has no narcotic properties.

High Pressure Nervous Syndrome (HPNS)

In dives greater than 600 fsw, HPNS may be present during descent and on the bottom. The diver will complain of tremor, dizziness, imbalance, nausea, dysmetria, and intermittent somnolence. The severity of HPNS is proportional to the speed of compression and the ultimate depth achieved (see Chapter 7).

Hypothermia/Hyperthermia

For long exposures in cold water, hypothermia may become a problem, particularly if inadequate thermal protection has been chosen. Confusion, lethargy, and inability to take corrective actions are the worrisome symptoms. Severe shivering may or may not be present depending on the thermal garment selected. On a very long cold exposure, nonfreezing cold injury to the hands and feet should be considered a possibility. In hot water suits, hypothermia can develop without the diver experiencing any sensations of cold. In the increasingly frequent instances of diving in very warm water, heat exhaustion or heat stroke may become a problem.

Occupational Hazards

On the bottom, trauma may occur from contact with hazardous marine life, an accident with tools, contact with debris from wreckage, or underwater blast. Aural injury may result from excessive noise levels, either externally or within the helmet itself. In semi-closed and closed-circuit units, it may be possible to get a caustic slurry of CO absorbent on the face, in the mouth, in the nose, or in the hypopharynx. Electrical shock occasionally occurs in military and commercial diving. There may also be exposure to radiation, as well as various chemical and microbiological pollutants in the water. The effects of these latter agents are generally delayed until after surfacing.

Counterdiffusion

Switching from breathing one gas mixture to another on the bottom can cause problems. If a diver has breathed a nitrogen-oxygen mixture at depth for a significant period of time and then is suddenly shifted to a helium-oxygen mixture, the diver is at risk for developing symptoms of DCS even though no change of ambient pressure occurred. This condition has been termed "deep tissue isobaric counterdiffusion" and is associated with skin rash, joint pains, and circulating venous gas bubbles. A second type of dangerous gas switch at depth involves a diver in a dry helium-oxygen filled DDC deeper than 200 fsw who begins to breathe a nitrogen-oxygen mixture. Differential diffusion of nitrogen and helium across the skin leads to bubble formation within the skin and eventually venous gas embolism. This condition is termed "superficial isobaric counterdiffusion."

Drowning

Drowning is an ever present possibility on the bottom, particularly in diving systems that do not employ a helmet. The precipitating event is generally some incident that impairs consciousness—i.e., hypoxia, hypercapnia, hypothermia, oxygen toxicity, contaminated gas supply, electrical shock.

Medical Problems During Ascent

The following medical problems should be considered during ascent.

Barotrauma

Ascent may be slowed by a ball valve-like obstruction in the outlet of one of the paranasal sinuses. This is a relatively infrequent occurrence. Gas trapped in the sinus is prevented from escaping by the ball valve action of a redundant mucosa, polyp, or cyst. Pain is the predominant symptom. The diver can usually be titrated to the surface by alternately descending and ascending. When the maxillary sinus is involved, an ischemic neuropraxia of the infraorbital nerve may occur with attendant neurological findings.[11, 12]

When one or both ears fail to vent properly during ascent, ABV may result. Onset of ABV is sudden and is often preceded by a feeling of fullness in one or both ears. Relief can be achieved by descending a few feet. This maneuver is diagnostic. In a number of individuals, the facial nerve is exposed to middle ear pressure as it traverses the temporal bone. If the middle ear fails to vent during ascent, an ischemic neuropraxia of the facial nerve may occur, resulting in unilateral facial palsy of the peripheral type (i.e., including paralysis of the forehead musculature). Generally 10 to 30 minutes of overpressure is necessary for symptoms to occur. ABV often coexists. Full facial function returns 5 to 10 minutes after the overpressure is relieved. An excellent review of this condition is given by Molvaer and Eidsvik.[13]

Vertigo secondary to a perilymph fistula incurred during descent may not actually appear until ascent. Such a delayed presentation appears fairly often.

Facial emphysema has been reported during ascent in individuals with healing facial fractures or with a recent history of dental extractions.[14] Pain in a tooth, aerodontalgia, may be experienced during ascent.

Hypercapnia

Carbon dioxide retention is considerably less likely during ascent than during the bottom phase because the diver is essentially at rest. The one exception is a completely exhausted CO_2 absorbent bed. This condition is most likely to cause problems in the late phases of the decompression.

Hypoxia

Hypoxia may occur during ascent if the mixed gas or oxygen injectors of semi-closed or closed-circuit equipment have partially failed, if a diver fails to purge a 100 per cent oxygen rebreather thoroughly before ascending, or if the oxygen content of the supply gas mixture is too low for the intended depth.

Contaminated Gas

Ascent is the most likely phase for the occurrence of CO poisoning in air diving because the oxygen partial pressure is decreasing and sufficient time has elapsed for CO uptake. Problems with new contaminants may be experienced during ascent if the diver is shifted to a new gas mixture for decompression. This diagnosis can usually be made by shifting the diver to an alternative source of that gas mixture.

Cerebral Arterial Gas Embolism (CAGE)

CAGE is most likely in an inexperienced diver making an emergency ascent. A finite number of cases occur, however, in apparently healthy, experienced divers ascending at normal rates. Symptoms are expected in the final stages of the ascent when the greatest expansion of trapped intrapulmonary gas occurs. Gas embolism should be high on the list of diagnostic possibilities if neurological symptoms, especially loss of consciousness, occur while the diver is ascending to a shallow decompression stop or the surface. Other stigmata of pulmonary barotrauma such as pneumomediastinum or pneumothorax will not usually be apparent until the diver surfaces.

Decompression Sickness

DCS under pressure either in the water or in a chamber is a possibility at any point during the ascent but is most likely at the terminal decompression stops. DCS under pressure is quite unusual for most ordinary dives unless the decompression is very long or inadequate. It is, however, quite common on saturation dives and deep (>300 fsw) nonsaturation dives. While the diver is in the water, it may be difficult to differentiate DCS from other conditions. The diagnosis becomes easier when the classic symptoms, such as joint pain, occur and when the decompression requirements have been substantial. Vertigo and/or tinnitus and hearing loss that appear within a few minutes of switching a decompressing helium-oxygen diver to air deeper than 100 fsw should be regarded as DCS. One case of inner ear DCS has been reported with an air change as shallow as 60 fsw.[15]

Oxygen Toxicity

Two separate phases of the ascent must be considered in evaluating the risk of oxygen toxicity during ascent: Phase 1, the initial ascent phase, including decompression stops during which the original gas source is used; and Phase 2, any decompression stops during which 100 per cent oxygen or oxygen-enriched gas mixtures are used to accelerate the decompression. Oxygen toxicity is very unlikely to develop during Phase 1 of the ascent because the oxygen partial pressure is decreasing. The probability of oxygen poisoning is also less during this phase because the diver's exercise level and CO_2 production are less than on the bottom. The one exception is the diver who was on the verge of a convulsion on the bottom; a convulsion triggered by the rapidly falling oxygen partial pressure may occur during the early ascent (the "off" phenomenon).

Once oxygen or oxygen-rich mixtures are breathed in the water to accelerate decompression (Phase 2), oxygen toxicity becomes a very real possibility. Indeed most decompression procedures have a whole set of rules to deal with this contingency. The "up ten and shift" and emergency surface decompression rules used by the U.S. Navy are typical.[2] The problem for the on-site physician is to distinguish oxygen toxicity from the host of other conditions that may develop at an oxygen decompression stop, conditions that require interventions different than those for oxygen toxicity. The differential diagnosis includes ABV, CAGE, DCS, hypercapnia from exhausted absorbers, a contaminated gas supply, and hypoxia from having shifted to the wrong gas mixture. The most important clue to diagnosis is the time of onset of symptoms. Oxygen toxicity requires time to develop. It becomes the most likely cause for symptoms as the time at the stop lengthens. In contrast, ABV and hypoxia should present on ascent or within one minute of arrival at the stop and completing the gas shift. CAGE should also present very shortly after arriving at the stop and should be excluded as a diagnosis after 10 minutes at the stop. DCS may present at any time during the stop but is most likely during the initial phases of the stop, because hyperbaric oxygen is a specific therapy for DCS. Hypercapnia from an exhausted absorber or a contaminated source of hyperoxic gas may lead to a symptom complex similar in presentation and time course to oxygen toxicity. These conditions can be distinguished from oxygen toxicity by shifting to an alternate source of hyperoxic gas and by going on an open-circuit mode of operation bypassing the CO_2 absorber.

Blowup

Blowup is a special problem that occasionally confronts medical personnel. The diver loses buoyancy control by overinflation of a buoyancy compensator or dry suit and makes a rapid uncontrolled ascent to the surface. If no decompression has been omitted, such individuals should be watched closely for emerging signs of pulmonary barotrauma. If decompression has been omitted but the individual remains asymptomatic, the diver should be returned immediately to pressure for further decompression. If gas embolism or DCS develop, the individual should be recompressed and treated on the appropriate therapeutic table. Rules for dealing with blowup are contained in various diving manuals.[1, 4]

Medical Problems After Surfacing

Medical problems that may arise after the diver has surfaced include hypoxia, hypercapnia, oxygen toxicity, ABV, IEBT, CAGE, pneumothorax, pneumomediastinum, pneumoperitoneum, DCS, hypothermia, hyperthermia, and various forms of dermatitis. The key to separating these various conditions is the nature of the presenting symptom and its time of onset after surfacing (Table 23–4).

Hypoxia

Hypoxia with loss of consciousness may occur immediately upon surfacing or during any period following surfacing in which the diver continues to breathe from the UBA. The greatest risk occurs in situations when divers must perform heavy exercise (e.g., swimming against a current) in semi-closed or closed-circuit gear. Hypoxia, however, may also occur in open-circuit systems if gas switches are performed on surfacing or if the oxygen content in the original supply gas is too low to allow surfacing. Rapid recovery from hypoxia will take place as soon as the diver breathes ambient air.

TABLE 23–4. Differential Diagnosis of Conditions Presenting After Surfacing by Time of Onset

TIME OF ONSET FOLLOWING SURFACING		
<2 min	2–10 min	>10 min
DCS	DCS	DCS
Hypothermia	Hypothermia	Hypothermia
IEBT	IEBT	IEBT
CAGE	CAGE	
Pneumothorax	Pneumothorax	
Pneumomediastinum	Pneumomediastinum	
Alternobaric vertigo		
Hypercapnia		
Hypoxia		
Oxygen toxicity		
CO poisoning		

Hypercapnia

In some older styles of free-flow air helmets and associated dress, it is not possible to climb a ladder out of the water without first securing the air supply. If the air supply is not secured, the arms will balloon out as soon as the spring-loaded exhaust valve becomes clear of the water. In these systems, CO_2 excess may occur while the diver climbs the ladder and walks to the dressing stool. Cerebral and respiratory symptoms of hypercapnia will clear rapidly once the diver breathes ambient air.

Oxygen Toxicity

An oxygen-induced seizure may occur within the first 1 to 2 minutes following surfacing from an oxygen breathing decompression stop (the "off" phenomenon). A seizure developing more than two minutes after surfacing should not be ascribed to this cause.

Alternobaric Vertigo

ABV should be present at the moment of surfacing or very shortly thereafter. Vertigo that develops more than two minutes after surfacing should not be considered ABV.

Pulmonary Barotrauma

Conditions associated with pulmonary barotrauma (i.e., pneumomediastinum, pneumothorax, pneumoperitoneum, and CAGE) should become apparent on or shortly after surfacing. The rapid onset of neurological signs followed by unconsciousness upon surfacing is highly suggestive of CAGE. Pulmonary barotrauma generally should not form part of the differential diagnosis of those symptoms that begin more than 10 minutes after the diver is on the surface.*

---

*Pneumoperitoneum is a very rare and generally asymptomatic condition, usually associated with pulmonary barotrauma. Since it may arise from a ruptured viscus, however, the first manifestation may be abdominal pain and signs of peritonitis arising some period of time after completion of the dive.

Decompression Sickness

DCS may occur upon surfacing but is most commonly delayed in onset. When neurological symptoms or signs arise more than 10 minutes following surfacing, DCS is the most likely diagnosis.

Inner Ear Barotrauma

When auditory-vestibular symptoms are the sole neurological symptoms arising 10 minutes after surfacing, IEBT must be considered in addition to DCS. Most forms of IEBT should have been manifest on surfacing, although minor impairments may have gone unnoticed until more than 10 minutes after surfacing. In addition, in IEBT with perilymph fistula, the diver may first become symptomatic after heavy lifting or straining. Thus, symptoms can occur well after surfacing. The differential diagnosis of DCS versus IEBT is discussed in the section on the differential diagnosis of vertigo.

Hypothermia

Hypothermia with mental clouding, nonresponsiveness, and semi-automatic behavior may be present following surfacing. Symptoms may worsen when the afterdrop in core body temperature occurs. For divers requiring decompression, the condition must be differentiated from DCS, which also may be associated with similar mental changes. Core body temperature measurement is diagnostic.

Dermatitis

Various forms of dermatitis may be seen following the dive. All are unusual. They include such conditions as sea bather's eruption, sea louse dermatitis, soapfish dermatitis, sponge dermatitis, seaweed dermatitis, and dermatitis from chemical contaminants present in the water. Excellent discussions are given by Fisher[16] and Sims.[17]

SUMMARY

Table 23–5 summarizes the problems that may be expected during the various phases of an air SCUBA dive to 130 fsw. This will be the most common form of diving encountered by the average physician or diving medical technician. For dives to a greater depth on air, a greater risk of narcosis, DCS, and hypercapnia can be expected. The latter risk will be equipment dependent. Once mixed gas systems are elected, hypercapnia (due to absorbent failure), hypoxia (due to wrong gas selection or gas injector failure), and oxygen toxicity (due to violation of oxygen limits) may be added to the list.

Other Medical Problems

Otitis Externa

Otitis externa is a very common and important condition that can adversely affect diving operations. It is a particularly troublesome problem for saturation divers who are continuously exposed to a hot, humid environment for many weeks. Up to 50 per cent of man-hours available for diving may be lost due to this condition. Severe cases are associated with pain, fever, lymphadenopathy, and inability to bite or chew. In the saturation environment, systemic antibiotics and local measures may barely be able to control the infection once it has begun. Prevention is of paramount importance. One regimen that has achieved great success is a twice-daily irrigation of the external ear canal with 1 per cent acetic acid/aluminum acetate solution.[18]

Sea Sickness

Sea sickness is another very common and debilitating problem on diving operations. Vomiting into masks and regulators can be extremely dangerous because of the possibility of pulmonary aspiration or laryngospasm. Sea sickness in small boats can be minimized by refraining from going below deck, by finding a spot on the deck which has the least motion, by fixing on the horizon, and by entering the water quickly once the boat is at anchor. To be effective, antimotion drugs generally must be taken in advance of the stimulus. A recurring concern with drug therapy is interference with diver performance and confusion of side effects of the drug(s) with symptoms of DCS or CAGE. Current recommendations include transdermal scopolamine or scopolamine 0.3 to 0.6 mg PO in conjunction with dextroamphetamine 5 to 10 mg PO. Two studies of psychomotor and side effects of Transderm-Scop during diving in a dry hyperbaric chamber have been reported.[19, 20] No alterations in psychomotor performance were noted, but there were side effects of fatigue, difficulty concentrating on tasks, and blurred vision. Further evaluation of these drugs in open water is required.

TABLE 23–5. Potential Medical Problems Associated with Each Phase of a 130 fsw Air SCUBA Dive

	DESCENT	ON BOTTOM	ASCENT	AFTER SURFACING
Aural and sinus barotrauma	Most likely injury	Impossible except for delayed perilymph fistula	Most likely injury	Impossible except for delayed perilymph fistula
Hypercapnia	Unlikely	Unlikely unless: —CO_2 in air —excessive regulator resistance —skip breathing	Unlikely	Not possible
Carbon monoxide poisoning	Unlikely —inadequate time for uptake —increased pO_2 protects	Unlikely —increased pO_2 protects	Most likely time —adequate uptake time —loss of pO_2 protection	Unlikely
Alternobaric vertigo	Possible	Possible immediately after arrival on bottom	Most likely time	Within first 2 min only
Nitrogen narcosis	Slight, aggravated if descent rapid	Slight	None	None
DCS	Not possible	Not possible	Rare	Most likely time
Occupational injury	Possible	Most likely time	Possible	Possible
CAGE	Not possible	Not possible	Possible in late stages	Possible—symptom onset within 10 min of surfacing
Pneumothorax, pneumomediastinum	Not possible	Rare, usually associated with ditch and don exercises	Possible in late stages	Possible—symptom onset within 10 min of surfacing

Sunburn

Sunburn is also a very common and painful sequela of open water diving operations. It is exacerbated by windy conditions. Recently, the connection between sunburn and skin cancer has been reemphasized. Sunburn can be prevented by the proper use of clothing and the active use of sunscreens containing para-amino benzoic acid or other absorbents of 290 to 320 nanometer ultraviolet radiation. A sunscreen with a skin protection factor (SPF) appropriate to the individual susceptibility should be used. A water insoluble sunscreen with an SPF of 29 and 18-hour protection is now available for individuals with the fairest skin.

DIFFERENTIAL DIAGNOSIS

The previous section reviewed the medical disorders that could be anticipated during various phases of the dive. A great deal of diagnostic information is gained simply by knowing at what point in the dive the problem occurred. This section will provide further information on the differential diagnosis of several common presenting complaints.

Musculoskeletal Pain

The differential diagnosis of musculoskeletal pain following a dive generally centers around two possible causes, traumatic injury and DCS.* Decompression sickness pain is generally described as a deep dull ache or deep "boring" sensation, although it may be throbbing in nature. It most commonly involves the shoulders or elbows on short duration dives and the knees on long duration dives. However, any synovial joint may be affected. In tunnel workers, Lam and Yau[21] report involvement of more than one site in 54 per cent of 793 cases. The sensation of discomfort may extend well beyond the joint into the surrounding muscle and indeed the joint may not be the primary focus of the complaint. The pain tends to be relatively insensitive to movement and usually lacks a trigger point. The area is not usually tender to palpation. Factors that favor a diagnosis of DCS include (1) the clear onset of pain

*In the Indo-Pacific, the severe generalized musculoskeletal pain that is produced by envenomenation by certain jellyfish (so called "Irukandji stings") may be confused with severe DCS.

after a dive at or near the no-decompression limit or following a dive having a decompression requirement, (2) the lack of known injury to that region either before or during the dive, (3) the involvement of more than one site, (4) the presence of other signs of DCS, and (5) gradually increasing severity of pain. Even in the presence of prior trauma, however, decompression sickness often cannot be excluded with certainty because of the tendency for DCS to develop in previously injured areas. Relief of pain by the application of a blood pressure cuff to the affected joint may suggest DCS.

In many instances it is impossible to distinguish between traumatic injury and DCS, and in those instances a diagnostic test of pressure is indicated. The victim is recompressed to 60 fsw (18 msw) breathing oxygen for a period of 20 to 30 minutes. If no relief is obtained, the condition is regarded as traumatic and the individual is returned to the surface and treated accordingly. If significant relief is obtained, the condition is regarded as DCS and the hyperbaric treatment is continued.

Focal Neurological Dysfunction

With the exception of vertigo and hearing loss, the onset of focal neurological signs following decompression almost always indicates the presence of either DCS or CAGE. Before either of these diagnoses are entertained, however, several forms of traumatic nerve injury should be ruled out. These conditions include an isolated facial nerve injury secondary to middle ear overpressure, an isolated infraorbital nerve injury secondary to maxillary sinus overpressure, brachial plexus injury secondary to shoulder harnesses or shoulder trauma, and lateral femoral cutaneous nerve injury (meralgia paresthetica) secondary to heavy weight belts. All of these conditions are relatively uncommon.

It is generally considered important to attempt to distinguish CAGE from DCS. This is because conventional treatment of CAGE calls for recompression to 165 fsw (50 msw), while standard treatment of DCS employed in most centers calls for recompression to only 60 fsw (18 msw). Unfortunately, as discussed below, it will be impossible to tell the two conditions apart in many instances.

The manifestations of CAGE usually begin during ascent or immediately after surfacing. In a review of 188 cases derived from submarine escape training and diving activities, Pearson[22] noted that cases exhibiting coma as the dominant manifestation developed within 30 seconds to 1 minute of surfacing. Those cases showing a variety of lesser focal signs all developed within five minutes, with the singular exception of one case that required 8 minutes. A delay of more than 10 minutes between surfacing and the onset of symptoms is generally not consistent with the diagnosis of CAGE.

DCS may also begin during ascent or immediately after surfacing. Such a rapid onset is not unusual, particularly in fulminant forms of the disease involving major disruptions of spinal cord or cerebral function. In an analysis of 1070 major cases of Type II DCS, Francis and colleagues[23] noted that 50 per cent of the cases presented within the first 8 minutes of surfacing. In an analysis of 100 DCS cases, Erde and Edmonds[24] noted 22 cases of cerebral involvement presenting within the first 3 minutes of surfacing. An additional four cases presented between 3 and 10 minutes. Three spinal cases were noted in the first 3 minutes on the surface, with an additional five cases presenting between 3 and 10 minutes. Minor focal neurological signs, on the other hand, tend to be delayed and have a slower time course for evolution, similar to the time course for Type I DCS. Focal neurological signs presenting 10 minutes after surfacing are likely to be DCS; those presenting within 10 minutes could represent either CAGE or DCS.

Gas embolism usually presents with an onset of neurological manifestations that suggest brain involvement, such as vertigo, visual disturbances, unilateral sensory and motor changes, convulsions, and stupor or loss of consciousness. Only 10 per cent of cases show bilateral sensory or motor changes.[22] Relatively rapid spontaneous recovery may occur. A lucid interval is occasionally seen. Coexisting signs of pulmonary barotrauma such as pneumomediastinum or pneumothorax are helpful in supporting the diagnosis, when present. Hemoptysis, if present, also helps support the diagnosis.

Neurological DCS usually presents with focal manifestations that suggest spinal cord or peripheral nerve involvement, such as nerve or nerve root distribution sensory losses, paraparesis or paraplegia, loss of bladder and bowel function, and the Brown-Séquard syndrome. Loss of sensory and motor function is often patchy and, in contrast to air embolism, bilateral involvement is common. When spinal long tracts are disrupted, a distinct motor and sensory level related to the spinal segments will be present. Unfortunately, a wide variety of cerebral symptoms may also be the primary manifestation of DCS. These symptoms frequently have a rapid onset and are difficult to distinguish from CAGE. Recent surveys have suggested that up to 30 per cent of cases of Type II neurological DCS may involve the brain.[23, 24] Cerebral DCS symptoms include confusion, personality changes, amnesia, aphasias, scotomata, visual field defects, headache, dizziness, motor or sensory disturbances involving only one limb, and a variety of cerebellar signs such as ataxia. Focal or generalized seizures and loss of consciousness may occur. The acute onset of stocking or glove anesthesia in DCS may be indicative of cortical involvement, although a spinal lesion is also possible.

Neurological signs of DCS will regress without treatment, but the rate of regression is significantly slower than for CAGE. A weak differential diagnostic point is that headache is a more prominent feature of DCS than CAGE. Coexisting signs and symptoms such as musculoskeletal pain and skin rashes can help support the diagnosis of DCS. The absence of these correlates does not argue against DCS, however. In a recent survey of U.S. Navy divers, Torrey and colleagues[25] observed coexisting arthralgia in only 21 per cent of Type II neurological cases. Erde and Edmonds[24] observed musculoskeletal involvement in 38 per cent of cerebral cases, in 27 per cent of spinal cases, and in 64 per cent of peripheral nerve cases.

The depth and time of the dive are often very helpful in distinguishing CAGE from DCS. Dives well inside no-decompression limits, especially those associated with emergency ascents (e.g., out-of-air) or emergency ascent training, are most likely to result in CAGE. Dives in which the diver made a normal ascent, but had a large amount of required decompression or omitted a large amount of decompression, are most likely to result in DCS. This is not an iron-clad rule, however, as some fulminant cases of spinal cord DCS have occurred inside the no-decompression limits.

It is worth noting that CAGE and DCS may coexist. When decompression has been omitted through emergency ascent, DCS could follow right on the heels of CAGE. Also there is evidence from both animal experiments and human cases that CAGE may predispose to the development of spinal cord DCS in situations where cord involvement would not ordinarily be expected.[26]

Because the manifestations of CAGE and DCS overlap so much, it is not always possible to distinguish between them clearly. This is not likely to have serious consequences if two points are kept in mind: (1) treatment by recompression benefits patients with both diseases, and (2) it is always the prerogative of the physician to recommend alteration of the treatment tables if the clinical response of the patient is unsatisfactory.

From the standpoint of focal neurological symptoms, a special diagnostic pitfall for the uninitiated is the occurrence of intense numbness in the fingertips while a diver is breathing oxygen during decompression or during recompression treatment. This condition does not represent DCS or CAGE but rather peripheral oxygen toxicity. This numbness will subside several hours after oxygen breathing is discontinued. This numbness does not herald the onset of CNS oxygen toxicity, and oxygen breathing need not be discontinued when it occurs.

Chest Pain and Dyspnea

Chest pain is fairly uncommon in diving, but its presence can pose diagnostic dilemmas. The nature and location of symptoms, the time of onset during the dive, and the physical examination are the key features in the differential diagnosis. The following conditions should be considered.

Pulmonary Decompression Sickness (Chokes). Theoretically, chokes may begin at any point after the diver leaves bottom, but it is most likely to occur after surfacing. In some instances, symptom onset may be delayed for several hours after surfacing. Symptoms consist of progressively worsening substernal burning pain or feeling of distress, paroxysmal cough, and shortness of breath. These symptoms are greatly aggravated by deep inspiration and by smoking. Tachypnea is invariably present. An EKG may show a peaked P wave, right axis deviation, and evidence of right ventricular strain. For chokes to be present, a severe decompression stress is usually required (i.e., either a large amount of required decompression was omitted or a very long and arduous decompression was undertaken). Often other stigmata of DCS will develop and aid in making the diagnosis. Erde and Edmonds[24] reported that 52 per cent of patients with respiratory symptoms had coexisting musculoskeletal symptoms, while 91 per cent had one or more findings relating to the CNS or inner ear.

Spinal Cord Decompression Sickness. Back pain followed by lancinating radicular or dull girdle-like chest pain presenting shortly after surfacing often herald the onset of paralytic spinal cord DCS. Such a condition is often seen following dives requiring only minimal decompression. Pneumothorax should quickly be ruled out. Usually other stigmata of evolving spinal cord DCS, such as numbness and weakness, appear rapidly and aid in making the diagnosis.

Pulmonary Oxygen Toxicity. The symptoms of pulmonary oxygen toxicity are quite similar to those of chokes but develop with a very much slower time course. During most conventional diving, the dose of oxygen delivered to the lung is inadequate to produce pulmonary oxygen toxicity, and the diagnosis can be excluded on that basis. If the exposure to oxygen has been sufficiently long to cause pulmonary oxygen toxicity, this condition can be distinguished from chokes by its very gradual onset and the absence of other stigmata of DCS. In some instances, DCS may not be a possibility. Pulmonary oxygen toxicity is most likely to be seen when the diver is in the chamber breathing oxygen. Chokes, on the other hand, is most likely to occur after the diver is on the surface breathing air. The computation of unit pulmonary toxicity dose (UPTD) or other quantitative indices of oxygen toxicity risk[27] give an estimation of whether pulmonary oxygen toxicity is likely in a given situation.

Pneumomediastinum. Symptoms associated with pneumomediastinum first appear during or after ascent, although the genesis of the problem may have started on the bottom during ditch and don exercises. The principal symptom is a substernal ache or tightness. Occasionally the pain may be sharp. Radiation to both shoulders, the back, or the neck may be present.[28] The discomfort is often aggravated by deep breathing, coughing, swallowing, moving the neck and trunk, or by lying flat. There may be a change in the quality of the voice. Dyspnea is present in more severe cases and subcutaneous crepitation may be felt over the clavicles. In contrast to chokes, progressively worsening cough and shortness of breath do not accompany the pain. Examination of the chest may reveal subcutaneous crepitus above and below the clavicles, decreased heart sounds, decreased area of cardiac dullness, and a crunching or crackling sound on auscultation (Hamman's sign). There may be some precordial tenderness. A chest x-ray is diagnostic.

Pneumothorax. Simple pneumothorax may occur as a consequence of lung overinflation, but it is considerably less common than pneumomediastinum. It should be suspected when there is pleuritic pain, especially when it is located over the more lateral aspects of the chest wall. Decreased or absent breath sounds and tactile fremitus, increased resonance to percussion, tracheal deviation to the affected side, and decreased chest wall motion on the affected side aid in making the diagnosis. These signs may be difficult to elicit in a small pneumothorax. An erect chest x-ray in full expiration or a lateral decubitus x-ray will be required. Tension pneumothorax may result from lung overinflation during ascent or it may occur as a result of recompression therapy for a patient with simple pneumothorax. The dominant manifestations of tension pneumothorax are those of circulatory collapse (arterial hypotension, cyanosis, dyspnea, and tachypnea) rather than chest pain. Tracheal deviation away from the affected side, absent breath sounds, bulging interspaces, distended neck veins, and hyperresonance of the affected side may be present.

Myocardial Ischemia. Unusually severe or prolonged substernal or precordial chest pain may be indicative of myocardial ischemia. Two possibilities exist: (1) the pain is the manifestation of underlying coronary artery disease, an anginal attack unrelated to the diving environment per se, or (2) the pain is the result of coronary artery gas embolism associated with pulmonary barotrauma. While not a common manifestation of pulmonary barotrauma, involvement of the coronary arteries has been documented in man[29] and a recent study suggests that involvement may be more prevalent than previously thought.[30] Other stigmata of pulmonary barotrauma with neurological involvement should be present. An EKG is essential for ruling out this possibility.

Anxiety-Hyperventilation Syndrome. This condition is not uncommon in novice divers and may produce shortness of breath and substernal tightness. The other characteristic findings of the syndrome such as lightheadedness; dizziness; numbness of the hands, feet, and perioral area; and carpal pedal spasms, along with a positive Chvostek's sign, help make the diagnosis. The diagnosis of anxiety hyperventilation should not be accepted until pneumomediastinum and chokes have been ruled out.

Trauma. Injury to the chest wall is always a possibility on any working dive. A history of injury and local tenderness or evidence of trauma will establish this diagnosis. Trauma to the respiratory muscles may occur during long dives when the breathing resistance is high. Following the dive, the diver will complain of generalized chest wall soreness.

Loss of Consciousness

The differential diagnosis of unconsciousness rests heavily on the phase of the dive when the problem occurred, the hazards present in the surrounding environment, the type of equipment employed, the nature of the prodromal symptoms, and the abruptness with which consciousness is lost. In many instances it will not be possible to establish the diagnosis with certainty. The following conditions should be considered.

Hypoxia. This is perhaps the most common cause of unconsciousness in diving and is an especially strong possibility when semi-closed and closed-circuit breathing systems are being used. Any phase of the dive may be involved. Gradual impairment of consciousness with attendant euphoria is the usual presentation with semi-closed and closed-circuit breathing sets and results from gradual depletion of oxygen in the breathing loop. In open-circuit demand systems, the loss of consciousness will be abrupt if a gas shift is involved and only slightly more gradual if the diver is ascending shallower than allowed for the gas mixture.

Hypercapnia. Carbon dioxide accumulation is unlikely to produce an abrupt loss of consciousness during any phase of the dive. Lesser symptoms of restlessness, lightheadedness, dizziness, weakness, confusion, a throbbing frontal or bitemporal headache, nausea, and sometimes a feeling of breathlessness or suffocation usually appear before narcotic levels of CO_2 are attained. The brightness, color, or shapes of objects may be distorted. If warning symptoms go unnoticed or unheeded, frank loss of consciousness will supervene. When the build-up of CO_2 is rapid, the warning period may be brief. The bottom and ascent phases of the dive are most commonly involved. A special syndrome called "shallow water blackout" has been recognized with the use of 100 per cent oxygen rebreathers. For reasons that are not entirely clear, accumulation of CO_2 in the rebreathing bag due to a faulty absorber does not trigger the usual compensatory hyperpnea in some individuals. The arterial CO_2 partial pressure rises rapidly in these individuals, causing them to lose consciousness.[31] The typical setting is one of a young, inexperienced, but highly motivated diver undergoing initial training with the apparatus. The loss of consciousness typically appears early in the dive, often during or after a period of hard work. The depth of the exposure ranges between 10 and 25 fsw, too shallow to incriminate oxygen toxicity. Approximately 50 per cent of divers will not experience (or will not remember) warning signs prior to the loss of consciousness.

Oxygen Convulsions or Syncope. Syncope or convulsion with abrupt loss of consciousness is often the first sign of CNS oxygen toxicity. The depth of the dive, the oxygen partial pressure, the length of exposure, the exercise level, and the degree of CO_2 retention all influence the probability of oxygen poisoning. When the oxygen partial pressures have been below 1.3 ata, convulsions or syncope are very unlikely. This can be used as a differential diagnostic point. The occurrence of prodromal symptoms such as irritability, involuntary muscle twitching, narrowing of the visual fields, nausea, auditory hallucinations, or vertigo followed by abrupt loss of consciousness in a hyperoxic environment strongly suggests oxygen poisoning. The sudden loss of consciousness upon moving a diver from a high oxygen partial pressure environment to a low oxygen partial pressure environment could also represent oxygen toxicity (the "off" phenomenon), although the presence of a hypoxic gas mixture must be ruled out. In an oxygen seizure, a single expiratory sigh or cry is commonly heard as the paroxysm begins.

Trauma. Trauma to the head or other serious injuries may cause abrupt loss of consciousness on the bottom. Trauma is especially likely when the diver is working around a wreck or platform or operating from a diving bell. This cause is usually self-evident.

Contaminated Gas. Gas contaminated with CO or hydrocarbons may produce unconsciousness if concentrations are sufficiently high. There will generally be a preceding period of increasing cerebral symptoms due to the pulmonary uptake and circulatory distribution of the offending agent to the brain and other body tissues. This rate will be accelerated by exercise. The likelihood of unconsciousness from CO poisoning is maximal during ascent, since there has been adequate time for uptake during the bottom phase and the oxygen partial pressure, which was helpful in maintaining oxygen transport and in preventing dissolved CO from attaching to hemoglobin and cytochromes, is rapidly decreasing. With CO intoxication, the diver may first experience tingling in the fingers and toes, and a "tight" feeling across the forehead. This will be followed by increasing confusion, euphoria, throbbing at the temples, headache, nausea, weakness, dizziness, and tinnitus. Loss of muscle control and dimming or blurring of vision may be experienced before the loss of consciousness. Intermittent convulsions and Cheyne-Stokes breathing may then be observed. One case has been reported in which CO poisoning was misinterpreted as CAGE.[32] With other contaminants, the problem is most likely to be experienced on the bottom. The specific symptom pattern with other contaminants will depend on the specific contaminant. In some instances, it will be possible to shift gas sources. Disappearance of symptoms following the shift strongly suggests the presence of contaminated gas. This can be confirmed by analysis of the questionable gas.

Cerebral Arterial Gas Embolism. CAGE is an unlikely cause of loss of consciousness until the final stages of ascent and surfacing are reached. Then it becomes one of the major diagnostic possibilities. Loss of consciousness is abrupt and often not preceded by a prodrome other than perhaps some vague feeling of chest discomfort or pain. Loss of consciousness occurs during the actual ascent itself or within the first few minutes of reaching the decompression stop or the surface. Unconsciousness late in a decompression stop or more than 10 minutes after surfacing is unlikely to be gas embolism. The presence of hemoptysis may help suggest this diagnosis.

Electric Shock. Electric shock may be severe enough to cause unconsciousness. Onset is abrupt. The victim may cry out one or more times before losing consciousness. The setting is usually a military or commercial dive, rather than a sport dive, and the problem generally occurs during the bottom phase. The hazards of underwater electrical shock have been reviewed by Bove.[33]

Postural Hypotension. Divers who have intravascular volume depletion from extended dives in cold water or who are peripherally vasodilated from hot water suits may experience dizziness and lightheadedness when climbing back into and standing inside a deep diving bell (PTC). The sudden loss of the hydrostatic support provided by the water leads to postural hypotension. Momentary unconsciousness may occur.

Hyperventilation. Excessive hyperventilation, particularly in inexperienced, anxious divers, can produce lightheadedness and dizziness. By itself, it will rarely lead to unconsciousness. Numbness of the hands, feet, and perioral area, and the presence of obvious hyperpnea, carpal pedal spasms, and a positive Chvostek's sign aid in the diagnosis. It is a controversial point whether performance of a vigorous Valsalva maneuver by a hyperventilating diver (for example to equalize middle ear pressure) would be sufficient to convert a simple disturbance of consciousness to a loss of consciousness in the water. The phenomenon is well known on dry land, but in the water there are circulatory factors that protect venous return to the heart. It is a possibility requiring further investigation.

Vasodepressor Syncope. Fainting (vasodepressor syncope or vasovagal reaction) is a debatable cause of loss of consciousness in divers.[31] The increased central blood volume during immersion is thought to protect against the hypotension and subsequent fall in cerebral blood flow. In very warm water, however, some of this protection may be lost as vasodilation reduces the extent to which central blood volume is increased. The author knows personally of two cases of syncope in subjects immersed in 35°C water. In each instance, syncope was related to flushing an indwelling arterial catheter. To make the diagnosis of vasodepressor syncope, there should be a clear antecedent cause (e.g., pain). If the diver is recovered from the water quickly, significant bradycardia should be present. Hunger, fatigue, and hangover predispose to vasodepressor syncope.

Cardiac Arrhythmia. A serious cardiac arrhythmia leading to confusion and helplessness, frank loss of consciousness, or even death is an ever present possibility in the water as it is on land. In the water, several factors may make an arrhythmia more likely. These include a dilated right heart from an increased central blood volume, increased circulating catecholamine levels, activation of autonomic nervous system reflexes by cold exposure, and occasionally respiratory acidosis from CO_2 retention. Several situations have been described in which arrhythmias have been implicated.[31] One example is the diver swimming back to base after completion of a shallow no-decompression air dive. He fails to keep up with his companions, complains of fatigue and perhaps breathlessness, calmly requests help, then passes out and sinks. The time on the surface is too long for the diagnosis of CAGE. In another situation, an open-circuit air SCUBA diver on a shallow dive signals to buddy breathe, but rejects the regulator when offered, then passes out. His cylinder contains an ample amount of air and no contaminants are found. Unless the diver is being monitored at the time of the event (a rare situation even in commercial and military diving), the arrhythmia diagnosis will have to be made by exclusion. Of the suspected cases, only a few will show evidence of coronary occlusion at autopsy. Suspicion of an arrhythmia should be raised when loss of consciousness occurs without obvious explanation in a middle-aged diver on a working dive in cold water, especially if the diver has had a history of cardiac disease and is taking cardiac or antihypertensive drugs.

Nitrogen Narcosis. Nitrogen narcosis can produce severe disturbances of consciousness and even loss of consciousness on air dives deeper than 300 fsw (90 msw). At lesser depths, however, euphoria, poor judgment, and impaired performance can be expected, but not loss of consciousness.

Hypothermia. Moderate hypothermia is occasionally seen in divers. The diver may appear confused, perform assigned tasks in a robot-like manner, or fail to respond to verbal commands. Outside of an accidental or uncontrolled exposure of a diver to cold water, however, hypothermia sufficient to induce unconsciousness would not be expected. The diagnosis of hypothermia can be made from a knowledge of the environmental exposure, the gradual onset of symptoms, the absence of other known causes for the disturbance in consciousness, the cold blue skin, and a rectal temperature below 35°C.

Hyperthermia. Heat exhaustion or even frank heat stroke can develop following dives in hot water. The diver is also at risk of developing these conditions during recompression therapy in hot climates, especially where the chamber is exposed to direct sunlight. Heat exhaustion will lead to symptoms of mild confusion but not loss of consciousness. Heat stroke, on the other hand, is characterized by confusion, delirium, disorientation, seizures, and eventual coma. There may be focal neurological signs. Hyperthermia should be suspected as a reason for loss of consciousness when the water temperature is greater than 35°C. Heat stroke can be diagnosed from knowledge of the environmental conditions, the presence of hot, dry skin, hypotension, and a rectal temperature above 40°C.

Decompression Sickness. Complete loss of consciousness from DCS is unusual. More often, the practitioner will encounter cases of DCS with collapse and semi-consciousness. The diagnosis of DCS should be entertained when the decompression obligation has been extensive, and the condition presents late in the decompression or after surfacing. Collapse and complete or partial loss of consciousness occurring more than 10 minutes after leaving the water constitute a presumptive diagnosis of DCS. Almost all other causes can be eliminated by this time.

Vertigo

Vertigo is common in diving and the average physician or diving medical technician can spend many anxious moments trying to sort out the probable cause. There are many different medical conditions associated with vertigo and the differential diagnostic list is very long. In this section only conditions unique to diving will be discussed.

When confronted with the general complaint of dizziness, it is first necessary to establish whether true vertigo is actually present. This is done by eliciting a history of a sensation of motion. The patient feels he is moving or that the environment is moving around him. Vertiginous symptoms are generally described as whirling, spinning, rotating, tilting, rocking, or undulating. Oscillopsia may be present. True vertigo in the diving setting is most often accompanied by pallor, sweating, nausea, and, occasionally, vomiting.

Vertigo may be caused by lesions of the membranous labyrinth, the eighth cranial nerve, or the vestibular nuclei and their central connections. In most diving instances, these lesions will be destructive in nature, leading to loss of function. Vertigo thus results from the unopposed signals emanating from the normal side. Many sophisticated tests are available to distinguish between peripheral, eighth nerve, and central lesions including audiometry, stapedius reflex measurements, electronystagmography with caloric, rotational, and optokinetic testing, and saccadic and smooth eye pursuit testing. These tests are described in detail by Baloh and Honrubia,[34] and their clinical application in diving problems is illustrated by Caruso and colleagues.[35] Unfortunately, few if any of these sophisticated tests will be available to the diving physician. In the field, the diagnosis will rest almost exclusively on the history (i.e., at what point in the dive the problem occurred) and the physical examination.

Physical Examination in Vertigo

The physical examination should be used to establish the presence of a vestibular disorder and to attempt to distinguish between a central and a peripheral vestibular lesion. This distinction is important because central lesions will always require recompression therapy, whereas some peripheral lesions (e.g., inner ear barotrauma) may not. Unfortunately, the various tests to distinguish central from peripheral findings may not always yield 100 per cent accurate results. Some central lesions may behave like peripheral ones and vice versa. Nevertheless, these tests should always be performed and interpreted in the context of the patient's overall presentation. The following examinations should be done.

Examination of General Balance. When positive, general tests of balance such as the Romberg, past pointing, tandem walking, and clock walking tests suggest the presence of a vestibular disorder. In a peripheral vestibular lesion, the Romberg test will be positive with the patient falling to the side of the lesion. Past pointing to the affected side will also occur. These general tests of balance are nonspecific with regard to localization.

Examination for Spontaneous Nystagmus. The presence of spontaneous nystagmus indicates the presence of a vestibular disorder. In acute peripheral labyrinthine lesions, spontaneous horizontal nystagmus is generally present, with the fast component directed to the side opposite the lesion.* The amplitude and frequency of the nystagmus will increase when the eyes are directed 30° from the midline in the direction of the fast component and will decrease when the eyes are directed 30° from the midline in the opposite direction. In mild cases, nystagmus may be present only when gaze is directed toward the fast component. If visual fixation is broken, for example through the use of Frenzel lenses, the amplitude of the nystagmus will be enhanced. In mild peripheral involvement, spontaneous nystagmus may appear only when visual fixation is abolished. Enhancement of nystagmus by loss of visual fixation is characteristic of a peripheral lesion. In a central lesion, spontaneous nystagmus is unchanged or inhibited when visual fixation is abolished. Peripheral labyrinthine nystagmus involves both eyes (i.e., is always conjugate) and both eyes beat in the same direction. The presence of spontaneous vertical nystagmus is always a sign of a CNS process.

Examination for Positional Nystagmus. Peripheral labyrinthine vertigo will generally be exacerbated by head movement. Indeed after the initial insult has subsided, vertigo and nystagmus may only occur following changes in head position. Tests for positional nystagmus therefore should always be made. In the Nylén-Bárány test for positional nystagmus (also called the Hallpike maneuver) the patient's head is first rotated 45° to the right or left, the patient then is rapidly moved from the seated to the supine position, and the head is allowed to hang over the edge of the examining table by 45°. The eyes are kept open and in midposition. In a peripheral labyrinthine lesion, nystagmus appears after a latency period of 2 to 10 seconds, reaches a crescendo in 2 to 10 seconds, and then rapidly subsides. The duration of the nystagmus is approximately 30 seconds. The nystagmus is horizontal and rotary in nature and beats toward the affected ear when it is placed lowermost. The nystagmus is usually accompanied by intense vertigo. When the affected ear is uppermost, no nystagmus or vertigo is seen. If the test is repeated immediately, the resultant nystagmus is generally diminished or absent, indicating fatigability of the response.

When the Hallpike maneuver is performed in vertigo secondary to CNS causes, a different pattern emerges. The nystagmus starts immediately (i.e., has no latency), generally persists as long as the head remains in the dependent position (or at least for a minute), and is associated with little or no vertigo. Nystagmus is seen in both right and left head positions and the rapid component is generally directed upward in both cases. The direction may be variable, however, and may be upward, downward, or changing. This central type of response does not fatigue.

In addition to the Hallpike maneuver, the patient should be examined for the presence of sustained spontaneous nystagmus that appears only in certain head positions. The direction of this nystagmus is variable. Failure of spontaneous positional nystagmus to suppress with visual fixation should suggest a central disorder.

Examination of Eye Pursuit. Saccadic eye pursuit and smooth eye pursuit should be normal in peripheral labyrinthine lesions. The presence of overshooting or undershooting of the target during saccadic pursuit testing or the presence of frequent corrective saccades during smooth pursuit testing is suggestive of a central lesion. When spontaneous nystagmus is present, it may be difficult for the uninitiated to separate these two types of eye movement.

Examination for Associated Hearing Loss. Associated tinnitus and/or neurosensory hearing loss suggest a peripheral lesion. Vertigo and hearing loss generally do not coexist in a central disorder.

Examination for Associated Neurological

*A useful mnemonic is "COWS," which stands for cold opposite, warm same. Although it applies to the results of caloric testing, it can also be used to describe the behavior of a paretic or dead (cold) labyrinth or an irritated (warm) labyrinth.

Findings. Convulsions, unconsciousness, and cranial nerve findings (with the exception of findings related to the eighth nerve) are not found in peripheral labyrinthine lesions.

Table 23–6 summarizes the differential diagnosis of central and peripheral vertigo in diving.

Differential Diagnosis of Vertigo

Determination of the etiology of the diver's vertigo generally rests on the phase of the dive in which the vertigo first became manifest, the duration of the attack, and the nature of the associated symptoms. The following conditions should be considered in the differential diagnosis of vertigo.

Caloric Vertigo. Rupture of the tympanic membrane causes violent vertigo lasting up to 1 minute when cold water enters the middle ear space. This condition generally occurs during descent, but may occur at any depth because of underwater blast, sonar, or other shock wave. Generally, the diver knows exactly what happened. Examination reveals a ruptured tympanic membrane. Vertiginous symptoms should be absent at the time of the examination.

Unilateral external ear canal obstruction generally produces a mild and relatively short-lived episode of caloric vertigo shortly after entering cold water. Examination shows an obstructed external canal secondary to cerumen or otitis externa. Vertigo is caused by cold water gaining access to one ear and not the other. Vertiginous symptoms should be absent at the time of the examination.

Alternobaric Vertigo. ABV of descent generally lasts less than 1 minute and often follows a forceful Valsalva maneuver by a subject with difficulty clearing. ABV of ascent generally lasts only seconds but may persist up to 10 minutes. Approximately 3 per cent of cases will have durations between 10 and 60 minutes and 1 per cent, durations between 60 minutes and 10 hours.[36] ABV of ascent always starts while the diver is moving upward in the water column and is usually associated with fullness or pain in the affected ear. Immediate relief of symptoms by descent is diagnostic. The risk factors for ABV have been reviewed recently by Molvaer and Albrektsen.[37]

Inner Ear Barotrauma with Perilymph Fistula. IEBT with perilymph fistula is characterized by the sudden onset of sustained vertigo in a subject who has experienced difficulty clearing ears during descent. It usually presents during descent or shortly after reaching the bottom. However, the onset of vertigo may be delayed until after surfacing when a small fistula is suddenly enlarged or the perilymph loss is suddenly increased by straining at stool or lifting heavy weights. A perilymph fistula may also develop during ascent secondary to a large overpressure in the middle ear.

A small perilymph fistula may lead only to a complaint of unsteadiness or ataxia while walking or to a complaint of episodic vertigo related to changes in head position, sneezing, or coughing. A large fistula produces steady vertigo, at least initially. Perilymph fistula is usually associated with a sensation of fullness, deafness, and tinnitus or a sensation of bubbling in the affected ear. The tinnitus may be described as

TABLE 23–6. Differential Diagnosis of Central and Peripheral Vertigo in Diving

	PERIPHERAL	CENTRAL
Symptoms	1. Generally intense with nausea and vomiting	1. May be intense, but often milder
	2. Generally affected by head movement; one head position may be critical	2. Only slightly responsive to head movement
Spontaneous nystagmus	1. Horizontal or rotatory, never vertical	1. All forms possible
	2. Suppresses with visual fixation	2. Unchanged or enhanced by visual fixation
	3. Gaze direction dependent	3. May be gaze direction dependent
	4. Always conjugate	4. May be disconjugate
Positional nystagmus	1. 2–10 sec latency period	1. No latency
	2. Short lived	2. Generally persists
	3. Positive when affected ear down	3. Positive when either ear down
	4. Direction of nystagmus fixed	4. Direction changing
	5. Response fatigues on repeat testing	5. Response does not fatigue
Saccadic and smooth eye pursuit	Normal	Abnormal
Associated auditory findings	Frequent	Very infrequent
Neurologic examination	Normal*	Abnormal

*Peripheral labyrinthine lesions in DCS and CAGE may be associated with an abnormal neurological exam.

roaring. Although cases have been reported in which coexisting auditory involvement was absent,[38–40] involvement of the auditory mechanism is common. The hearing loss is neurosensory in nature. In one series, only five cases of normal hearing were observed in 40 proven fistula cases.[38] The hearing loss may be described as fluctuating in intensity. Sounds may be perceived as distorted and there may be loudness intolerance.[38] Speech discrimination scores less than 80 per cent were observed in 75 per cent of the cases in one series.[38] A small improvement in hearing may be reported when the affected ear is kept up. Vertigo and nystagmus associated with positional testing are of the peripheral type described earlier.[38]

A fistula test may prove helpful in establishing the diagnosis. To perform the test, a good seal of the external ear canal is obtained with a pneumatic otoscope. Several puffs of air are then delivered. A positive response is obtained when a forced deviation of the eyes away from the side of the stimulus is observed. This may or may not be followed by a few beats of nystagmus. Frenzel lenses are helpful in reducing the suppressive effect of occular fixation and to aid in observing the response. This test has proved positive in approximately 25 to 40 per cent of known fistula cases.[38, 39] However, a significant false-positive rate ranging from 10 to 20 per cent has also been reported.[39, 41] Using impedance audiometry to generate precise pressure fluctuations and ENG to record the results, Daspit and colleagues[41] reported a diagnostic accuracy of 90.8 per cent. A false-positive and false-negative rate of 4.5 per cent each was observed. Unfortunately, this testing is not available in the field.

When symptoms of IEBT first appear during ascent or after surfacing, CAGE or DCS must be ruled out. This is considered important since inappropriate recompression might cause further damage in IEBT.[42] In practice, the distinction may be very difficult to make. The differential diagnostic points are summarized in Table 23–7. The diagnosis of perilymph fistula should be considered if (1) there is a clear history of difficulty equalizing middle ear pressure and there is otoscopic evidence of middle ear barotrauma, (2) the dive did not require decompression, (3) no emergency ascent was involved, (4) coexisting auditory signs are present, (5) there are no other focal neurological signs, and (6) other stigmata of DCS such as musculoskeletal pain are absent. If the onset was delayed 10 minutes after surfacing, CAGE can be ruled out.

Inner Ear Barotrauma Without Perilymph Fistula. This condition presents under conditions essentially identical to perilymph fistula and with comparable symptoms, but no fistula can be demonstrated on surgical exploration of the middle ear. When this condition first appears during or following ascent, CAGE and DCS must be ruled out, as above.

Decompression Sickness. Vertigo is a common manifestation of DCS. Dizziness, vertigo, or symptoms relating to the vestibular mechanism are reported in 4.4 to 18 per cent of the cases reported in various series.[23, 43, 44] In deep nonsaturation helium-oxygen decompression, vertigo may dominate the picture of clinical DCS.[45] Vertigo may occur from lesions affecting the labyrinth, the eighth cranial nerve, or the central vestibular nuclei and their connections. More than one site may be involved.[35] Vertigo may present after the long pull to the first stop on deep dives, with deep gas switches from helium to air, or during the later stages of a particularly arduous decompression,[46] but it occurs most commonly some time after surfacing. One case reported by Farmer and co-workers[46] occurred 206 minutes after surfacing. Vertigo bends is often, but not invariably, associated with tinnitus and neurosensory deafness in the affected ear. In 16 cases of inner ear DCS manifesting vertigo, Farmer[46] noted coexisting auditory symptoms in six. Other stigmata of DCS (i.e., rashes, limb pain, hypesthesia, paresis, or chokes) are variously present. In 23 cases of inner ear DCS reported by Farmer,[46] 5 (22 per cent) had other symptoms of DCS, generally pain. In 18 cases with inner ear symptoms, Erde and Edmonds[24] noted coexisting musculoskeletal symptoms in 33 per cent. Before the diagnosis of inner ear DCS is made, IEBT and gas embolism must be ruled out (Table 23–7).

Cerebral Arterial Gas Embolism. The sudden onset of vertigo during ascent or within 10 minutes of surfacing may be a sign of CAGE. Central vestibular mechanisms are most commonly involved, although isolated embolization of the internal auditory artery or its vestibular branches may occur. Pearson reports that vertigo was a presenting symptom of 22 of 100 gas embolism cases.[22] Vertigo secondary to gas embolism is infrequently associated with tinnitus and neurosensory hearing loss. It is most often accompanied by other rapidly evolving focal neurological signs. The patient may rapidly become unconscious. Subcutaneous supraclavicular crepitus may be present suggesting pulmonary barotrauma as the etiology. Hemoptysis

TABLE 23–7. Differential Diagnosis of Vertigo Following Surfacing

	ABV	IEBT	DCS	CAGE
Onset	Within 2 min	Anytime	Anytime	Within 10 min
Duration	Usually short, less than 10 min	Persistent	Persistent	Persistent
Associated neurological findings	Never*	Never	Possible	Common
Decompression stress required†	No	No	Yes	No
Difficult clearing/evidence of MEBT	Not required	Generally present	Not required	Not required
Coexisting auditory signs	Unusual	Very common (88%)	Common (38%)	Less common
Nystagmus	Peripheral	Peripheral	Central or peripheral	Central or peripheral
Fistula test	Unknown	May be positive	Unknown	Unknown

*Except alternobaric facial palsy.

†Sufficient time has elapsed on the bottom to allow for inert gas absorption. For sensitive individuals, this may be inside the no-decompression limits.

is an inconstant sign but when present can help support the diagnosis. The differential diagnosis includes DCS and IEBT. Severe DCS may be ruled out if the dive was well within the no-decompression limits. IEBT should be considered in the absence of focal neurological signs (Table 23–7). Parell and Becker[47] report one case in which CAGE and a documented perilymph fistula occurred simultaneously.

CNS Oxygen Toxicity. CNS oxygen toxicity may lead to the sudden onset of vertigo while the diver is breathing a high oxygen partial pressure on the bottom or during decompression stops. Vertigo may or may not be associated with other symptoms of oxygen toxicity such as nausea, tunnel vision, or muscular twitching. The vertigo rapidly abates when the oxygen partial pressure is lowered, allowing the diagnosis to be made.

Isobaric Counterdiffusion. This type of sustained vertigo occurs under two conditions: (1) at stable depths of approximately 600 fsw or greater when the diver breathes nitrogen or neon while his body is surrounded by helium,[48] and (2) during decompression from deep nonsaturation helium-oxygen dives when a transition from a helium-oxygen to air environment is made deeper than 100 fsw.[46] The first condition has only existed in the experimental laboratory and is unlikely to be experienced in a diving operation unless a mistake in gas switching is made. The vertigo has not been associated with auditory findings. The second situation is more likely to be seen, as deep air shifts are commonplace. In four such cases, Farmer[46] noted coexisting auditory findings in one. Care must be taken to distinguish true vertigo from the intense nitrogen narcosis that can be experienced with a sudden shift from helium-oxygen to air. If true vertigo is present, the diver should be restored to the complete helium environment, recompressed, and the condition treated as DCS.

Nitrogen Narcosis/High Pressure Nervous Syndrome. Dizziness and unsteadiness may be associated with nitrogen narcosis and HPNS. In the latter case, the cerebellum appears to be the target organ. Neither condition is associated with true vertigo.[15]

Hearing Loss

Complaints of tinnitus and hearing loss in diving are commonplace. When confronted by a complaint of hearing loss, stuffiness of the middle ear, or tinnitus, it is first necessary to determine whether a true hearing loss exists. In the clinic, this is best done by pure tone audiometry; in the field, tuning forks, watches, and the whispered and spoken voice must be used. If hearing loss is discovered, it is imperative next to determine whether this loss is conductive or neurosensory, as neurosensory losses may require more urgent therapeutic intervention. In the clinic, audiometry is used to make this determination. Tuning forks must be used in the field.

Three tuning fork tests are useful in distinguishing conductive from neurosensory losses: the Rinne test, the Weber test, and the Schwabach test. A 512 Hz fork should be used to start. In the Rinne test, the tuning fork is struck and placed firmly on the mastoid of the ear to be tested. When the patient no longer hears the vibrating fork, it is placed 2 cm opposite to the auditory meatus until the sound disappears. The test may also be performed by alternatively placing the fork on the mastoid and opposite the meatus until the sound disappears in one of the two locations. Normally, the fork is heard longer and more intensely by air conduction than by bone conduction. A conductive loss is present if the air conduction time is less than the bone conduction time, or if the sound is heard more intensely by bone conduction than air conduction. If a conductive loss is found, the result should be confirmed with a 1024 Hz fork. The 512 Hz fork will indicate that bone conduction is greater than air conduction when the conductive loss is 20 db or greater; the 1024 Hz fork, when the conductive loss is 25 db or greater.

In the Weber test, the tuning fork is struck and placed in the center of the patient's forehead, and the patient indicates the ear in which sound is heard best. In a conductive loss, hearing is better in the affected ear. In a neurosensory loss, hearing is better in the normal ear. In the Schwabach test, the examiner compares his hearing by bone conduction to the patient's affected ear. In a conductive loss, the patient hears longer. In a neurosensory loss, the examiner hears longer. Table 23–8 summarizes the tuning fork tests.

Tuning fork tests may be very difficult or impossible to conduct adequately in a noisy shipboard environment. When such tests are not possible, the presence of middle ear barotrauma by otoscopic examination may suggest a conductive loss but does not absolutely rule out the possibility that the loss is neurosensory in nature.

In the clinic, pure tone audiometry with air and bone conduction should be used to assess whether conductive or neurosensory hearing loss is present. In addition, a wide variety of specialized tests are available to pinpoint the location of a lesion in neurosensory losses as either cochlear or retrocochlear. These tests include speech reception threshold and speech discrimination, Békésy audiometry, the alternate binaural balance test for recruitment, the short increment sensitivity index (SISI), tone decay, acoustic reflex tests, auditory evoked response tests, and various tests for central auditory function. These tests are described in detail by Katz[49] and their use in diving cases is illustrated by Caruso and colleagues.[35]

Conductive losses are the most common losses in diving cases, and in most instances the etiology can be confirmed by otoscopic examination. The major conditions that lead to conductive hearing loss in diving are severe middle ear squeeze with or without tympanic membrane rupture, obstruction of the external ear canal by cerumen or severe otitis externa, disarticulation of the auditory ossicles or dislocation of the stapes foot plate secondary to middle ear barotrauma, and serous otitis media.

The major conditions that leads to neurosensory hearing loss in diving are noise trauma, IEBT, DCS, and gas embolism. Recently, neurosensory hearing loss has been reported as a consequence of CO poisoning.[50]

Noise trauma by far is the most common cause of neurosensory hearing loss in divers. Transient auditory threshold shifts of 20 to 30 db lasting up to 24 hours are not uncommon after noisy dives.[51] Tinnitus is usually present. Comparison of pre- and post-dive audiograms will reveal the extent of the loss. Usually the diagnosis is straightforward and can be made on the basis of high noise levels during the dive and the absence of other probable causes. Repetitive noise trauma will lead to permanent neurosensory losses. Most divers show such changes. The auditory frequencies above 4000 Hz are the most commonly affected.

IEBT (with or without perilymph fistula) presents as tinnitus, a feeling of ear blockage, and neurosensory hearing loss, often but not invariably accompanied by vertigo. The tinnitus may be described as roaring. Three patterns of hearing loss have been observed: (1) a flat line, i.e., a major loss across all frequencies from 250 to 8000 Hz, (2) a linear decrease in auditory acuity as frequency increases, or (3) a relative preservation of auditory acuity at the lower frequencies with a precipitous fall off at higher frequencies.[40, 52–54] One case of midfrequency loss concentrated at 1000 Hz has been reported.[55] Speech discrimination may be very poor.[38, 40] A fistula test may be positive. From the literature it is not possible to ascertain the percentage of

TABLE 23–8. Comparison of Various Tuning Fork Tests to Determine the Type of Hearing Loss

TYPE OF LOSS	RINNE	WEBER	SCHWABACH
None	AC>BC	Midline	Equal
Conductive loss	BC>AC	Lateralizes to poor ear	Patient hears longer
Neurosensory loss	AC>BC	Lateralizes to good ear	Examiner hears longer

AC = Air conduction; BC = bone conduction

cases that will present as an isolated hearing loss, i.e., hearing loss without accompanying vertiginous symptoms. From the differential diagnostic viewpoint, it can be said that isolated hearing loss is not uncommon and the absence of vertiginous symptoms should not dissuade one from this diagnosis. Auditory symptoms related to IEBT may begin during descent, during ascent, or after surfacing. DCS and gas embolism must be ruled out in those cases that occur during ascent or after surfacing. As in the differential diagnosis of vertigo, this can be done when a history of difficulty equalizing middle ear pressure is present, when other stigmata of DCS and gas embolism (e.g., joint pain or other neurological signs) are absent, when the depth and time of the dive are within no-decompression limits, and, in the case of gas embolism, when the symptoms begin more than 10 minutes after surfacing (see also Table 23–7). The absence of middle ear barotrauma on otoscopic examination does not rule out the possibility of IEBT.[56]

DCS is a common cause of neurosensory hearing loss in divers. Tinnitus and hearing loss occur during or following ascent from a dive, most commonly a deep dive requiring a fair amount of decompression. The hearing loss may be partial or complete. There is no characteristic audiometric pattern. Vertigo is often but not invariably present. The other stigmata of DCS are frequently present and aid in making this diagnosis.

Gas embolism of the internal auditory artery may present as the sudden onset of tinnitus and deafness during ascent or within 10 minutes of surfacing from any dive. It is usually associated with vertigo. Other focal neurological deficits are also generally present, representing the effects of emboli to other locations. This condition may be very difficult to distinguish from DCS. A short or shallow dive, symptom onset within 10 minutes of surfacing, and the absence of joint pain or skin rash favor this diagnosis.

Diving may also be associated with disruptions in central auditory processing while pure tone audiometry remains intact.[35] Such lesions will almost always reflect the sequelae of DCS or CAGE.

SUMMARY

Most diving operations will be free of major medical problems if medical personnel select the divers and equipment carefully and engage in meticulous pre-dive planning. Each phase of the dive should be carefully evaluated and comprehensive contingency plans established. Such an exercise may result in different equipment being chosen or different approaches being taken. Once an operation is underway, medical personnel should be vigilant to detect incipient problems. Intimate familiarity with the equipment and knowledge of what may go wrong during each phase of the dive are essential ingredients for effective monitoring of diving operations.

Once a problem has occurred, the nature of the presenting complaint and the phase of the dive in which the symptoms first became apparent will be the most important clues to diagnosis and treatment. Barotrauma of the ears and paranasal sinuses will be the most common complaint, followed by sea sickness, sunburn, and various traumatic and envenomation injuries. Depending on the tables used, DCS will occur in approximately 1 per cent of dives requiring decompression; the deeper and longer the dive, the more likely its occurrence. Oxygen toxicity may occur when oxygen limits are approached or exceeded. Carbon dioxide intoxication and contaminated gas episodes will be infrequent. Pulmonary barotrauma will be relatively infrequent, but evidence for this condition should always be sought whenever respiratory or neurological symptoms are present.

REFERENCES

1. U.S. Navy Diving Manual, Vol. I—Air Diving. Revision 1, NAVSEA Publication 0994-LP-001-9010, June 1985.
2. U.S. Navy Diving Manual, Vol. II—Mixed Gas Diving. Revision 2, NAVSEA Publication 0994-LP-001-9020, October 1987.
3. Morrison JB, Reimers SD: Design principles of underwater breathing apparatus. *In* Bennett PB, Elliott DH (eds): The Physiology and Medicine of Diving. 3rd Ed. San Pedro, CA, Best Publishing Company, 1982.
4. NOAA Diving Manual: Diving for Science and Technology. 2nd Ed. National Oceanic and Atmospheric Administration, U.S. Department of Commerce, 1979.
5. Hayes P: Thermal protection equipment. *In* Rey L (ed): Arctic Underwater Operations. London, Graham and Trotman, Ltd, 1985.
6. Proceedings of the International Symposium on the Hazards of Diving in Polluted Waters. Jacoby M (ed): NOAA National Undersea Research Program Tech. Rep. TR-89-1, 1989.
7. Traver RP: Interim protocol for diving operations in contaminated water. Environmental Protection Agency Project Summary. EPA/600/S2-85/130, August 1986.
8. Molvaer OI: Inner ear barotrauma. Proceedings of the

10th Congress of the European Undersea Biomedical Society, 1984, pp 410–419.
9. Craig AB: Underwater swimming and loss of consciousness. JAMA 179:255–258, 1961.
10. Gerhardt T, Göthert M, Malorny G, Wilke H: Zur Frage der Toxicität von Kolenoxid bei Atmung von CO-luftgemischen unter erhöhtem Druck (On toxicity of carbon monoxide in man breathing mixtures of CO and air at elevated pressure.) Int Arch Arbeitsmed 28:127–140, 1970.
11. Idicula J: Perplexing case of maxillary sinus barotrauma. Aerosp Med 43:891–892, 1972.
12. Neuman T, Settle H, Beaver G, Lineaweaver PG: Maxillary sinus barotrauma with cranial nerve involvement: Case report. Aviat Space Environ Med 46:314–315, 1975.
13. Molvaer OI, Eidsvik S: Facial baroparesis: A review. Undersea Biomed Res 14(3):277–295, 1987.
14. Leitch DR: Unusual case of emphysema. Br Med J 1:383, 1969.
15. Farmer JC: Diving injuries to the inner ear. Ann Otorhinol Laryngol 86(Suppl 36):1–20, 1977.
16. Fisher AA: Atlas of Aquatic Dermatology. New York, Grune and Stratton, 1978.
17. Sims JK: Dangerous marine life. *In* Shilling CW, Carlston CB, Mathias RA (eds): The Physician's Guide to Diving Medicine. New York, Plenum Press, 1984.
18. Thalmann ED: A prophylactic program for the prevention of otitis externa in saturation divers. Navy Experimental Diving Unit Research Rep 10–74, 1974.
19. Schwartz HJC, Curley MD: Transderm scopolamine in the hyperbaric environment. Undersea Biomed Res 12(1)(Suppl):36, 1985.
20. Williams TH, Wilkinson AR, Davis FM, Frampton CMA: Effects of transcutaneous scopolamine and depth on diver performance. Undersea Biomed Res 15(2):89–98, 1988.
21. Lam TH, Yau KP: Manifestations and treatment of 793 cases of decompression sickness in a compressed air tunneling project in Hong Kong. Undersea Biomed Res 15(5):377–388, 1988.
22. Pearson RR: Diagnosis and treatment of gas embolism. *In* Shilling CW, Carlston CB, Mathias RA (eds): The Physician's Guide to Diving Medicine. New York, Plenum Press, 1984.
23. Francis TJR, Pearson RR, Robertson AG, et al: Central nervous system decompression sickness: Latency of 1070 human cases. Undersea Biomed Res 15(6):403–417, 1988.
24. Erde A, Edmonds C: Decompression sickness: A clinical series. J Occup Med 17:324–328, 1975.
25. Torrey SA, Webb SC, Zwingelberg KM, Biles JB: Comparative analysis of decompression sickness: Type and time of onset. J Hyperbar Med 2:55–62, 1987.
26. Neuman TS, Bove AA: Severe refractory decompression sickness resulting from combined no-decompression dives and pulmonary barotrauma: Type III decompression sickness. *In* Bove AA, Bachrach AJ, Greenbaum LJ (eds): Underwater and Hyperbaric Physiology IX. Bethesda, Undersea and Hyperbaric Medical Society, 1987.
27. Harabin AL, Homer LD, Weathersby PK, Flynn ET: An analysis of decrements in vital capacity as an index of pulmonary oxygen toxicity. J Appl Physiol 63(3):1130–1135, 1987.
28. Munsell WP: Pneumomediastinum: A report of 28 cases and review of the literature. JAMA 202(8):129–133, 1967.
29. Harveyson KB, Hirschfeld BEE, Tonge JI: Fatal air embolism resulting from the use of a compressed air diving unit. Med J Aust 1:658–660, 1956.
30. Smith RM, Neuman TS: Evidence for coronary artery air embolism associated with cerebral air embolism in diving accidents. Undersea Biomed Res 14(2)Suppl:17, 1987.
31. Lanphier EH (ed): The Unconscious Diver: Respiratory and Other Contributing Factors. 25th Undersea Medical Society Workshop. Bethesda, Undersea Medical Society, Sept, 1980.
32. Furgang FA: Carbon monoxide intoxication presenting as air embolism in a diver: A case report. Aerosp Med 43(7):785–786, 1972.
33. Bove AA: Underwater hazards and the physiology of electric shock. *In* Underwater Electrical Safety Practices. Washington, DC, National Academy of Sciences, 1976, pp 93–114.
34. Baloh RW, Honrubia V: Clinical Neurophysiology of the Vestibular System. Philadelphia, F.A. Davis, 1979.
35. Caruso VG, Winkelmann PE, Correia MJ, Miltenberger GE: Otologic and otoneurologic injuries in divers: Clinical studies on nine commercial and two sport divers. Laryngoscope 87:508–521, 1977.
36. Lundgren CEG, Tjernstrom Ö, Örnhagen H: Alternobaric vertigo and hearing disturbances in connection with diving: An epidemiologic study. Undersea Biomed Res 1(3):251–258, 1974.
37. Molvaer OI, Albrektsen G: Alternobaric vertigo in professional divers. Undersea Biomed Res 15(4):271–282, 1988.
38. Healy GB, Friedman JM, Strong MS: Vestibular and auditory findings of perilymph fistula: A review of 40 cases. Trans Am Acad Ophthalmol Otolaryngol 82(1):44–49, 1976.
39. Singleton GT, Post KN, Karlan MS, Buck DG: Perilymph fistula: Diagnostic criteria and therapy. Ann Otol Rhinol Laryngol 87:797–803, 1979.
40. Freeman P, Tonkin J, Edmonds C: Rupture of the round window membrane in inner ear barotrauma. Arch Otolaryngol 99:437–442, 1974.
41. Daspit CP, Churchill D, Linthicam FH: Diagnosis of perilymph fistula using ENG and impedance. Laryngoscope 90:217–223, 1980.
42. Farmer JC: Inner ear injuries in diving—differential diagnosis of inner ear decompression sickness and inner ear barotrauma. *In* Bachrach AJ, Matzen MM (eds): Underwater Physiology VII, Proceedings of the Seventh Symposium on Underwater Physiology. Bethesda, Undersea Medical Society, 1981.
43. Rivera JC: Decompression sickness among divers: An analysis of 935 cases. Milit Med 129:314–334, 1966.
44. Slark AG: Treatment of 137 cases of decompression sickness. J Roy Naval Med Serv 50:219–225, 1965.
45. Bühlmann AA, Waldvogel W: The treatment of decompression accidents. Helv Med Acta 33:487–491, 1967.
46. Farmer JC, Thomas WG, Youngblood DG, Bennett PB: Inner ear decompression sickness. Laryngoscope 86:1315–1327, 1976.
47. Parell GJ, Becker GD: Conservative management of inner ear barotrauma resulting from SCUBA diving. Otolaryngol Head Neck Surg 93(3):393–397, 1985.
48. Lambertsen CJ, Gelfand R, Peterson R, et al: Human tolerance to He, Ne, and N_2 at respiratory gas densities equivalent to HeO_2 breathing at depths to 1200, 2000, 3000, 4000, and 5000 feet of seawater. Aviat Space Environ Med 48:843–855, 1977.
49. Katz J: Handbook of Clinical Audiology. 3rd ed. Baltimore, Williams and Wilkins, 1985.

50. Baker SR, Lilly DJ: Hearing loss from acute carbon monoxide intoxication. Ann Otorhinol Laryngol 86:323–328, 1977.
51. Molvaer OI, Gjestland T: Hearing risk damage to divers operating noisy tools underwater. Scand J Work Environ Health 7(4):263–270, 1981.
52. Kanzaki J: Idiopathic sudden progressive hearing loss and round window membrane rupture. Arch Otorhinolaryngol 243:158–161, 1986.
53. Pullen FW: Round window membrane rupture: A cause of sudden deafness. Trans Am Acad Ophthalmol Otolaryngol 76:1444–1450, 1972.
54. Pullen FW, Rosenberg GJ, Cabeza CH: Sudden hearing loss in divers and fliers. Laryngoscope 89:1373–1377, 1979.
55. Butler FK, Thalmann ED: Report of isolated midfrequency hearing loss following inner ear barotrauma. Undersea Biomed Res 10(2):131–134, 1983.
56. Freeman P, Edmonds C: Inner ear barotrauma. Arch Otolaryngol 95:556–563, 1972.

Chapter 24

Medical Evaluation for Diving

JEFFERSON C. DAVIS

Some medical and emotional conditions are permanently or temporarily disqualifying for all compressed gas diving: sport, commercial, naval, scientific, hyperbaric chamber, or caisson. Special circumstances of certain types of diving may allow greater leniency than more rigorous or isolated diving modes. The examining physician must know the type of diving planned as well as the specific conditions that may represent hazards in the diving environment. Commercial, naval, scientific, caisson, and hyperbaric chamber divers are generally examined and certified according to a set of standards set forth by the employer or agency involved. There are no regulations or standards for sport divers except those set forth by training agencies for acceptance of students into scuba classes. Once trained, a sport diver usually decides personally whether or not it is safe to dive and may never undergo a diving physical examination. Sport divers may argue that decisions regarding fitness to dive involve only themselves but that is not really true. Fellow divers may be endangered by trying to rescue a disabled diver; and prolonged and expensive use of medical facilities and personnel are required to transport and treat ill or injured divers from remote diving locations. Further, in our litigious society when a coincidental medical event occurs during diving or causes an accident, the fact that the diver alone decided to dive is often forgotten. Survivors, or the diver, and their attorney may point liability action toward all others concerned: those who provided equipment or training, those who conducted the dive, fellow divers, and personnel in medical facilities who tried successfully or unsuccessfully to treat the diver.

Medical examinations for professional divers are usually performed by fully trained military or civilian diving medical officers. Medical considerations for commercial divers are provided in Chapter 25. Sport divers may either have no examination or may be examined by a physician with little or no formal training in diving medicine. Because the key element is correlating medical conditions with the underwater environment, it is preferable that examining physicians have formal training in diving medicine and that they dive themselves in order to have personal experience with diving conditions.

Some considerations in evaluating sport diving candidates according to the type of diving are shown in Table 24–1.

While the preceding comments and Table 24–1 appear to rather clearly separate types of diving, it must be noted that there are exceptions. For example, some scientific professional divers have special areas of knowledge and may be able to do their underwater work under conditions limited to conservative diving situations. Leniency in some areas of medical standards may be allowed by an employer. However, employers must be cautious about accepting new divers or continuing with those with significant disorders because of legal and worker's compensation considerations.

It should be recognized that even sport scuba diving means different things to different people. A new diver may be disqualified if there is even a slight risk for diving because of findings

---

This chapter is derived from Davis JC (ed): *Medical Examination of Sport Scuba Divers*, with permission of Medical Seminars, Inc., San Antonio, 1986.

TABLE 24–1. Factors to Consider in Examinations for Sport Scuba Diving

FAVORABLE TO SPORT DIVING	UNFAVORABLE TO SPORT DIVING
1. Sport diver can choose the time and water conditions for a dive. Professional divers cannot predict such choices.	1. Medical examination may or may not be required.
2. Strenuous labor is usually not required in sport diving. Professional divers must dive where needed and must often perform heavy work.	2. There are no standards for training of examining physicians.
3. The best sport diving is at shallow depths. There is no need to exceed 60 to 80 fsw. Professional divers may work at great depths.	3. There may be no review of medical findings by experienced diving physicians.
4. There should be no financial or peer pressure to require the sport diver to dive on days of even minor illness.	4. Professional diving is usually under supervision of an experienced master diver. Sport diving supervision is variable.
	5. Sport diving may be in remote locations without access to modern emergency medical care or recompression chambers.
	6. There are no upper age restrictions on sport divers. Healthy older divers may continue safely, but the risk of incapacitating illness does increase with age.

on medical history or physical examination. The same rigid recommendations should be applied to most sport divers who develop conditions for which scuba diving introduces any risk. For sport divers without employers or agencies responsible for diving, the physician can only make recommendations. There are no standards or laws governing medical fitness for sport diving, but the physician who renders medical opinions must realize possible legal implications. Thus, advice must be slanted toward conservatism and, if a specific physician does not feel fully competent to advise on a given condition, the diver should be referred to a more knowledgeable diving medicine specialist or specialist in the specific area of concern.

Professional underwater photographers and explorers represent a population of divers who may have no employer-employee relationship (and hence there are no legal ramifications) but for whom diving is in fact their livelihood. Such divers should be provided with all available information on the risks of diving with certain conditions; but, ultimately, they will make their own decision about continued diving.

Clinical chapters of this book provide detailed information to help with decisions in specific organ systems. This chapter is based upon a consensus report of a multispecialty group of physicians who dive.[1] It is not intended to represent a standard or regulation but rather is a set of guidelines and a rationale upon which to base recommendations. In examination of professional divers, any conflict between this material and standards set forth by an employer must be resolved totally according to the latter.

Other chapters of this book provide clinical details and recommendations by organ system, and lists of absolute and relative contraindications are available.[2] The following provides a brief rationale on common problems and recommendations not covered elsewhere under specific organ systems (see Chapter 21, Cardiovascular Disorders and Diving; Chapter 18, Ear and Sinus Problems in Diving; Chapter 19, Neurological Consequences of Diving; and Chapter 20, Pulmonary Disorders and Diving).

PSYCHIATRY

We begin with the most difficult and elusive subject for most examiners. There are generally no objective tests with absolute end points, and disability can be disguised by a clever diving candidate. Naval and commercial diving schools rely on a rigorous training program to exclude those whose emotional makeup would present risks in diving. Formal psychological testing has proved less valid than observations by an experienced diving instructor. Instructors can best judge the student's comfort under water and ease of handling equipment, stressful situations during training, and interpersonal relationships. The large number and sometimes lesser experience of sport diving instructors, along with a shorter and less demanding training program, may make this selection process less effective. An examining physician who understands and has personally experienced the stresses of diving can seek clues to psychological fitness during medical examination. Experience has shown that the examiner can focus attention to seek out potential problems in diving by watching for several common behavior patterns.

The Panic-Prone Individual

The diving candidate should be questioned about previous recreational activities. Those who do not include water activities such as swimming, snorkeling, or breath-hold diving may be afraid of water. The most common cause of death in sport scuba divers is panic with ineffective behavior if an emergency situation develops under water. The prospective diver who is comfortable and "at home" in the water is far less likely to panic. Panic-prone individuals often have other phobias such as claustrophobia, a fear of new situations, or a lack of self-confidence. The examiner should ask questions to seek evidence of past anxiety attacks, hyperventilation episodes, or fainting. Candidates may describe terrifying childhood claustrophobic events or episodes of asthma, fainting, or seizures under highly stressful situations. Such individuals should be disqualified from diving because an event under water would surely result in drowning and risk to buddy divers in rescue attempts. Panic-stricken divers under water represent a tremendous hazard to other divers in the area; they can mindlessly rip equipment from buddy divers or forcefully defeat rescue efforts and cause multiple drownings.

Some apprehension is normal, but those who are basically comfortable in the water can respond to training and can gain confidence to handle underwater emergencies in a purposeful manner. Those who are terrified of water cannot be relied upon to respond fully for training and must be eliminated from diving. When such people manage to "tough it out" through diver training, they go out into the world as certified divers and represent even greater hazards by demonstrating counterphobic behavior.

The Counterphobe

This type of person has a deep-seated fear of the water, perhaps unknown to others. In an attempt to be more normal or to boost feelings of self-confidence, this individual may decide to attempt diving to overcome the fear of water. A candidate will attempt to hide such fears from the examining physician and diving instructor. Questions about anxiety-provoking events in the history and careful observation during training may offer the only life-saving hope to exclude this individual from diving. The counterphobe is likely to panic in an emergency situation.

The "Dragooned," Reluctant Diver

Savage[1] described this situation for which the examining physician can make a significant contribution to diving safety. Diving candidates should always be interviewed alone, away from spouse, parents, or friends, so that the individual's true feelings about diving can be determined. The questioning should begin with the candidate's real motivation for diving and questions regarding previous aquatic activities thoroughly explored. If it becomes clear that the examinee has little interest in diving but is doing it to please someone else, the physician must warn the individual and others concerned. The physician will be doing the individual a great service and may avert future tragedy. No one should take up diving unless personally motivated to do so. Motivation to please a spouse or parent without equal motivation by the individual is *extremely dangerous*, and medical clearance must not be granted.

The Buccaneer

This headstrong, self-centered, impetuous individual will not or cannot follow directions. In diving, the buccaneer will be recognized as one who regularly dives deeper and longer than directed by the divemaster. In sport diving, such individuals have caused many cases of decompression sickness in buddy divers or divemasters who have had to violate their own safe dive plan to go down after them. They will be inadequate buddy divers, ignoring, as they do in life generally, the needs of others. As in all other dealings with such self-centered, selfish individuals, little can be done in practical terms except to try to avoid them either as dive buddies or in hiring practice.

Psychotic Disorders

While it is unlikely that an active psychotic patient would apply for diving training, the affective psychoses may be difficult to detect. Initial examination during a period of remission or development of psychosis in a trained diver could be extraordinarily dangerous.

Inquiry should seek the type of medications the candidate has taken as well as psychiatric care in the past. A history of taking phenothiazines, haloperidol, antidepressant drugs, or lithium may be evoked. The social and work history as well as a flat affect may be diagnostic. Obviously, a psychiatric patient trying to pass a diving medical examination may not be entirely truthful.

Patients requiring psychotropic medications should be disqualified. Psychoactive drugs may cause somnolence or may provoke extrapyramidal crises that could incapacitate a diver under water. (Note: Compazine, a phenothiazine, has been used at 5 mg doses to combat nausea or seasickness. It has been known to cause oculogyric crisis in some individuals even at this low dose and must not be used for this purpose). Any drug that induces somnolence may enhance the effects of nitrogen narcosis.

Due to the relapsing and recurring nature of the psychoses, approval of such patients to dive during a period of remission may grant a permanent license to dive and may endanger a diving partner at some later date.

Alcohol and Drug Abuse

The examining physician must recognize that many applicants or active divers will be found to be users of alcohol or other drugs, if only in a recreational setting.

When the applicant is an addict or heavy user, there is no problem in the decision to exclude them from diving. The problem lies in recreational or social use, and the medical decision must rest on a question of ability and willingness to control behavior. Does the diver who is an admitted user of alcohol or other drugs have the common sense and the ability to abstain before and during surface intervals when diving?

Clues may be found in the history, even though it may be of questionable reliability. Does the applicant use alcohol or drugs every day? How intense is the use? Can the individual do without the substance when the occasion demands? Does drug or alcohol use interfere with daily living? Have there been arrests or occupational problems because of alcohol or drugs? Has the person required formal drug or alcohol treatment?

Alcohol

Alcohol interferes with memory, judgment, perception of danger, and reaction time. It impairs coordination and, like hypoxia, it causes indifference to these impairments by the individual.[3] For these and other reasons it is clear that diving under the influence of alcohol is very dangerous. The diver must never be allowed to enter the water after even small amounts of alcohol have been taken. Furthermore, diving during a hangover state may predispose to decompression sickness because of dehydration.

Since it is unlikely that a serious diving candidate will present for medical examination while intoxicated, detection of excessive drinking is difficult. Verification by examination of driving arrest records, school and work records, and interviews with family and friends may be required.

The diagnosis of chronic alcoholism is defined in various ways. As it relates to diving, we are interested in two major facets:

- Have there been any organic changes?
- Can the individual control drinking?

There may be end-organ damage detectable by laboratory testing, as well as cognitive deficits and changes in social and occupational functioning.

Obviously the chronic alcoholic must be disqualified from diving of any type. The remaining question is whether or not a recovered alcoholic can resume diving. If the candidate has abstained for at least one year and has a social and occupational record reflecting successful adjustment, consideration could be given for clearance to dive. A word of caution is that fatty liver has been suggested as a predisposition to serious decompression sickness. Examination for return to diving should include liver function studies.

Other Nonprescription Drugs; Marijuana and Other Hallucinogens

Cannabis intoxication is characterized by tachycardia, euphoria, altered sense of time and self, intensified perceptions, indifference, conjunctival injection, anxiety, suspiciousness, paranoid ideation, and impaired judgment. These may progress to actual delusions. Hallucinogenic drugs are not compatible with diving. Heroin, barbiturates, PCP (sernyl, phencyclidine, angel dust), cocaine, and amphetamines are all obviously incompatible with diving.

NEUROLOGY

Migraine (see Chapter 19)

Head Injuries

The main considerations for returning to diving after head trauma are residual neurological deficits, which would interfere with performance, and the risk of post-traumatic seizures. The risk is related directly to the severity of the injury. A history of intracranial hemorrhage, brain contusion, seizures that occur soon after the injury, or prolonged unconsciousness or amnesia all raise the risk of post-traumatic seizure disorders.[4]

Amnesia that lasts for four weeks or longer is

evidence of severe brain damage and should always cause disqualification. A more common question among a population of active, otherwise healthy scuba divers is return to diving after less severe head trauma. A guide from aviation medicine follows: With even momentary amnesia or unconsciousness, there is brain damage, but if all other studies are normal, including stress EEG (photic/sleep deprived/hyperventilation) with no anticonvulsant medication, diving could be considered after six weeks. With longer periods of amnesia, a guide is that based on the above studies; return to diving is possible after six months following one week of amnesia, nine months following two weeks of amnesia, and one year following three weeks of amnesia.

For the diving physician faced with borderline or difficult decisions, the best course is to combine his/her knowledge of the stresses of diving with the best predictions of the attending neurosurgeon/neurologist to arrive at the best recommendation to the diver.

Seizure Disorders

Because of the risk of drowning and the serious risk to would-be rescuers, major or minor seizure disorders are absolutely disqualifying for diving, regardless of control by anticonvulsant medication. The attack may be preceded by a warning or aura that is usually momentary and may be a motor, sensory or emotional change, indicating the part of the brain where the discharges start. The typical periodic breath-holding during the tonic and clonic phases of a major seizure make rescue (bringing the diver to the surface) an especial risk for pulmonary overpressure accident, with resulting pneumothorax or arterial gas embolism.

A history of episodes of unconsciousness early in life should evoke evaluation. Information about such episodes must be obtained from parents, a family doctor, or medical records. Neurological evaluation at the time of the episodes may have included EEG, but normal EEG would not overrule a good clinical impression that the attack was due to epilepsy. A history of epileptiform seizures in childhood is disqualifying for diving unless there is good evidence that they were simple febrile seizures.

According to the National Institutes of Health Consensus Statement on febrile seizures, when two or more of the following are present with febrile seizures, there is a 13 per cent risk of subsequent nonfebrile seizures: (1) abnormal neurological examination; (2) prolonged (greater than 15 minutes) or focal seizure or one associated with transient or permanent neurological deficit; (3) a family history of nonfebrile seizures. In our opinion, the following types of seizures occurring only in early childhood need not disqualify a person from scuba diving:

- Simple febrile seizures for which the history and physical closely adhere to the criteria described in the NIH statement.
- Seizures occurring during the neonatal period in children who are ultimately normal neurologically. These seizures might be due to perinatal hypoxia, hypocalcemia, hypoglycemia, or intracranial bleeding. This would not apply to a child with an underlying condition that would predispose the patient to further seizures.
- Seizures secondary to sepsis or meningitis without subsequent neurological sequelae.
- Seizures secondary to drug ingestion.
- Seizures secondary to breath-holding spells.
- Seizures post–head trauma in a child who is ultimately normal neurologically and has a normal EEG.

It is mandatory that a patient with a history of any of the above seizures of early childhood have a completely normal neurological examination. In addition, an EEG and/or a neurological consultation may be indicated. Syncope, feelings of faintness, sweating, and pallor can occur in otherwise normal subjects under conditions of great emotional stress, repulsive sights, or in hot, stuffy conditions if combined with hypoglycemia or other physiological stresses. Because maintenance of useful consciousness under water is so important, syncope-prone individuals who suffer unexplained or repeated episodes should be disqualified.

Herniated Nucleus Pulposus

If there are no neurological or physical impairments, diving can be allowed but with caution about further injury from climbing, lifting, tank donning, and so forth. With any neurological manifestations, diving should be avoided until after successful surgery. After about three months following successful disc surgery below L1-L2 with no complications, diving may be resumed. Most low back disc surgery is below L1-L2 at the level of the cauda equina and does not involve the spinal cord. Some neurological consultants consider uncomplicated cervical surgery from an anterior approach not to be disqualifying for diving. In either case, neurological deficit post-surgery should cause rejection for diving.

Spine Injury With or Without Cord Damage With Full Recovery

The diver must be advised that there is suspicion of an increased incidence of spinal cord decompression sickness after spinal trauma. These observations have not been correlated and there is no proof, but if diving is undertaken it may be at increased risk. In our opinion, a history of spinal cord trauma with neurological deficit should be cause for disqualification, with or without residual deficit. A history of Guillain-Barré syndrome, Brown-Séquard syndrome, degenerative joint disease as seen with spinal stenosis, and cervical disc disease with peripheral signs are all considered disqualifying.

History of Cerebrovascular Accident

A history of cerebrovascular accident should be cause for disqualification. Even though function has apparently been restored, the likelihood of loss of neural reserve and possible local CNS hypoperfusion make serious CNS decompression sickness more likely. History of transient ischemic attack is also disqualifying.

Trigeminal Neuralgia

Patients with a "trigger zone" in the face mask contact area could suffer attacks during diving or donning diving gear.

Disposition of Divers Afflicted with Dysbaric Cerebral Gas Embolism or CNS Decompression Sickness

A troublesome problem for physicians arises when a diver who has incurred gas embolism or CNS decompression sickness attempts to return to diving. Although data that directly bear on the advisability of further diving after CNS injury are sparse, several points can be considered. If the initial neurological deficit completely cleared within about 24 hours with or without therapy, it is possible that virtually no irreversible nerve cell damage occurred. In focal brain ischemia, a state of neuronal paralysis can exist for hours during which there is potential for complete recovery if normal blood flow can be restored.[5] This circumstance has been termed the "ischemic penumbra," and it is associated with local blood flow rates ranging from about 12 to 20 ml/100 g/min (normal about 50 ml/100 g/min). The spinal cord certainly can enter a similar state, although the relevant blood flows would be lower. Transient ischemic attacks (TIAs) are related to this state, and the defined upper limit for resolution of symptoms and signs in TIAs is 24 hours. On this basis, one might be justified in viewing an individual who suffered neurological decompression sickness and whose neurological deficit cleared completely with or without recompression therapy in roughly 24 hours as not very different from normal. Opinions differ, and some consultants would recommend against diving after any neurological decompression illness event.

The existence of a persistent neurological deficit raises another issue. There is some evidence that regions of the central nervous system that have suffered some degree of irreversible damage are selectively vulnerable to further damage under circumstances of decreased blood flow. One mechanism for partial recovery in zones of ischemic nerve cell damage involves the reinnervation of synapses on dendrites by collateral sprouting of surviving axons. This compensatory mechanism ought to be less effective in subsequent episodes of ischemia as the reserve is depleted. Also, blood flow in zones of ischemic CNS damage may remain at subnormal levels with impaired ability of the vascular bed to adjust its resistance to changes in perfusion pressure (autoregulation), and, hence, the zones stand at increased risk during states that cause further lowering of local blood flow.

Based on these considerations, it would seem prudent to advise an individual with sequelae from CNS injury to not resume diving. An individual choosing to dive anyway should be apprised of the increased vulnerability of the affected region to further lowering of local blood flow. The above is quoted from Hallenbeck.[6]

Intracranial Tumors, Vascular Disease, Aneurysms

Whether or not diving could be allowed after successful surgery for benign intracranial tumors, vascular disease, or aneurysms depends on freedom from seizures, normal EEG, and individual evaluation by the neurosurgeon/neurologist. Some knowledgeable neurosurgeons advise against diving after any of the above surgery.

Peripheral Neuropathy

Patients with peripheral neuropathy deserve individual evaluation regarding underlying disorders and functional disability that could interfere with diving activities. In general, disqualification must be advised because of inability to differentiate neuropathy from decompression sickness in diving. Also any sensory loss could result in severe, undetectable trauma (e.g., cuts on coral or other objects) while diving. The wound-healing impairment in peripheral neuropathy would make such injuries in the water especially dangerous.

OPHTHALMOLOGY

Because the eye is a liquid and incompressible system, it is relatively unaffected by pressure changes in diving. It is important that the candidate have visual acuity and visual fields adequate for safe conduct on a boat or shore diving site for underwater orientation. Near vision adequate to read the pressure gauge, watch, compass, decompression tables, and depth gauge is necessary. Visual acuity correction compatible with the diving mask may be accomplished by several means:

1. Contact lenses. While soft contact lenses are preferred to allow free inert gas exchange, hard contact lenses should be no problem within the depth ranges of sport scuba diving.
2. Correction lenses ground into the diving face plate. Cylinder correction for astigmatism is not available.
3. Lenses cemented to the face plate.
4. Special braces to hold corrective lenses can be wedged in the mask or strapped to the head.

Special considerations regarding common ocular disorders can be summarized as follows:

1. The existence of glaucoma or ocular hypertension does not preclude diving as long as adequate visual acuity and visual fields exist. The use of Timoptic eye drops can affect heart rate and response to stress. A candidate using Timoptic should be cleared by a cardiologist for diving. Laser trabeculoplasty for treatment of glaucoma is not considered a contraindication for diving. Until further data are available, diving after a filtering bleb should be avoided.
2. Retinal detachment that has been repaired or laser photocoagulation of a retinal hole is not considered a contraindication to diving.
3. Color vision deficiency is not disqualifying for the sport diver. Color perception is changed at depth with the loss of red perception by about 50 to 60 feet of sea water.
4. Patients with cataracts who still have adequate vision may dive. However, cataract surgery does introduce some special considerations. Aphakia with a high plus spectacle correction will not lend itself to practical lens placement in front of the eyes due to diving face plate location. If contact lens correction of visual acuity in aphakia can be achieved, there is no problem with diving after wound healing is secure. Pseudophakia (lens implant) should represent no problem in scuba diving, although there is a special note of caution to alert the nondiving ophthalmologist of the ever present risk of a pressure imbalance between the air space in the diver's face mask and the surface of the eye. Unless the diver actively exhales through the nose into the face mask during descent in water, a significant negative pressure in the face mask can occur. Forgetting this maneuver is more common among new scuba diving students. Its consequences in relationship to the known long duration (months) for corneal wounds to achieve maximum strength must be considered before allowing a patient who has had ocular surgery, including penetrating keratoplasty, to dive. This pressure imbalance (face squeeze) can occur in breath-hold free diving with a face mask as well as in scuba diving. Until further data are available, we believe this risk should permanently disqualify a person who has had radial keratotomy.

ENDOCRINOLOGY

Diabetes Mellitus

A diagnosis of diabetes mellitus can be made according to the guidelines of one of several criteria. The decisions on whether or not sport diving can be recommended range between two obvious situations: *from the absolutely disqualifying evidence of end-organ disease, ketoacidosis, or frequent signs or symptoms of hyperglycemia or hypoglycemia,* to those with mild abnormalities of glucose metabolism, fully controlled by weight loss and dietary control, who can be cleared for diving. Between those two extremes we find a large percentage of those with insulin-dependent diabetes mellitus (IDDM) with great variation in adequacy of control of their diabetes. It is this variation that produces controversy and differences of opinion about whether or not insulin-dependent diabetics can or cannot scuba dive. Those who favor approving well-controlled diabetics point out the world-class athletes who are diabetics. Those conservative diving medicine physicians who adhere to the widely accepted rule that IDDM is disqualifying for scuba diving do so with the admonition that an insulin reaction under water could very well result in drowning and serious risk for buddy divers in rescue attempts.

Currently the most widespread recommendation of diving medicine physicians is to disqualify those with IDDM for diving of any type. It is known that some IDDM patients do dive successfully. On the other hand, every physician who has been present during insulin reactions can attest to the rapid onset and impairment of judgment, and diving physicians can quickly see how very dangerous such a reaction would be under water. The concern of diving medicine physicians is that if the doors were opened—that is, if we said IDDM patient may dive at will—hypoglycemic accidents and drowning under water would begin to occur with regularity. For now, we must say no diving for those with insulin dependent diabetes mellitus or with non–insulin-dependent diabetes mellitus if there is a history of hypoglycemic episodes. For the future, we believe endocrinologists specializing in diabetes mellitus will be able to identify for us a set of selection criteria to allow well-controlled diabetics to dive.

Thyroid Disorder

The diversity of presenting manifestations can make thyroid dysfunction difficult for the nonendocrinologist to recognize. Besides cardiovascular effects, CNS manifestations can be of considerable significance to diving safety. Laboratory diagnosis and treatment are quite specific and effective, and as soon as good control is ensured, return to diving can be recommended.

GASTROINTESTINAL TRACT AND ABDOMINAL WALL

There are both absolute and relative contraindications to diving. Most of the relative contraindications are diseases that have acute exacerbations and then long periods of stability and quiescence, such as peptic ulcer disease or the many forms of inflammatory bowel disease. There are several reasons why a patient should not dive with these or similar diseases in an active state. Scuba diving is a sport often enjoyed in remote areas where there is frequently minimal or no definitive medical care available. Many dives are made from boats, and sometimes any medical care is hours away. The fluid and electrolyte losses that can occur with acute exacerbations of these disease processes can render the individual more susceptible to decompression sickness and to heart syndromes in the tropical climates to which divers often travel.

Absolute contraindications to diving center around conditions that could cause air trapping from gas expansion during ascent from depth and those that increase the risk of vomiting under water. The magnitude of these risks is understood when we remember that a gas volume of 250 ml trapped in a viscus at 100 fsw will expand to over 1000 ml upon ascent to sea level. We should also remember that vomiting under water has led to drowning and to panic ascents with pulmonary barotrauma and air embolism.

Esophagus

Esophageal diverticula are disqualifying for diving because of the risk of aspiration of pooled secretions. Significant free gastroesophageal reflux is disqualifying because of the likelihood of aspiration and reflux of gastric contents into the diver's regulator. Because of the weightlessness under water, many of the normal protective mechanisms against reflux are lost.

Achalasia is disqualifying because of the likelihood of pooling of secretions and food in the proximal esophagus. Paraesophageal or incarcerated sliding hiatal hernia are absolute contraindications for diving. There is risk of massive overdistention of the gastric remnant in the hernia with rupture on ascent. A nonsymptomatic or minimally symptomatic sliding hiatal hernia is not disqualifying.

Gas bloat syndrome, post–hiatal hernia repair, can lead to gastric rupture on ascent. Patients who have had hiatal hernia surgery and can belch are not at risk and should be able to dive. Those who are unable to belch and are therefore unable to relieve gastric dilation due to aerophagia should not be cleared to dive.

Stomach

Partial chronic gastric outlet obstruction of a high grade is a disqualifying factor due to the risk of overdistention of the stomach on ascent.

Severe post-gastrectomy dumping syndrome is disqualifying because of the risk of prostration at depth. A dumping syndrome that is mild and well controlled with diet alone is not necessarily a contraindication as long as the patient does not eat prior to diving.

Small and Large Intestine

Small bowel obstruction, either chronic or recurring and acute, is a contraindication to diving due to the possibility of rupture or strangulation of the bowel as gases expand during ascent. After surgical correction of an obstruction, the individual may dive after at least 6 months free of symptoms and if studies show no evidence of residual partial obstruction.

Uncomplicated small or large bowel diverticulae should pose no problem in diving. A continent ileostomy, for example, a Koch pouch, is a disqualifying factor because air trapping could not be relieved without stomal catheterization. There is considerable risk of rupture of the pouch during ascent due to gas expansion. Planned exterocutaneous fistulae such as ileostomy or colostomy are not disqualifying. The only exception is the continent procedure as discussed above.

Hepatobiliary

Significant fatty liver is disqualifying because of the danger of inert gas excess and rupture of fat cells due to bubble formation, with resulting serious decompression sickness complicated by fat embolism. Stable biliary tract disease is not a contraindication to diving. For example, the presence of gallstones is not a contraindication to diving unless symptomatic. Biliary-enteric anastomoses are not disqualifying; although they allow air into the biliary tract, they also allow free egress of air.

Abdominal Wall

Any abdominal hernia that could have bowel present in the sac is disqualifying for diving until successfully repaired. This includes incisional, inguinal, and umbilical hernias. The first reason is that the risk of incarceration is significantly increased because of the need to lift and carry heavy scuba tanks and other diving gear. The second reason is the danger of air trapping in the contents of the hernia which could lead to strangulation when air expansion occurs during ascent.

Return to diving after abdominal surgery is generally safe after the incision is healed without hernia and if the surgeon would allow the individual to return to other athletic endeavors such as tennis.

VARICOSE VEINS AND PERIPHERAL ARTERIAL INSUFFICIENCY

Varicose veins without significant venous insufficiency and skin changes represent no problem. During scuba diving, venous return is excellent. However, coral cuts under water are known to produce indolent, infected wounds even in normal tissue, and with stasis skin changes such injuries could be especially dangerous.

ORTHOPEDIC DISORDERS

Trauma and Acute Inflammatory Conditions

The reasons to disqualify a person for diving during the period of incompletely healed fracture or acute inflammation are the immobility and loss of dexterity with a cast, even if made of newer water-compatible materials. Also inert gas uptake and elimination at a fracture site is impaired, and bubble formation is more likely to occur during decompression. Climbing into boats and the physical aspects of diving require good mobility and strength.

A diver who has suffered a musculoskeletal injury, either fracture, sprain, or dislocation, or who has bursitis, tendinitis, or other inflammatory process, should not return to diving until the part has returned to full range of motion and strength. No residual pain should be present which could impair the diver's ability to perform in diving emergencies or which could be confused with limb bends. With these, as well as with all orthopedic considerations, the examining physician must know the particular arrangements and stresses of diving equipment. For example, the location and weight-bearing of straps on the back pack would make diving with residual pain or instability of fractures of the clavicle or ribs painful and dangerous should a rib fracture be forced by stress to puncture the parietal pleura during a dive. A pneumothorax at depth becomes a life-threatening tension pneumothorax with pleural gas expansion during ascent.

Amputation

Amputees have been successfully trained to dive. Many unilateral upper or lower extremity amputees dive successfully with special equipment such as corrosion-resistant prostheses or specially designed fins. Bilateral amputees have been trained to dive, but they require close buddy cooperation.

Scoliosis

Scoliosis need not be an absolute disqualification, but there must be *normal pulmonary function*, and the severity must not interfere with the wearing of diving gear to represent a risk of spinal trauma due to straps and heavy compressed air tanks.

Artificial Devices

Artificial joints, plates, screws, or other internal fixation devices need not preclude diving if well healed and secure and if full range of motion and strength is present.

Aseptic Bone Necrosis

A diver who has aseptic bone necrosis from any cause, whether related to previous diving with dysbaric osteonecrosis or due to other causes, must be advised of the possible increased risk of progression due to compressed gas diving. Dysbaric osteonecrosis is exceedingly rare among sport divers, but the diver must be apprised of the increased risk of disability and then must make his own decision. Divers should be warned that juxta-articular lesions are the most significant because progression with destruction of joint function is possible.

Developing Epiphyseal Plates

An unknown risk concerns developing epiphyseal plates of children. There are no data on gas uptake and elimination to suggest whether or not there is risk of damage to young divers. Most agencies require a minimum age of 14 to 16 years for scuba training for other reasons of maturity, strength, and equipment fitting (see Chapter 14).

ORAL AND MAXILLOFACIAL/ DENTAL CONSIDERATIONS

Prerequisites

Ability to fit and hold a scuba mouthpiece. Edentulous patients may dive with appropriate devices if comfortable.

Contraindications

Status post–major oral surgery with any osseous or soft tissue deformity that would interfere with scuba mouthpiece fitting is a contraindication.

Special Considerations

Divers with prosthesis, i.e., full dentures or partial dentures should be handled on an individual basis. Stability of a partial denture with a scuba mouthpiece would vary. In an emergency, airway obstruction could be a problem. Advanced periodontal disease with loose teeth may be a problem with a scuba mouthpiece, as would osteomyelitis or osteoradionecrosis.

Temporomandibular joint dysfunction syndrome could be aggravated by a mouthpiece. Endodontically treated teeth should be no problem, but teeth undergoing treatment (e.g., root canal) could cause tooth squeeze due to changing pressures. Extremely broken down and badly carious teeth are a contraindication.

Orthodontic appliances and custom scuba mouthpieces are available which can be adjusted by the diver's dentist or orthodontist so as not to impinge on the orthodontic appliances. Any successful tooth replacement or subperiosteal frame implant should withstand normal biting forces and represent no problem in diving.

MEDICATIONS AND DIVING

In general regarding significant medications, it is not only the drug but also the underlying disease requiring medication that disqualifies. A diver who requires antihistamines, vasoconstrictors, and nasal sprays to clear the ears for an acute upper respiratory infection (URI) or chronic rhinosinusitis should not dive. Aside from the drowsiness and possible tachycardia induced by such drugs, it is possible that the combination of nitrogen narcosis and antihistamines may decrease alertness more than either alone.

Another example is antibiotics. While the drug itself is usually of no known concern, the underlying disease is the question. For example, tetracycline for bronchitis is part of the contraindication for diving because of the risk of bronchospasm and local air trapping, but tetracycline for chronic prostatitis presents no known problem for the diver except for photosensitivity. Other drugs must be used with caution because of unknown possible synergism with the diving environment. The problems of cardiovascular drugs have been presented. Amphetamines combined with nitrogen narcosis have produced bizarre behavior.

DERMATOLOGY

Since the skin is the body's main direct exposure to the water and all environments associated with diving, many factors can affect the skin during diving. Pre-existing skin disorders that could be aggravated by some aspect of diving include:

1. Any acute or chronic dermatitis that would be made worse by prolonged submersion or by wearing tight rubber wet suits must be cause for disqualification.
2. Allergic reactions to dyes in wet suits or face masks can usually be managed by changing material or by using nonpigmented rubber or silicone equipment.
3. Diving is usually done in hot, sunny environments, hence those with sun allergies or those taking photosensitivity medication such as tetracycline must be warned to use extreme caution. All divers should be cognizant of the serious sunburn possible while snorkeling or while on dive boats or beaches.

OBSTETRICS AND GYNECOLOGY

Pregnancy

With conflicting studies in animal experimentation, *the female who is pregnant must be advised of possible significant risks to the unborn fetus.* Further studies may elucidate inert gas uptake and elimination in fetal tissues and the risk of bubble formation, but current evidence makes pregnancy a contraindication for compressed gas diving to any depth at any time during pregnancy. We do not recommend that pregnancy be terminated for a female who dives during pregnancy, but prenatal ultrasonography may be indicated to rule out fetal malformations.

Special Considerations

- Menses need not disqualify unless the diver is uncomfortable on the dive day.
- Contraceptive pills need not disqualify, but a question remains of possible severe complications if decompression sickness should occur due to hypercoagulability of the blood.
- Intrauterine devices represent no known problem in diving.
- Tampons represent no known problem in diving.

MISCELLANEOUS

Many times, physicians are confronted with borderline or grey areas for consideration of fitness for diving. For legal, safety, and financial reasons, such questions rarely present in the military or commercial diving medicine areas, but among sport divers decisions may be quite difficult. The following comments must be seen against the background that there are no laws or regulations to prohibit a sport diver continuing against medical advice. However, the physician must protect against legal action by documenting conservative, yet sensible, recommendations.

An examiner can be too lenient or too rigid. A physician who does not understand the likely fatal outcome and risk to other divers of sudden loss of consciousness at depth during a scuba dive may see no problem with diving by a well-controlled seizure disorder patient, an insulin-dependent diabetic patient, or other syncope-prone individuals. An obstetrician who does not know the life-threatening risk of underwater vomiting, which might occur with morning sickness, the conflicting data on inert gas uptake by the fetus with risk of bubble formation and fetal malformation, and the possible trauma associated with diving equipment could fail to warn the pregnant female to avoid diving during pregnancy. These examples of excessive leniency are usually based on lack of diving medicine knowledge and experience by the physician.

On the other hand, the examining physician can be so rigid that any medical problem leads to disqualification. The nondiving physician may disqualify many candidates because "scuba diving is too dangerous and is not necessary." This would be analogous to a nonskiing physician who forbade all patients to ski because of the "unnecessary" risk of fractures, serious spinal injuries, and death.

DIVING FOR THE PHYSICALLY HANDICAPPED

An admirable trend in programs for physically handicapped patients has been to increase their activities and generally let the patient feel equal to nondisabled counterparts. Spinal cord wheelchair athletes are an exceptional example, and similar trends have been extended to diabetics, asthmatics, and epileptics.

Scuba diving introduces very unique and specific risks that lead to the restrictions set forth in this chapter. Sudden alterations of consciousness under water can lead to drowning or serious pulmonary overpressure accidents during rescue to the surface.

With the exception of bronchial asthma and seizure disorders, which all diving medicine specialists agree are absolutely disqualifying for any compressed gas diving, differences of opinion prevail. In an attempt to allow courageous diabetic and wheelchair athletes to pursue all activities, emotional debates develop. Perhaps a middle ground is possible and has already been instituted in the case of paraplegic divers. There could be a distinct separation between unrestricted diver certification and "therapeutic diving training."

In the opinion of this author it is unfair for a diver with known coronary artery disease, diabetes mellitus, seizure disorder, bronchial asthma, history of spontaneous pneumothorax, or psychiatric disease to be issued a diver certification that can be presented to a diving operation for clearance to go diving.

The University of Rhode Island fatality statistics[7] for diving show that a high percentage of fatal scuba diving accidents are due to diver panic, drowning, barotrauma, lack of physical fitness for diving, or coincidental medical events. Obviously, the next major drop in the already declining fatality rate in diving must come through excluding those who are medically or emotionally unfit.

REFERENCES

1. Davis JC (ed): Medical Examination of Sport Scuba Divers. Medical Seminars, Inc., San Antonio, 1986.
2. Hickey DD: Outline of medical standards for divers. Undersea Biomed Res 11(4):407–432, 1984.
3. Mohler SR: Civil aviation medicine. *In* DeHart RL (ed): Fundamentals of Aerospace Medicine. Philadelphia, Lea and Febiger, 1985, p 686.
4. Annegers JF, Grabow JD, Groover RV, et al: Seizures after head trauma: A population study. Neurology 30:683–689, 1980.
5. Astrup J, Symon L, Branston NM, Lassen NA: Cortical evoked potential and extracellular Kt and Ht at critical levels of brain ischemia. Stroke 8:51–57, 1977.
6. Hallenbeck JM: Neurological disorders and diving. *In* Davis JC (ed): Hyperbaric and Undersea Medicine. San Antonio, Medical Seminars, Inc., 1979.
7. McAniff JJ: U.S. Underwater Diving Fatality Statistics, 1983-1984. Washington, DC, U.S. Department of Commerce, NOAA Undersea Research Program, 1986.

Chapter 25

Physical Examination of Divers

PAUL G. LINAWEAVER
and ALFRED A. BOVE

A diver entering an aquatic environment is at a great disadvantage with regard to propulsion and protection against heat loss. Both activities require high energy expenditure. The diver breathes gas of increased density with equipment designed to maintain adequate exchange of oxygen, carbon dioxide, and inert gases, utilizing a cardiorespiratory system that has been altered as a result of exposure to this altered environment. The diver must accommodate to changes in gas volume and pressure in anatomical spaces to prevent morbid changes and must function within narrowly defined limits imposed by the effects of the partial pressure of gases, which cause toxic, narcotic, stimulatory, and gas solubility alterations to bodily functions.

Because of the obligatory stresses of underwater exposure, an individual must possess certain physical and physiological attributes and must be devoid of certain limitations or conditions to function safely in this unique environment. The physical requirements and limitations fall into two major categories. The first are those that concern everyone exposed to pressure, whether in a wetsuit, in a deep-sea rig, in a caisson, or during sport diving. The second major category that defines limitations or influences requirements is the type of diving to be undertaken. The following types of diving are decreasingly stringent in physical requirements although not necessarily in potential risk: military diving, commercial diving, scientific and technical diving, semiprofessional diving, recreational (sport) diving.

MILITARY DIVING

Divers of the uniformed services must meet stringent physical standards for enlisted service and even more stringent standards for officer status. Additional restrictions are then applied for diving status and are typified by U.S. Navy standards.[8] These strict standards are necessary, since military diving may be under combat conditions and may be performed in arduous, dangerous situations, such as salvage in the open sea, disposal of explosive ordnance, clandestine operations, or the extremely urgent nature of rescue and assistance in escape from a sunken submarine. Military divers may use compressed air or semiclosed or closed-circuit mixed-gas scuba; closed-circuit oxygen apparatus; deep-sea gear, with both air and helium-oxygen mixtures supplied; or advanced bell and saturation systems. Military divers have no choice of the duty they perform, as is the case of a commercial diver who can simply quit or the recreational diver who can dive when and where he pleases. Therefore, excellent physical fitness among military divers must be assured without question.

COMMERCIAL DIVING

Commercial diving activities range from shallow work (underwater construction, cleaning ship hulls, marine salvage) to the deep diving of offshore petroleum and gas exploration and production which poses the greatest risk. Many deep-diving operations are carried out hundreds of miles from shore with minimal medical and support facilities. Inclement weather may hamper medical attention or evacuation of a casualty. One estimate gives an annual fatality rate (not actual number of deaths) of offshore employment, other than diving, at 22 fatalities per 10,000 persons and that of offshore diving, for the year 1974, at 111 fatalities per 10,000 persons. This is contrasted to the general construction industry and mining industry—approximately 2.6 fatalities per year per 10,000 persons engaged. These figures come primarily from experience in the North Sea and the Gulf of Mexico.[1] In these geographical areas there is governmental oversight to ensure reasonable adherence to prudent safety precautions and safe diving techniques. In more remote areas, however, and particularly in those around the underdeveloped countries, conditions are considerably worse.

Selection criteria for employment in commercial diving are strict, not only because of the hazardous and heavy labor conditions involved, but also because the risk of litigation for injuries incurred during work or for aggravated injury is extremely high for the employer and third-party insurers. As a result, commercial diving firms in the United States are extremely selective, in terms of physical standards, in screening potential divers. Commercial divers utilize the entire spectrum of diving modes—from compressed air scuba to deep saturation mixed gas. They may be expected to go from one type of diving to another and from employer to employer for a variety of reasons. When passed "fit," a diver is physically qualified for all types of diving unless a specific limitation has been imposed.[2]

In the recent past certain state occupational safety and health organizations (e.g., CAL-OSHA) required commercial divers to have annual physical examinations and re-examination after an illness or injury of more than 72 hrs or after an episode of unconsciousness related to diving activity.[3] Although the tests and examinations required are explicit, the standards set by these regulatory agencies are vague concerning the criteria for fitness, thus leaving the responsibility for selection to the employer and the examining physician.

SCIENTIFIC AND TECHNICAL DIVING

Individuals who use diving in scientific or technical work in the marine environment are usually associated with universities or other laboratories and enjoy an excellent safety record. Their activities are generally in shallow water, and they work under strict rules and regulations established by their local diving regulatory body, such as a university diving safety board. Most scientific divers are required to have annual physical examinations that are quite comprehensive. Their diving mode is primarily shallow air, but many use techniques of mixed gas and even bottom habitat saturation.

SEMIPROFESSIONAL DIVING

So-called semiprofessional divers are self-employed divers, such as the divers for California abalone and sea urchin, the operators of dive shops and dive-boat enterprises, and those part-time marine handymen who clean boat bottoms and change propellers. This group has no standards with regard to physical requirements or training, and they are not under any regulatory control. In some areas such divers do not enjoy a favorable safety record.

RECREATIONAL DIVING

Recreational or sport divers represent the largest group of individuals engaged in underwater activity. They number in the millions. Most have had good basic training supervised by recognized training agencies such as the YMCA, National Association of Underwater Instructors (NAUI), the Professional Association of Diving Instructors (PADI), and others. Most of those so trained have not had physical examinations, although most have answered health questionnaires. Positive answers on these questionnaires require an individual to have clearance by a physician before training. This questionnaire is used primarily as legal protection for the dive shop operator, instructor, or sponsoring training agency, and true physical evaluations are recommended but not required. Each agency has an appropriate medical form (see Appendix 3) when an examination is required. The dropout rate is high after initial sport diver training in spite of the considerable investment in equipment and training courses.

The exact population at risk and their frequency of diving is essentially unknown. Treatment statistics,[4] however, do indicate a much higher incidence of serious conditions than is seen among professional or military divers (Tables 25–1 and 25–2). Numerous factors influence these data, and further elaboration is not undertaken here.

DIVER PHYSICAL EXAMINATION

Physical examination of divers requires a knowledge of the physiology of diving and a fundamental understanding of the type of work in which the individual diver will be engaged. The examiner must be an astute clinician to elicit a careful history and to perform an equally careful physical examination to detect disqualifying or potentially hazardous conditions. There must be consistency in the application of findings and clinical judgment concerning the certification or disqualification of divers. The physician must consider himself a member of a team responsible for the health and safety of divers and must be knowledgeable in all aspects of diving medicine.

A careful history is of utmost importance. There is little disagreement among experts about which specific conditions would automatically disqualify a potential diving candidate, whether for recreational or commercial endeavors. These are discussed as the chapter progresses.

The physical examination should be conducted with the goal of detecting signs of absolute, relative, or temporary disqualifying conditions. Lastly, the physician has a distinct responsibility to the diver, as a patient, in terms of preventive medicine. He should look carefully for the signs of excessive smoking, which can be injurious to the individual: nicotine-stained fingers, chronic hyperemic pharynx, chronic cigarette cough. He should look also for evidence of substance abuse: tremor, alcohol odor on the breath. In addition, poor muscle tone, lack of conditioning, and obesity and other evidences of dietary indiscretion should prompt the physician to advise the diver-patient in constructive fitness programs.

The diving candidate that the physician will most often encounter is the sport diver. Any condition present that could hurt the diver or result in injury to his buddy diver should be considered disqualifying. The buddy-diver system is the universally recognized practice of pairing scuba divers for mutual safety and implies that each of the pair is fully capable of providing effective aid to the other in any emergency. The physician may be called upon to determine the fitness of a commercial diver or to examine a candidate for one of the many schools that train commercial divers. For this reason, commercial standards in some detail, as well as general standards, are presented in this chapter and in Chapter 24. An individual can spend as much as $4000 or invest two years of time in studying to become a commercial diver. He should know, at the outset, his employability chances from the physical point of view.

In considering the specifics of the physical examinations and selection criteria for diving, we have sought advice and comments from a heterogeneous group of diving medical experts to make the opinions stated herein as universally acceptable as possible.

Age

It is difficult to set a minimum age for diving; individual variation in development, strength, maturity, and intelligence is too wide. By practice 18 years is the accepted minimum age for commercial diving in the United States, and it is the age mandated by regulation in the United Kingdom and other jurisdictions. At the other end of the age scale, to begin a commercial diving career after the age of 30 is a doubtful venture and should be discouraged because of the reluctance of commercial diving companies to hire older individuals. Susceptibility to diving accidents, such as an increased incidence of decompression sickness, has been documented

TABLE 25–1. Typical Types of Diving Accidents Treated

TREATMENT FACILITY	TYPE I DCS %	TYPE II DCS %	AIR EMBOLISM %
University of Southern California, Catalina Island	13	54	33
Pearl Harbor, Hawaii, civilian facility	48	52	[a]
Grand Cayman, British West Indies	19	38	45
U.S. Navy, military facility	89	11	[a]

[a] = Not recorded.
Data obtained by personal communication.

TABLE 25–2. Summary of Number of All Underwater Fatalities, by Year

PURPOSE OF UNDERWATER ACTIVITY	FATALITIES													
	1970		1975		1980		1981		1983		1985		1987	
	M	F	M	F	M	F	M	F	M	F	M	F	M	F
Nonprofessional, underwater	99	11	123	8	98	11	88	15	104	6	81	7	75	12
Professional, scuba diving	3	0	4	0	14	0	6	0	8	0	9	0	8	0
Professional, surface-supplied air or mixed gas	6	0	8	0	6	0	8	0	4	0	4	0	4	0
On military duty	0	0	1	1	0	0	0	0	0	0	1	0	0	0
Skindiving	18	1	16	1	19	1	19	1	25	1	8	1	9	0
Totals, M + F	138		162		149		137		148		111		108	

M = Male; F = Female.
From McAniff JJ: U.S. Underwater Fatality Statistics, 1986–1987. Report No. URI-SSR-89-20. Washington, DC, National Oceanic and Atmospheric Administration, 1989.

for increasing age.[4] Careful attention to the neuromuscular, pulmonary, and cardiovascular condition of the diver is recommended for both commercial and sport divers. The U.S. Navy permits only supervisory activity for divers older than 45. For most diving activities, physiological age is more important than chronological age.

Sex

Special considerations for women in diving are discussed in Chapter 13.

Body Build

Obesity represents a hazard to divers because of the common lack of adequate physical condition in obese individuals and because inert gas exchange and its relationship to decompression sickness are modified unfavorably. Body weight that is 20 per cent over ideal weight should at least temporarily disqualify commercial, scientific, and military divers. With average skin-fold thickness measurements from the midtriceps, subscapular, and sacroiliac areas, the estimate of percentage of total body fat can be obtained from several nomograms. Total body fat of less than 22 per cent in males and of less than 28 per cent in females is desirable.

Specific abnormalities of organ systems are addressed in individual chapters and are presented here only briefly.

Nervous System

The examiner should perform and document in detail the result of the neurological examination. Reflexes, including deep tendon reflexes and superficial abdominal and cremasteric reflexes, must be tested, and the presence or absence of abnormal reflexes should be elicited and documented. Motor strength and cutaneous, vibratory, and position sense must be described. Documentation is extremely important. The post-dive evaluation of a diving accident may reveal changes from the baseline data indicating a serious condition that might otherwise go unrecognized and thus untreated. Chapter 19 provides further details on the neurological evaluation.

Ear, Nose, Throat

The anatomical and functional interrelationship between the ear structures and the conducting airways of the nose, pharynx, and air spaces of the head makes the otorhinolaryngological evaluation extremely important in assessing a candidate's ability to dive.

The examiner must look closely for patent nasal pharyngeal airways and note the presence of obstructive polyps or turbinates, purulent discharge, or the inflammatory atrophic mucosa of the habitual nose-drop user. Most important, the individual must prove his ability to move the tympanic membrane during a Valsalva maneuver. Careful examination of the external ear canals and tympanic membranes is, therefore, essential in a diving physical examination.

Electronystagmography, tympanometry, and audiometry should be done prior to consideration of requalification following the repair of round window fistula, although most experienced otorhinolaryngologists believe that this lesion is absolutely disqualifying. In this regard, initial and annual audiograms are required of all commercial divers, and some companies require baseline electronystagmograms on preplacement physical examinations.

There are no prescribed standards for hearing acuity. For commercial diving, unilateral deafness (defined as an average of 80-db loss at 500, 1000, and 2000 Hz), or an average 40-db bilateral loss in the speech range (250 to 3000 Hz) should probably disqualify. In the case of commercial divers, annual audiometry is recommended for hearing conservation programs under state and federal guidelines. Because of gas flow characteristics, many hyperbaric chambers and diving helmets have noise levels in the decibel range that can produce occupational hearing loss.[6]

Examination of the oropharynx should reveal good oral hygiene and the absence of extensive dental caries or significant gingival disease. Improperly filled teeth may be the cause of dysbaric odontalgia, which can only be determined by the application of pressure. If present, reconstruction of the suspect restoration is required. The candidate should demonstrate the ability to securely hold a mouthpiece. Dental prostheses that could obstruct the diver's airway should not be considered disqualifying for any type of diving, but the prostheses should not be worn during diving. A commercial diver may be temporarily disqualified until his oral hygiene is corrected, since very often work is carried out in locations where dental care either is not available or is substandard.

Eyes

Visual standards are quite specific for military divers and for scientific divers under the jurisdiction of the National Oceanic and Atmospheric Administration (NOAA).[7, 8] There are no standards for the commercial divers in the United States. Commercial divers under the jurisdiction of the United Kingdom and Norway require as a minimum acceptable standard for uncorrected distant vision 6/36 for o.d. and o.s. and 6/24 for o.u. This corresponds to 20/120 and 20/80 Snellen, respectively. For near vision, Jaeger 16 for each eye separately and Jaeger 15 for both eyes together, corresponding to 20/100 and 20/90, respectively, are required. A more reasonable approach would be to consider binocular visual efficiency (BVE) as a limiting criterion at 80 per cent efficiency. Table 25–3 illustrates and describes how to derive the BVE percentage rating.[8]

Color vision tests should be performed using standard techniques, such as the pseudoisochromatic plate test available in several forms or the Farnsworth-New London Navy lantern test. Color-deficient divers should not needlessly be disqualified unless they will be required to perform tasks that involve color-coded electrical or compressed gas circuits. In questionable cases testing for demonstrated ability should be performed.

Respiratory System

Avoidance of pulmonary overpressurization is a primary concern of all engaged in diving, and especially of those responsible for selection of diving candidates, because of the potential seriousness of the triad of pathological pulmonary conditions that can result in injury from diving.[9] The triad consists of pneumothorax, mediastinal emphysema, and traumatic arterial gas embolism, the last named being the most serious of the triad. In traumatic arterial gas embolism, the dissection of gas into the pulmonary veins and then directly into the arterial circulation, and usually to the central nervous system or the systemic arteries (including the coronaries), causes immediate obstruction of blood flow. Survival times of tissues beyond this obstruction have a finite limit, roughly 4 to 10 minutes. Immediate recompression therapy of air embolism casualties is indicated.

In the history, general information should be obtained regarding asthma or wheezing, smoking habits, occupational exposure, presence of dyspnea, cough, quantity and characteristics of sputum, and pulmonary or bronchial infections.

Inquiry should be made regarding the history of the following specific conditions, which may be absolute or relative contraindications to diving.

- Spontaneous pneumothorax, absolute
- Pneumothorax due to trauma, relative
- Pneumothorax, subcutaneous or mediastinal emphysema, or arterial gas embolism due to pulmonary overpressurization incidents, relative to circumstances
- Thoracotomy, relative to circumstances and outcome
- Established diagnosis of chronic pulmonary disease, whether obstructive, restrictive, neoplastic, or suppurative, absolute
- Asthma, allergic, nonallergic, absolute if established

Chest Examination

In examining the chest, the examiner should be looking for evidence of conditions that would contraindicate diving as well as a general assessment of the health and function of the

TABLE 25–3. Binocular Visual Efficiency Computation*

LEFT EYE	RIGHT EYE							
	20/20	20/30	20/40	20/50	20/70	20/100	20/200	20/400
20/20	100	98	96	94	91	87	80	76
20/30	98	92	90	88	85	81	74	69
20/40	96	90	84	82	79	75	68	64
20/50	94	88	82	77	73	70	62	58
20/70	91	85	79	73	64	60	53	49
20/100	87	81	75	70	60	49	42	38
20/200	80	74	68	62	53	42	20	16
20/400	76	69	64	58	49	38	16	3

*Instructions: Using the corrected Snellen vision in the right eye, find the appropriate vertical column and come down to the horizontal line that corresponds to the corrected vision in the left eye. The number where these columns meet is the corrected binocular visual efficiency (BVE) expressed in percentage.

pulmonary system. Several specific items should be looked for during inspection. During inspiration is there equal expansion bilaterally or intercostal or lower rib retraction? Are accessory muscles of respiration being used? Are there surgical scars to suggest thoracotomy, placement of chest tubes, or penetrating wounds of the chest? The expansion of the chest should be measured with a measuring tape at the nipple level, the descent of the diaphragms should be percussed, and the result documented. On auscultation, the usual signs of bronchial or parenchymal disease should be listened for specifically over each major lobe area during forced expiration for evidence of bronchoconstriction, and expiration should be timed. Disqualifying lesions, such as pulmonary cysts, bullae, atelectasis, parenchymal and pleural abnormalities, and solid lesions, such as tumors and granulomata, cannot be detected by physical examination and are best detected by chest radiograph. Military, commercial, and most scientific or technical divers are required to have 14 × 17 posterior-anterior (PA) and lateral chest roentgenography initially. The frequency for follow-up chest radiograph examination varies widely, depending on the diving regulations that apply to the particular diver: ordinary military divers, triennially; saturation and experimental military divers, annually; California OSHA (CALOSHA), biennially; United Kingdom and Norway, annually; most companies belonging to the Association of Diving Contractors, annually. Sport divers should have a PA and lateral chest radiograph examination initially, but it is not required by most training agencies. The authors will not certify any diver as being fit initially unless the examinee has had a normal 14 × 17 PA chest radiograph within a year, interpreted either personally or by a radiologist who understands the physical requirements of diving.

The need for pulmonary function tests is at the discretion of the examining physician for commercial divers under United States jurisdiction. It is recommended, and is required by the United Kingdom and Norway, that at each examination a forced vital capacity (FVC) and a 1-sec forced expired volume ($FEV_{1.0}$) be measured. A value of less than 80 per cent of the predicted FVC or a ratio of the actual $FEV_{1.0}$/FVC of less than 70 per cent should disqualify. Other special tests such as xenon studies and methacholine challenge may be required under certain conditions.[10] If arterial blood gas analysis is considered necessary by the physician, then the diver's fitness is suspect at the outset.

Cardiovascular System

Ordinary diving activities are strenuous, requiring high oxygen consumption and therefore high cardiac output. The physician must determine whether cardiac abnormalities are present, and if so whether they are hemodynamically significant.

Although candidates for commercial, scientific, or other occupational diving positions are usually in good health, it is incumbent upon the examining physician to ensure that no serious cardiac disease exists in the diving candidate. The history thus becomes extremely important since a serious illness like coronary artery disease may exhibit no clues of its existence in the physical examination. Similarly, presence of an atrial septal defect, a disqualifying abnormality (see Chapter 21), may be determined by history if the diagnosis has been established but is often difficult to detect by physical examination.

The approach to the examination of the cardiovascular system in diving candidates should include a careful history to detect the presence of congenital heart disease, coronary disease, valvular heart disease, rheumatic heart disease, hypertension, and peripheral vascular disease. A family history of these disorders should be recorded, and the use of drugs for cardiovascular disorders should be noted.

Examination of the cardiovascular system usually begins with inspection of the venous and arterial system, the chest, and abdomen. Abnormal pulsations in any area, but especially in the neck or abdomen should be noted. The motion of the precordium should be minimal except in thin subjects in whom the apical impulse can sometimes be observed. Venous distention should be noted, and evidence of compromised circulation especially of the extremities should be sought. Retinal arteries should be examined with an ophthalmoscope. Edema is usually due to circulatory abnormalities, and, if noted, careful assessment of venous pressure should be done.

Palpation of all accessible arterial pulses should be done and recorded, as should palpation over the abdominal aorta. Palpation of the precordium should be oriented to localizing the apical impulse and detecting abnormal palpatory signs.

Auscultation of the heart should include a careful determination of the timing and quality of the first and second heart sounds, detection of third or fourth heart sounds, and timing and characterization of all murmurs.

Examination of the peripheral arterial and venous systems should also include auscultation. Localized bruits for example may indicate atherosclerotic narrowing or presence of an arteriovenous shunt. An important habit is to listen over surgical scars where an occasional iatrogenic A-V fistula may be detected.

A careful examination of the cardiovascular system will always provide the necessary clues for diagnosing organic heart disease. In general, it is unlikely that a significant cardiac anatomical abnormality will be undetected on physical examination. Notable exceptions to this general concept are mitral stenosis, atrial septal defect, and early coronary artery disease. The current state of diagnostic testing in cardiology provides a powerful adjunct to the physical examination.

Adjunctive Studies

The complete cardiac evaluation should include a PA and lateral chest radiograph and a resting electrocardiogram, although these studies are unlikely to demonstrate an abnormality in the age group of diving candidates (e.g., 18 to 35 yrs). The value of these records for baseline data essential for later comparison demands their acquisition. Cognizance of normal variation in the ECG is necessary when reading it in this population.

When concerns are raised from the physical examination, other diagnostic studies are also useful. These can include echocardiography for assessment of cardiac valves, ventricular size and function, and cardiac hypertrophy; perfusion studies with radio-labelled tracers for assessment of myocardial perfusion; and exercise testing to determine cardiovascular reserve. Combined perfusion and exercise studies are often used to determine whether coronary disease is present.

Rarely, cardiac catheterization may be needed to exclude congenital or coronary disease when other data suggest their presence.

Musculoskeletal System

There are no universally accepted criteria for determining fitness for diving from an orthopedic point of view. As with other systems, consideration must be given to whether the diver will be in a decompression situation that uses mixed gases as opposed to shallow sport or professional diving with air. Any condition that significantly compromises blood supply to the musculoskeletal system should render a diver unfit.

A careful history should be elicited of injuries, cervical or lumbar spine degenerative disease, documented osteonecrosis, and fractures.

With the exception of osteonecrosis, there are no other absolutely disqualifying musculoskeletal abnormalities. Diver candidates with prior lumbar or cervical disk disease may find difficulty in obtaining employment as a diver due to medical-legal concerns of many employers. Serious restriction in range of motion of a joint or extremity, or limited use of an extremity due to musculoskeletal abnormality may disqualify divers from specific types of employment.

Of course, metabolic disorders of the musculoskeletal system, such as idiopathic myoglobinuria, and other inherited biochemical abnormalities, such as myothenia gravis and scleroderma, exclude a candidate from commercial diving.

Examination of the musculoskeletal system should include testing, range of motion of all extremity joints, documentation of structural abnormalities of bone or muscle, and examination of the spine to rule out cervical or lumbar disk disease.

Adjunctive studies usually involve x-ray ex-

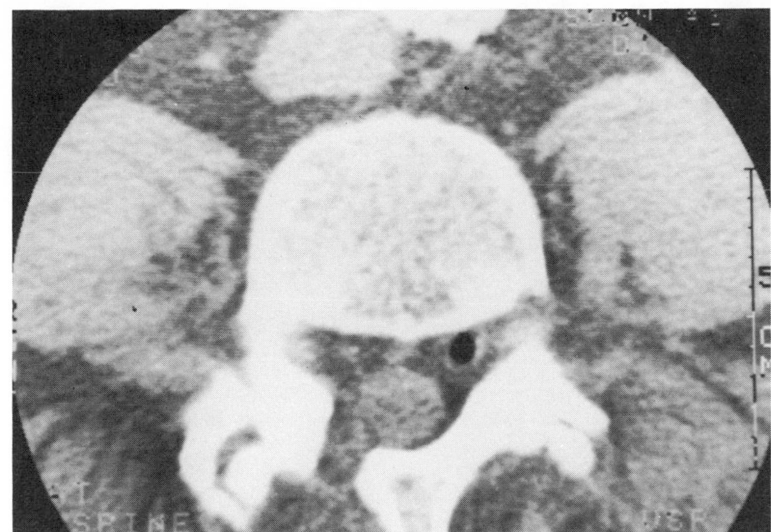

FIGURE 25–1. Extruded disk fragment containing gas visualized from CT scan of vertebral column. Black circle is a gas pocket. (Courtesy of G. Perlmutter, M.D.)

amination of long bones and the shoulder, hip, and knee joints to rule out osteonecrosis.[10] Specific protocols for these examinations are required in most countries.

The spinal column can be studied in detail using computed tomography (CT) or magnetic resonance imaging (MRI) to evaluate the status of the intervertebral disks and joints (Figure 25–1).

SPECIAL STUDIES REQUIRED FOR DIVERS

In addition to the history and physical examination, NOAA requires (and is considered a reasonable minimum) the following laboratory or special tests for government sponsored divers: initial 14 × 17 PA chest radiograph; initial standard 12-lead electrocardiogram; initial and annual audiogram to American National Standards Institute (ANSI) standards; initial tests of visual acuity and color vision; initial and annual hematocrit, hemoglobin, white blood count, and routine urinalysis. Bone and joint radiographs are required initially and triennially for those commercial divers engaged in dives outside the no-decompression depth-time limits. The use of the protocol established by the British Medical Research Council Decompression Sickness Registry is required. Many diving contractors have additional requirements: an initial electroencephalogram and electronystagmogram; initial and annual pulmonary function tests (usually FVC and $FEV_{1.0}$); stress electrocardiography initially and re-examination after reaching a certain age level, usually age 30. Many of the diving contractors require the use of chemistry panels, particularly to look for evidence of alcoholic hepatitis, and stress indicators, such as cholesterol and uric acid levels. Recently, they have also been insisting on a urinalysis for chromatographic drug screening for evidence of drug abuse.

REFERENCES

1. Grorud HF, Bol C: Hazards of offshore operations and control. *In* Galtung FL, et al (eds): Automation in Offshore Oil Field Operations. New York, Elsevier-North Holland, 1976.
2. Linaweaver PG: Physical examination requirements for commercial divers. J Occup Med 19:817–818, 1977.
3. OSHA and USCG: Commercial diving operations, medical requirements. Fed Regist 42(141):Article 1910.41, 1977.
4. Rivera JC: Decompression sickness among divers: An analysis of 935 cases. Milit Med 129:314–334, 1964.
5. McAniff JJ: U.S. Underwater Fatality Statistics, 1980–1983. Report no. URI-SSR-86-18. Washington, DC, National Oceanic and Atmospheric Administration, 1986.
6. Summitt JF, Reiners SD: Noise: A hazard to divers and hyperbaric personnel. Aerosp Med 42:1173–1177, 1971.
7. National Oceanic and Atmospheric Administration: NOAA Diving Manual. Washington, DC, U.S. Department of Commerce, 1975.
8. U.S. Navy: Physical examinations. *In* Manual of the Medical Department. Washington, DC, U.S. Department of the Navy, 1980, p 117.
9. Linaweaver PG: Injuries to the chest caused by pressure changes, compression and decompression. Am J Surg 105:514–521, 1963.
10. Linaweaver PG: Physical examination requirements for commercial divers. J Occup Med 19:817–818, 1977.

APPENDICES

Appendix 1

Pressure Conversion Table

Multiply This Unit → / To obtain ↓	KG/CM²	ATA*	ATM†	BAR	TORR (mm Hg)	LBS/IN²	METERS SEA WATER (msw)	FEET SEA WATER (fsw)	PASCAL‡ (Pa)
KG/CM²	1.00	1.00	1.0033	1.020	1.36×10^{-3}	7.031×10^{-2}	0.1026	3.124×10^{-2}	1.02×10^{-5}
ATA	1.00	1.00	1.033	0.9807	1.36×10^{-3}	7.031×10^{-2}	0.1026	3.124×10^{-2}	1.02×10^{-5}
ATM	0.9678	0.9678	1.00	1.013	1.316×10^{-3}	6.805×10^{-2}	9.921×10^{-2}	3.024×10^{-2}	0.987×10^{-5}
BAR	0.9807	0.9807	1.013	1.00	1.333×10^{-3}	6.895×10^{-2}	1.0052×10^{-1}	3.064×10^{-2}	1.040×10^{-5}
TORR (mm Hg)	735.5	735.5	760	750.1	1.00	51.71	75.40	23.00	7.502×10^{-3}
LBS/IN²	14.22	14.22	14.70	14.50	1.934×10^{-2}	1.00	1.458	0.4445	1.45×10^{-4}
METERS SEA WATER (msw)	9.76	9.76	10.08	9.95	1.33×10^{-2}	0.6859	1.00	0.3048	0.898×10^{-4}
FEET SEA WATER (fsw)	32.01	32.01	33.07	32.64	4.38×10^{-2}	2.250	3.281	1.00	3.264×10^{-4}
PASCAL (Pa)	9.807×10^{4}	9.807×10^{4}	1.01×10^{5}	1×10^{5}	1.333×10^{2}	6.895×10^{3}	1.005×10^{4}	3.064×10^{3}	1.00

*A technical atmosphere is equal to 1 kg/cm².
†A standard atmosphere is equal to pressure of a 760 mm mercury column of density 13.5951 g/cm³.
‡A pascal is defined as one newton/M².

Appendix 2

Conditions for Which Disqualification is Recommended

1. Tympanic membrane perforation or aeration tubes
2. Inability to autoinflate the middle ears
3. External ear exostoses or osteomas adequate to prevent external ear canal pressure equilibration
4. Meniere's disease or other chronic vertiginous conditions; status post-surgery, such as subarachnoid endolymphatic shunt for Meniere's disease
5. Stapedectomy and middle ear prosthesis
6. Chronic mastoiditis or mastoid fistula
7. Any oral or maxillofacial deformity that interferes with retention of the mouthpiece
8. Corrected near visual acuity not adequate to see tank pressure gauge, watch, decompression tables, and compass under water. Uncorrected visual acuity not adequate to see the diving buddy or locate the boat in case corrective lenses are lost under water
9. Radial keratotomy or other recent ocular surgery
10. Claustrophobia of a degree to predispose to panic
11. Suicidal ideation
12. Psychosis
13. Significant anxiety states
14. Severe depression
15. Manic states
16. Alcoholism
17. Mood-altering drug use
18. Improper motivation for diving
19. Episodic loss of consciousness
20. History of seizures (history of seizures in early childhood must be evaluated individually)
21. Migraine
22. History of cerebrovascular accident or transient ischemic attack
23. History of spinal cord trauma with neurological deficit—whether fully recovered or not
24. Demyelinating process
25. Brain tumor with or without surgery
26. Intracranial aneurysm or other vascular malformation
27. History of neurological decompression sickness with residual deficit
28. Head injury with sequelae
29. History of intracranial surgery
30. Sickle cell disease
31. Polycythemia or leukemia
32. Unexplained anemia
33. History of myocardial infarction
34. Angina or other evidence of coronary artery disease
35. Unrepaired cardiac septal defects
36. Aortic stenosis or mitral stenosis
37. Complete heart block
38. Fixed second degree heart block
39. Exercise-induced tachyarrhythmias
40. Wolff-Parkinson-White (WPW) syndrome with paroxysmal atrial tachycardia or syncope
41. Fixed rate pacemakers
42. Any drugs that inhibit the normal cardiovascular response to exercise
43. Peripheral vascular disease, arterial or venous, adequate to limit exercise tolerance
44. Hypertension with end-organ finding—retinal, cardiac, renal, or vascular
45. History of spontaneous pneumothorax
46. Bronchial asthma (history of childhood asthma requires special studies)
47. Exercise or cold air–induced asthma
48. Chronic obstructive pulmonary disease
49. X-ray evidence of pulmonary blebs, bullae, or cysts
50. Insulin-dependent diabetes mellitus. Diet- or oral medication–controlled diabetes mellitus if there is a history of hypoglycemic episodes
51. Any abdominal wall hernia with potential for gas trapping until surgically corrected
52. Paraesophageal or incarcerated sliding hiatal hernia
53. Sliding hiatal hernia if symptomatic due to reflux esophagitis
54. Pregnancy

Appendix 3

Medical Examination Forms

MEDICAL HISTORY
(To be completed by applicant)

Name ______________________ Age _____ Sex _____ Date ________
Address ______________________ Phone ______________________

1. Having you had previous experience in diving?
   Yes _____ No _____
2. When driving through mountains or flying do you have trouble equalizing pressure in your ears or sinuses?
   Yes _____ No _____
3. Have you ever been rejected for service, employment, or insurance for medical reasons?
   Yes _____ No _____
   (If yes, explain under remarks or discuss with doctor.)
4. When was your last physical examination?
   Date __________ Results ______________________
5. When was your last chest x-ray?
   Date __________ Results ______________________
6. Have you ever had an electrocardiogram?
   Yes _____ No _____
   Date __________ Results ______________________
7. Have you every had an electroencephalogram (brain wave study)?
   Yes _____ No _____
   Date __________ Results ______________________
8. Do you smoke?
   Yes _____ No _____
   If so, how much? ______________________

(Check the blank if you have, or ever have had, any of the following. Explain under remarks, giving dates and other pertinent information, or discuss with doctor.)

9. _____ Frequent colds or sore throat
10. _____ Hay fever or sinus trouble
11. _____ Trouble breathing through nose (other than during colds)
12. _____ Painful or running ear, mastoid trouble, broken eardrum
13. _____ Hardness of hearing
14. _____ Asthma or bronchitis
15. _____ Shortness of breath after moderate exercise
16. _____ History of pleurisy
17. _____ Collapsed lung (pneumothorax)
18. _____ Chest pain or persistent cough
19. _____ Tiring easily
20. _____ Spells of fast, irregular, or pounding heartbeat
21. _____ High or low blood pressure
22. _____ Any kind of "heart trouble"
23. _____ Frequent upset stomach, heartburn or indigestion, peptic ulcer
24. _____ Frequent diarrhea or blood in stool
25. _____ Anemia or (females) heavy menstruation
26. _____ Bellyache or backache lasting more than a day or two
27. _____ Kidney or bladder disease; blood, sugar, or albumin in urine
28. _____ Broken bone, serious sprain or strain, dislocated joint
29. _____ Rheumatism, arthritis, or other joint trouble
30. _____ Severe or frequent headaches
31. _____ Head injury causing unconsciousness
32. _____ Dizzy spells, fainting spells, or fits

33. ______ Trouble sleeping, frequent nightmares, or sleepwalking
34. ______ Nervous breakdown or periods of marked nervousness or depression
35. ______ A phobia for closed-in spaces, large open places, or high places
36. ______ Any neurological or psychological condition
37. ______ Train, sea, or air sickness or nausea
38. ______ Alcoholism or any drug or narcotic habit (including regular use of sleeping pills, benzedrine, and so forth)
39. ______ Recent gain or loss of weight or appetite
40. ______ Jaundice or hepatitis
41. ______ Tuberculosis
42. ______ Diabetes
43. ______ Rheumatic fever
44. ______ Any serious accident, injury, or illness not mentioned above (describe under remarks, give dates)
45. ______ Dental bridgework or plates
46. ______ Susceptibility to panic
47. ______ Pain from altitude or flying
48. ______ What sports or exercise do you regularly engage in? ______________________________

Remarks: ______________________________

____

Signature of applicant

MEDICAL EXAMINATION

(This form and the medical history form are retained by the physician for his/her records.)

A. Height ______ (in.) Weight ______ (lbs.)
Blood Pressure ______ Pulse ______
Vision: Right eye Left eye
uncorrected ______ ______
corrected ______ ______

B. **Medical History:** Is there a significant past history that would disqualify the applicant from scuba diving? (See medical history form.)
Yes ______ No ______
Remarks: ______________________________

C. **Examination:** (Check following items. If abnormal, give details below.)

	Normal	Abnormal
1. General appearance (including obesity, gross defects, postural abnormalities)	______	______
2. Head and neck	______	______
3. Eyes	______	______
4. Nose and sinuses	______	______
5. Ears (including otitis, perforation)	______	______
6. Mouth and throat	______	______
7. Spine	______	______
8. Lungs and chest	______	______
9. Heart	______	______
10. Abdomen	______	______
11. Inguinal ring (males)	______	______
12. Genitalia (males)	______	______
13. Anus and rectum	______	______
14. Extremities	______	______
15. Skin reactions or eruptions	______	______
16. Nervous system	______	______
17. Psychiatric (including apparent motivation for diving, emotional stability, claustrophia)	______	______

Explanation of abnormals: ______________________________

____

D. **Test Results:**

All applicants: Chest x-ray(s) ________________

As indicated: EKG ________________ V.C. and FEV1 ________________ Audiogram ________________

Hematocrit ________________ Urinalysis ________________ Other ________________

E. **Final Impression** (circle one):

Approval: I find no defects that I consider incompatible with diving.

Conditional Approval: I do not consider diving in this person's best interests but find no defects that present marked risk. I have discussed my impression with him/her.

Disapproval: This applicant has defects that, in my opinion, constitute unacceptable hazards to his/her health and safety in diving.

________________ ________________

Date *Signature of physician*

(The form below is to be completed and returned to the examinee if evidence of medical examination is required.)

Impression (circle one):

I have examined ________________ and reached the following conclusion concerning his/her fitness for diving:

Approval: I find no defect that I consider incompatible with diving.

Conditional Approval: I do not consider diving in this person's best interests but find no defects that present marked risk. I have discussed my impression with him/her.

Disapproval: This applicant has defects that, in my opinion, constitute unacceptable hazards to his/her health and safety in diving.

Signature of Physician: ________________

Address: ________________

Date: ________________

Appendix 4

United States Navy Oxygen Treatment Tables

TREATMENT TABLE 5. Oxygen Treatment of Type I Decompression Sickness*

1. Treatment of Type I decompression sickness when symptoms are relieved within 10 minutes at 60 feet and a complete neurological exam is normal.
2. Descent rate — 25 ft/min.
3. Ascent rate — 1 ft/min. Do not compensate for slower ascent rates. Compensate for faster rates by halting the ascent.
4. Time at 60 feet begins on arrival at 60 feet.
5. If oxygen breathing must be interrupted, allow 15 minutes after the reaction has entirely subsided and resume schedule at point of interruption (see Section 8.12.4.1).
6. If oxygen breathing must be interrupted at 60 feet, switch to Table 6 upon arrival at the 30 foot stop.
7. Tender breathes air throughout unless he has had a hyperbaric exposure within the past 12 hours in which case he breathes oxygen at 30 feet in accordance with Section 8.12.5.7.

Depth (feet)	Time (minutes)	Breathing Media	Total Elapsed Time (hrs:min.)
60	20	Oxygen	0:20
60	5	Air	0:25
60	20	Oxygen	0:45
60 to 30	30	Oxygen	1:15
30	5	Air	1:20
30	20	Oxygen	1:40
30	5	Air	1:45
30 to 0	30	Oxygen	2:15

TABLE 5 DEPTH/TIME PROFILE

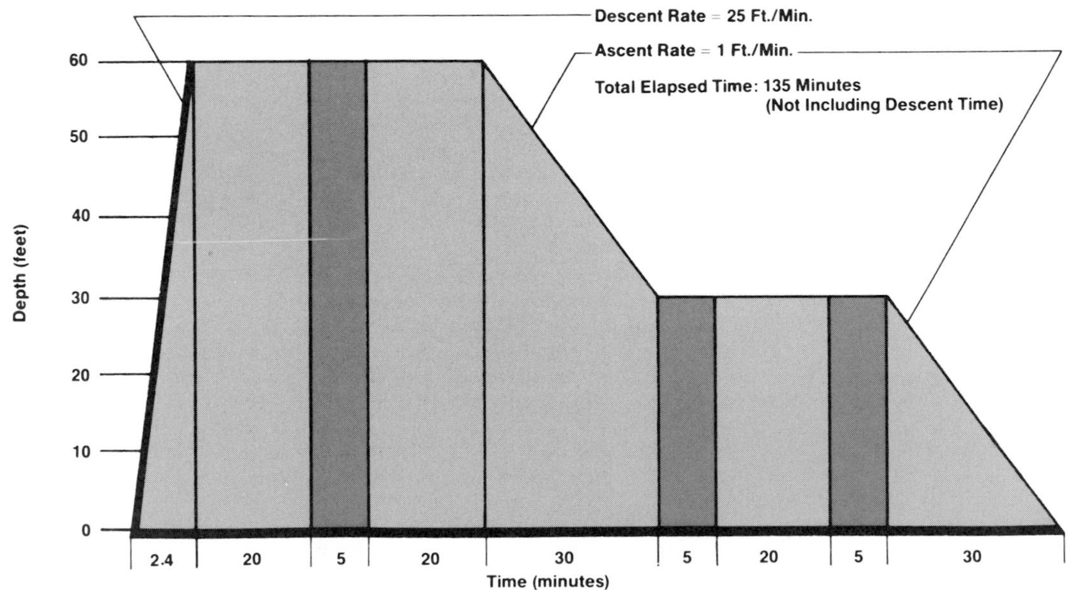

*Many diving physicians use Table 6 for Type I decompression sickness and exclude Table 5 from any initial therapy.

TREATMENT TABLE 6. Oxygen Treatment of Type II Decompression Sickness

1. Treatment of Type II or Type I decompression sickness when symptoms are not relieved within 10 minutes at 60 feet.
2. Descent rate — 25 ft/min.
3. Ascent rate — 1 ft/min. Do not compensate for slower ascent rates. Compensate for faster rates by halting the ascent.
4. Time at 60 feet begins on arrival at 60 feet.
5. If oxygen breathing must be interrupted, allow 15 minutes after the reaction has entirely subsided and resume schedule at point of interruption.
6. Tender breathes air throughout unless he has had a hyperbaric exposure within the past 12 hours in which case he breathes oxygen at 30 feet in accordance with Section 8.12.5.7.
7. Table 6 can be lengthened up to 2 additional 25 minute oxygen breathing periods at 60 feet (20 minutes on oxygen and 5 minutes on air) or up to 2 additional 75 minute oxygen breathing periods at 30 feet (15 minutes on air and 60 minutes on oxygen), or both. If Table 6 is extended only once at either 60 or 30 feet, the tender breathes oxygen during the ascent from 30 feet to the surface. If more than one extension is done, the tender begins oxygen breathing for the last hour at 30 feet during ascent to the surface.

Depth (feet)	Time (minutes)	Breathing Media	Total Elapsed Time (hrs:min.)
60	20	Oxygen	0:20
60	5	Air	0:25
60	20	Oxygen	0:45
60	5	Air	0:50
60	20	Oxygen	1:10
60	5	Air	1:15
60 to 30	30	Oxygen	1:45
30	15	Air	2:00
30	60	Oxygen	3:00
30	15	Air	3:15
30	60	Oxygen	4:15
30 to 0	30	Oxygen	4:45

TABLE 6 DEPTH/TIME PROFILE

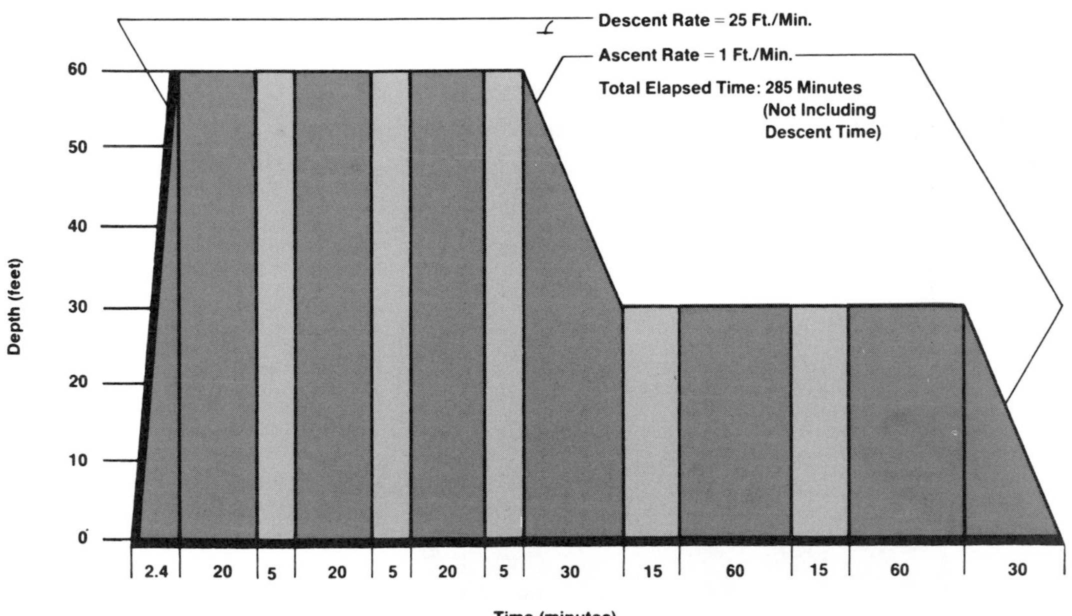

TREATMENT TABLE 6A. Initial Air and Oxygen Treatment of Arterial Gas Embolism

1. Treatment of arterial gas embolism where complete relief obtained within 30 min. at 165 feet. Use also when unable to determine whether symptoms are caused by gas embolism or severe decompression sickness.
2. Descent rate — as fast as possible.
3. Ascent rate — 1 ft/min. Do not compensate for slower ascent rates. Compensate for faster ascent rates by halting the ascent.
4. Time at 165 feet — includes time from the surface.
5. If oxygen breathing must be interrupted, allow 15 minutes after the reaction has entirely subsided and resume schedule at point of interruption (see Section 8.12.4.1).
6. Tender breathes oxygen during ascent from 30 feet to the surface unless he has had a hyperbaric exposure within the past 12 hours in which case he breathes oxygen at 30 feet in accordance with Section 8.12.5.7.
7. Table 6A can be lengthened up to 2 additional 25 minute oxygen breathing periods at 60 feet (20 minutes on oxygen and 5 minutes on air) or up to 2 additional 75 minute oxygen breathing periods at 30 feet (15 minutes on air and 60 minutes on oxygen), or both. If Table 6A is extended either at 60 or 30 feet the tender breathes oxygen during the last half at 30 feet and during ascent to the surface.
8. If complete relief not obtained within 30 min. at 165 feet, switch to Table 4. Consult with a Diving Medical Officer before switching if possible.

Depth (feet)	Time (minutes)	Breathing Media	Total Elapsed Time (hrs:min)
165	30	Air	0:30
165 to 60	4	Air	0:34
60	20	Oxygen	0:54
60	5	Air	0:59
60	20	Oxygen	1:19
60	5	Air	1:29
60	20	Oxygen	1:44
60	5	Air	1:49
60 to 30	30	Oxygen	2:19
30	15	Air	2:34
30	60	Oxygen	3:34
30	15	Air	3:49
30	60	Oxygen	4:49
30 to 0	30	Oxygen	5:19

TABLE 6A DEPTH/TIME PROFILE

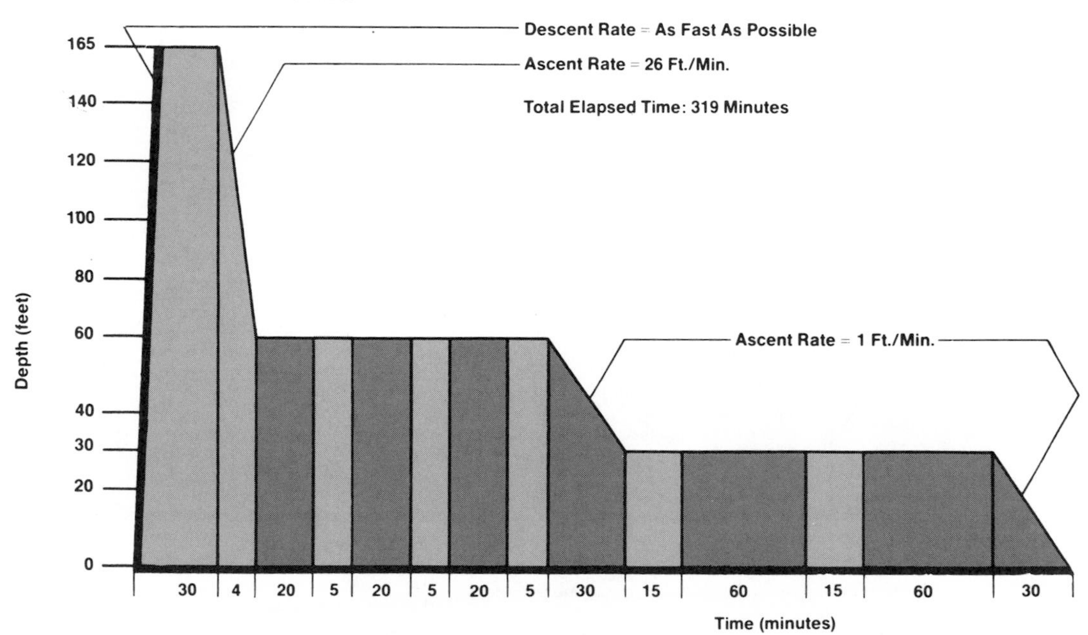

TREATMENT TABLE 7. Oxygen/Air Treatment of Unresolved or Worsening Symptoms of Decompression Sickness or Arterial Gas Embolism

1. Used for treatment of unresolved life threatening symptoms after initial treatment on Table 6, 6A, or 4.
2. Use only under the direction of or in consultation with a Diving Medical Officer.
3. Table begins upon arrival at 60 feet. Arrival at 60 feet accomplished by initial treatment on Table 6, 6A or 4. If initial treatment has progressed to a depth shallower than 60 feet, compress to 60 feet at 25 ft/min to begin Table 7.
4. Maximum duration at 60 feet unlimited. Remain at 60 feet a minimum of 12 hours unless overriding circumstances dictate earlier decompression.
5. Patient begins oxygen breathing periods at 60 feet. Tender need breathe only chamber atmosphere throughout. If oxygen breathing is interrupted no lengthening of the table is required.
6. Minimum chamber O_2 concentration 19%. Maximum CO_2 concentration 1.5% SEV (12 mmHg). Maximum chamber internal temperature 85°F (Section 8.12.5.4).
7. Decompression starts with a 2 foot upward excursion from 60 to 58 feet. Decompress with stops every 2 feet for times shown in profile below. Ascent time between stops approximately 30 sec. Stop time begins with ascent from deeper to next shallower step. Stop at 4 feet for 4 hours and then ascend to the surface at 1 ft/min.
8. Ensure chamber life support requirements can be met before committing to a Treatment Table 7.
9. See Section 8.12.3.5 for details.

TREATMENT TABLE 7 DEPTH/TIME PROFILE

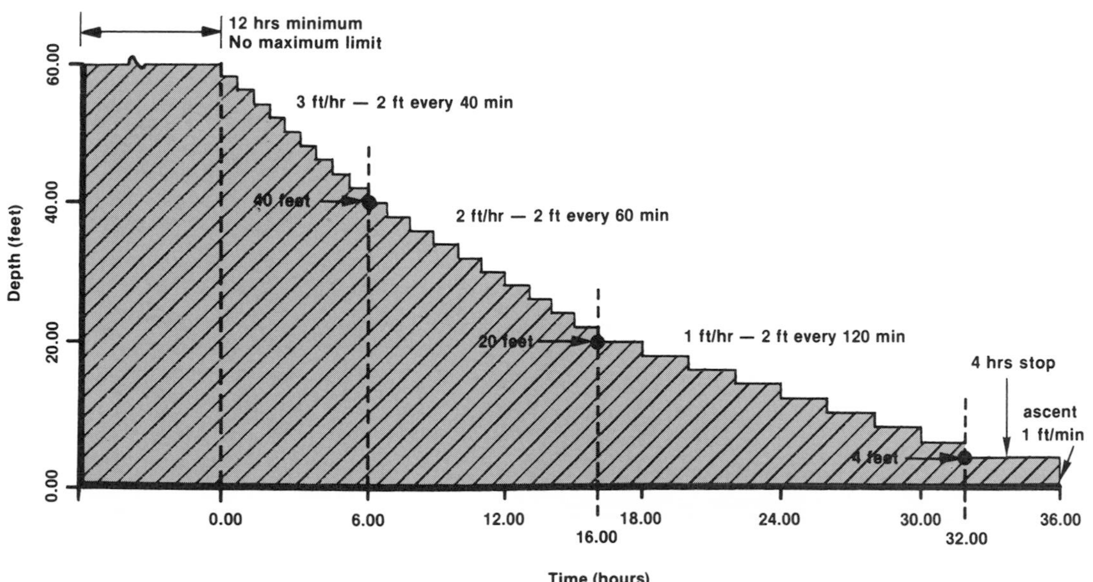

Appendix 5

Considerations for Diving Medicine Physician's Kit for Remote Locations

EQUIPMENT
Sphygmomanometer
Stethoscope
Otoophthalmoscope
Oropharyngeal airway
Endotracheal tubes, scope, blade
Foley catheters, 18–22 gauge
Syringes and needles
Venous cannula
Tourniquet
Intravenous infusion sets
Scissors, disposable scalpels
Bandage materials
Ace bandages
Sterile gloves
DRUGS AND FLUIDS
Normal saline and lactated Ringer's solution
Injectable dexamethasone
Sodium bicarbonate ampuls
Local anesthetic injection
Aspirin tablets
Domeboro® otic solution
Cortisporin® otic solution
Antibiotic ophthalmic solution
Afrin® nasal spray
Benadryl® for injection and capsules
Topical steroid cream
Topical antibiotic ointment
Hibiclens® surgical soap
Antacid tablets
Bactrim DS® tablets
Diazepam injection
Baby ear syringe
White vinegar

Index

Note: Page numbers in *italics* refer to illustrations; page numbers followed by t refer to tables.